The Major Histocompatibility System in Man and Animals

Contributors

E.D. Albert H. Balner N. Cohen N.H. Collins C.S. David M.E. Dorf W.R. Duncan A.F. Geczy D. Götze H. Grosse-Wilde E. Günther K. Hála P. Iványi J. Klein O. Štark J.W. Streilein H.M. Vriesendorp A.L. de Weck

Editor

Dietrich Götze

With 23 Figures

Springer-Verlag Berlin Heidelberg New York 1977

Prof. Dr. DIETRICH GÖTZE
The Wistar Institute for Anatomy and Biology
36 Street at Spruce, Philadelphia, Pa. 19104/USA

ISBN-13: 978-3-642-95295-1 e-ISBN-13: 978-3-642-95293-7
DOI: 10.1007/978-3-642-95293-7

Library of Congress Cataloging in Publication Data. Main entry under title: The major histocompatibility system in man and animals. Includes bibliographies and index. 1. Histocompatibility. I. Albert, Ekkehard. II. Götze, Dietrich, 1941.– QR 184.3.073. 599′.02′9. 77-1134.

Contents

Chapter 4

The Major Histocompatibility System of Cattle, Pig, Rabbit, and Syrian Hamster

Chapter 5

The Major Histocompatibility System of the Guinea Pig. A.F. Geczy and A.L. de Weck. With 1 Figure

Chapter 6

The Major Histocompatibility System of the Rat (Ag-B or H-1 System).
E. GÜNTHER and O. ŠTARK

Chapter 7
The Major Histocompatibility System of the Mouse. C.S. David. With 3 Figures

Chapter 8
The Major Histocompatibility System of the Chicken. K. Hála

Chapter 9

Major and Minor Histocompatibility Systems of Ectothermic Vertebrates.
N. COHEN and NANCY H. COLLINS. With 1 Figure

Chapter 10

Evolution and Function of the Major Histocompatibility System: Facts and Speculations. J. KLEIN. With 4 Figures

List of Contributors

E.D. ALBERT, Polikinderklinik der Universität, Pettenkofer Straße, D-8000 München

H. BALNER, Primate Center TNO, 151, Lange Kleiweg, NL—Rijswijk ZH

N. COHEN, Department of Mikrobiology, Division of Immunology, The University of Rochester, School of Medicine and Dentistry, Rochester, New York 14642, USA

N.H. COLLINS, Department of Mikrobiology, Division of Immunology, The University of Rochester, School of Medicine and Dentistry, Rochester, New York 14642, USA

C.S. DAVID, Department of Genetics, Washington University School of Medicine, St. Louis, Mo. 63110, USA

M.E. DORF, Harvard Medical School, Boston, USA

W.R. DUNCAN, Department of Cell Biology, University of Texas, Southwestern Medical School, Dallas, Texas 75235, USA

A.F. GECZY, Institute for Clinical Immunology, Inselspital, CH-3006 Bern

D. GÖTZE, The Wistar Institute for Anatomy and Biology, Philadelphia, Pa. 19104, USA

H. GROSSE-WILDE, Institut für Hämatologie, GSF, Abt. Immunologie, D-8000 München

E. GÜNTHER, Max-Planck-Institut für Immunbiologie, D-7800 Freiburg

K. HÁLA, Institute of Experimental Biology and Genetics, Czechoslovak Academy of Science, Prague, CSSR

P. IVÁNYI, Central Laboratory Blood Transfusion Service, Plesmanlaan 125, NL-Amsterdam

J. KLEIN, Department of Microbiology, The University of Texas, Southwestern Medical School, Dallas, Texas 75235, USA

O. Štark, Charles University, Faculty of General Medicine,
Department of Biology, Albertov 4, Prague 2, CSSR

J.W. Streilein, Department of Cell Biology, University of Texas,
Southwestern Medical School, Dallas, Texas 75235, USA

H.M. Vriesendorp, Radiobiological Institute GO-TNO, 151, Lange Kleiweg,
NL-Rijswijk ZH

A.L. de Weck, Institute for Clinical Immunology, Inselspital, CH-3006 Bern

Introductory Remarks

The Major Histocompatibility System

Dietrich Götze

The concept of a "Major Histocompatibility Gene" was first introduced by Snell and collaborators in 1956 to make a distinction between gene(s) associated with acute rejection of allogeneic tissue and tumor grafts, from those which control chronic rejection of normal allogeneic tissue grafts and usually do not cause rejection of tumor grafts. The latter were called "Minor Histocompatibility Genes." Today, we know that, in most species, there is not only one gene, but a cluster of genes, whose products are involved in acute (strong) transplantation reactions. This genetic region is therefore called the Major Histocompatibility Gene Complex (MHC) or System (MHS). It represents the most polymorphic and multiallelic genetic system known to date in mammals.

Genes of this complex control the expression of alloantigens (H-antigens) on the cell surface, as well as levels of some serum proteins. This antigenic system was first described in the mouse by Gorer in 1936, after its existence had been predicted some time earlier by Haldane who postulated such antigens in order to explain why tumors of one inbred strain of mice were not accepted by members of another inbred strain. This phenomenon was observed in the first decade of this century by Jensen and Loeb, and was shown to be controlled by dominant genes by Tyzzer and Little and Tyzzer.

Our current understanding of the genetics, biology, and physiology of the MHS is primarily the results of the fundamental and ingenious work of Little, Gorer, and Snell who developed the ideas, materials, and methods that led to the identification and the thorough genetic analysis of the MHS (H-2 complex) in the mouse. The development of genetically defined inbred strains of mice by Little led to the formal expression of the laws of transplantation: (1) tumor grafts exchanged between members of the same inbred line (syngeneic) are accepted; (2) tumor grafts exchanged between members of two different lines (allogeneic) are uniformly rejected; and (3) tumor grafts placed from parental lines to F_1 hybrids of two lines are accepted, but transplants in the opposite direction are not.

The work of Gorer led to the recognition that the acceptance or rejection of a tumor graft was the direct result of antigenic structures present on the cells and tissue which, if different between recipient and donor, caused the recipient to destroy the graft. Gorer also demonstrated that the relevant antigenic structures, later called histocompatibility or H-antigens, can be identified by serological methods.

Snell developed the concept, and initiated the production, of congenic mouse lines. Analysis using congenics formed the basis for current knowledge about the genetics and biology of histocompatibility in general and, in particular, the genetic fine structure of the MHS, its relevance in transplantation biology, immune response, immune cell differentiation, susceptibility to diseases, embryonic development, and cell biology.

The link-up of the laws of transplantation revealed by the tumor studies with the rejection mechanism of normal tissue suggested by early experiments of Little and Johnson, and Bittner was extended by Medawar in the mid-forties using simple skin-grafting techniques. Medawar was able, furthermore, to show that the transplantation reaction represented an immune response by the recipient to the H-gene products of the donor. He and his colleagues Billingham and Brent thereby established the modern approach to allotransplantation of organs and tissue.

The next important finding was the discovery of leukocyteagglutinins by Dausset and Miescher in 1956, and the attempt to define leukocyte groups using pregnancy sera or post-transfusion sera by Payne and van Rood. This led to the characterization of the human equivalent of the mouse MHS, the HLA (Human Leukocyte Antigen) system.

Clinical pressures to attempt organ transplantation as a therapeutic tool have led to further intensive efforts at understanding the genetic fine structure, gene action, regulation, and evolution of the MHS not only in the mouse (the dominant animal model of basic immunogenetically oriented research) but also in man and other species relevant for the advancement of human clinical transplantation. As the result of these efforts, it is now recognized that the biological importance of the MHS lies not only in its pre-eminent role in affecting allograft survival, but also in the control of a large array of biological phenomena, including immune responsiveness, development and susceptibility to diseases. The MHS may be thought of as a genetic region important in the determination of cell surface structures, and thereby in cell-interaction such as those involved in morphogenesis and the maintenance of individuality and selfintegrity.

The discovery of the MHS's involvement in the regulation of host defense mechanisms not only led to new speculations concerning the biological role of this system, but also gave it a further dimension beyond transplantation biology. This all started with several discoveries made in the last decade; in 1964, Lilly and collaborators found that susceptibility to Gross virus in mice is controlled by genes within the MHS (Rgv-1 locus); in 1965, Benacerraf and McDevitt showed independently that the antibody response to synthetic polypeptides was genetically controlled, and that the controlling genes, called Ir (Immune response) were located within the MHS. Also in 1964, both Bain and collaborators and Bach and Hirschhorn observed that, in an *in vitro* mixture of lymphocytes derived from two different individuals, transformation and proliferation of these cells occurred and that this blast transformation (mixed leukocyte culture reaction, MLR) was controlled, again, by genes of the MHS which code for lymphocyte activating determinants (LAD). These genes were closely linked to, or even identical with, Ir genes.

In 1974, Doherty and Zinkernagel demonstrated that the MHS is also implicated in the control of the cellular (cytotoxic) reaction to virus-infected isogeneic cells or tissue. They provided evidence that this control was mediated by H-gene products. Shearer and collaborators, Bevan, and Simpson and Gordon extended this finding, demonstrating that H-genes not only control the immune reaction to virus-infected cells but also against isogeneic chemically modified or minor H-antigen-different cells or tissue. H-genes appear, in general, to be involved in the reaction against cells or tissue displaying modified Self.

Another major aspect of the MHS has emerged rather slowly and was at first little noticed; Shreffler and Owen discovered in 1963 that the level of a serum protein (serum substance, Ss) was controlled by the MHS in mice. This serum protein was shown later to be the complement component C4, after Demant and his collaborators had already observed in 1973 that the quantity of Ss protein in the serum related to the complement activity. Meanwhile, it was realized that other complement components are also controlled by genes closely linked to the MHS in different species: C4 and C2 which form the C3-convertase enzyme of the classical pathway, and factor B which represents the C3-convertase of the properdin pathway. In addition to these components there is a locus closely linked to the MHS of mice which controls the ontogenic expression of the C3b-receptor on macrophages and B lymphocytes.

Taken together, three classes of genes can be distinguished within the MHS: *Class I* consists of genes which are involved in the immune response to cell-bound antigens, like virus-infected cells, chemically modified cells or otherwise-altered cells, and which control the expression of target antigens in the transplantation reaction. These are the so-called H-antigens. *Class II* consists of genes which are involved in the antibody response to soluble antigens, so-called Ir genes with their products most likely identical to Ia (*I*mmune response gene *a*ssociated) antigens and lymphocyte activating determinants. *Class III*, finally, consists of genes which control the expression of certain components of the complement system, particularly those which are involved in the activation of C3, the merging point of the classical and properdin pathway.

Although it is assumed that the actual binding of antigens is due to immunoglobulin (or Ig-like) receptors whose controlling genes are not linked to the MHS, and which can be demonstrated on the surface of B and T lymphocytes, the MHS gene products apparently facilitate the recognition of antigens by T cells and, are thereby involved in the interaction of immunocompetent cells whose cooperation is necessary for the final, specific differentiation process mandatory to produce an effective immune response.

Thus, in the cellular immune response, *cytotoxic T* cells are generated which specifically recognize the cell-bound antigen *together* with their own H-gene products, as the cell-mediated cytotoxic activity requires identity

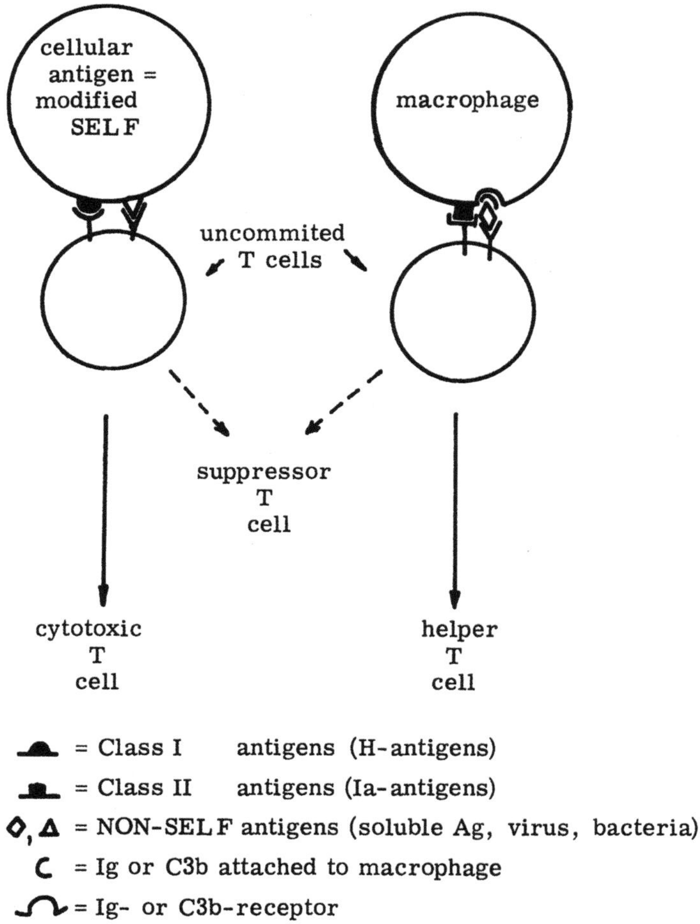

Fig. 1

at the H-loci of the MHS between the effector T cells and the stimulator cells. In the humoral response, it appears that the antigens have to be presented together with certain Ir-gene products to be recognized by *helper* (or *suppressor*) *T* cells presented by macrophages (or B cells) in order to become activated and to bring about the final differentiation of B cells into IgG-producing plasma cells and into memory cells since, again, identity at the Ir-genes between the interacting cells is necessary for these reactions (Figure 1). T cells possessing only recognition units for Self might be tolerized in the thymus as argued by Jerne.

The products of MHS genes apparently serve as SELF determinants, in both the cellular and the humoral immune responses. The interaction of T cells and SELF determinants alone does not lead to activation. However, the concomitant recognition of SELF and NON-SELF (e.g., an infectious agent) induces differentiation to active killer, helper, or suppressor cells. The transient, yet continuous, interaction of T cells with SELF-determinants might be considered as the essence of immunological surveillance (Burnet). Disturbances of this regulatory mechanism may be the basis for the explanation of the linkage of certain MHS genotypes with susceptibility to infectious and autoimmune diseases.

The third class of MHS gene, coding for enzymes necessary in the early steps of the complement reaction chain, might be viewed as an auxiliary component in antigen processing, facilitating the concomitant presentation of NON-SELF antigens with SELF-determinants. The C4 and C2 complement components are the key components of the classical pathway for activation of C3 to C3b under conditions where antibodies, particularly IgM antibodies which are produced early and without the interacting help of T cells, are present. The properdin system of which factor B is a crucial component, becomes activated even without immunoglobulins in cases where bacteria are the infectious agent. This pathway also results in the activation of C3 to C3b which is then bound to the bacteria. The C3b-IgM-Ag as well as the C3b-bacterium complex can now be opsonized through C3b-receptors or Fc-receptors by macrophages, probably the first step in antigen-processing by macrophages.

The enormous genetic and phenotypic complexity and extreme polymorphism of the MHS may become comprehensible if we consider the functional interaction of the MHS gene products as acceptors for SELF-specific receptors whose encoding genes (variable region genes, V-genes) are not linked to the MHS and are believed to exist in a diversity even greater than the MHS. Since the V region (specific binding site) of B and T cells are probably identical and the SELF as well as NON-SELF-determinants on the cell surface are detected by structures carrying those V gene products, one might expect that T cells have the same V gene repertoire as that for immunoglobulins. T cells, therefore, possess numerous recognition units for SELF. In fact, the antigenic complexity—and also the allelic polymorphism of H-genes—might be a direct image of the degree of diversity of the V gene pool in the population. The more V genes, the more numerous are structures with the potential to serve as recognizable determinant.

In general terms, the MHS may merit its importance in that it is the counterpart of the specific receptor system necessary to guide and guard differentiation, in the particular situation described above, the specific differentiation of the cellular elements involved in immune responsiveness. A mechanism as described above for the interaction of cells regulated by the concomitant appearance of SELF and NON-SELF and its recognition might, in principle, be identical for other biological systems requiring symbiosis of single cells and, therefore, differentiation processes, i.e., compatibility between certain tissues at certain stages. It is known that, in the mouse, embryonic development (differentiation) is largely controlled by genes closely linked to the MHS, the T-t complex; this complex is considered by some to act as the functional ontogenic precursor of the MHS.

The analysis of the MHS focuses, therefore, on the very essence of individuality and embodies determinants of morphogenesis, differentiation, immunologic responsiveness, susceptibility to a wide variety of diseases including neoplastic diseases and perhaps, even reproduction. Suice in mice the MHS appears to influence sex partner preference as recently demonstrated by Boyse and his colleagues.

It will be necessary to analyze this highly complex genetic region in different species in order to find out the exact mechanism involved in the operation of these genetic controls and their expression on the surface of cells. Each may have the potential to provide a special model for investigating a particular problem related to applied human biology: clinical transplantation, pathogenesis of infectious, allergic, and autoimmune diseases, ontogenic malformations, embryology, or basic science: phylogeny, ontogeny, molecular and population genetics, developmental biology, cell physiology, and biochemistry.

This book was, therefore, designed to provide a comprehensive summary of the available data on the Major Histocompatibility System for all of the species in which detailed analysis has been attempted. I wish to express my gratitude to all contributors, and to Springer-Verlag, for having both the courage and the persistence to undertake this venture.

Chapter 1

The Major Histocompatibility System in Man*

E. ALBERT and D. GÖTZE

1. Introduction

The knowledge about the major histocompatibility system (MHS) in man has evolved in very close interrelationship with the pioneer work in the mouse model with an intensive exchange of methodology and "ideology" concerning the analysis of serologic data. As will be documented in this book there is a remarkable analogy between the histocompatibility systems of many mammalian species, most notably of mouse and man. This is expressed in a phrase coined by Jean Dausset: "The mouse has never lied" relating to the fact that most of the systems found in the mouse H-2 complex (the MHS of the mouse) have also been described for man and other species. These analogies are in marked contrast to the widely different experimental approaches used for histocompatibility research in both species. Through the pioneer work of Gorer and Snell (Gorer 1938, 1961; Snell 1948, 1953) it has become possible to use inbred strains of mice, which allows the detailed genetic characterization of a relatively restricted number of H-2 haplotypes (i.e., chromosomes carrying the H-2 region) using a limited number of recombinants. In man one is faced with an outbred population containing an almost unlimited number of different haplotypes representing a very large number of recombinations. Therefore the laws of population genetics have to be utilized in the analysis of serologic data in an outbred species. As history has shown, both types of basic approaches have provided contributions that were essential for reaching today's state of knowledge about the major histocompatibility complex in both species.

2. Serologically Defined Histocompatibility Antigens

2.1 Historical Remarks

The history of the HLA system begins with the description of the antigen MAC (today: HLA-A2) by Dausset 1958. The definition was based on the reaction pattern of leuko-agglutinating antibodies found in the sera of parous women. Using similar methods, van Rood (1962) soon thereafter found the first allelic system consisting of the two specificities 4a and 4b. In the follow-

* This work was partially supported by NIH grant CA-10097 and DFG grant SFB-37-B6 and by SFB-37-B1, B2 as well as by grant A1-92/9/10 of Deutsche Forschungsgemeinschaft.

ing years the pioneering work of an international group of investigators (Bodmer, Batchelor, Çeppellini, Payne, Terasaki, Amos, Kissmeyer-Nielsen, Dausset, van Rood, Walford) led to the recognition of the HLA system as one autosomal region consisting of at least two separate loci (HLA-A and HLA-B) with a series of multiple alleles at each of these loci. This formulates the basic genetic model of the HLA system which was generally accepted at the 4th International Histocompatibility Workshop in 1970 (Joint Report 1970). This concept was enlarged by the addition of a third locus (AJ = HLA-C) with five mutually exclusive alleles (Sandberg et al. 1970; Mayr et al. 1973; Bernoco et al. 1973). Thus the serologically defined HLA antigens (the "classical" HLA antigens) are coded for by a highly polymorphic system of three closely linked loci: HLA-A, B and C.

2.2 Serology

The definition of HLA-A, B, and C locus antigens is generally accomplished by a microcytotoxicity test using lymphocytes separated from peripheral blood by the flotation method first described by Böyum (1968). Two standard modifications of the microcytotoxicity test are currently in use: the NIH technique as first described by Terasaki and McClelland (1964) and a technique introduced by Kissmeyer-Nielsen and Kjerbye (1967). In both tests, lymphocytes are incubated with antisera in 1-μl quantities under a film of mineral oil to prevent evaporation. In the Terasaki technique the reaction mixture is incubated a total of 90 min at room temperature while in Kissmeyer-Nielsen's (KN) test incubation for only 60 min takes place at 37° C. The source of complement is fresh-frozen rabbit serum which in the KN test is mixed with an equal volume of fresh human AB serum. The two techniques operate at slightly different levels of sensitivity; the NIH test is more sensitive. It is clear that the selection of antisera has to take into account the sensitivity of the test procedure. Under these conditions HLA typing can be performed with equally good results in both techniques.

Antisera for HLA typing are obtained basically in two different ways: (1) from parous women, who develop antibodies against HLA antigens of fetal lymphocytes, which enter the maternal bloodstream during pregnancy and (2) from volunteers who have been immunized with a skin graft and booster injection of buffy coat cells from donors selected so that they would differ from the recipient only by one antigen (Thorsby and Lie 1968). Another very effective means of immunization is by repeated transfusions of small amounts of whole blood. (Ferrara et al. 1973). With these immunization procedures it is of critical importance to find the optimal time for procurement of serum before the antiserum becomes too broadly reactive.

2.3 The Definition of HLA Antigens

Today's well-defined HLA antigens are the product of a development which started with the analysis of a large number of cell samples from unrelated

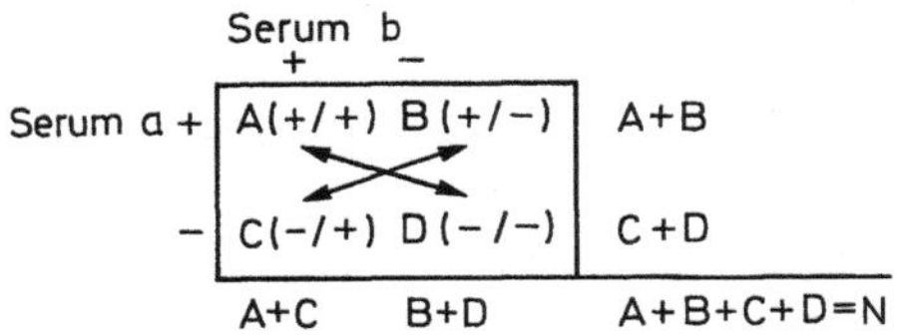

Fig. 1.1

individuals tested with many different undefined antisera. The resulting reaction patterns were analyzed by 2×2 comparison of pairs of antisera where each serum was compared with all others—a gigantic amount of calculations, which could best be managed with the help of the computer. The significance of similarity—or dissimilarity—of two sera can best be measured with a χ^2 test based on the 2×2 contingency table (Fig. 1.1). (Cavalli-Sforza and Bodmer 1971).

The χ^2 is calculated as

$$\chi^2 = \frac{(|AD - BC|)^2 \cdot N}{(A+C) \cdot (B+D) \cdot (A+B) \cdot (C+D)}.$$

In the case of a small sample size it is advisable to introduce a correction (Yate's correction) leading to the slightly more conservative formula

$$\chi^2 = \frac{(|AD - BC| - N/2)^2 \cdot N}{(A+C) \cdot (B+D) \cdot (A+B)(C+D)},$$

where a value of 3.84 for one degree of freedom corresponds to a probability (p value) of 0.05 that the similarity or dissimilarity in the reaction pattern of two sera is due to chance alone. Likewise a χ^2 of 6.63 corresponds to $p = 0.01$ and a χ^2 of 10.83 to $p = 0.001$. It should be noted that the χ^2 value is dependent on the absolute value of the expression $(AD - BC)$. If $B \cdot C$ (the product of the discordant reactions $(+/-)$ and $(-/+)$) is greater than $A \cdot D$, there is a negative association between these two sera. The degree of association—positive or negative—is measured by the correlation coefficient

$$r = \sqrt{\frac{\chi^2}{N}}.$$

Using these methods one was able to select groups of sera which were highly associated suggesting that they all contained antibodies directed against the same antigen. Therefore one was justified to conclude that cell samples that reacted positively with all sera of such a highly associated group indeed carry the "antigen" corresponding to the "antibody" common to all sera of the group. Thus it was possible to define "antigens" even with multispecific sera. It is clear that this type of definition is an operational one. Frequently enough "antigens" were found to be of compound nature, a problem which will be returned to in the section on "cross-reactivity".

2.4 The Genetic Organization of HLA-A, B, and C Antigens

Soon after the definition of the first HLA antigens it became obvious that these antigens were inherited as simple co-dominant mendelian traits. In addition it could be shown that practically all of these antigens are governed by one single autosomal region (Dausset et al. 1967). This was the conclusion drawn from the fact that in any given family there are no more than four different types of children. Schematically, if the diploid chromosomes of the parents are designated as A/B for the father and C/D for the mother, there are four possible combinations: AC, AD, BC, BD since each child inherits one paternal and one maternal chromosome. Further it was observed that certain antigens, such as HLA-A1 and HLA-A2, are never coded for by the same chromosome: In families in which one parent is positive for A1 and A2 and the other parent has neither antigen (a double back-cross situation) these antigens are never present together in one child nor are there any children possessing neither antigen. It was further demonstrated that there were two groups of antigens showing this allelic behavior among themselves while one antigen of one group is inherited in coupling with one antigen of the second group of alleles. This led to the concept of two closely linked loci with multiple alleles (Dausset et al. 1968; Bodmer et al. 1966; Kissmeyer-Nielsen and Kjerbje 1967a). This assumption was further supported by the fact that when tested in an unrelated population the antigens in each of these groups displayed a negative association among each other

Table 1.1. Listing of the Officially Recognized HLA-A, B, C and D Antigens with the New WHO Nomenclature (WHO Terminology Report 1976)

New	Previous	New	Previous	New	Previous	New	Previous
HLA-A1	HL-A1	HLA-B5	HL-A5	HLA-CW1	T1	HLA-DW1	LD 101
HLA-A2	HL-A2	HLA-B7	HL-A7	HLA-CW2	T2	HLA-DW2	LD 102
HLA-A3	HL-A3	HLA-B8	HL-A8	HLA-CW3	T3	HLA-DW3	LD 103
HLA-A9	HL-A9	HLA-B12	HL-A12	HLA-CW4	T4	HLA-DW4	LD 104
HLA-A10	HL-A10	HLA-B13	HL-A13	HLA-CW5	T5	HLA-DW5	LD 105
HLA-A11	HL-A11	HLA-B14	W14			HLA-DW6	LD 106
HLA-A28	W28	HLA-B18	W18				
HLA-A29	W29	HLA-B27	W27				
HLA-AW19	Li	HLA-BW15	W15				
HLA-AW23	W23	HLA-BW16	W16				
HLA-AW24	W24	HLA-BW17	W17				
HLA-AW25	W25	HLA-BW21	W21				
HLA-AW26	W26	HLA-BW22	W22				
HLA-AW30	W30	HLA-BW35	W5				
HLA-AW31	W31	HLA-BW37	TY				
HLA-AW32	W32	HLA-BW38	W16.1				
HLA-AW33	W19.6	HLA-BW39	W16.2				
HLA-AW34	Malay 2	HLA-BW40	W10				
HLA-AW36	Mo	HLA-BW41	Sabell				
HLA-AW43	BK	HLA-BW42	MWA				

while they were positively associated with some antigens of the other group. Finally, the finding of families with recombination between the two loci (Kissmeyer-Nielsen et al. 1969) led to the general acceptance of the two-locus (HLA-A and HLA-B) model of the HLA system (Joint Report 1970). Later this concept had to be enlarged by a third locus (HLA-C) which is very closely linked with the HLA-B locus (Sandberg et al. 1970; Mayr et al. 1973; Bernoco et al. 1973). Through intensive antibody screening and immunizations a considerable number of allelic specificities at the three HLA loci were defined. In Table 1.1 the presently recognized antigens are listed with the new WHO nomenclature agreed upon in Aarhus in 1975 (WHO-IUIS Terminology Committee 1975).

2.5 Phenotype and Gene Frequencies

The distribution of HLA antigens was tested in large populations of unrelated individuals in order to establish the phenotype and gene frequencies. Table 1.2 lists the phenotype and gene frequencies of 16 HLA-A, 26 HLA-B and 5 HLA-C antigens in the European Caucasian population as determined by the 6th International Histocompatibility Workshop in 1975 (Joint Report 1975). The gene frequencies can be determined by a number of different ways. The most simple estimate is through the formula $g=1-\sqrt{1-f}$, where g is the gene frequency and f the phenotype frequency as a fraction of one. This formula assumes that the tested population is in Hardy-Weinberg equilibrium, which is generally the case if there is no selection based on HLA types (Albert et al. 1973a). Other methods for gene frequency estimates include the maximum likelihood method (Yasuda and Kimura 1968), the minimum χ^2 method (Albert et al. 1973), and the gene counting method in materials where family typing is available for deduction of genotypes. It has been shown by Albert et al. (1973a) that all these methods generally yield virtually identical results. It is therefore justified to use the most simple method (the square root formula) for gene frequency estimates. This, however, is not true for samples of individuals with HLA associated diseases, where alternate methods have been devised.

Table 1.2 shows that only a relatively small fraction of the gene frequency at the HLA-A and B loci is still unaccounted for, whereas there is a considerable part of the gene frequency at the HLA-C locus still serologically undetected (the serologically undefined genes are summarized under the term "blank").

As in all blood-group polymorphisms the genes of the HLA system show a markedly different distribution in different ethnic groups. The gene frequencies of HLA-A and B locus antigens in Japanese and Negro populations are given in Tables 1.3 and 1.4. It can be seen that in the Oriental population there is a comparatively low degree of polymorphism. The antigens HLA-A2, A9, B5, and BW40 are particularly common. In the Negroid populations there is a more diverse picture, while it is obvious that a considerable proportion of the HLA-A and B antigens in Negroes are still to be discovered.

Table 1.2. Phenogype and Gene Frequencies of the Central European Caucasian Population ($n=964$) (Joint Report 1976)

Antigen New	Old	Phenotype Frequency in Percent	Gene Frequency	
HLA-A1	HL-A1	26	0.140	HLA-A
A2	HL-A2	44	0.252	
A3	HL-A3	26	0.140	
A9	HL-A9	23	0.123	
AW23[a]	W23	7	0.036	
AW24[a]	W24	16	0.083	
A10	HL-A10	15	0.078	
AW25[b]	W25	4	0.020	
AW26[b]	W26	10	0.051	
A11	HL-A11	10	0.051	
A28	W28	7	0.036	
A29	W29	5	0.025	
AW30	W30	4	0.020	
AW31	W31	7	0.036	
AW32	W32	7	0.036	
AW33	W19.6	2	0.010	
A blank		–	0.053	
HLA-B5	HL-A5	11	0.057	HLA-B
B7	HL-A7	19	0.100	
B8	HL-A8	17	0.089	
B12	HL-A12	22	0.117	
B13	HL-A13	7	0.036	
BW35	W5	19	0.100	
BW40	W10	10	0.051	
B14	W14	7	0.036	
BW15	W15	13	0.067	
BW38	W16.1	4	0.020	
BW39	W16.2	6	0.030	
BW17	W17	8	0.041	
B18	W18	12	0.062	
BW21	W21	6	0.030	
BW22	W22	4	0.020	
B27	W27	10	0.051	
TT	TT	1	0.005	
407	407	5	0.025	
BW41	Sabell	2	0.010	
BW37	TY	5	0.025	
HR	HR	1	0.005	
KSO	KSO	0	0.000	
BW42	MWA	1	0.005	
B blank		–	0.018	
HLA-CW1	T1-AJ	7	0.036	HLA-C
CW2	T2-170	10	0.051	
CW3	T3-UPS	23	0.123	
CW4	T4-315	21	0.111	
CW5	T5	12	0.062	
C blank		–	0.617	

[a] Included in HLA-A9.
[b] Included in HLA-A10.

Table 1.3. Phenotype and Gene Frequencies of HLA-A, B and C Antigens in the Japanese Population (n=416) (Joint Report 1976)

Antigen	Phenotype Frequency in Percent	Gene Frequency	Antigen	Phenotype Frequency in Percent	Gene Frequency
HLA-A1	3	0.015	HLA-CW1	33	0.181
A2	45	0.258	CW2	4	0.020
A3	3	0.015	CW3	41	0.232
A9	58	0.352	CW4	6	0.030
A10	17	0.089	CW5	3	0.015
A11	24	0.128	C blank		0.522
A28	6	0.030			
A29	2	0.010			
AW30	3	0.015			
AW31	6	0.030			
AW32	7	0.036			
AW33	4	0.020			
A blank		0.002			
HLA-B5	34	0.188			
B7	11	0.057			
B8	1	0.005			
B12	15	0.078			
B13	5	0.025			
B14	2	0.010			
BW15	14	0.073			
BW16	7	0.036			
BW17	4	0.020			
B18	2	0.010			
BW21	3	0.015			
BW22	16	0.083			
B27	4	0.020			
BW35	19	0.100			
BW37	4	0.020			
BW40	31	0.169			
BW41	2	0.010			
BW42	11	0.057			
KSO	0	–			
B blank		0.044			

2.6 Haplotype Frequencies

As discussed above, HLA antigens belonging to the different loci are inherited in coupling forming the haplotype. Each individual possesses two haplotypes, a paternal and a maternal one. For example, a common HLA genotype would be composed of the haplotypes HLA-A2, B12, and HLA-A3, BW35. If the antigens of the HLA-C locus are also included, these haplotypes could be: HLA-A2, B12, CW5 and HLA-A3, BW35, CW4. Thus every individual can express up to six different HLA antigens belonging to three loci. Often enough the typing results yield only information about five, four or even

Table 1.4. Phenotype and Gene Frequencies of HLA-A, B and C Antigens in the African Black Population ($n=411$) (Joint Report 1976)

Antigen	Phenotype Frequency in Percent	Gene Frequency	Antigen	Phenotype Frequency in Percent	Gene Frequency
HLA-A1	9	0.046	HLA-CW1	0	–
A2	22	0.117	CW2	24	0.128
A3	10	0.051	CW3	15	0.078
A9	23	0.123	CW4	22	0.117
A10	15	0.078	CW5	6	0.030
A11	0	–	C blank		0.647
A28	23	0.123			
A29	17	0.089			
AW30	36	0.200			
AW31	4	0.020			
AW32	4	0.020			
AW33	5	0.025			
AW36	3	0.015			
A blank		0.093			
HLA-B5	4	0.020			
B7	18	0.094			
B8	7	0.036			
B12	16	0.083			
B13	4	0.020			
B14	9	0.046			
BW15	6	0.030			
BW16	4	0.020			
BW17	33	0.181			
B18	10	0.051			
BW21	2	0.010			
BW22	1	0.005			
B27	1	0.005			
BW35	14	0.073			
BW37	0	–			
BW40	2	0.010			
BW41	2	0.010			
BW42	16	0.083			
B blank		0.223			

fewer antigens, making it impossible to distinguish on a phenotypic level between homozygosity for certain antigens on one side and the presence of a serologically unaccounted antigen. To solve this question it is necessary to study the inheritance of the antigens in the family or to calculate the probability for a given genotype, a method to be discussed below.

Since the haplotype is the unit of inheritance it is logical to express the distribution of HLA genes in a given population as the matrix of haplotype frequencies. Haplotype frequencies can be determined by haplotype counting in parents of families which have been genotyped. Unfortunately, there is a certain proportion of families in which an unequivocal deduction of haplo-

Table 1.5

	Phenotype	Genotype
Father	HLA-A1, A10, B8, B18	A1, B8/A10, B18
Mother	HLA-A2, A9, B12	A9, B12/A2-X or A2, B12
Child 1	HLA-A1, A9, B8, B12	A1, B8/A9, B12
Child 2	HLA-A9, A10, B12, B18	A10, B18/A9, B12
Child 3	HLA-A1, A9, B8, B12	A1, B8/A9, B12

ιypes is not possible. Since one would introduce a considerable bias by omitting such families from analysis, it is necessary to tally unclear phenotypes according to the most probable genotypes (maximum likelihood procedure). For example, in the family given in Table 1.5 there is no segregation for the maternal haplotypes and the phenotype of the mother shows only three antigens—HLA-A2, 9, B12 (the C locus is omitted for the sake of simplicity).

It is therefore unclear whether the mother is homozygous for HLA-B12 (A9, B12/A2, B12) or whether she possesses a serologically undefined antigen of the HLA-B locus (A9, B12/A2, BX). The decision will be made on statistical grounds on the basis of the relative frequencies of the haplotypes in question in the population under study.

Thus, assuming a first count of equivocal haplotypes had yielded a frequency of 0.050 for A2, B12 and 0.020 for A2, BX, we can formulate that only two geotypes are possible for the mother:

$$p(2,\ 12/9,\ 12)+p(2,\ X/9,\ 12)=1.0 \tag{1}$$

which can be reduced to

$$p(2,\ 12)+p(2,\ X)=1.0. \tag{2}$$

From the preliminary haplotype frequencies (hf) we can write

$$\frac{p(2,\ 12)}{p(2,\ X)}=\frac{hf(2,\ 12)}{hf(2,\ X)}=\frac{0.05}{0.02} \tag{3}$$

and transform to

$$p(2,\ X)=0.4\ p(2,\ 12). \tag{4}$$

This can be introduced in (2) to give

$$p(2,\ 12)+0.4\ p(2,\ 12)=1.0$$

$$p(2,\ 12)=0.714.$$

From (2) we can determine $p(2,\ X)=1-0.714=0.286$. In the haplotype counting which then includes also the uncertain haplotypes the genotype of the mother in our example is scored as one haplotype A9, B12 and 0.714 haplotype A2, B12 as well as 0.286 haplotype A2, X. In this way all unclear haplotypes can be accounted for on the basis of probability calculations.

Table 1.6. HLA-A, B Haplotype Frequencies in the Caucasian Population ($n = 4302$). Albert et al. 1976b

	HLA A1	HLA A2	HLA A3	HLA A9	HLA A10	HLA A11	HLA A28	HLA A29	HLA AW 30/31	HLA AW 32	Blank	Total
HLA-B5	65	243	82	74	44	76	50	4	15	2	74	729
HLA-B7	112[b]	328[b]	638[a]	151	45	36	17	30	15	18	59	1449
HLA-B8	798[a]	110[b]	32[b]	31[b]	1	18	14	7	10	10	1[b]	1032
HLA-B12	15[b]	538[a]	82[b]	155	72	10[b]	65	124[a]	9	34	84	1188
HLA-B13	28	104	30	43	10	15	7	4	32	7	34	314
HLA-B14	24	60	9	30	2	7	22	8	10	11	73[a]	256
HLA-BW15	47	422[b]	90	79	19	14	21	4	6	16	27	745
HLA-BW16	30	17[b]	41	44	44	6	13	0	9	5	20	229
HLA-BW17	122[a]	144	33	26	21	15	5	14	9	11	23	423
HLA-B18	5	121	41	45	124[a]	35	16	7	16	4	24	438
HLA-BW21	22	67	30	46	18	8	3	3	7	8	14	226
HLA-BW22	10	40	20	28	12	25	0	2	2	1	13	153
HLA-B27	35	177[a]	52	54	16	23	18	10	6	18	11	420
HLA-BW35	40[b]	136[b]	333[a]	93	26	138[a]	27	17	24	5	71	910
HLA-BW40	32[b]	280[a]	89	75	17	19	30	4	20	36	59	661
Blank	133	252	51[b]	91	99	60	48	0	23	44	26	827
Total	1518	3039	1653	1065	570	505	356	238	213	230	613	10,000

Frequencies are given as numbers per 10,000.

[a, b] Significant linkage disequilibrium is indicated by [a] (positive delta) and by [b] (negative delta) $p = <0.001$.

It is also possible to calculate the haplotype frequency from the phenotype data on the basis of a 2×2 contingency table using a formula given by Mickey (Joint Report 1970) or by Mattiuz et al. (1970). This formula can also be extended to the calculation of three-point haplotype (e.g. HLA-A, B, C) frequencies based on the $2 \times 2 \times 2$ contingency table of the phenotype data (Piazza 1975). It is quite important to note however that for such calculations it is necessary to analyze fairly large populations ($m = 500$) in order to obtain a reasonably accurate estimate.

The matrix of haplotype frequencies of a Caucasian population is given in Table 1.6. It can be seen that certain haplotypes are relatively frequent whereas a majority of haplotypes is rather infrequent. The most common haplotypes in the Caucasian race are HLA-A1, B8; A2, B12; and A3, B7. It has been shown that the haplotype frequencies are quite characteristic for certain ethnic groups.

Table 1.7 lists the most common haplotypes of a Japanese and a Negroid population to demonstrate the large degree of variation between populations.

2.7 Linkage Disequilibrium

Analysing the frequency of certain haplotypes it was noted that some haplotypes are much more frequent than one would expect on the basis of the gene frequencies of the antigens involved. If two loci are separable by recombi-

Table 1.7. Frequent HLA-A, B Haplotypes in the Japanese and Negro Populations (Albert et al. 1972d)

		Japanese	Negroes
Frequent in Japanese	HLA-A9, B5	0.0073	0.0012
	A2, BW40	0.0044	0.0015[a]
	A9, BW40	0.0052	0.0006
	A10, BW40	0.0027	0.0004
	A9, B7	0.0036[a]	0.0021
	A2, BW35	0.0033	0.0029
	A2, BW15	0.0027	0.0003
	A11, BW22	0.0015[a]	0.0000
Frequent in Negroes	HLA-A28, BW17	0.0000	0.0027
	AW31, BW35	0.0007	0.0025
	A2, B12	0.0008	0.0025
	A2, BW17	0.0000	0.0020
	AW31, BW17	0.0005	0.0018

[a] Significant linkage disequilibrium.

nation—as has been shown for HLA-A and B—one can assume that evolution has provided an infinite number of recombinations between these loci so that the alleles of the two loci are associated at random, i.e. they behave as independent traits. This situation is termed linkage disequilibrium.

If the probabilities of two independent events are p and q then the probability of joint occurrence is p·q. Translated into HLA terms this means that the frequency of joint occurrence on one chromosome (haplotype) of any HLA-A allele with any HLA-B allele would be expected to be equal to the product of the gene frequencies of the two alleles involved. For example, the haplotype HLA-A1, B8 is expected to have a frequency of $g_{(1)}0.15 \times g_{(8)}0.1 = 0.015$. In reality, however, the haplotype A1, B8 is counted as 0.079, which is highly significantly more than the expected frequency. Classically the difference between expected and observed haplotype frequency is determined as the linkage disequilibrium parameter or delta value. Since this parameter is frequency-dependent the proportion of h obs/h exp has been offered as a more useful measure of the linkage disequilibrium, where h obs is the observed and h exp the expected haplotype frequency. The value for this "delta ratio" lies above one for positive linkage disequilibria and below one for negative delta values. As is demonstrated in Table 1.6 there is considerable linkage disequilibrium between HLA-A and B. It must be borne in mind that many haplotypes are so rare that even in the large populations investigated the deviations are not statistically significant. It can be seen in Table 1.9 that most but not all frequent haplotypes (see Table 1.6) have a high linkage disequilibrium (such as HLA-A1, B8; A2, B12; A3, B7; A3, BW35). Conversely there are some relatively rare haplotypes with a very high linkage disequilibrium (A29, B12; A1, B17; A33, B14; A30, B13). On the level of the unrelated population linkage disequilibrium expresses itself in the form of an association of two alleles of two different closely linked loci. The observations made on the properties of linkage disequilibrium in the HLA-A, B system serve as a model for the relationship between HLA-A, B and other closely linked loci such as HLA-D, Bf and disease-susceptibility genes. The reasons for linkage disequilibrium are not known. It may be explained by a number of different mechanisms including selection, migration and mixture of populations as well as genetic drift. Selection has been favored by Bodmer (1972) and Bodmer (1973) while Degos and Dausset (1974) discussed the effects of mixtures of populations which can lead to linkage disequilibrium. In considering the degree of linkage disequilibrium it can be noted that the positive deviations are much stronger than the negative ones, which is in agreement with the assumption that the primary deviation is in the positive direction while the negative values are secondary effects. In other words, one strongly positive deviation is compensated by a large number of small negative deviations from linkage equilibrium. It must be stressed that the recombination frequency between HLA-A and B is so low (approximately 0.85 percent) (Svejgaard et al. 1971) that once a linkage disequilibrium has been established by any means, it will take a very large number of generations until recombination can establish linkage equilibrium. Therefore it is possible that we are dealing here with the late effects of a selection mechanism that took place hundreds of generations ago. On the other hand, the great biological importance of the HLA region makes it quite conceivable that selection is still acting on the products of the HLA genes.

2.8 Cross-Reactivity

One of the major obstacles to understanding HLA serology is the existence of a phenomenon which is generally—and somewhat inaccurately—referred to as "cross-reactivity." In early immunization experiments it was observed that antisera which were produced between donor and recipient pairs differing only for one known HLA antigen (e.g., donor HLA-A2, A3, B7, B12 and recipient HLA-A2, A3, B8, B12), reacted not only with all individuals positive for HLA-B7 but also with individuals positive for HLA-B27 and BW22, although it was clear that the immunizing cell did not carry these additional antigens. When an attempt was made to eliminate this additional activity by absorption with cells from a B27-positive, B7-negative individual, all activity—including the anti-HLA-B7 reactivity—was eliminated. The same results were obtained when BW22 positive cells were used for absorption. Thus it was first assumed that this phenomenon is due to cross-reactivity based on biochemical similarity of the respective antigens. This notion, however, was contradicted by the fact that there are anti-HLA-B7 sera which cannot be absorbed with HLA-B27 and/or BW22. It was found that this type of "cross-reactivity" was a general phenomenon involving—in some way—all known HLA-A and HLA-B antigens. There are several "families" of "cross-reacting" antigens such as HLA-A1, A3, A11 or HLA-A2, A28 at the HLA-A locus and HLA-B7, B27, BW22 or HLA-B5, BW35, BW15, B18 to name only the most outstanding examples (Mittal et al. 1972a; Mueller-Eckhardt et al. 1972). This pattern of "cross-reactivities" was not only found in sera which were produced by planned immunization but also in sera from multiparous women, where it was shown that antibodies directed at two or more "cross-reacting" antigens tend to occur together in sera from unselected multiparous women (Albert et al. 1973d) thereby confirming cross-reactivity patterns observed in absorbtion experiments (Mittal et al. 1972b). The groups of cross-reacting antigens always involve a number of alleles belonging to the same locus, which is also confirmed by the experience that antibodies directed at antigens belonging to different loci can in general quite easily be separated by absorption. Titration experiments of antisera containing antibodies directed against a group of cross-reacting antigens revealed that most of these sera have one "main" specificity which is relatively high-titered (this specificity corresponds to the antigens present on the immunizing cells) while the other "cross-reacting" specificities generally have a low titer (Albert et al. 1973d). A similar result was obtained when weak antisera were concentrated with the effect that previously undetected "cross-reacting" antibodies became apparent after concentration. These experiments suggest that there are several antibody populations with different specificities present in these "cross-reacting" sera (Albert et al. 1973d), a notion which was shown to be correct by absorption-elution experiments (Mueller-Eckhardt et al. 1972; Colombani et al. 1969, 1970), clearly demonstrading the existence of different antibody populations in sera, which, according to classical cross-absorption criteria, would have been classified as "monospecific."

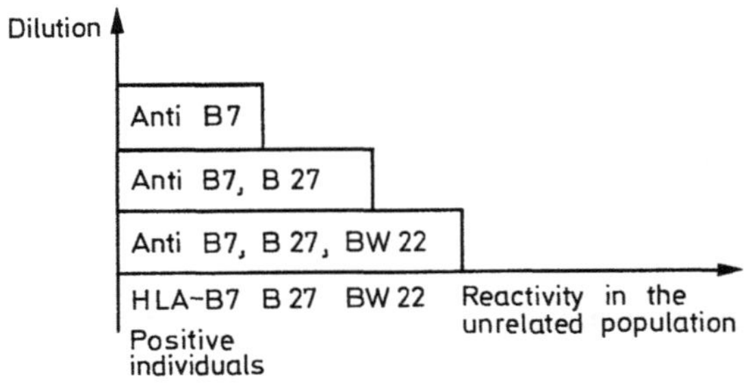

Fig. 1.2

Figure 1.2 describes schematically how the mixture of different antibody populations in a cross-reacting serum may be imagined: The vertical axis describes the test sensitivity and the antibody titer while the horizontal axis reflects the reactivity in the population. Since the antibodies are cumulative in their cytotoxic activity, it can be seen that the removal by absorption of one of the antibody populations may render the serum negative, while a sublytic concentration of antibodies remains in the absorbed serum.

Experiments using Fab fragments of HLA antibodies as blocking factors showed that different antibodies directed at the same cross-reacting group of antigens react with different sites on the cell surface (Legrand and Dausset 1973). With these experiments, Dausset's much earlier prediction (Ivanyi and Dausset 1966), that HLA antigens are probably of compound nature containing several antigenic factors, was shown to be correct.

After it had been established that HLA antigens are composed of a number of highly associated antigenic factors with different immunogenicity, the question arose whether these antigenic factors reside on the same or on different molecules. Kourilsky et al. (1972) showed in capping experiments that the antigenic sites corresponding to the different "cross-reacting" antibody populations reside together on the same molecule.

From these data the old problem of serology (Hirschfeld et al. 1965)—"simple antigen and complex antibodies or simple antibody and complex antigens?"—may be answered with: "Complex antigens *and* complex antibodies." In other words, it is clear that the HLA antisera contain a mixture of different antibody populations and the HLA antigens are composed of a number of different antigenic sites of the same molecule. On the genetic level this may be translated into the existence of one gene with a number of mutational sites coding for one polypeptide chain exhibiting several antigenic sites. The different antigenic factors making up one "antigen" are highly associated in the random population so that one could speak of an "intragenic" linkage disequilibrium. Thus the varying degrees of cross-reactivity between HLA antigens can be explained in terms of the sharing of varying numbers of antigenic factors. These conclusions are not restricted to HLA-A and B locus antigens. They may very well serve as a model for the fine structure of HLA-C and D locus antigens.

3. Lymphocyte-Defined Antigens

3.1 Historical Remarks

In an attempt to devise an *in vitro* measure of histocompatibility, lymphocytes from different individuals were cultured together and it was found that the degree of blast transformation after several days of culture was indeed related to the incompatibility for transplantation antigens (Bach and Hirschhorn 1964). This test was developed (Bach et al. 1967) into what is today referred to as mixed lymphocyte culture (MLC), where the blast transformation is measured by the uptake of radioactive thymidine. Since it became necessary to analyze the two-way MLC (A–B) in the form of two one-way reactions (A–B and B–A), one of the two lymphocyte samples involved was blocked from blast transformation by means of irradiation or treatment with mitomycine (Bach and Voynow 1966), indicated by the suffixes "x" and "m" respectively. Thus a simple MLC between A and B consists of the following reactions:

A + Bm (A = responder, Bm = stimulator)
B + Am (B = responder, Am = stimulator)
A + Am } Controls
B + Bm }

3.2 Genetics of MLC

Investigations among unrelated individuals showed that only a very small proportion of pairs (less than 1 in 500) of randomly chosen individuals have a negative MLC reaction (i.e., do not produce mutual stimulation) (Mempel et al. 1973a). In contrast, among pairs of siblings there was mutual nonstimulation in approximately 25 percent (Bach et al. 1969). If nonstimulation is taken as proof of identity for "MLC-antigens" then these data lead to the conclusion that one single autosomal region with a large number of different alleles is responsible for the expression of the MLC antigens. When it was discovered that HLA-A, B-identical siblings generally do not stimulate each other in MLC (Bach et al. 1969), it was frist assumed that the HLA-A, B antigens could be the structures responsible for stimulation in MLC. This assumption, however, proved to be wrong, when it was demonstrated that unrelated HLA-A, B-identical individuals showed mutual MLC stimulation in 9 out of 10 pairs (Mempel et al. 1973). Further evidence was provided by exceptional families in which HLA-identical siblings do stimulate in MLC, while HLA-different siblings do not (Yunis and Amos 1971; Mempel et al. 1972). This led to the conclusion that "MLC-antigens" are coded for by a separate locus closely linked to HLA-B. It then became necessary to devise methods for the identification of single alleles of this MLC locus (now HLA-D). The following scheme was developed (Mempel et al. 1973a and b, van den Tweel et al. 1973): Under the assumption that absence of MLC stimulation indicates identity for HLA-D antigens, "typing cells" were selected which are homozygous for an HLA-D antigen. These homozygous typing cells (HTC) are tested in MLC with the cells under study. The typing procedure is based on the assumption that an immunologically competent cell will not be stimulated by an antigen which the cell itself possesses. Thus if a cell heterozygous for the HLA-D-antigen A (A/X) meets in the MLC a cell which is homozygous for a (A/A), then A/X cannot find any foreign antigen on A/A and is therefore not stimulated, whereas A/A recognizes X in A/X as foreign and will react with a stimulation.

A/X + (A/A)m → no stimulation
A/A + (A/X)m → stimulation

This type of one-way nonstimulation is therefore characteristic for the presence of an HLA-D antigen, which is defined by a homozygous reference cell. (For definition of typing response, see p. 142ff.)

In a system as polymorphic as HLA-D it is obviously quite difficult to find homozygous individuals. One approach was to utilize the linkage disequilibrium which exists between HLA-A, B and HLA-D (Albert et al. 1973a, c). In families where the parents share one HLA-haplotype, some children are HLA-identical with one of their parents and some children are homozygous for the shared haplotype as is demonstrated below:

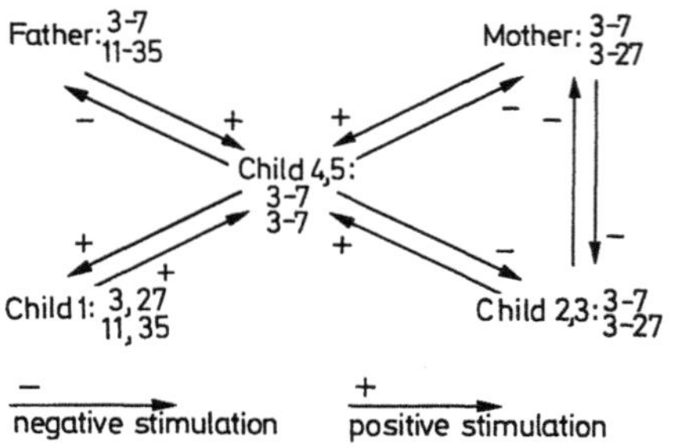

Due to the linkage disequilibrium between HLA-A, B and HLA-D it may be expected that approximately 1 in 10 of such HLA-A3, B7 homozygotes should also be homozygous for the HLA-D antigen (DW2) which is associated with A3, B7. Homozygosity for HLA-DW2 in child 4 and 5 could be proved by the fact that children 2 and 3 showed no stimulation with the mother, whereas children 4 and 5 gave one-way nonstimulation with both parents and with siblings C_2 and C_3.

Another way to find HLA-D-homozygous individuals is by testing the offspring of cousin marriages (van den Tweel et al. 1973) where the chance for homozygosity is 1 in 16. These two approaches have been instrumental in the collection of a fair number of homozygous typing cells which were used at the 7th International Histocompatibility Workshop to identify six tentative HLA-D specificities (HLA-DW1, DW2, DW3, DW4, DW5, DW6) (Joint Report MLC 1976). Thus it had become possible, by using a battery of typing cells, to determine the distribution of a number of HLA-D antigens in an unrelated population. The investigation of the relationship between HLA-A, B, C and HLA-D revealed a variety of associations, mainly between HLA-B and HLA-D locus antigens, reflecting a considerable degree of linkage disequilibrium between HLA-B and HLA-D as had been predicted from the finding that 10 percent of the pairs of HLA-A, B-identical unrelated individuals did not stimulate each other in MLC, while less than one in 500 random pairs are MLC-negative. The very characteristic HLA-A, B, D haplotypes with strong linkage disequilibrium are:

A3, BW35, DW1
A3, B7, DW2
A1, B8, DW3
A2, B12, DW4 (Grosse-Wilde et al. 1976).

Obviously the definition of these HLA-D antigens is still rather preliminary and it is becoming apparent that some of the DW "antigens" will be subject to splitting and redefinition. In addition, evidence is mounting that there are inclusion phenomena suggesting the existence of "cross-reactivity" also for HLA-D antigens (Dupont et al. 1973). Furthermore, there is evidence for the existence of at least one more locus within the human MHC coding for structures, which cause weak, but definite stimulation in MLC: In some families with recombination between HLA-A and B there is some stimulation associated with the chromosomal fragment carrying HLA-A (Thorsby et al. 1973; Thomas, E.D. personal communication).

3.3 "Primed Lymphocyte Typing"

Lymphocytes which are cultured can be stimulated repeatedly and show a clear second-set reaction after *in vitro* priming in a regular MLC. This property of specific recognition of the priming antigen was used by Sheehey et al. (1975) as well as by Fradelizi and Dausset (1975) for the positive identification of MLC antigens. It was shown that these antigens are either identical or very highly associated with the HLA-D antigens defined by homozygous typing cells. One of the major advantages of the PLT test is that specific reagents can be produced quite easily by choosing haploidentical family members for mutual priming.

	Responder	Stimulator	Specificity of PLT cell
Father A/B Mother C/D C_1 A/C	Father (A/B)	C_1 (A/C)	Anti-C
	C_1 (A/C)	Mother (C/D)	Anti-D
	Mother (C/D)	C_1 (A/C)	Anti-A
	C_1 (A/C)	Father (A/B)	Anti-B

Fig. 1.3. Schematic description of PLT priming in a family

It can be seen that four different PLT cells can be produced in any family of two parents and one child (C_1). This is in marked contrast to the very cumbersome search for homozygous typing cells in random families and those with cousin marriages. The PLT test has one more potentially very important advantage over the "regular" MLC typing using HTCs: Specific restimulation can be obtained in as little as 12 to 24 hr, whereas a regular MLC test takes at least 5 days. Thus it is possible to include the PLT testing in the donor selection for kidney transplantation, a measure which can be expected to improve the clinical results.

A third advantage of the PLT method lies in the fact that the test is based on the positive identification of an antigen; in the HTC method an antigen is defined by a lack of reactivity. It is clear that positive identification lends itself much better to the analysis of the very complex MLC antigens under study. The complexity of these antigens is quite clearly demonstrated by the cross-reactivity of PLT's with some of the unrelated control cells (Bach et al. 1976), a situation which is strongly reminiscent of the cross-reactivity phenomena observed in HLA-A, B, C serology. With all these improvements in the technique it has to be borne in mind that the reactivity pattern of a PLT depends not only on the antigens of the priming cell but also on the antigenic make up of the responding cell. If there is a considerable degree of "cross-reactivity" between different MLC antigens, most likely—as in serology—due to the sharing of antigenic factors, then we must expect that the cells from different responders primed with the same homozygous cell should react differently when tested in a random population. Let the homozygous stimulating cell have the MLC antigen A with the antigenic factors a, b, c, d, e, and f and the responding cell B the antigen B with the factors c, d, e, f, g, h, while the responding cell C has the factors e, f, g, h, i, and k. After priming with A, the PLT B should react with all antigens possessing the factors a and/or b, while the PLT C is expected to react with the antigens possessing one or more of the factors a, b, c, d. Thus the reaction pattern of B is included in C. It is even possible that different PLT's primed with the same cells would recognize antigenic factors associated with two allelic HLA-D antigens. Therefore PLT's have to be selected for their discriminatory power and for their specificity. In analogy to classical HLA serology there are broadly reacting PLT's and PLT's with a more restricted reaction pattern. Effective PLT typing can only be obtained with a highly selected panel of primed cells, where—again as in HLA-A, B serology—more than one reagent is needed for the definition of one antigen.

4. Serological Definition of B-Cell-Specific Alloantigens

4.1 Historical Remarks

Soon after the definition of MLC antigens using HTC's, it was attempted to define the same antigens serologically (van Leeuwen et al. 1973) in analogy to the results obtained in the mouse with antisera directed at immune response-associated (Ia-) antigens (Sachs et al. 1975a, b), which were shown to inhibit the MLC in a specific fashion. Since mouse Ia antigens are predominantly expressed on B-lymphocytes and not on platelets, techniques were developed in which B-cell-enriched lymphocytes are tested in a modified cytotoxicity test with platelet-absorbed antisera (van Rood et al. 1975b).

4.2 Methodology

A number of different techniques have been developed for the preparation of a B-cell-enriched cell suspension. The most widely used method is the rosetting of T-cells with sheep erythrocytes and the separation of T-cell rosettes from B-cells by Ficoll gradient centrifugation. A new method of B-cell typing, recently described by van Rood, utilizes a fluorescent double-staining technique in which B-cells are marked with FITC-coupled anti-immunoglobulin and cytotoxicity is demonstrated by a staining of killed cells with ethidium bromide (van Rood et al. 1975). In this way unseparated T- + B-cell suspensions can be tested and read using a filter combination permitting red and green fluorescence to be observed simultaneously.

4.3. Genetics of B-Cell Alloantigens

It was shown that many HLA-A,B antisera contain antibodies directed at B-cell-specific alloantigens. A number of distinct antigenic groups of B-cell-specific alloantigens were defined by classical "clustering" techniques (J. Bodmer et al. 1976; Ting et al. 1976). Some of these Ia-like antigens revealed a very strong association with HLA-D antigens as determined by MLC typing, suggesting identity or very close linkage of the corresponding genes. Interestingly, these associations involve those HLA-A, B, D-haplotypes which are known for strong HLA-A, B and HLA-B*, D-linkage disequilibrium such as HLA-A1,B8,DW3, HLA-A3,B7,DW2 or HLA-A3,BW35,DW1. On the other hand there is mounting evidence for the existence of human B-cell-specific alloantigens, which can be quite clearly separated from HLA-D both in population and family data (Ting et al. 1976) as well as in studies in recombinant families (Albert et al. 1977a). In addition, there is evidence for B-cell-specific alloantigens which segregate independently of HLA (Legrand and Dausset 1975a, b). Since typing for HLA-D-associated B-cell-specific antigens could be used for the selection of unrelated MLC-identical individuals, this method might prove very important for donor selection in kidney and bone marrow transplantation. Therefore a major collaborative effort is under way to elucidate the system(s) of human B-cell-specific alloantigens and their relationship to HLA-D and the other genes of the MHC (7th International Histocompatibility Workshop to be held in Oxford in 1977).

The present knowledge about the genetics of human B-cell-specific alloantigens may be summarized as follows: Most but not all B-cell-specific alloantigens are coded by HLA-linked genes. At least two loci, each with multiple alleles, are assumed to exist. One of these loci is either identical or very closely linked with HLA-D. The observation of inclusion phenomena (Albert et al. 1977; Legrand and Dausset 1975b) in serological reaction patterns strongly suggests the existence of "cross-reactivity" based on complexity of antigens, quite in analogy to that observed for HLA-A and B antigens.

5. Cell-Mediated Cytotoxicity

5.1 Methodology

In an attempt to study the development of effector cells *in vitro*, Lightbody et al. (1971) developed a test which measures the cytotoxic effect of lymphocytes immunized in a mixed leukocyte culture on various targets. Cells from individuals A and B are cultured in a regular one-way MLC where the stimulating cell population is treated with mitomycine or irradiation (indicated by the subscript $_m$ or $_x$ respectively). After 6 days of culture, the lymphocytes are mixed in varying effector: target cell ratios (25:1 or 50:1) with ^{51}chromium-labeled lymphocytes, which had been transformed into blasts by a 3-day culture with phytohemaglutinin (PHA). After a 4-h incubation the amount of ^{51}Cr in the supernatant is measured. The results are expressed as percent specific release which is determined as

$$\frac{\text{experimental release—spontaneous release}}{\text{maximal release—spontaneous release}} \times 100$$

where the maximal release is obtained by repeated freezing and thawing of labeled cells. A simple schematic experiment is given below:

MLC	MLC cpm	Target	Specific killing
A+Bm	10,000	B	50 percent
		A	5 percent
		C	26 percent
A+Am	500	A	10 percent
		B	5 percent
		C	5 percent
B+Am	15,000	A	55 percent
		B	4 percent
		C	5 percent
B+Bm	600	A	5 percent
		B	10 percent
		C	5 percent

5.2 Genetics of CML

It is indicated in this theoretical experiment that the effector cells react specifically with the immunizing cells, although there is occasional "cross-reactivity" with third-party cells reflecting the sharing of antigens (in this case between B and C). Both the specific target antigens and the cross-reacting antigens detected by CML are linked with HLA (Goulmy et al. 1976; Sondel and Bach 1976). In families with different types of recombinations Eijsvoogel et al. (1972, 1973a, b, c) were able to show (1) that production of cytotoxic effector cells occurs only in the presence of a significant proliferative response caused by differences at the HLA-D locus, (2) that effector cells can only be generated if the stimulating cells differ in the HLA-A and/or B loci from the responder, and (3) that the target structures hit by the cytotoxic cells are coded in the HLA-A and/or B loci or at very closely linked loci. Recently, Kristensen and Grunnet (1976) presented evidence that favors the assumption that separate but very closely linked loci with high linkage disequilibrium to HLA-A and B code for the CML target structures. The situation becomes less clear when results of *in vivo* primed effector cells (direct CML) are analyzed. Mawas et al. (1973a, b) observed after immunization with skin grafts and bone marrow transplants target structures associated with HLA and, in addition, structures coded by HLA-independent loci. In spite of these complexities the assay of CML has provided information about the genetic basis of the transplantation reaction, where the MLC may be understood as a model of the afferent limb with antigen recognition and the CML as the efferent part with the generation of cytotoxic cells aimed at the destruction of the graft.

6. Tissue Distribution of HLA Antigens

Antigens controlled by the HLA-A or B locus are detectable on the membrane of almost all cells in the organism. HLA-C antigens have been more exactly defined only recently and therefore no data are available about their presence on cells or tissue other than lymphocytes.

The antigens can be identified on the external cell membrane mainly by (a) classical serological methods, such as agglutination, lymphocytotoxicity, absorption, and by inhibition of these reactions; and by (b) labeling methods, either as a direct test with ^{125}iodine, fluorescein, or ferritin-labeled anti-HLA antibodies (Kourilsky et al. 1971) or with hybrid antibodies (anti-IgG coupled with, e.g., ferritin antibodies) (Hämmerling et al. 1968), or as an indirect "sandwich" technique using labeled anti-human immunoglobulins.

HLA antigens are also present on internal cell membranes: Manson (1972), Wilson and Amos (1972), and Lewis et al. (1974) isolated microsomal lipoprotein fractions from cells that exhibited inhibitory capacity of anti-HLA sera.

6.1 HLA-A and -B Antigens

6.1.1 Cells

The cells which have been most thoroughly investigated in this regard are lymphocytes, which possess by far the highest content of HLA antigens of all cells or tissues. Labeling techniques have revealed that there are at least 10^3 to 10^4 HLA determinants per specificity per lymphocyte (Sanderson and Welsh 1974; Giphart et al. 1975b). Generally, there seems to be no difference in the HLA content of lymphocytes from different origins, i.e., peripheral blood, lymph nodes, thoracic duct (Patel 1971), or spleen (Götze, *unpublished*); thymus lymphocytes, however, appear to possess fewer HLA antigens than peripheral blood lymphocytes when tested by the quantitative absorption technique (Götze, *unpublished*; Dumble and Whittingham, 1975).

Also, B-lymphocytes appear to carry more HLA antigens than T-lymphocytes, and the latter more than thymocytes.

Of blood elements—such as granulocytes, neutrophils, basophils, and eosinophils (Bialek et al. 1966; Thorsby 1969; Giphart et al. 1975b), monocytes (Kourilsky et al. 1971; Giphart et al. 1975b), platelets (Bialek et al. 1966; Heinrich et al. 1974; Haynes et al. 1974; Svejgaard et al. 1971a), and reticulocytes (Harris and Zervas 1969; Silvestre et al. 1970)—all possess HLA molecules. Although Cook (1974), Harris and Zervas (1969), and Silvestre et al. (1970) could not detect HLA antigens on red blood cells, others demonstrated that erythrocytes carry very small quantities (Seaman et al. 1967; Morton et al. 1969, 1971; Doughty et al. 1973; Nordhagen and Orjasaeter 1974; Reekers et al. 1975) that were detectable only by very sensitive techniques (e.g., autoanalyzer, saline-18° C agglutination, or indirect antiglobulin test in low ionic strength buffer containing 30 percent bovine serum albumin).

Fibroblasts isolated from skin possess HLA antigens, as indicated by their ability to bind anti-leukocyte antibodies (Melief et al. 1967; Miggiano et al. 1971). Also, fibroblasts in culture possess HLA antigens (Thorsby and Lie, 1968; Sasportes et al. 1971; Goldstein and Singal, 1972; Brautbar et al. 1973a, b). Endothelial cells have been reported to carry HLA antigens (Moraes and Stastny, 1975; Gibofsky et al. 1975).

The question remains as to whether human spermatozoa carry HLA antigens. Piazza et al. (1969), Fellous and Dausset (1970), Kerek and Afzelius (1972), and Halim et al. (1974) were able to detect by cytotoxicity that anti-HLA sera kill sperms, although Seigler and Metzgar (1970) did not succeed in absorbing HLA leukagglutinins with human spermatozoa. Some authors (Fellous and Dausset 1970; Halim et al. 1974) have concluded that HLA antigens show a haploid expression on sperms. This conclusion was drawn from the observation that only about 50 percent of sperms were killed in the direct complement-dependent cytotoxicity test, when testing was done for one specificity only; however, about 80 percent of the sperms were killed when they were tested for two specificities of the same locus. Because of the limitations of the complement-dependent cytotoxicity test (antigen density, complement activation, lysability) and the use of only operationally monospecific anti-HLA sera, this question should not be considered solved. Many HLA alloantisera may contain antibodies against B-cell-specific (Ia-like, see Chapter 7) antigens which may be identical to lymphocyte-activating determinants, whose presence has been established on the surface of sperms in a haploid expression (Festenstein et al. 1976; Halim and Festenstein 1975).

6.1.2 Cultured Cells

Continuous lymphoid cells in culture (Rogentine and Gerber 1969, 1971; Dick et al. 1972; Ferrone et al. 1971; Pellegrino et al. 1972), fibroblasts (Brautbar et al. 1973a, b; Thorsby and Lie 1968), and malignant cells (Evans and Pegrum 1973; Schlessinger and Amos 1971; Walford et al. 1971; Harris 1973) have been shown to possess HLA antigens; during some malignancies, however, a decrease or loss of HLA antigens has been reported (Bertrams et al. 1971; Seigler et al. 1971; van Rood and van Leeuwen 1971). So far, there seems to be only one exception: The cultured cell line DAUDI, derived from a Burkitt lymphoma, apparently does not express HLA antigens on its surface (Nilsson et al. 1974; Poulik et al. 1974). Interestingly, these cells also lack the expression of β_2-microglobulin. When DAUDI cells are hybridized with cells expressing β_2-microglobulin, however, the HLA type of DAUDI cells reappear. It seems possible, therefore, that β_2-microglobulin may be involved in the expression of HLA antigens. On cells which are diploid and have a limited life span in tissue culture (normal fibroblasts), i.e., they usually survive for approximately 40 successive generations, Sasportes et al. (1971) and Goldstein and Singal (1972) found that HLA antigens were decreasingly detectable after 30 or so generations, and that in the generations prior to "crisis," first the B locus antigens and then all HLA antigens disappeared. In contrast, Brautbar et al. (1973a, b) could not observe any difference in the expression of HLA antigens up to the last generation of fibroblasts of embryonic or adult (from different organs) origin. These discordant results might be attributable to the different techniques for detecting HLA antigens that were used in these studies. While Brautbar et al. (1973a, b) tested the presence of HLA antigens by quantitative absorption (Pellegrino et al. 1971), the former investigators tested the presence of HLA antigens by the direct cytotoxicity test, which depends not only on antigen density—which influences the complement activation—but also on the lysability of the cells; a well-known expression of this is the cytotoxic-negative-absorption-positive (CYNAP) phenomenon, described by Ferrone et al. (1967). These data may indicate that aging accompanies an alteration of the outer cell membrane, and thereby affects the "physiological" characteristics of the cells.

6.1.3 Tissue

During the investigation of tissues for the presence of HLA antigens, few attempts have been made to study different kinds of cells of one tissue. As a result, our knowledge is limited concerning the tissue distribution of HLA antigens. It appears, however, that HLA antigens are expressed in almost all tissue with only quantitative differences (Berah et al. 1970): the spleen carries most HLA antigens, followed by the lung, the liver, the intestine, the kidney (McKenzie and Morris 1971; Douglas et al. 1971), and the heart, in that order. Human brain was found to be incapable of absorbing HLA antibodies.

The placenta appears to be rich in HLA antigens (Bruning et al. 1964); trophoblasts, however, do not expose accessibly HLA antigens, although tumors originating from trophoblasts (e.g., chorionepithelioma) possess HLA antigens (Loke et al. 1971). Currie and Bagshawe (1967) found that maternal lymphocytes exerted a profound cytotoxic effect on trophoblast cells cultured after trypsinization from the fetus. Treatment of early mouse trophoblastic cells with neuraminidase revealed normal histocompatibility antigens (Currie et al. 1968). Trophoblasts, therefore, might possess HLA antigens that are not accessible under regular conditions. Human fetal cells grown in culture (monolayers) were shown by Seigler and Metzgar (1970), who used a mixed agglutination technique, to possess HLA antigens. Fetal cells were tested from as early as 6 weeks after conception up to parturition. Tissue culture cells of 15-week-old fetus organs—skin, brain, thymus, lung, spleen, stomach, gut, adrenal gland, and kidney—reacted with anti-leukocyte sera (which were, however, not operationally monospecific). These studies indicate only that HLA antigens can be detected under tissue culture conditions; they do not indicate the presence and quantitative distribution of HLA antigens *in vivo*. On the other hand, Pellegrino et al. (1970) were able to extract HLA antigens from fetal tissue which inhibited specifically anti-HLA antibody reactivity in a pattern consistent with the phenotype of the antigen donor (parents).

6.1.4 Body Fluids

Van Rood and his colleagues (1970 and 1971) found that normal plasma after concentration was able to block HLA-antibody activity specifically, i.e., antibodies directed against the plasma donor's antigens. The presence of HLA antigens in plasma was later confirmed by several groups (Charlton and Zmijewski 1970; Schultz and Shreffler 1972; Aster et al. 1973; Miyakawa et al. 1973a; Billing et al. 1973; Billing and Terasaki 1974; Billing and McMillan 1975; Oh et al. 1975; Pellegrino et al. 1974; Allison et al. 1976; Giphart et al. 1975a). Reisfeld and his collaborators were able to isolate certain HLA antigens from serum (*see below*). HLA antigens have also been found in the urines both of normal healthy individuals (Reisfeld et al. 1976, 1977; Bernier et al. 1976) and of patients with tubulopathies (Robert et al. 1974). Seminal plasma has been reported to contain HLA antigens (Singal et al. 1971; Mittal 1975). Dawson et al. (1974a) and Kachru and Mittal (1975) were able to detect HLA antigens in colostrum and milk.

6.2 HLA-D or Lymphocyte Activating Determinants

HLA-D gene products are defined by their ability to stimulate incompatible, allogeneic (or xenogeneic) lymphocytes. There are no systematic data available on the different cells and tissues with stimulating capacity. Among blood cells, lymphocytes are the best stimulator cells (Alter and Bach 1970); in human, B-cells as well as T-lymphocytes stimulate (Lohrman et al. 1974); also, monocytes are able to induce a lymphoblastic response (Marshall et al. 1966; Hirschberg et al. 1976). In contrast, granulocytes have been reported to suppress stimulation (Johnson et al. 1971; Ragab and Cowan 1973). Platelets are unable to stimulate allogeneic lymphocytes. Fibroblasts lack the ability to induce transformation and proliferation (Schellekens and Eijsvoogel, 1970). On the other hand, it appears that epithelial cells (Cochrum et al. 1971; Levis and Miller 1972; Hirschberg and Thorbsy 1975), endothelial cells (Hirschberg et al. 1974), and spermatozoa can stimulate (Halim and

Festenstein 1975; Festenstein et al. 1976). According to the latter authors, sperms appear to express HLA-D determinants haploid. Also, cells of continuous lymphoid lines are able to stimulate lymphocytes in culture (Hardy et al. 1969; Netzel et al. 1975a).

This tissue distribution of lymphocyte-activating determinants is similar to that observed for B-lymphocyte-specific antigens, whose controlling genes are linked to the HLA-D locus (Legrand and Dausset 1975a, b; Solheim et al. 1975; Terasaki et al. 1975; van Rood et al. 1975a, b, 1976a, c; Winchester et al. 1975a, b; Bodmer et al. 1975a, b; Fellous et al. 1975; Gosset et al. 1975). Antisera against those antigens specifically inhibit allogeneic stimulation. This coincidence of tissue distribution might be taken as additional suggestive evidence for the identity of HLA-D determinants and B-lymphocyte-specific antigens whose controlling genes are linked to HLA.

7. Surface Distribution of HLA Antigens

The membrane consists of a fluid bilayer in which many different proteins or glycoproteins are embedded (Singer and Nicolson 1972). In order to elucidate the topographical and molecular relationship or association of different HLA gene products in this fluid membrane, the capping method first introduced by Taylor et al. (1971) and Loor et al. (1972) (membrane rearrangement) has proved to be the most elegant approach. In this technique, the addition of bivalent antibodies against the determinants carried by one set of molecules causes rearrangement of the immune complexes into aggregates (patches) or caps when the procedure is performed at room temperature or 37° C (de Petris and Raff 1973). Antigen association can be presumed if capping of one set of molecules by specific antibodies also causes capping of the other molecules (i.e., cocapping). As mentioned, the process of capping is temperature-dependent; it requires that the cell be metabolically active (since it is inhibited by azide, cyanide, hexamide and other metabolic inhibitors), and that the antibody (or other aggregate-causing reagents, such as lectins or antigens) is at least bivalent. (Monovalent Fab fragments do not induce cap formation.) Under these conditions the fluorescinated antibody bound to its antigen first shows an even and diffuse distribution over the surface which remains when the reaction takes place at 0° C (Kourilsky et al. 1971). After warming, the fluorescein label aggregates to spots and patches which move to the uropod of the cell to form a cap. These aggregates eventually become internalized by pinocytosis or may be released as antibody-antigen complexes into the medium (Amos et al. 1970; Loor et al. 1972; Miyajima et al. 1972; Cullen et al. 1973; Jacot-Guillarmod et al. 1975). In order to analyze whether another antigen is associated with the first antigen, the cells which had capped the first antibody are reincubated with (rhodamine-labeled) antibodies against a second set of antigens under conditions which prevent cap formation. If both labels are found in the same polar cap, it is likely that the first antibody cocapped both antigens. In contrast, if both antigens are not associated, the second antibody will be found evenly diffused over the cell surface.

Instead of labeling cells with a second antibody, they may be tested, after incubation with the first antibody, by direct cytotoxicity for the presence or absence of the second antigen (lysostrip, Miyajima et al. 1972; Cullen et al. 1973).

With these methods HLA antigens of the A, B, and C locus were shown to be independent molecules in the membrane (Preud'homme et al. 1972; Kourilsky et al. 1972; Cullen et al. 1973; Neauport-Sautes et al. 1973, 1974; Solheim et al. 1973; Solheim and Thorsby 1974; Mayr et al. 1973; Mayr 1974, 1975; Bismuth et al. 1974; Pierres et al. 1975). Identical results were obtained when indirect staining methods were employed (Bernoco et al. 1973). Also, β_2-microglobulin capping has been shown to result in cocapping of HLA antigens (Poulik et al. 1973; Östberg et al. 1974). However, when HLA antigens were capped first, β_2-microglobulin was found in the cap as well as diffusely distributed over the cell surface. These data indicated that HLA is, indeed, associated with β_2-microglobulin but that not all β_2-microglobulin is linked to HLA antigen molecules. In agreement with this is the finding that there are in the range of 10^6 to 10^7 β_2-microglobulin sites versus only about 10^5 HLA sites on the surface of a human lymphocyte (Sanderson and Welsh 1974; Giphart et al. 1975b; Nilsson et al. 1974; Ferrone et al. 1975). In contrast, antisera for B lymphocytes which are able to inhibit MLR (and which are most probably recognizing HLA-D determinants) have been found to cause rearrangement of antigens not associated with β_2-microglobulin (Solheim et al. 1975; Bodmer et al. 1975a). Stripping the membrane of β_2-microglobulin did not alter the lysability for HLA-D antibodies (Bodmer et al. 1975a), indicating that "B-cell specific determinants" are not associated with β_2-microglobulin.

8. Biochemistry

Efforts to biochemically characterize histocompatibility antigens started as early as 1957 by Kandutsch and Reiner-Wenck (1957). The elucidation of the molecular structure of these antigens, however, was hampered by the fact that they are intrinsic components of the fluid bilayer lipid membrane of cells, and therefore, are in their native form insoluble. The first step for isolation, purification, and structural analysis, therefore, was to separate the individual macromolecules assembled in the membrane and keep them in solution. A variety of solubilization procedures have been used such as mechanical, physicochemical, and chemical disruption of cells and biochemical (proteolytic) release of these antigens from the cell surface.

8.1 Localization of H Antigens and Source for Their Purification

Detailed investigations summarized in the previous sections indicate that the major portion of H antigens are arrayed on the cell surface although the investigations of Manson (1972), Wilson and Amos (1972), and Lewis et al. (1974) may suggest that relatively great antigenic activity is associated with the internal membrane system.

Of all the tissue or cells of the organism, blood cells, especially lymphocytes and platelets, carry more H antigens than any other tissue; in fact, in relation to surface area, platelets appear to have the highest density of HLA-A and HLA-B antigens (Giphart et al. 1975b; Dumble and Wittingham 1975). The quantity of HLA (A and B) antigen molecules on the cell surface has been estimated by antibody binding studies at 10^4 to 10^5 per lymphocyte (Sanderson and Welsh 1974; Giphart et al. 1975b); biochemical isolation studies suggest that these molecules may represent about 1 percent or less of the surface proteins of lymphocytes (Springer et al. 1974; Turner et al. 1975).

The following tissues have been employed for the isolation and purification of HLA antigens: spleen (Sanderson and Batchelor 1968; Snary et al. 1975; Etheredge and Najarian 1971), peripheral blood lymphocytes (Rapaport et al. 1967; Etheredge et al. 1973), platelets (Bernier et al. 1974; Pellegrino et al. 1974; Uhlenbruck et al. 1973), liver (Wilson and Amos 1972), serum (Billing et al. 1973; Pellegrino et al. 1974; Oh et al. 1975), and urine (Reisfeld et al. 1976, 1977; Bernier et al. 1976). The development of continuous lymphoid cell lines derived from normal donors (Moore et al. 1967; Levy et al. 1968; Papermaster et al. 1969, 1972; Choi and Bloom 1970), however, has contributed significantly to the progress made within the last few years because such cell lines provide large quantities of genetically uniform cellular material (Reisfeld et al. 1970, 1971b; Strominger et al. 1974; Cresswell et al. 1973; Miyakawa et al. 1971a). In addition, these cultured lines of lymphoblastoid cells carry 5 to 13 times as many HLA antigens as peripheral blood lymphocytes (Papermaster et al. 1972; McCune et al. 1975).

8.2 Assays Monitoring Activity of Soluble HLA Antigens

There are two principal methods for monitoring the activity of solubilized HLA antigens: (a) inhibition of the cytotoxicity of specific HLA antisera, and (b) the binding or the inhibition of binding of soluble HLA antigens to specific alloantisera, with subsequent immunoprecipitation with anti-Ig sera.

8.2.1 Inhibition of Lymphocytotoxicity

These assays are based on the ability of soluble HLA antigens to combine specifically with HLA antibodies and to prevent subsequent antibody activity as measured by the killing of target cells in the lymphocytotoxic test either by ^{51}Cr release (Wigzell 1965; Sanderson 1964), or by microdye exclusion (Mittal et al. 1968; Pellegrino et al. 1973). If the antigen is solubilized by detergents, it is necessary to use protein-rich buffers (30 percent albumin or fetal calf serum) in the test in order to prevent unspecific detergent-mediated lysis (Dawson et al. 1973; Springer et al. 1974).

In order to compare data from different experiments and from different antigen preparations, the inhibition dose and specificity ratio parameters have proved to be extremely useful (Sanderson 1968; Kahan et al. 1971; Pellegrino et al. 1973).

The inhibition dose (ID_{50}) represents the amount of soluble HLA antigen, expressed in μg of protein, required to halve the cytotoxic activity of the specific anti-HLA serum at the last dilution causing $\geqq 80$ percent killing. The specificity ratio (SR) is the relationship between (a) the amount of soluble HLA antigen preparation required for 50 percent inhibition of the cytotoxicity of an indifferent antiserum directed against HLA determinants undetected in the phenotype of cells used for the extraction, and (b) the amount required to inhibit the specific antiserum. While ID_{50} indicates the serologic potency of soluble HLA antigens, SR reflects their immunologic specificity.

8.2.2 Binding or Inhibition of Binding of Soluble HLA Antigens by Specific Alloantisera

The binding of soluble HLA antigens by specific or indifferent antisera and the subsequent precipitation of immune complexes by anti-Ig sera or by protein A-bearing staphylococci (Cullen and Schwartz 1976), or the subsequent separation of the immune complex, as by gel filtration (Cresswell et al. 1973; Sanderson and Welsh 1974; Springer et al. 1974), is usually performed as a qualitative procedure for isolating antigens with different specificities. Pressman and his collaborators (Miyakawa et al. 1972, 1973b; Tanigaki et al. 1973b; Katagiri et al. 1974), however, have developed a radioimmunoassay to quantitatively monitor antigenic activity. In this assay, the HLA activity is determined by the inhibition of direct binding of a standard iodine-labeled antigen by corresponding antisera by the (cold) antigen preparation to be assayed. The sample is incubated with a given amount of specific HLA alloantiserum for 2 hr at room temperature. Then, the radiolabeled antigen (standard) is added. The ratio of antiserum to labeled antigen is such that about 50–70 percent of the radiolabel is precipitated in the absence of inhibitor that could be bound in antibody excess. After the mixture is stored cold overnight, anti-human gamma globulin is added in slight excess; the precipitate is washed and the radioactivity is measured and compared to the control without inhibitor.

8.2.3 Inhibition of Platelet Complement Fixation

A little-used method for monitoring HLA antigenic activity is the inhibition of platelet complement fixation (Colombani et al. 1970b). In this assay, the inhibition of complement fixation by platelet-antibody reaction can be measured by the quantitative lysis of sheep red blood cells sensitized by hemolytic antibodies. The results can be scored automatically with a microscope densitometer (D'Amato et al. 1971). However, the complement fixation test is only approximately 1/20 as sensitive as the microcytotoxicity test (Svejgaard et al. 1967), and good typing reagents for complement fixation are difficult to find.

8.3 Extraction Procedures

In order to separate H antigens from the membrane and from other membrane constituents and to solubilize them in aqueous solvents, widely different techniques have been employed: mechanical or physicochemical disruption of cells, such as sonication (Pellegrino et al. 1970; Kahan and Reisfeld 1971; Reisfeld and Kahan 1970; Kahan et al. 1968), hypotonic lysis and freezing and thawing (Haughton 1964; Davies 1966; Rapaport et al. 1967; Mann et al. 1969a, b), and nitrogen pressure decompression (Hunter and Commerford 1961; Del Villano et al. 1968; Avis 1969; Manson 1972; Wilson et al. 1972); the use of salts such as TIS (Tris salt of 2-hydroxy-3,5-di-iodobenzoic acid) and EDTA (Mann 1972b) or 3 M potassium chloride (Reisfeld et al. 1971a, b; Etheredge et al. 1973); autolysis (Davies 1966; Davies 1968; Colombani et al. 1970b); proteolytic enzyme procedures, especially with papain (Nathenson and Davies 1966; Nathenson and Shimada 1968; Sanderson and Batchelor 1968; Mann et al. 1969b, 1971; Miyakawa et al. 1971a, b; Tanigaki et al. 1971; Sanderson and Welsh 1972; Cresswell et al. 1973, 1974b), release in some cases the H antigens with virtually all their immunologic activity intact though not in their native form; ionic detergents, such as sodium deoxycholate (Metzgar et al. 1967; Snary et al. 1974; Dawson et al. 1974b); and nonionic detergents, such as Triton, Brij and NP-40 (Kandutsch 1960; Kandutsch and Stimpfling 1963; Hilgert et al. 1969; Schwartz et al. 1973; Springer et al. 1974; Dautigny et al. 1973; Strominger et al. 1974; Springer et al. 1974; Bernier et al. 1974), which are thought to release the antigens in their native form.

8.3.1 HLA-A and -B Antigens Isolated From Cell Membranes: Purification Procedures and Physicochemical Properties

8.3.1.1 Proteolytic Cleavage

The release of HLA antigens by proteolytic (papain) digestion can be performed with whole cells or purified membranes (Cresswell et al. 1973; Turner et al. 1975). Whole cells are used if the cells are internally radiolabeled with ^{3}H- or ^{14}C-amino acids or ^{3}H-carbohydrates prior to the solubilization of antigens. Cells are suspended at $3–5 \times 10^{7}$ per ml of medium, consisting of medium, consisting of Hank's salts, basal medium vitamins, 2 mM glutamine and 4 percent Ficoll (plus 0.2 percent glucose, when labeled with radioamino acids, or 0.1 percent Bacto-amino acids and 0.025 percent sodium pyruvate, when labeled with radiocarbohydrates). For solubilization, papain (60 µl, 32 mg/ml, Worthington) and L-cysteine (150 µl, 10 mM, in phosphate-buffered saline) are added, and after 45 min at 37° C with repeated mixing, digestion is terminated by the addition of 140 µl of 50 mM sodium iodoacetate in phosphate-buffered saline. The cells are removed by centrifugation at 400 *g* for 5 min. The supernatant solution is kept in an ice bath for 1–2 hr and the flocculent precipitate that forms is removed by low speed centrifugation. The supernatant is then applied to a column of Sephadex G-150 and eluted with 0.15 M NaCl-0.01 M Tris-HCl (pH 8.2).

For the preparation of HLA antigens on a larger scale, the digestion is performed on purified membranes: cells are lysed by freezing and thawing, and after removal of cell debris by low speed centrifugation, crude membranes are pelleted by centrifugation at 105,000 *g* for 1 hr. Membranes are purified by zonal centrifugation on a 5 to 30 percent gradient of sucrose with a 50 percent sucrose cushion, at 30,000 rpm for 1 hr. Membranes are then suspended in 0.01 M Tris-HCl, pH 8.2 at a concentration of 10 mg of protein per ml. To this suspension, 2 mg/ml of papain in the presence of 5 mM cysteine are added and digestion proceeds at 37° C for 30 min; it is terminated by addition of 6.5 mM sodium iodoacetate. The membranes are then removed, the supernatant solution is dialyzed against 5 mM Na_2HPO_4 (pH 6.0), and the mixture is chromatographed on carboxymethylcellulose in the same buffer. The HLA antigen is not bound. Further purification involves gel filtration on Sephadex G-150 and DEAE-cellulose chromatography; using a pH and molarity gradient, HLA-A2 and HLA-B7, 12 were found to separate in this last step (Cresswell et al. 1974b; Turner et al. 1975; Tanigaki et al. 1974a, 1975). The purification procedure produces glycoproteins which usually show several antigen fractions (when analyzed under non-dissociating conditions on polyacrylamide gel electrophoresis) with molecular weights of 45,000, 82,000, and larger (Mann et al. 1969a, b; Rask et al. 1974). After dissociation in sodium dodecylsulfate (SDS) and urea or guanidine, the HLA antigens are found to have a molecular weight of between 34,000 and 31,000 (Strominger et al. 1974; Springer et al. 1974; Turner et al. 1975; Cresswell et al. 1974b; Tanigaki et al. 1971, 1974a; Nakamuro et al. 1975; Terhorst et al. 1976; Peterson et al. 1974; Mann et al. 1969b; Sanderson 1968). In addition, a small molecule with an approximate molecular weight of 11,500 is usually found in equimolar amounts. This small molecule has been shown to represent β_2-microglobulin (Rask et al. 1974; Grey et al. 1973; Miyakawa et al. 1973b; Nakamuro et al. 1973; Poulik et al. 1974; Strominger et al. 1974; Peterson et al. 1974; Tanigaki et al. 1973a and 1974b; Cresswell et al. 1973, 1974a, b; Springer et al. 1974; Reisfeld et al. 1975). It is assumed that β_2-microglobulin, which is noncovalently bound to HLA-A or -B antigens, is associated with the larger polypeptide (approximately 34,000); this would signify a molecule of about 45,000 (86,000 to 96,000 for a dimeric, more than 120,000 for a polymeric aggregate). The papain-solubilized and purified HLA antigens carry a carbohydrate portion with a molecular weight of about 3000 (Sanderson et al. 1971; Parham et al. 1974; Terhorst et al. 1976).

8.3.1.2 Hypertonic Salt Extraction

Cells are dispersed in phosphate-buffered saline, pH 7.4, containing 3 M KCl (20 ml/10^9 cells); then, the cell suspension is gently agitated on a rotary shaker for 16 hr at 4° C. The resulting viscous extract is centrifuged overnight at 163,000 *g*. Lipid layers are siphoned off, and the supernatant fluid is dialyzed against 3 changes of 200 vol each of isotonic saline. Gelatinous material, which is largely DNA, is removed by centrifugation at 1500 *g* for 20 min. The supernatant fluid is then salted out with ammonium sulfate (0.5 saturation), dialyzed against 0.1 M Tris-HCl buffer, pH 7.8, and passed over a Concanavalin A (Con A)-Sepharose column. HLA antigens can be eluted with 0.1 M Tris-HCl, 0.15 M NaCl, pH 7.0, since they are not bound (about 40 percent of contaminating glycoproteins are removed by this procedure, however). The antigenically active elution fractions are then concentrated (to about 10 to 20 mg protein/ml) and subjected to preparative polyacrylamide gel electrophoresis (system "B" of Rodbard and Chrambach 1971). Elution is performed at a flow rate of 0.8 ml/min with a Tris-HCl buffer (0.138 M Tris, 0.18 M HCl, pH 8.2) containing 5 percent sucrose. Fractions eluting at R_f 0.78–0.80 exhibit specific antigenic activity (Ferrone et al. 1975).

This purification results in molecules of a homogeneous molecular size (Reisfeld et al. 1971a; Papermaster et al. 1972) with a sedimentation coefficient $s_{20,w}$ of 2.3 and a molecular weight of 31,000 (Reisfeld et al. 1971b, 1973). The KCl-extracted HLA antigen appears to be a pure protein and does not react with periodic acid-Schiff (PAS) reagent, suggesting that it contains less than 1 percent carbohydrate (Reisfeld et al. 1973). Some highly purified KCl-solubilized HLA antigens lack an association with β_2-microglobulin (Poulik et al. 1974; Ferrone et al. 1975).

8.3.1.3 Detergents

Detergents are thought to dissociate HLA antigens from the membrane in their native form. Both kinds of detergent, ionic and nonionic, have been successfully employed.

8.3.1.3.1 Ionic Detergent Sodium Deoxycholate

Cells suspended in Eagle's minimal essential medium (MEM) (5×10^7 to 2×10^8 cells per ml of MEM) are disrupted at 0° C by extrusion at a rate of about 400 ml/hr through a small orifice under pressure of about 750 psi against a syringe-loaded ball. Under these conditions, about 90 percent of the cells have lost their viability and almost all HLA antigenic activity is present in the membrane fraction, which is prepared at 4° C by differential centrifugation and subsequent centrifugation on a continuous or discontinuous sucrose density gradient (density between 1.1 and 1.2 g/cm^3). HLA antigenic material is recovered with the plasma membrane marker, 5′-nucleotidase, in the leading edge of the protein peaks (sucrose density of 1.14 g/cm^3).

The purified membrane is dissolved (4 mg membrane protein per ml) in 1 percent sodium deoxycholate in 10 mM Tris-HCl buffer, pH 8.2, for 30 min at room temperature, followed by centrifugation at 100,000 *g* for 1 hr. The supernatant fraction, containing about 90 percent of the membrane protein together with HLA antigen is then fractionated on *Lens culinaris* phythemagglutinin covalently attached to Sepharose. About 10 percent of the added protein is bound to the column and can be eluted with methyl-α-D-manno-pyranoside. In this eluted fraction, about 80–90 percent of the added HLA antigenic activity is recovered. Sodium deoxycholate can be removed from the preparation on Amberlite XAD-2.

In this way purified HLA antigens are slightly polydisperse on sucrose density gradient centrifugation and have sedimentation coefficients $s_{20,w}$ of 5.15 (HLA-A) and 4.55 (HLA-B). Reduction with 2-mercaptoethanol does not affect the sedimentation rate. Under the assumption that deoxycholate is bound to HLA antigens (assuming 0.57 g [HLA-A] and 0.38 g [HLA-B] per g protein on the basis of data obtained with erythrocyte membrane proteins [Helenius and Simmons 1972]) the rates of sedimentation correspond to those for proteins with molecular weights of about 54,000 for HLA-A and 45,200 for HLA-B antigens, respectively. (If no detergent is bound to the purified antigens, the molecular weights will be 88,000 and 73,000, respectively.) It is assumed that the higher molecular weights of the deoxycholate-purified HLA antigens compared with papain-solubilized or nonionic detergent-solubilized antigens (*see below*) result from membrane components attached to the hydrophobic portion of the HLA molecule (Snary et al. 1975). The use of lectin adsorbents implies that HLA molecules contain carbohydrates; in some experiments up to 25 percent of the serologic activity is not bound to lectin-Sepharose, indicating that part of the HLA molecules lack carbohydrate (or contain carbohydrate not bound by lectin-Sepharose).

8.3.1.3.2 Nonionic Detergents

8.3.1.3.2.1 NP-40. The concentration of NP-40 usually applied to solubilize HLA antigens is in the range of 0.1 to 0.5 percent (vol/vol). After incubation of the cell-NP-40 mixture for 15 to 30 min at 4° C, insoluble material is removed by high speed centrifugation (165,000 *g* for 90 min).

Purification of the antigens has been accomplished by (a) immunoprecipitation with specific antisera and goat (or rabbit) anti-human-Ig sera, followed by SDS-urea (7.5–5 percent) polyacrylamide gel electrophoresis (PAGE) of previously isotopically labeled antigens (either enzymatically with lactoperoxidase and Na ^{125}I on the intact cells [Marchalonis et al. 1971] or internally [see above] by incorporation of ^{3}H- or ^{14}C-labeled amino acids or carbohydrates). The radioactive fraction can be cut out of the gel and eluted for further analysis; (b) gel filtration on Sephadex G-200 ion exchange chromatography (Rask et al. 1974; Peterson et al. 1974); (c) electrofocusing after removal of NP-40 by dialysis on Diaflo membranes (PM-10, Amicon) (Dautigny et al. 1973); (d) preparative polyacrylamide electrophoresis in the presence of detergent (with 0.05 M Tris-HCl, 0.38 M glycine buffer, pH 8.3, as electrophoresis buffer and 0.35 M Tris-HCl buffer, pH 8.3, as elution buffer, both containing 0.3 percent NP-40); or (e) filtration on Sepharose 6B in the presence of detergent (0.05 M Tris-HCl, 0.15 M NaCl buffer, pH 7.3, containing 0.3 percent NP-40) (Bernier et al. 1974). Except for the preparation obtained by procedure (a), all other procedures described yield only partially purified HLA antigen molecules.

HLA antigens solubilized by NP-40 and isolated by these various techniques appear to vary in their physical properties. Rask et al. (1974) found that their preparations had a molecular weight of approximately 70,000 when estimated by gel filtration procedures under physiologic buffer conditions; a molecular weight of about 150,000 was found in the presence of detergent. When the same material was analyzed by gel filtration in 6 M guanidine-HCl after reduction and alkylation, a predominant component with a molecular weight of nearly 50,000 was found; in addition, materials migrating in the gel indicate molecular weights of 34,000, 23,000, and 17,000 were also observed. Peptide maps of each of these components led the authors to assume that the various components are parts of the 50,000–molecular weight species and that they arose by proteolysis.

Dautigny et al. (1973) and Bernier et al. (1974) found, when they solubilized HLA antigens with NP-40 from platelet membranes and purified them by electrofocusing, preparative polyacrylamide gel electrophoresis, or filtration on Sepharose B, that the antigens consist of two glycoproteins (PAS-positive) with approximate molecular weights of 45,000 and 90,000 under dissociation conditions; under nondissociating conditions in the presence of NP-40, HLA antigens were found to have an average molecular weight of 200,000 to 400,000. NP-40 solubilized and purified HLA antigens also seem to be associated with β_2-microglobulin (Rask et al. 1974; Grey et al. 1973; Poulik et al. 1974; Strominger et al. 1974).

8.3.1.3.2.2 *Brij*. The most extensive studies on nonionic detergent-solubilized HLA antigens from lymphoid cells have been carried out by Springer et al. (1974), who extracted the antigen from purified membranes with Brij-99. Membranes were prepared by freeze-thawing and hypotonic washing of cultured lymphoblasts. The membranes were resuspended in sodium-Tris (hydroxymethyl)methyl-2-ethanesulfonate (NaTES) buffer, pH 7.5. To this suspension was added a 10 percent Brij-99 solution in a 2:1 (w/w) ratio of detergent to protein. Insoluble material was removed by centrifugation at 100,000 *g* for 1 hr. The supernatant was either purified by adsorption to a *Lens culinaris* lectin-Biogel A-5m column (elution with a 0.2 percent methyl-α-D-mannoside gradient) and then applied, or applied directly to a Biogel A-5m (200–400 mesh) column equilibrated with 0.01 M NaTES (pH 7.5), 0.14 M NaCl, 0.1 percent Brij-99, 0.02 percent NaN_3. HLA antigens are eluted at the leading edge of the included protein peak. The antigenically active fractions are concentrated by adsorption to a DEAE-cellulose (DE-52) column in 0.01 M NaTES, 0.1 percent Brij-99, and eluted with 0.25 NaCl added to the same buffer.

The lectin-purified material is contaminated with at least 50 percent non-HLA protein as determined by PAGE in SDS. Two prominent bands can be found at positions indicating proteins with molecular weights of 44,000 and 12,000. Under nonreducing conditions, an additional polypeptide appears with a molecular weight of 82,000. This large polypeptide can be split into a single polypeptide fraction with a molecular weight of about 44,000 upon reduction, suggesting that at least a part of HLA antigens exist—when solubilized—as dimers linked together by disulfite bridges (Springer et al. 1974; Strominger et al. 1974; Cresswell and Dawson 1975).

If the solubilized membrane antigen is applied directly to Biogel A-5m column, the HLA antigens are eluted at the leading edge of the included protein peak at a position that indicates a molecular weight of about 460,000; most probably this moiety represents a complex between the detergent micelle and HLA antigens. HLA antigens purified by NP-40 or Brij are glycoproteins, at least in the majority, and are associated with a small molecular weight component which appears to be identical to β_2-microglobulin (Rask et al. 1974; Poulik et al. 1974; Springer et al. 1974; Strominger et al. 1974). In general, it appears that HLA molecules after solubilization consist of two polypeptide chains: one larger, with a molecular weight in the range of 29,000 to 55,000, depending upon the solubilization procedure employed, and one smaller with a molecular weight of approximately 12,000, which appears to be identical with β_2-microglobulin. When solubilized enzymatically, different HLA specificities show different behavior on electrophoresis mobility and ion exchange chromatography; HLA-A2 seems to have the least acidic pI and HLA-B7 the more acidic. The pI of the different specificities ranges from 4.6 to 6.3 (Turner et al. 1975; Parham et al. 1974; Dautigny et al. 1973). On the other hand, after hypertonic salt extraction or NP-40 solubilization, HLA antigens appear to be homogeneous, not only with respect to their molecular weights but also their electric charges, i.e., the various specificities are not separable by electrophoresis or ion exchange chromatography (Reisfeld et al. 1971a; Reisfeld et al. 1973; Dautigny et al. 1973).

8.3.2 Chemical Composition

8.3.2.1 Carbohydrate Moiety

Although there is still some controversy over the presence of carbohydrates on the HLA antigen molecule, it is clear that HLA antigens solubilized by certain methods do possess carbohydrate residues (Mann et al. 1969b; Sanderson et al. 1971; Parham et al. 1974; Terhorst et al. 1976; Snary et al. 1974; Dawson et al. 1974b; Bernier et al. 1974; Cresswell et al. 1973, 1974b; Springer et al. 1974). Some researchers, however, were not able to detect carbohydrates associated with HLA antigens after solubilization by sonication (Kahan and Reisfeld 1971) or KCl extraction (Reisfeld et al. 1971a; Ferrone et al. 1975). Also, Dawson et al. (1974b) found carbohydrate-free HLA antigens after solubilization with sodium deoxycholate.

Detailed studies on the carbohydrate structure of HLA gene products have been undertaken only recently. Papain-solubilized HLA antigens have been analyzed for their carbohydrate component in more detail by Sanderson et al. (1971), Parham et al. (1974), and Terhorst et al. (1976).

Purified HLA antigens display a heterogeneity upon isoelectric focusing and isotachyphoresis (Turner et al. 1975; Parham et al. 1974). Thus, upon isoelectric focusing in 6 M urea, three bands are usually observed in the pI range of 6.3 and 6.1 for HLA-A2 and in the range of pI 5.3 and 5.1 for HLA-B7, 12. After treatment with neuraminidase, the bands migrate toward the pI 6.3 (HLA-A2) and the pI 5.3 (HLA-B7, 12) positions, respectively (Parham et al. 1974). These findings indicate that HLA antigens contain 1 to 3 sialic acid residues per molecule, with the species containing two residues predominant in the papain-solubilized product.

The neuraminidase-treated HLA antigens still react with their specific antibodies; it appears, therefore, that the sialic acid residues are not involved in immunologic specificity. When Sanderson et al. (1971) treated partially purified (about 35 percent) HLA antigens with pronase and separated the digest on Sephadex G-50 columns, they found the carbohydrate to elute in one molecule. Since only one major peak was found, they deduced that carbohydrates occur as a single unit, or as a few units in close proximity on the peptide chain since, otherwise, smaller and presumably more carbohydrate fractions should have been observed. The composition of the carbohydrate moiety was analyzed by Sanderson et al. (1971), and more recently by Terhorst et al. (1976). In both studies, quite similar results were obtained when compared, assuming the protein portion to be 29,000 in molecular weight: the material was found to consist of 3 to 1 sialic acid, 3 mannose, 1 fucose, 4 galactose, and 4 glucosamine residues per molecule with no glucose or N-acetyl-galactosamine present. These residues add up to a molecular weight of about 3000 (roughly 10 percent of the whole molecule). No differences in that composition have been found for HLA antigens with different serologic specificities of either the A or B series in the studies by Terhorst et al. (1976); in the earlier study by Sanderson et al. (1971), differences had been reported, but a much less purified preparation had been used. As yet, no data are available regarding the possible structure and linkage of the carbohydrate residues, except that sialic acids are known to be terminal residues.

8.3.2.2 *Protein Moiety*

As a general feature, it appears that HLA antigens consist of two polypeptide chains, one "heavy" with a molecular weight in the range of 34,000 (papain) to 44,000 (Brij, NP-40) to 55,000 (sodium dodecylsulfate), and one "small" with a molecular weight of 11,500, identified as β_2-microglobulin.

8.3.2.2.1 *HLA (Heavy Chain)*

As outlined above, the HLA gene products are molecules of different sizes in molecular weight, depending upon the solubilization procedure employed. The procedures which result in lower molecular weight substances are those involving proteolytic (autolysis, papain) and/or otherwise degrading procedures (KCl). This indicates that those HLA molecules in solution do not represent the actual molecule as it is integrated in the membrane although their antigenic sites are intact. On the other hand, the exceedingly high molecular weight substances found after detergent solubilization might result from the binding of detergent micelles and detergent-facilitated aggregate formation, or might occur after removal of the detergent, due to insolubility in aqueous solutions.

The difference of size for the papain- and Brij (or NP-40)-solubilized HLA antigens has been demonstrated as resulting from the papain degradation. When the Brij-solubilized 44,000 molecular weight glycoprotein is subjected to hydrolysis by papain, two antigenically intact products could be found: one with a molecular weight of 39,000 which, after further digestion, converted to the second, a 34,000 size molecule. Sequence analysis of the N-terminal amino acids of the 44,000 and 34,000 molecules revealed that they were the same; therefore, during papain digestion, degradation takes place on the COOH-terminal end (Springer and Strominger 1976). Amino acid analysis of the three polypeptides (44,000, 39,000, and 34,000) revealed that the 39,000 molecule had lost a high proportion of hydrophilic amino acids with a summarized polarity of 64 percent; upon degradation of the 39,000 to the 34,000 molecule, a high proportion of hydrophobic amino acids were lost (with a polarity of about 21 percent). Consistent with this data are findings that the 44,000 and 39,000 molecules bind to detergent micelles and chromatograph at a high molecular weight in gel filtration, while the 34,000 molecule does not bind detergents (Springer et al. 1974). These data suggest that the penultimate (hydrophobic) COOH-terminal peptide might be responsible for the anchorage of the HLA antigen in the membrane.

The COOH-terminal, hydrophilic peptide is presumably present in the aqueous phase either inside the cell spanning the membrane, or outside, if the COOH-terminus is U-shaped. The hydrophobic and hydrophilic portion of the COOH-terminal might be called Fm (membrane fragment); the papain-released portion with the HLA antigenic determinants might be designated Fs (soluble fragment). The molecular size of KCl-extracted antigens (31,000) appears to be nearer the size of papain-released antigens than that of detergent-solubilized molecules; they also tend apparently not to aggregate in aqueous solutions and appear to be highly hydrophilic (Reisfeld and Kahan 1970). Therefore, one might assume that they are released during the extraction by autolytic activities (Mann 1972a) which, though they may act differently than papain, nevertheless include the cleavage of peptides that carry the carbohydrate moiety (which could be at the N-terminal part of the molecule or close to the membrane adjacent part), or include the action of carbohydrolases (which would explain the pure proteinaceous nature of this antigen). Such an assumption is disputed by Reisfeld and his collaborators (Reisfeld and Kahan 1971; Oh et al. 1974; Ferrone et al. (1975).

The amino acid compositions of papain-released and purified HLA antigens with different specificities and from both segregant series show a high degree of similarity (Terhorst et al. 1976; Tanigaki et al. 1975; Mann et al. 1971). The data suggest that there are a few more acidic amino acids than basic amino acid residues; this difference is larger for the B7 antigen than for the A2 antigen as one would expect on the basis of electrophoretic and ion exchange separation data obtained earlier (Parham et al. 1974; Colombani et al. 1970b; Mann et al. 1969b; Turner et al. 1975; Tanigaki et al. 1971; Sanderson 1968). The overall differences seem to indicate that various HLA antigenic molecules may not differ in more than 20 to 30 residues (which could be enough, however, to account for the observed antigenic polymorphism). Papain-solubilized antigens of both series contain four half-cystine residues, as do KCl-solubilized antigens (Terhorst et al. 1976; Tanigaki et al. 1975; Ferrone et al. 1975), forming two intramolecular loops (Strominger et al. 1974). Whether detergent-solubilized (Brij) HLA antigens possess one cystein more, as suggested by Strominger et al. (1974) and Springer and Strominger (1976), is not clarified yet. Recently, the first 25 N-terminal amino acid positions of several papain-released and purified HLA antigens have been reported by Strominger and his colleagues (Terhorst et al. 1976): HLA-A2 antigens isolated from two different cell lines had a completely identical sequence. But also, HLA-A2 and B7 differered only at one position (see Table in Chapter 10). HLA-B12 may differ in three positions from HLA-A2, and possibly, in at least two positions from HLA-B7. Further analysis of ^{3}H-carboxymethylated HLA-molecules gave no indication of the presence of cysteine residues within the first 40 positions. This finding makes unlikely the possibility that HLA antigens are homologues of immunoglobulin molecules, as had been suggested by several investigators (Cunningham and Berggard 1974; Peterson et al. 1972; Strominger et al. 1974). Bridgen et al. (1976) sequenized the first 16 position of deoxycholate-solubilized and by gel filtration, lectin-Sepharose 4B and ethanol precipitation (66 percent vol/vol) purified HLA-A1, 2, B8, 13 antigens. Amino acid sequences were determined employing an automatic solid-phase sequencer using high specific activity ^{35}S-labeled phenyl-isothiocyanate (2 percent vol/vol). Although these authors analyzed a mixture of antigens, by comparison with the above-described sequence of HLA-A2 and HLA-B7, they found two amino acid differences for the B antigens and one for the A antigens, i.e., B8, 13 differed from B7 in position 8 (Tyr for Phe) and 10 (Ser for Thr), whereas HLA-A1, 2 showed a difference only for position 13 (Val for Ser). The A and B series differed in at least five positions. Considering that a mixture of four antigens was analyzed, an average amino acid exchange of one to two per antigen within the 16 positions might be estimated (Table 1.8).

It appears that the differences at position 9 is locus-specific. It might be assumed that the other differences (6, 8, 10, 13) are related to the antigenic specificities.

At least 10 of the N-terminal 16 residues are apparently constant for both the A and B locus antigens, and all of the amino acid variations correspond to single nucleotide base changes. This restricted heterogeneity is consistent with the suggestion that A and B genes arose from a common ancestral gene by duplication (Bodmer 1972).

Table 1.8. N-Terminal Amino Acid Sequences of HLA-A and HLA-B Antigens and β_2-Microglobulin

Antigen specificity	Residue No. 1	2	3	4	5	6	7	8	9	10	11	12
A2[a]	Gly	Ser	.	Ser	Met	Arg	Tyr	Phe	Phe	Thr	Ser	Val
A1, A2[b]	.	Ser	.	Ser	Met	Arg	Tyr	Phe	Phe	Thr	Ser	Val
B7[a]	Gly	Ser	.	Ser	Met	Arg	Tyr	Phe	Tyr	Thr	Ser	Val
B12[a]	Gly	Ser	.	Ser	Met	Val	Tyr	Phe	Tyr	Thr	Ala	Val
B8, B13[b]	.	Ser	.	Ser	Met	Arg	Tyr	Tyr	Tyr	Ser	Ala	Val
β_2-mg[c]	Ile	Val	Glu	Leu	Leu	Glu	Ser	Gly	Gly	Gly	Leu	Val

[a] From Terhorst et al. (1976): papain-solubilized, molecular weight of 31,000.
[b] From Bridgen et al. (1976): deoxycholate-solubilized, molecular weight of 43,000.
[c] From Cunningham et al. (1973).

8.3.2.2.2 β_2-Microglobulin (Light Chain)

β_2-microglobulin was first isolated by Berggard and Bearn (1968) form the urine of patients with tubular proteinurias. It has a molecular weight of 11,600 and can be found in small amounts in the serum (1.8 mg/ml), cerebrospinal fluid (1.7 mg/ml), and urine (0.1 mg/24 hr urine) (Ferrone et al., 1975). The complete primary structure has been determined by Cunningham and his collaborators (1973). It consists of 100 amino acid residues, with two cysteine residues at positions 25 and 81, forming a single disulfite loop. There are no free sulfhydryl groups and no carbohydrates. Genetically, β_2-microglobulin is coded for by a gene located at the human chromosome 15, and, therefore, is not linked to genes controlling HLA antigens (Goodfellow et al. 1975).

On the basis of partial amino acid sequence data, Smithies and Poulik (1972) and Peterson et al. (1972) already noted a striking homology (about 30 percent) of β_2-microblobulin with the third constant region domain of the γ-chain (C_3H) of the myeloma protein Eu. From this observation it was suggested that β_2-microglobulin represents a free immunoglobulin domain possibly serving an effector function similar to that of the C_3H domain of γ-1 chains of IgG (Peterson et al. 1972; Cunningham et al. 1973).

A link between β_2-microglobulin and HLA was first made by Nakamuro et al. (1973) after Poulik and Motwani (1972) and Fanger and Bernier (1973) demonstrated the protein on the surface of lymphocytes. Nakamuro and his colleagues found an 11,000-dalton fragment, the "HLA common structure" (without HLA specificity!) from papain-solubilized HLA antigens which behaved electrophoretically identical to a fragment isolated from spent culture medium (Nakamuro et al. 1975) which, in turn, had been shown to possess the amino acid composition of the urinary β_2-microglobulin (Miyakawa et al. 1973b). Tanigaki et al. (1973a, 1974b) then demonstrated that the "HLA

Residue No.												
13	14	15	16	17	18	19	20	21	22	23	24	25
Ser	Arg	Pro	Gly	.	Gly	Glu	.	.	Phe	Ile	Ala	Val
Ala	Arg	Pro	Gly									
Ser	Arg	Pro	Gly	.	Gly	Glu	.	.	Phe	Ile		Val
Ser	Arg	Pro	Gly	.	Gly	Glu	.	.	Phe	Ile	Ala	Val
Ser	Arg	Pro	Gly									
Glu	Pro	Gly	Gly	Ser	Leu	Lys	Leu	Ser	Cys	Ala	Ala	Ser

common structure" fragment possessed the same first 24 amino acid residues as β_2-microglobulin. In the following years, it was often demonstrated that the HLA antigens solubilized by either papain or detergents all consisted either of a larger polypeptide chain (mol.-wt. 32,000 for papain-solubilized, or 44,000 for detergent-solubilized) and a small polypeptide chain (11,600) which could be dissociated from the larger under denaturing conditions (urea, SDS, guanidine). The small polypeptide was identified as β_2-microglobulin by immunologic (Tanigaki et al. 1973a; Cresswell et al. 1974a; Poulik et al. 1974; Strominger et al. 1974; Rask et al. 1974) and immunochemical methods (Peterson et al. 1974; Grey et al. 1973; Cresswell et al. 1973; Poulik et al. 1974), as well as by its amino acid composition (Nakamuro et al. 1973; Tanigaki et al. 1975; Terhorst et al. 1976) and partial amino acid sequence (Smithies and Poulik 1972; Peterson et al. 1972). Usually, the two polypeptide chains are present in a 2.6:1 to 1.9:1 molecular weight ratio (Cresswell et al. 1973), corresponding to a 1:1 molar ratio.

The β_2-microglobulin does not possess HLA antigenic specificity (Peterson et al. 1974; Poulik et al. 1974; Miyakawa et al. 1973a; Reisfeld et al. 1975), and Poulik with his colleagues (1974) found that not all HLA antigenic specificities prepared from cell extracts show an association with β_2-microglobulin, regardless of the method of solubilization. On the other hand, the majority of β_2-microglobulin on the cell membrane does not appear to be associated with HLA antigens, since only about 10 percent of β_2-microglobulin might be found in association with HLA.

At this time, there is no clue to the biological function of this association, if indeed it is not merely fortuitous. However, several far-reaching hypotheses have been advanced: because of the similarity of β_2-microglobulin and the C_3H domain of IgG, it was suggested that the former might serve as a link between histocompatibility and the immune system (Peterson et al. 1972;

Cunningham and Berggard 1974). One hypothesis even went so far as to suggest an immunoglobulin-like structure (and function) for histocompatibility antigens with two heavy (HLA) and two light (β_2 mg) chains (Strominger et al. 1974). This theory postulated that the H system was derived from an ancestor gene common with the immunoglobulin system (Cunningham and Berggard 1974; Strominger et al. 1974). Doubts exist that the H antigens are arranged as dimers in the cell membrane (*see below*) and it appears unlikely from the (although still partial) sequence data that HLA antigens have a structural similarity to immunoglobulins. Other data may suggest a function of β_2-microglobulin in the expression of surface proteins, including HLA.

8.3.3 Dimeric or Monomeric Structure of HLA Antigens in the Cell Membrane

When HLA antigens are solubilized by detergent, in general, substances are found under dissociating but not reducing conditions which exhibit a molecular weight of about 82,000 to 88,000 upon SDS polyacrylamide electrophoresis (Cresswell and Dawson 1975; Strominger et al. 1974). When this large molecule was again analyzed after being reduced, only 44,000 molecular weight substances could be detected, suggesting a dimeric structure of the HLA antigens with two heavy chains linked together by disulfide bonds. Amino acid analysis, however, did not reveal unequivocally the presence of a free sulfhydryl group or five half-cysteine molecules per HLA molecule but only four (*see below*).

In addition, Snary et al. (1975) solubilizing HLA antigens in deoxycholate under nonreducing conditions found no indication for the presence of HLA dimers when the molecular weight was estimated by gel filtration (Ultragel AcA 34, Sephadex G-200, G-150, or Sepharose 6B), and sucrose density gradient centrifugation in 0.5 to 1.0 percent deoxycholate (Snary et al. 1974). These authors assumed that the previously reported findings suggesting a dimeric structure could have been caused by aggregation through disulfite interchange promoted by storage, and by a sulfhydryl-disulfite interchange enzyme present in the endoplasmatic reticulum.

8.3.4 Antigenic Sites of the HLA Glycoprotein

For a long time the question was unresolved as to whether the antigenic sites reside in the protein or carbohydrate portion of the HLA molecule. Today it appears certain that HLA antigenic specificity is determined by the protein portion. Thus, the HLA antigen solubilized by chaotropic salt extraction does not contain detectable carbohydrates, yet it is antigenic because of its capacity to bind to specific antibodies and it is immunogenic because it elicits specific antibody production in rabbits (Ferrone et al. 1972, 1973). Removal of carbohydrates from the purified HLA molecule does not lead to any change in the antibody binding capacity for the HLA specificities measured (Parham et al. 1974), and there is evidence that HLA molecules with different serologic specificities possess the same carbohydrate composition

(Terhorst et al. 1976). On the other hand, protein denaturants affect antigenic activity as, for example, 6 M urea, low pH (below 3), or proteolytic digestion reduces or abolishes antibody binding capacity (Turner et al. 1972; Shimada and Nathenson 1969).

8.3.5 One Locus-One Glycoprotein

Mann et al. (1969b) found, upon gel filtration of papain-solubilized material, separation of A and B HLA antigens into two peaks. Colombani et al. (1970) also separated, upon DEAE-cellulose ion-exchange chromatography, HLA antigen specificities obtained from membrane-rich extracts by autolysis. Turner et al. (1975) were able to separate HLA specificities upon CM-cellulose chromatography and isoelectric focusing. Cresswell et al. (1973, 1974b) were able to separate HLA-B7 and A2 antigen-bearing molecules of the same size by forming soluble immune complexes and separating them by gel filtration. Sanderson and Welsh (1974), testing the capacity of papain- and detergent-solubilized HLA molecules to complex with specific HLA antibodies, presented evidence also for the molecular independence of the antigens of the two HLA segregant series. Similarly, Fahey and collaborators (Thieme et al. 1974) showed that all four HLA antigenic specificities from a cell line (RPMI 4265) of an heterozygous donor resided on separate molecules.

With the successive immunoprecipitation procedure, Springer et al. (1974) demonstrated that detergent (Brij-99)-solubilized HLA antigens are precipitable independently. Dautigny et al. (1973) obtained separation of HLA-B7 and HLA-A2 specificities by electro-focusing of NP-40-solubilized antigens form platelets. HLA-A2 eluted mainly at a pH between 5.5 and 6.5, whereas HLA-B7 eluted below pH 5.0. Similar results were obtained by Turner et al. (1975). These data, together with the results obtained by redistribution experiments (*see* Section 2 *above*) fully confirm the separability of the HLA gene products on the lymphocyte membrane.

8.4 HLA-A and B Antigens in the Serum and Urine

Today it is well documented that HLA antigens exist in a soluble state in both serum (Charlton and Zmijewski 1970; van Rood and van Leeuwen 1970; van Rood et al. 1971; Miyakawa et al. 1972; Schultz and Shreffler 1972; Aster et al. 1973; Billing et al. 1973; Billing and Terasaki 1974; Billing and McMillan 1975; Pellegrino et al. 1974; Oh et al. 1975; Reisfeld et al. 1976; Allison et al. 1977) and urine (Reisfeld et al. 1977; Bernier et al. 1976; Reisfeld et al. 1976).

8.4.1 Serum HLA

HLA antigenic activity appears to be associated with the high density lipoprotein (HDL) fraction of the serum (Aster et al. 1973; Billing and McMillan 1975; Reisfeld et al. 1976; Allison et al. 1977) and can be prepared by polyanion precipitation with sodium phosphotungstate and $MgCl_2$, followed by ultracentrifugal flotation (Burstein et al. 1970; Allison et al. 1977). Upon column chromatography of HDL purified in this manner, the HLA antigenic activity (HLA-A9) is eluted in a volume indicating a molecular weight of approximately 170,000; after delipidation with sodium deoxycholate, the HLA activity is recovered upon gel filtration (Ultragel AcA 34) in a position that indicates a protein with a molecular weight of about 100,000. Under dissociating conditions, this antigenic active fraction moved, upon SDS polyacrylamide electrophoresis, to a position signifying 45,000; the same results were obtained by specific immunoprecipitation. HDL-associated HLA antigens are associated with β_2-microglobulin (Allison et al. 1977) and contain 2 to 4 percent carbohydrates (Billing et al. 1973). From these data, it was concluded that serum HLA exist as a single 45,000 molcular weight chain associated with β_2-microglobulin (12,000) and boundary lipid attached to the membrane-binding domain (Allison et al. 1977).

8.4.2 Urinary HLA Antigen

HLA antigenic activity is not only found in the urine of patients with nephrotic syndromes but also in the urine of normal individuals. For purification, standard biochemical procedures have been applied, such as ion exchange chromatography (DEAE-cellulose) and preparative polyacrylamide electrophoresis; apparently, isoelectric focusing does not yield satisfactory results (Reisfeld et al. 1977). The purified urinary HLA antigen (HLA-A9) has a molecular weight of 38,000 and is associated with β_2-microglobulin (Reisfeld et al. 1977), although some researchers have been unable to detect such an association in a similar preparation isolated from urine (Bernier et al. 1976). Since urinary HLA is adsorbed to ConA-Sepharose, it appears to contain carbohydrates.

8.5 HLA-C Antigens

Antigens of the third segregant series (HLA-C) have not been investigated biochemically in such detail as A and B antigens. Rask et al. (1974) found no difference with regard to the molecular weight for HLA-C and A/B antigens when the antigen was anlayzed after papain-solubilization by specific immunoprecipitation and polyacrylamide gel electrophoresis under dissociating and reducing conditions: two components were found, one with a molecular weight of 33,000 and the other with 12,000 (probably β_2-microglobulin). Wernet et al. (1975), analyzing NP-40 solubilized HLA-C antigens by immunoprecipitation procedures, found major polypeptide chains with molecular weights of about 45,000 and 12,000. The larger molecule could be found, however, only if the precipitate was not dialyzed but immediately electrophoresed; otherwise, only a molecule was found at a position that indicated protein with a molecular weight of approximately 28,000. From these data, HLA-C antigens appear to be similar to HLA-A or -B antigens on the molecular basis, but they are more easily degraded.

8.6 HLA-D Antigen (B-Cell-Specific, HLA-D Locus-Linked Gene Products)

There are no data available on the biochemical structure of HLA-D gene products. However, in recent years a growing number of laboratories have reported alloantisera reacting predominantly with B-lymphocytes and inhibiting specifically the HLA-D-controlled mixed lymphocyte culture reaction, suggesting that the determinants recognized by these antibodies might reside on HLA-D gene products. Immunochemical analysis using those sera for specific precipitation of NP-40 solubilized membranes revealed that the antigenic determinants reside on moieties with a molecular weight of between 55,000 and 70,000 under nonreducing conditions; after reduction and alkylation, two molecular size classes of 30,000 and 26,000 molecular weight, respectively, can be identified. No small molecular weight substances (12,000) were found, suggesting that B-cell-specific HLA-D-associated antigens are not complexed with β_2-microglobulin (Wernet and Kunkel 1975). Similar results were reported by Billing et al. (1976): Papain digests of surface membranes (extracted anigens and sodium deoxycholate) were purified by QAE-A50 Sephadex and Concanavallin A-Sepharose 4B-chromatography, and preparative sodium dodecylsulfate polyacrylamide gel electrophoresis under nonreducing conditions. The antigenic activity was revovered from position on the gel corresponding to a molecular weight of 58,000 for the papain-released and of 65,000 for the detergent-extracted antigen. After reduction, two bands were detectable, one with an apparent molecular weight of 27,000 and another of 35,000. The same authors could obtain identical results with a B-cell-specific serum from rabbits immunized with papain-solubilized antigens of spleens form lymphoma patients. With the same kind of xenogeneic serum which inhibited stimulation in mixed lymphocyte cultures and reacted with B-cells only (Cresswell and Geier 1975), Strominger and his collaborators (Kaufman, *personal communication*) could obtain similar data.

9. Linked Loci and Mapping of the HLA Region

The HLA region was concordantly assigned to chromosome 6 by three different sets of data: Lamm et al. (1971) discovered the linkage of PGM_3 (third isoenzyme of phosphoglucomutase) with HLA by the classical method of linkage analysis in families. These data were confirmed by experiments with somatic cell hybrids providing evidence for synteny (presence of two loci on one chromosome, not necessarily detectable by classical linkage analysis) between HLA and PGM_3 (von Someren et al. 1974). Using the same techniques, Jongsma et al. (1973) had been able to assign PGM_3 and thereby also HLA to chromosome 6. This was again confirmed by direct evidence found by Lamm et al. (1974) in a family with a large pericentric inversion on chromosome 6, where seven of seven family members who carry the inversion also possess the HLA haplotype A2, B12 (identical by descent).

In studies of cultures of ovarian teratomas the PGM_3 locus was found to be linked to the centromere of chromosome 6 (Ott et al. 1975), while Lamm et al. (1972) had in linkage studies placed the PGM_3 locus on the side of HLA-B. These data result in the order of:

Centromere — PGM_3 — HLA-D — B — C — A

In 1974, Allen found a close linkage between HLA and the GBG ploymorphism (glycin-rich glycoprotein or properdin factor B or recently renamed Bf) which is the proactivator of the complement component C3 and which marks the start of the "alternate pathway" of complement activation. Although there is still conflicting evidence as to the relative map position of the Bf locus (Raum et al. 1976; Sucin-Foca et al. 1976; Rittner et al. 1975; Albert et al. 1976; Olaisen et al. 1975; Lamm et al. 1976; Hauptmann et al. 1976) the most likely position for Bf is between HLA-B and D. The alleles of the Bf locus have been found to be in pronounced linkage disequilibrium with HLA-B (Albert et al. 1976, 1977b; Teisberg et al. 1975). Two more complement components are known to be linked with HLA: The gene for deficiency of C2 has been found to segregate with HLA-haplotypes (Fu et al. 1974), apparently in high linkage disequilibrium with HLA-A10, B18 and DW2 (Fu et al. 1975). Its map position was tentatively placed between HLA-D and PGM_3. The gene for deficiency of the complement component C4 was shown to be closely linked with HLA by Rittner et al. (1976). The exact map position, however, could not be determined as yet.

The polymorphism of the red cell glyoxalase (GLO) (Kömpf et al. 1975a) was found to be linked with HLA by Mayr et al. (1976), Bender and Grzeschik (1975), Weitkamp et al. (1976) and Kömpf et al. (1976). The map position of the GLO gene was determined in recombinant families to be located between HLA-B and PGM_3 (Mehra Khan et al. 1976; Pretorius et al. 1976; Weitkamp et al. 1976). Two more blood groups present on red cells and in serum Chido (Ch a− or Ch a+) (Middleton et al. 1974) and Rodgers (Rg a + or Rg a−) (Giles et al. 1976) are linked with HLA and are coded for by genes which are most likely very closely linked with HLA-B or C. Furthermore the genes for superoxide dismutase 2 (SOD-2), for malic enzyme 1 (ME1) (van Someren et al. 1974) and for urinary pepsinogen (Pg-5) (Ruddle and Gibblet 1975) are also located on chromosome 6. Information about the mapping of these genes in relation to HLA is not available. Thus the full linkage group on chromosome 6 most likely has the following order:

Centromere ... PGM_3 ... GLO ... C2—HLA-D—Bf—HLA-B—HLA-C ... HLA-A

⟵——⟶

Ch, Rg, C4

The recombination frequency between HLA-A and B is in the order of 0.85 percent (Svejgaard et al. 1971b) to 0.96 percent (Bijnen et al. 1976), between HLA-B and HLA-D approximately 1 percent (Netzel et al. 1976; Mickelson et al. 1976), between HLA-B and PGM_3 in the male 12.5 percent (Albert et al., *unpublished data*) to 15 percent (Lamm et al. 1972; Mayr et al. 1975) and in the female 35 percent (Mayr et al. 1975) to 40 percent (Lamm et al. 1972) and 45 percent (Albert et al., *unpublished*). The distance found between HLA and GLO in terms of recombination frequency varies in the male from 4 percent (Albert et al., *unpublished*) to 5 percent (Kömpf et al. 1976) and 7 percent (Weitkamp et al. 1976) while in the female it ranges from 6 percent (Albert et al., *unpublished*) to 7 percent (Weitkamp et al. 1976) and 10 percent (Kömpf et al. 1976). These data are compatible with a position of GLO between PGM_3 and HLA-D.

10. HLA and Transplantation

Originally it had been hoped that matching for HLA antigens would solve the problems presented by graft rejection. When the first larger series of kidney transplantations from unrelated donors were analyzed it became clear that matching for HLA antigens had very little effect on the clinical outcome (Mickey et al. 1971). Nevertheless there is undisputed evidence that HLA antigens play a role in graft rejection: (1) Kidney transplants from HLA-identical siblings have in all series reported so far a significantly better prognosis than transplants from siblings mismatched for one or two HLA haplotypes (Dausset et al. 1965; Dausset et al. 1969; Kissmeyer-Nielsen et al. 1970; Opelz and Terasaki 1972). Similarly, in bone marrow transplantation with very few exceptions only transplants from HLA-identical sibling donors have been clinically successful (Thomas et al. 1975; van Rood and van Leeuwen 1976a). (2) Antibodies reacting with HLA-antigens of the donor are produced as the result of skin or kidney graft rejection. (3) The presence of antibodies in the recipient's serum directed at donor HLA antigens (positive crossmatch) causes hyperacute rejection of the graft in over 80 percent of the cases (Terasaki et al. 1967; Patel and Terasaki 1969). (4) HLA antigens (SD) form the major targets in cell-mediated cytolysis (Eijsvoogel et al. 1973a, b, c; Goulmy et al. 1976).

From the discrepancy between good results of HLA matching in families and poor efficiency of matching in unrelated transplants it must be concluded that genetic systems closely linked with HLA-A and B play a significant role in graft rejection. Due to the close linkage between HLA-A and B these systems will be generally matched in HLA-identical siblings but mismatched in the unrelated population. On the other hand—as mentioned above there is evidence for the direct involvement of HLA-A and B (SD) antigens in graft rejection. Therefore both SD antigens and other HLA-linked systems are important for histocompatibility. It is quite obvious that the HLA-D locus could be one of these histocompatibility systems, because HLA-D antigens are responsible for proliferative response in MLC which is the prerequisite for the production of cytotoxic effector cells believed to be involved in the destruction (rejection) of the graft. Data from skin graft rejection by Koch et al. (1971, 1973) and preliminary results in kidney transplantation

(Cochrum et al. 1975) seem to support the importance of HLA-D incompatibility for graft rejection. Unfortunately, typing for HLA-D antigens is still a rather cumbersome procedure which cannot (yet) be used in the selection of transplant donors. It can be expected however, that both the PLT method and the serologic definition of HLA-D antigens could become feasible for an improvement of donor selection.

In spite of these considerations, the matching for HLA-A and B antigens at its present level of sophistication does show a beneficial effect even in unrelated transplants (van Hoof et al. 1972, 1974; Eurotransplant Annual Reports 1973, 1974, 1975). This effect is large enough to justify the considerable effort invested in international organ exchange systems (van Rood 1967, 1973). In the combined French and English data (Dausset et al. 1974), there is a overall correlation between HLA-A, B match and graft prognosis. The Eurotransplant data show a strong effect of HLA matching only in preimmunized patients with HLA antibodies, a group which is known to have a poorer graft prognosis than patients without HLA antibodies (van Rood et al. 1973). Since a positive crossmatch is a contraindication to transplantation, it must be assumed that the presence of cytotoxic antibodies indicates that this group of patients reacts strongly against an allogenic stimulus. Therefore these patients require particularly well-matched kidneys in order to have a successful graft.

Due to the extreme polymorphism of the HLA-A and B loci it is very difficult to obtain identity between donor and recipient for all four HLA-A and B antigens. Through international cooperation a fair number of these "full-house" identical transplants from unrelated donors have been performed with a particularly high success rate (Eurotransplant Annual Report 1975), so that it has become imperative to transport donor kidneys even for long distances to obtain such "full-house" matches whenever possible. The fact, that these four antigen-matched kidneys do so much better than e.g., three-antigen-matched kidneys, supports the expectation that the HLA-D and/or other closely linked systems play a major role in determining graft survival: Very common HLA-A, B phenotypes, such as A1, A3, B7, B8 are usually the result of HLA-A, B haplotypes with particularly strong linkage disequilibrium not only between HLA-A and B but also between B and D or B and Bf (Albert et al. 1973c, 1977b). Thus it can be assumed, that in this group which is selected on the basis of a high phenotype frequency there is a high proportion of cases not only matching for HLA-A and B but also for HLA-D and other closely linked systems by virtue of linkage disequilibrium.

Recently it has become apparent that graft prognosis is strongly influenced by a condition which is—at least presently—not connected with the HLA system: It has been observed by Opelz et al. (1972, 1973, 1974) and confirmed by others (Persijn et al. 1977), that patients who have never been transfused have a prognosis which is significantly worse than that of patients who have received one or more transfusions prior to transplantation. There is the possibility that transfusions can form the antigenic stimulus for the production of enhancing antibodies which protect the graft from rejection.

The importance of HLA matching for kidney transplantation can be summarized as follows: Selection of donors on the basis of HLA-A and B identity is highly successful in siblings, whereas in unrelated donor and recipient pairs there is only a small benefit from HLA-A, B compatibility, except in cases of "full-house" identity. In patients with cytotoxic antibodies matching is particularly important, because this group has *per se* a poor prognosis. The lack of pretransplant blood transfusions is associated with a very low graft survival. Matching for HLA-D antigens is not feasible for practical reasons, but it can reasonably be assumed that new techniques such as PLT and B-cell serology will overcome this problem and lead to an improved graft survival.

11. HLA-Disease Associations

11.1 Historical Remarks

The first association of any disease with HLA antigens was reported for Hodgkin's disease by Amiel (1967). It is ironic to note that even a large number of different studies have not been able to clearly establish whether there is an association with Hodgkin's disease and with which antigens (Amiel 1971; Bertrams et al. 1972; Bodmer 1973; Falk and Osoba 1971; Forbes and Morris 1970, 1972; Kissmeyer-Nielsen et al. 1971; Morris and Forbes 1971; Zervas et al. 1970). Nevertheless after these rather frustrating results, a number of HLA-disease associations have been found, which are reproducible and statistically beyond any doubt. The most outstanding examples were psoriasis (White et al. 1972; Sveijgaard et al. 1974b), celiac disease (Stokes et al. 1972; Falchuk et al. 1972) and ankylosing spondylitis (Brewerton et al. 1973a; Schlosstein et al. 1973). These reports were followed by a very large array of studies resulting in a considerable number of—by now–well-established HLA-disease associations and an even greater number of ambiguous reports.

11.2 Statistical Considerations

One major problem of HLA-disease studies is the assessment of statistical significance. It must be quite clearly stated that in a system as polymorphic as HLA the sample size must be considerable (50 to 100 persons) to detect a moderately strong association. When comparing a disease population with a control population there are two essential questions to be answered: (1) Are there any *significant* differences and (2) how strong is the association?

The significance of a difference can be judged using a simple χ^2 test as given below:

	Antigen-positive	Negative	Total
Patients	a	b	a+b
Controls	c	d	c+d
Total	a+c	b+d	a+b+c+d=N

$$\chi^2 = \frac{(|a \cdot d - b \cdot c| - N/2)^2 \cdot N}{(a+c) \cdot (b+d) \cdot (a+b) \cdot (c+d)},$$

where the expression $N/_2$ is the Yate's correction introduced to correct for discontinuity in small samples. The p values (probability of error) corresponding to the χ^2 values can be found in χ^2 tables such as those provided by Race and Sanger (1975). Since usually a large number (25–30) of HLA antigens are studied, it must be taken into account that among 20 comparisons one is expected to differ at a probability level of $^1/_{20} = 0.05$ by chance alone. Therefore it has become customary to multiply the p value by the number of comparisons made in the study. This safeguard is not necessary if the study serves to confirm a previously reported association.

The degree of association is generally given as the relative risk $\chi = \frac{a \cdot d}{b \cdot c}$ according to Woolf (1955), where a, b, c and d are taken from the 2×2 table used for the χ^2 calculations.

11.3 Groups of HLA-Associated Diseases

In Table 1.9 a list of diseases is given, which show an undisputed association with one or more HLA antigens. It can easily be seen that there are groups of diseases which have been known for a long time to be associated in some way. One such example is dermatitis herpetiformis and celiac disease (CD), both disorders caused by gluten sensitivity and known to occur together in families. There is an equally strong association with HLA-B8 in both diseases indicating the common genetic background. A similar situation exists for ankylosing spondylitis (AS), acute anterior uveitis, Reiter's syndrome, all of which are clinically associated and show the characteristic increase of HLA-B27. Another group of diseases comprises disorders with strong autoimmune features such as Addison's disease, myasthenia gravis and chronic aggressive hepatitis, all associated with HLA-B8. Thus the joint HLA association in each of these groups confirms that these diseases share genetic determinants coded for on chromosome 6.

Considering the list of diseases in Table 1.9, a number of common features come to light:

1. There is evidence for increased familial incidence in almost all disorders, as should be expected, if there is a moderately strong association with a genetic marker such as HLA. It is furthermore quite characteristic that in none of these diseases does the mode of inheritance follow a simple pattern. As will be discussed in more detail below, one is led to assume a dominant type of inheritance with a very low degree of penetrance. In addition, many of the HLA-associated diseases exhibit a strong preponderance of sex, e.g., ankylosing spondylitis (male to female 9:1) or celiac disease (female to male 2:1).
2. Immunologic mechanisms are suspected to play a major role in the pathogenesis of most HLA-associated diseases.
3. With very few exceptions, the strongest HLA associations are found for

Table 1.9. List of Well-Established HLA-Disease Associations

Disease	HLA Association	References
Celiac disease	B8	Albert et al. 1973b; Albert 1975; Albert et al. 1975a; Evans 1973; Falchuk et al. 1972; Gebhard et al. 1973; Granditsch et al. 1973; Harms et al. 1974; Ludwig et al. 1973; McDonald et al. 1965; McNeish et al. 1973; Mowbray et al. 1973; Shiner and Shmerling 1972; Stokes et al. 1972; Wank et al. 1974
Dermatitis herpetiformis	B8	White, A.G. et al. 1973a, b
Psoriasis	B13, BW17, BW38	Russell et al. 1973; Schoefinius et al. 1974; Scholz et al. 1974; Svejgaard et al. 1974b; White, S.H. et al. 1972
Ankylosing spondylitis	B27	Albert 1975; Albert et al. 1975; Brewerton et al. 1973a; Caffrey and James 1973; Dick et al. 1974; Schlosstein et al. 1973; Steinbauer-Rosenthal et al. 1974
Reiter's disease	B27	Arnason et al. 1972; Brewerton et al. 1973; Morris et al. 1974; Zachariae et al. 1973
Acute anterior uveitis	B27	Brewerton et al. 1973; Ehlers et al. 1974; Mapstone and Woodrow 1974
Juvenile rheumatoid arthritis	B27	Rachelewski et al. 1974; Albert et al. *unpublished data*
Myasthenia gravis	B8	Behan et al. 1973; Engelfriet et al. *personal communication;* Fritze et al. 1974
Addison's disease	B8	Platz et al. 1974
Chronic aggressive hepatitis	B8	Mackay and Morris 1972
Juvenile diabetes	B8 and BW15	Cudworth and Woodrow 1974; Nerup et al. 1974
Graves disease	B8	Grumet et al. 1974
Psoriatic arthritis	BW38, B13, BW17, B27	Brewerton et al. 1974
Multiple sclerosis	A3, B7, B18 and DW2	Bertrams et al. 1972; Bertrams and Kuwert 1972; Bertrams and Kuwert 1974; Bertrams et al. 1974; Degos and Dausset 1974b; Jersild et al. 1973a; Jersild et al. 1973b; Jersild et al. 1972; Jersild et al. 1973c; Naito et al. 1972

the antigens of the HLA-B locus. The fact that so many and different diseases are associated with antigens of the HLA-B locus makes it highly unlikely that the phenomenon is a merely coincidental finding. Rather, one is led to suspect a common mechanism by which these associations are brought about.

11.4 Models of HLA-Disease Associations

There are a number of different models for the explanation of HLA-disease associations:

1. It is conceivable that the HLA antigenic structure is by chance very similar or identical to the antigenic features of a pathogenic microorganism. Through selftolerance the microorganism could not be recognized as foreign and could therefore not be eliminated by immunologic means.
2. The HLA antigen could provide a binding site for pathogenic agents such as bacteria, virus, or other toxic substances and thus lead to the destruction of cells.
3. The most economical explanation is the assumption of genes which play a role in the pathogenesis in the disease and which are in close linkage with the HLA-B locus. The association on the population level could then be explained as a reflection of linkage disequilibrium as is almost regularly observed for closely linked systems.

Explanations 1. and 2. are somewhat unlikely, because not even in the strongest association observed do all patiens carry the respective antigen and not all carriers of the antigen suffer from the disease. Thus it is more likely that not the HLA antigens themselves but rather closely linked genes are directly involved with the pathogenesis of the disease. This is strongly supported by the fact that for some diseases it has been found that the antigens of the HLA-D locus are much more strongly associated with the disease than are the respective HLA-B antigens (Keuning et al. 1976). Such data have been provided for multiple sclerosis (Jersild et al. 1973a, b, c) celiac disease and for juvenile diabetes mellitus (Ryder and Sveijgaard 1976). It seems reasonable to assume that for many diseases such increased associations could be found when testing for HLA-D and other closely linked genes. Furthermore in multiple-case family studies it could be shown that the disease segregates with HLA haplotypes, which do not carry the antigens with which the disease is highly associated (Harms et al. 1974). This proves that the disease is associated with HLA in general and not only with a particular antigen. Or in other words: a gene involved in this disease is associated with HLA, but separable by recombination. Deduced from this evidence it is now generally accepted that for most if not all diseases the HLA antigens are not directly involved but rather are structures which are coded for by closely linked genes.

11.5 Genetic Considerations

In order to study further the mode of action of these HLA-linked "disease genes" it is necessary to investigate the inheritance of both HLA and the disease in multiple case families. This was done for AS (Albert et al. 1975a), for CD (Harms et al. 1974) and for juvenile diabetes (Cudworth and Woodrow 1974). It could be shown in AS and CD that all affected members of one family share at least one HLA haplotype but that by far not all family members who possess this haplotype are affected with the disease. This type of incomplete penetrance is best explained by the assumption of a susceptibility mechanism, which requires environmental factors for the expression of the disease. This concept is supported by the experience with twin data: In AS there is a high rate of concordance in monozygotic twins indicating a strong influence of genetic factors, whereas the existence of a number of discordant monozygotic twins proves the requirement for environmental factors. Thus if not even all monozygotic twins are concordant with respect to AS there is no reason to expect this from two siblings sharing one or two HLA haplotypes. Such environmental factors could be—e.g., in AS—certain bacteria or viruses, which in susceptible individuals could lead to arthritic disease. Indeed it is known that Reiter's syndrome develops frequently after a bout of "nonspecific" (i.e., nongonococcal) urethritis. Thus it can be concluded that the observed pattern of inheritance in HLA-associated diseases such as AS and CD can be explained by the coincidence of a dominant disease susceptibility gene with food components. The activity of the environmental factors could then easily be modified by sex or age or even other genetic factors. Family studies indicate that the weight of the HLA-linked disease susceptibility genes varies between different diseases: Whereas in AS and CD the HLA-linked gene must be of paramount importance, this is not so in psoriasis, where HLA-linked segregation of the disease can be observed only in relatively few families; in most cases psoriasis segregates independently from HLA (Albert et al. 1975a). These latter findings could, of course, also be due to heterogeneity of the "psoriasis" disease entity.

Investigations into a dominant or recessive type of inheritance of the HLA-linked susceptibility genes in AS and CD have led to results suggesting a dominant character: In both diseases there was a decrease in the number of homozygotes for the associated HLA-B antigen (B27 and B8 respectively) in the unrelated patient population (Albert et al. 1975a). In the case of a recessive mode one would expect to find a significant excess of homozygotes. The finding of a more dominant mode may give some hint about pathophysiologic mechanisms as dominance indicates a production of a deleterious gene product, a "too much" of reactivity, while recessive genes often code for the lack or the inefficient production of, e.g., enzyme activity. Considering the immunologic nature of most HLA-associated diseases it is not unreasonable that the HLA-linked susceptibility genes could well be defective immune response genes causing a derangement of immunoregulatory processes and thereby leading to autoimmune phenomena. This speculation is supported by the fact that immune response genes are suspected to map exactly in the region near the HLA-B and D loci, where most of the disease susceptibility genes can be tentatively mapped, based on the varying degrees of association with the alleles of the HLA-B and D loci. While the AS-susceptibility gene could be localized in the close proximity of HLA-B, one would expect the susceptibility genes for multiple sclerosis, celiac disease and diabetes mellitus more in the vicinity of HLA-D.

It may be an undue oversimplification to search for a common mechanism of action for the HLA-associated disease susceptibility genes. On the other hand, the fact that so many, so widely differing diseases are to a large extent genetically determined in what must be a very restricted part of the human genome (perhaps 2–3 centimorgans), suggests that these susceptibility genes affect a very basic regulatory function which may or may not be of immunologic nature. It is not surprising that immunologists would suspect an immunologic mechanism, perhaps seeing Helena in every woman.

The HLA disease associations pose the question about the biologic function of the MHC and at the same time they may hold the key to its understanding.

References

Albert, E.D. The significance of HL-A disease associations. *Z. Immunitaetsforsch., Exp. Klin. Immunol. 148*:382–383, 1975.

Albert, E.D., Andreas, A., McNicholas, A., Scholz, S., and Kuntz, B. B- and T-cell specific alloantigens in man. *Scand. J. Immunology, in press,* 1977a.

Albert, E.D., Harms, K., Schattenkirchner, M., Scholz, S., Steinbauer-Rosenthal, I., and Wank, R. HL-A antigens—genetic markers for disease susceptibility genes? *Int. Congr. Internal Med., 12th,* Karger, 1975a.

Albert, E.D., Harms, K., Wank, R., Steinbauer-Rosenthal, I., and Scholz, S. Segregation analysis of HL-A antigens and haplotypes in 50 families of patients with coeliac disease. *Transplant. Proc. 5,* No. 4: 1785–1789, 1973b.

Albert, E.D., Mempel, W., and Grosse-Wilde, H. Linkage disequilibrium between HL-A7 and the MLC Specificity Pi. *Transplant. Proc. 5,* No. 4:1551, 1973c.

Albert, E.D., Mickey, M.R., and Terasaki, P.I. Serology and genetics of Te58 (W18) and other specificities included in the 4c complex. *Tissue Antigens 2*:47–56, 1972a.

Albert, E.D., Mickey, M.R., and Terasaki, P.I. A new approach to crossreactivity in the HL-A system, *Int. Symp. Standardisation HL-A Reagents, 1972, Ser. Immunobiol. Standard. 18*:156–164, 1972b.

Albert, E.D., Mickey, M.R., and Terasaki, P.I. The use of computer programs for tissue typing and immunogenetic research. *Tissue Antigens II*: 173–181, 1972c.

Albert, E.D., Mickey, M.R., and Terasaki, P.I. Genetics of the HL-A system in four populations: Caucasians, Japanese, American Negroes and Mexican Americans. *Histocompatibility Testing 1972d*, pp. 233–340.

Albert, E.D., Mickey, M.R., and Terasaki, P.I. A new approach to crossreactivity in the HL-A system. *International Symposium on the standardisation of HL-A reagents, Copenhagen, 1973,* pp. 156–164, S. Karger, Basel, 1973d.

Albert, E.D., Mickey, M.R., Ting, A., and Terasaki, P.I. Deduction of 2140 HL-A haplotypes and segregation analysis in 535 families. *Transplant. Proc. 5,* No. 1:215, 1973a.

Albert, E.D., Rittner, Ch., Grosse-Wilde, H., Netzel, B., and Scholz, S. Recombination frequency and linkage disequilibrium between HL-A and Bf. *Histocompatibility Testing 1975,* pp. 941–944, Munksgaard, Copenhagen, 1976.

Albert, E.D., Rittner, Ch., Scholz, S., Kuntz, B., and Mickey, M.R. Three point association of HLA-A, B, Bf haplotypes deduced in 200 parents of 100 families. *Scand. J. Immunology,* in press. 1977b.

Albert, E.D., Scholz, S., Bertrams, J., Ewald, R.W., Seidl, S., Ratschko, W., and Westphal, E.: Representative HL-A haplotype frequencies of several german populations. *Z. Immun.-Forsch. 148*:367–371, 1975b.

Allen, F.H., Jr. Linkage of HL-A and GBG. *Vox Sang. 27*:382–384, 1974.

Allison, J.P., Pellegrino, M.A. Ferrone, S., Callahan, G.N., and Reisfeld, R.A. Biological and chemical characterization of HLA antigens in human serum. *J. Immunol.,* in press 1977.

Alter, B.J., and Bach, F.H. Lymphocyte reactivity in vitro. I. Cellular reconstitution of purified lymphocyte response. *Cell. Immunol. 1*:207–218, 1970.

Amiel, J.L. Study of the leucocyte phenotypes in Hodgkin's disease. *Histocompatibility Testing 1967*, pp. 79–81, E.S. Curtoni, P.L. Mattiuz, and M.R. Tosi, eds., Munksgaard, Copenhagen, 1967.

Amiel, J.L. Hodgkin's disease and HL-A. *Transplant. Proc. 3*, No. 3:1277, 1971.

Amos, D.B., Cohen, I., and Klein, W.J., Jr. Mechanisms of immunologic enhancement. *Transplant. Proc. 2*:68–69, 1970.

Arnason, B.G., Fuller, T.C., Lehrich, J.R., and Winn, J.H. Leukocyte antigens (HL-A) in multiple sclerosis. *Proc. Transplant. Soc. Congr.*, p. 8, 1972 (abstr.).

Aster, R.H., Miskovich, B.H., and Rodey, G.E. Histocompatibility antigens of human plasma. Localisation to the HLD-3 lipoprotein fraction. *Transplantation 16*:205–210, 1973.

Avis, P.J.G. Pressure homogenization of mammalian cells. *Subcellular Components*, pp. 1–14, G.D. Birnie and S.M. Fox, eds., Plenum Press, New York, 1969.

Bach, F.H., Albertini, R.J., Amos, D.B., Ceppellini, R., Mattiuz, P.L., and Miggiano, V.C. Mixed leukocyte culture studies in families with known HL-A genotypes. *Transplant. Proc. 1*:339–341, 1969.

Bach, F.H., Albertini, R.J., Klostermann, H., and Day, E. Evaluation of compatibility at the major histocompatibility locus in man. *Histocompatibility Testing*, pp. 55–65, Munksgaard, Copenhagen, 1967.

Bach, F.H., and Hirschhorn, K. Lymphocyte interaction: A potential histocompatibility test *in vitro*. *Science 142*:813–814, 1964.

Bach, F.H., Sondel, P.M., Sheehy, M.J., Wank, R., Alter, B.J., and Bach, M.L. The complexity of the HL-A LD system: A PLT analysis. *Histocompatibility Testing 1975*, pp. 576–580, Munksgaard, Copenhagen, 1976.

Bach, F., and Voynow, N.K. One way stimulation in mixed leukocyte cultures. *Science 153*:545–547, 1966.

Behan, P.O., Simpson, J.A., and Dick, H. Immune response genes in myasthenia gravis. *Lancet II*:1033, 1973.

Bender, K., and Grzeschik, K.H.: Assignment of the glyoxalase I (GLO) gene to chromosome 6 using man-mouse hybrids. Third Int. Conf. on Human Gene Mapping, Boston 1975. In: *Cytogenet. Cell Genet.* 1975.

Berah, M., Hors, J., and Dausset, J.J. A study of HL-A antigens in human organs. *Transplantation 9*:185–192, 1970.

Berggard, I., and Bearn, A.G. Isolation and properties of a low molecular weight β_2-globulin occuring in human biological fluids. *J. Biol. Chem. 243*:4095–4103, 1968.

Bernier, I., Dautigny, A., Colombani, J., and Jolles, P. Detergent solubilized HL-A antigens from human platelets. A comparative study of various purification techniques. *Biochim. Biophys. Acta 354*:82–90, 1974.

Bernier, I., Dautigny, A., Colombani, J., and Jolles, P. Investigations on human leukocyte antigens (HLA) from urine. *FEBS Letters 63*:320–322, 1976.

Bernoco, D., Cullen, S., Scudeller, G., Trinchieri, B., and Ceppellini, R. HL-A molecules at the cell surface. *Histocompatibility Testing 1972*, pp. 527–537, J. Dausset and J. Colombani, eds., Munksgaard, Copenhagen, 1973.

Bertrams, J., Kuvert, E., Böhme, U., Reis, H.E., Gallmeier, W.M., Wetter, O., and Schmidt, C.G. HL-A antigens in Hodgkin's disease and multiple myeloma. *Tissue Antigens 2*:41, 1972.

Bertrams, J., Kuwert, E., Fisenne, E. von, and Höher, P.G. Measles antibodies and HL-A antigens in multiple sclerosis. *Z. Immunitaetsforsch., Exp. Klin. Immunol. 147*:4, 1974.

Bertrams, J., and Kuwert, E. HL-A-antigen frequencies in multiple sclerosis: significant increase of HL-A 3, HL-A 10 and W 5 and decrease of HL-A 12. *Eur. Neurol. 7*:74, 1972.

Bertrams, J., Kuwert, E., and Liedtke, U. HL-A antigens and multiple sclerosis. *Tissue Antigens 2*:405, 1972.

Bertrams, J., and Kuwert, E. HL-A antigen segregation analysis in multiple sclerosis. *Lancet II*:43–44, 1974.

Bertrams, J., Kuwert, E., Gallmeier, W.M., Reis, H.E., and Schmidt, C.G. Transient lymphocyte HL-A loss in a case of irradiated M. Hodgkin. *Tissue Antigens 1*:105–108, 1971.

Bialek, J.W., Bodmer, W.F., Bodmer, J.G., and Payne, R. Distribution and quantity of leukocyte antigens in the formed elements of the blood. *Transfusion 6*: 193–205, 1966.
Bijnen, A.B., Schreuder, I., Giles, C.M., Los, W.R.T., Meera Khan, P., Volkers, W.S., and Rood, J.J. van. A study on genetic markers in families with a recombination in the HL-A region. J. Immunogenetics *3*: 171–183, 1976.
Bijnen, A.B., Schreuder, I., Meera Khan, P., Allen, F.H., Giles, C.M., Los, W.R.T., Volkers, W.S., Rood, J.J. van Linkage relationships of the Loci of the major histocompatibility complex in families with a recombination in the HLA region. *J. Immunogenet. 3*: 171–183, 1976.
Billing, R., and McMillan, M. The lipoprotein nature of serum HLA antigens. *Transplant. Proc. 7*, Suppl.: 227–231, 1975.
Billing, R.J., Mittal, K.K., and Terasaki, P.I. Isolation of soluble HL-A antigens from normal human sera by ion exchange chromatography. *Tissue Antigens 3*: 251–256, 1973.
Billing, R.J., Safani, M., and Peterson, P. Isolation and characterization of human B cell alloantigens. *J. Immunol. 117*: 1589–1593, 1976.
Billing, R.J., and Terasaki, P.I. Purification of HL-A antigens from normal serum. *J. Immunol. 112*: 1124–1130, 1974.
Bismuth, P., Neauport-Sautes, C., Kourilsky, M., Manuel, Y., Greenland, T., and Silvestre, D. Distribution and mobility of β_2-microglobulin on human lymphocyte membrane: immunofluorescence and immunoferritin studies. *J. Immunol. 112*: 2036–2046, 1974.
Bodmer, W.F. Evolutionary significance of the HL-A system. *Nature (London) 237*: 139–145, 1972.
Bodmer, W.F. Population genetics of the HL-A system retrospect and prospect. *Histocompatibility Testing 1972*, pp. 611–617, J. Dausset and J. Colobani, eds., Munksgaard, Copenhagen, 1973.
Bodmer, W.F., Bodmer, J., Adler, S., Payne, R., and Bialek, J. Genetics of 4 and LA human leukocyte groups. *Ann. N.Y. Acad. Sci. 129*: 673, 1966.
Bodmer, W.F., Bodmer, J.G., Cullen, P.R., Dick, H.M., Gelstorph, K., Harris, R., Lawler, S.D., McKintosch, P., and Morris, P.J. Ia antigens on chronic lymphocytic leukaemic lymphocytes: association between the reactions of VI Workshop Sera on CLL and lymphoid line cells. *Histocompatibility Testing 1975*, pp. 685–688, F. Kissmeyer-Nielsen, ed., Munksgaard, Copenhagen, 1975b.
Bodmer, W.F., Jones, E.A., Young, D., Goodfellow, P.N., Bodmer, J.G., Dick, H.M., and Steel, C.M. Serology of human Ia like type antigens detected on lymphoid lines. An analysis of the VI Workshop Sera. *Histocompatibility Testing 1975*, pp. 677–684, F. Kissmeyer-Nielsen, ed., Munksgaard, Copenhagen, 1975a.
Boyum, A. Separation of leukocytes from blood and bone marrow. *Scand. J. Clin. Lab. Invest. Suppl. 97*: 21, 1968.
Brautbar, C., Pellegrino, M.A., Ferrone, S., Reisfeld, R.A., and Hayflick, L. Fate of HL-A antigens in aging cultured human diploid cell strains. II. Quantitative absorption studies. *Expt. Cell Res. 78*: 367–375, 1973a.
Brautbar, C., Stanbridge, E.J., Pellegrino, M.A., Ferrone, S., Reisfeld, R.A., Payne, R., and Hayflick, L. Expression of HL-A antigens on cultured human fibroblasts infected with mycoplasma. *J. Immunol. 111*: 1783–1789, 1973b.
Brewerton, D.A., Caffrey, M., Hart, F.D., James, D.C.O., Nicholls, A., and Sturrock, R.D. Ankylosing spondylitis and HL-A27. *Lancet II*: 904–907, 1973a.
Brewerton, D.A., Caffrey, M., Nicholls, A., Walters, D., Oates, J.K., and James, D.C.O. Reiters disease and HL-A27. *Lancet II*: 996–999, 1973b.
Brewerton, D.A., Caffrey, M., Nicholls, A., Walters, D., Oates, J.K., and James, D.C.O. Acute anterior uveitis and HL-A27. *Lancet II*: 994–996, 1973c.
Brewerton, D.A., Nicholls, A., Caffrey, M., and Walters, D. HL-A27 and arthopathies associated with ulcerative colitis and psoriasis. *Lancet I*: 956–957, 1974.
Brigdon, J., Snary, D., Crumpton, M.J., Barnstable, C., Goodfellow, P., and Bodmer, W.F. Isolation and N-terminal amino acid sequence of membrane bound human HLA-A and HLA-B antigens. *Nature 261*: 200–205, 1976.
Bruning, J.W., Leeuwen, A. van, and Rood, J.J., va. Purification of leukocyte group substances from human placental tissue. *Transplantation 2*: 649–653, 1964.

Burstein, M., Cholnick, H.R., and Bortin, R. Rapid method for the isolation of lipoproteins from human serum by precipitation with polyanions. *J. Lipid Res. 11*:583–595, 1970.

Caffrey, M.F.P., and James, D.C.O. Human lymphocyte antigen association in ankylosing spondylitis. *Nature (London) 242*:121, 1973.

Cavalli Sforza, L.L., and Bodmer, W.F. *The Genetics of Human Populations.* Freeman, San Francisco, 1971.

Charlton, R.N., and Zmijewski, C.M. Soluble HL-A7 antigen: localization in the lipoprotein fraction of human serum. *Science 170*:636–637, 1970.

Choi, K.W., and Bloom, A.D. Cloning human lymphocytes in vitro. *Nature 227*:171–173, 1970.

Claussen, F., und Kober, E.: Beiträge der Zwillingsforschung zum Rheumaproblem. *Z. Rheumaforsch. 14*:145, 1955.

Cochrum, K.C., Main, R.K., and Kountz, S.L. A new matching technique: the mixed skin cell-leukocyte reaction (MSLR). *Surgery 70*:97–102, 1971.

Cochrum, K., Salvatierra, O., Jr., Perkins, H.A., and Belzer, F.O. MLC-Testing in renal transplantation. *Transplant. Proc. 7*, No. 1:659–662, 1975.

Colombani, J., Colombani, M., and Dausset, J. Cross-reactions in the HL-A system with special reference to the Da6 cross-reacting group. Description of HL-A antigens Da22, Da23, Da24 defined by platelet complement fixation: *Histocompatibility Testing 1970*, pp. 79–92, P.I. Terasaki, ed., Munksgaard, Copenhagen, 1970a.

Colombani, J., Colombani, M., Visa, D.C., Degani-Bernard, O., Dausset, J., and Davies, D.A.L. Separation of HL-A transplantation antigen specificities. *Transplantation 9*:228–239, 1970b.

Colombani, M., Colombani, J., Dastot, H., Mayer, S., Tongio, M.M., and Dausset, J. Définition de deux nouveaux antigènes du système HL-A: Da19 et Da20. Réactions croisées entre les antigènes Da19, Da20, HL-A5 et Da6. *Rev. franç. Étud. clin. biol. 14*:995, 1969.

Colombani, M., Colombani, J., Dastot, H., Meyer, S., Tongio, M.M., and Dausset, J. Définition de deux nonveaux antigènes du système HL-A: Da19 et Da20. Réaction croisée entre les antigènes Da19, Da20, HL-A5 et Da6. *Rev. Franc. Etud. Clin. Biol. 14*:995, 1969.

Cook, K.M. Distribution of HL-A antigens on blood cells. *Tissue Antigens 4*:202–209, 1974.

Coukell, A., Bodmer, J.G., and Bodmer, W.F. HL-A types of forty-four Hodgkin's patients. *Transplant. Proc. 3*, No. 3:1291, 1971.

Cresswell, P., Turner, M.J., and Strominger, S.J.L. Papain solubilized HL-A antigens from cultured human lymphocytes contain two peptide fragments. *Proc. Natl. Acad. Sci. 70*:1603–1608, 1973.

Cresswell, P., Springer, T., Strominger, J.L., Turner, M.J., Grey, H.M., and Nubo, R.T. Immunological identity of the small subunit of HL-A antigens and β_2-microglobulin and its turnover on the cell membrane. *Proc. Natl. Acad. Sci. 71*:2123–2127, 1974a.

Cresswell, P., Robb, R.J., Turner, M.J., Strominger, J.L. Papain solubilized HL-A antigens. Chromatographic and electrophoretic studies of the two subunits from different specificities. *J. Biol. Chem. 249*:2828–2832, 1974b.

Cresswell, P., and Geier, S.S. Antisera to human B lymphocyte membrane glycoproteins block stimulation in mixed lymphocyte culture. *Nature 257*, 147–149, 1970.

Cresswell, P., and Dawson, J.R. Dimeric and monomeric forms of HL-A antigens solubilized by detergent. *J. Immunol. 114*:523–525, 1975a.

Cudworth, A.G., and Woodrow, J.C. HL-A antigens and diabetes mellitus. *Lancet II*:1153, 1974.

Cullen, S.E., Bernoco, D., Carbonara, A.O., Jacot-Guittarmond, H., Trinchieri, G., and Ceppellini, R. Fate of HL-A antigens and antibodies at the lymphocyte surface. *Transplant. Proc. 5*:1835–1847, 1973.

Cullen, S.E., and Schwartz, B.D. An improved method for isolation of H-2 and Ia alloantigens with immunoprecipitation induced by protein A bearing staphylocci. *J. Immunol. 117*:136–141, 1976.

Cunningham, B.A., and Berggard, I. Structure, evolution and significance of β_2-microglobulin. *Transplant. Rev. 21*:3–14, 1974.

Cunningham, B.A., Wang, J.L., Berggard, I., and Peterson, P.A. The complete amino acid sequence of β_2-microglobulin. *Biochemistry 12*:4811–4822, 1973.

Currie, G.A., and Bagshawe, K.D. The masking of antigens on trophoblast and cancer cells. *Lancet I*:708–710, 1967.

Currie, G. A., van Doorwinck, W., and Bagshawe, K. B. Effect of neuraminidase on the immunogenicity of early mouse trophoblasts. *Nature (London) 219*: 191–192, 1968.
D'Amato, J., Hensen, E., and van Rood, J. J. The micro-complement fixation test. III. Automatic quantitative scoring with a microscope densitometer. *Tissue Antigens 1*: 171–177, 1971.
Dausset, J. Iso-Leuco-anticorps. *Acta Haematol. (Basel) 20*: 156–166, 1958.
Dausset, J., Rapaport, F.T., Ivanyi, P., and Colombani, J. Tissue allo-antigens and transplantation. *Histocompatibility Testing 1965*, pp. 63–69, Munksgaard, Copenhagen, 1965.
Dausset, J., Colombani, J., Legrand, L., and Feingold, N. Le deuxième sub-locus du système HL-A. *Nouv. Rev. Franc. Hematol. 8*: 861, 1968.
Dausset, J., Hors, J., Busson, M., Festenstein, H., Oliver, R. T. D., Paris, A. M. I., and Sachs, J. A. Serologically defined HL-A antigens and long-term survival of cadaver kidney transplants. *N. Engl. J. Med. 290*: 979–983, 1974.
Dausset, J., Ivanvi, P., Colombani, J., Feingold, N., and Legrand, L. The Hu-1 system. *Histocompatibility Testing 1967*, p. 189, Munksgaard, Copenhagen, 1967.
Dausset, J., Walford, R. L., Colombani, J., Legrand, L., Feingold, N., and Rapaport, F. T. The HL-A sub-loci and their importance in transplantation. *Transplant. Proc. 1*: 331, 1969.
Dautigny, A., Bernier, L., Colombani, J., and Jolles, P. Purification and characterization of HL-A antigens from human platelets, solubilized by the non-ionic detergent NP-40. *Biochim. Biophys. Acta 298*: 783–789, 1973.
Davies, D. A. L. Mouse histocompatibility antigens derived from normal and from tumor cells. *Immunology 11*: 115–125, 1966.
Davies, D. A. L. Isolation and purification of transplantation and tumorspecific antigens. *Transplantation 6*: 660–661, 1968.
Davies, D. A. L. The molecular individuality of different mouse H-2 histocompatibility specificities determined by single gen types. *Transplantation 8*: 51–70, 1969.
Dawson, J. R., Shasby, S. S., and Amos, D. B. Serologic assay fo HL-A antigens in the presence of detergents. *J. Immunol. 111*: 281–283, 1973.
Dawson, J. R., Shasby, S. S., and Amos, D. B. The serological detection of HL-A antigens in human milk. *Tissue Antigens 4*: 76–82, 1974a.
Dawson, J. R., Silver, J., Sheppard, L. B., and Amos, B. The purification of detergent-solubilized HL-A antigens by affinity chromatography with the hemagglutinin from lens culinaris. *J. Immunol. 112*: 1190–1193, 1974b.
Degos, L., and Dausset, J. Human migrations and linkage disequilibrium of HL-A system. *Immunogenetics 3*: 195–210, 1974a.
Degos, L., and Dausset, J. Histocompatibility determinants in multiple sclerosis. *Lancet I*: 307–308, 1974b.
Del Villano, B., Carp, R. I., Manson, L. A., and Defendi, V. Studies on the cellular distribution and purification of SV_{40} T antigens. *Transplantation 6*: 632–634, 1968.
Dick, H. M., Dick, W. C., Sturrock, R. D., and Buchanan, W. W. Inheritance of ankylosing spondylitis and HL-A antigen W27. *Lancet II*: 24–25, 1974.
Dick, H. M., Steel, C. M., and Crichton, W. B. HL-A typing of cultured peripheral lymphoblastoid cells. *Tissue Antigens 2*: 85–93, 1972.
Doughty, R. W., Goodier, S. R., and Gelsthorpe, K. Further evidence for HL-A antigens present on adult peripheral red blood cells. *Tissue Antigens 3*: 189–194, 1973.
Douglas, K. S., Perkins, H. A., Cockrum, K., and Dountz, S. L. Comparison of the HL-A phenotypes on lymphocytes and kidney cells determined by the fluorochromasia cytotoxicity assay. *J. Clin. Invest. 50*: 274–281, 1971.
Dumble, L., and Whittingham, S. Quantitative differences in histocompatibility antigens (HL-A) in populations of lymphocytes. *Histocompatibility Testing 1975*, pp. 761–766, F. Kissmeyer-Nielsen, ed., Munksgaard, Copenhagen, 1975.
Dupont, B., Jersild, C., Hansen, G. S.; Staub Nielsen, L., Thomsen, M., and Svejgaard, A. Multiple MLC (LD) determinants on the same HL-A haplotype. *Transplant. Proc. 5*: 1481–1487, 1973.
Ehlers, N., Kissmeyer-Nielsen, F., Kjerbye, K. E., and Lamm, L. HL-A27 in acute and chronic uveitis. *Lancet I*: 99, 1974.
Eijsvoogel, V. P., Bois, M. J. G. J. du, Meinesz, A., Bierhorst-Eijlander, A., Zeylemaker, W. P.,

and Schellekens, P. Th. A. The specificity and the activation mechanism of cell-mediated lympholysis (CML) in man. *Transplant. Proc. 5*: 1675–1678, 1973c.

Eijsvoogel, V. P., Bois, M. J. G. J. du, Melief, C. J. M., Groot-Kooy, M. L. de, Koning, C., Rood, J. J. van, Leeuwen, A. van, Toit, E. D., and Schellekens, P. T. A. Position of a locus determining mixed lymphocyte reaction (MLR), distinct from the known HL-A loci, and its relation to cell-mediated lympholysis (CML). *Histocompatibility Testing 1972*, pp. 501–508, J. Dausset and J. Colombani, eds., Munksgaard, Copenhagen, 1973a.

Eijsvoogel, V. P., Bois, R. du, Melief, C. J. M., Zeylemaker, W. P., Koning, L., and Groot-Kooy, L. de. Lymphocyte activation and destruction *in vitro* in relation to MLC and HLA-A. *Transplant. Proc. 5*: 415–420, 1973b.

Eijsvoogel, V.P., Rood, J.J. van, Toit, E.D., and Schellekens, P.T.A. Position of a locus determining mixed lymphocyte reaction distinct from the known HL-A loci. *Eur. J. Immunol. 2*: 413–418, 1972.

Engelfriet, C. P., Feltkamp, Th. E. W., Nijenhuis, L. E., Galama, S. M. D., Rijn, A. van, Loghem, E. van, Berg-Loonen, E. van den, Possum, A. van, and Loghem, J. van. HL-A phenotype and haplotype frequencies in patients with myasthenia gravis. *Personal communication.*

Etheredge, E. E., and Najarian, J. S. Solubilization of human histocompatibility substances. *Transplant. Proc. 3*: 224–226, 1971.

Etheredge, E. E., Shons, A. R., and Najarian, J. S. Solubilization of HL-A antigens from peripheral blood leukocytes. *Immunol. Comm. 2*: 141–149, 1973.

Eurotransplant Reports 1973, 1974, 1975. Eurotransplant foundation, Leiden, The Netherlands.

Evans, C. H., and Pegrum, G. D. The reactivity of leukaemic cells to HL-A typing cells. *Tissue Antigens 3*: 454–464, 1973.

Evans, D. A. P. Coeliac disease and HL-A 8. *Lancet II*: 1096, 1973.

Falchuk, J. M., Rogentine, G. N., and Strober, W. Predominance of histocompatibility antigen HL-A 8 in patients with gluten-sensitive enteropathy. *J. Clin. Invest. 51*: 1602, 1972.

Falk, J., and Osoba, D. HL-A antigens and survival in Hodgkin's disease. *Lancet II*: 1118, 1971.

Fanger, M. W., and Bernier, G. M. Subpopulations of human lymphocytes defined by β_2-microglobulin. *J. Immunol. 111*: 609–617, 1973.

Fellous, M., and Dausset, J. J. Probable haploid expression of HL-A antigens on human spermatozoon. *Nature 225*: 191–193, 1970.

Fellous, M., Mortchelewicz, F., Kalhoun, M., and Dausset, J. The use of lymphoid cell lines to define new B lymphocyte specificities, probably controlled by the MHC region. *Histocompatibility Testing 1975*, pp. 708–712, F. Kissmeyer-Nielsen, ed., Munksgaard, Copenhagen, 1975.

Ferrara, G.B., Tosi, R., Azzolina, G., Carminati, G., and Longo, A. Production of isoantisera for HL-A typing by planned immunization. A four year's experiment. International Symposium on Standardization of HL-A Reagents, Copenhagen 1972. *Symp. Ser. Immunobiol. Stand. 18*: 20–26, 1973.

Ferrone, S., Natali, P. G., Hunter, A., Terasaki, P. I., and Reisfeld, R. A. Immunogenicity of soluble HL-A antigens. *J. Immunol. 108*: 1718–1799, 1972.

Ferrone, S., Pellegrino, M. A., Götze, D., Mittal, K. K., Terasaki, P. I., and Reisfeld, R. A. Cytotoxic heteroantisera against soluble HL-A antigens. *Symp. Ser. Immunobiol. Stand. 18*: 218–223, 1973.

Ferrone, S., Pellegrino, M. A., and Reisfeld, R. A. A rapid method for direct typing for HL-A of cultured lymphoid cells. *J. Immunol. 107*: 613–615, 1971.

Ferrone, S., Pellegrino, M.A., and Reisfeld, R.A. A biological and chemical profile of histocompatibility antigens. *The Antigens III*, pp. 361–447, M. Sela, ed., Academic Press, New York-London, 1975.

Ferrone, S., Tosi, R. M., and Centis, D. Anticomplementary factors affecting the lymphocytotoxic test. *Histocompatibility Testing 1967*, pp. 357–360, E. S. Curtoni, P. L. Mattiuz, and R. M. Tosi, eds. Munksgaard, Copenhagen, 1967.

Festenstein, H., Halim, K., and Arnaiz-Villena, A. New HLA-D locus determinants detected by sperm lymphocyte culture. *Transplant. Proc., in press*, 1976.

Forbes, J. K., and Morris, P. J. Analysis of HL-A antigens in patients with Hodgkin's disease and their families. *J. Clin. Invest. 51*: 1156, 1972.

Forbes, J.F., and Morris, P.J. Leucocyte antigens in Hodgkin's disease. *Lancet II*:849, 1970.
Fradelizi, D., and Dausset, J. Mixed lymphocyte reactivity of human lymphocytes primed in vitro. I. Secondary response to allogenic lymphocytes. *Eur. J. Immunol. 5*:295–301, 1975.
Fritze, D., Herrman, Ch., Naeim, F., Smith, G.G., and Walford, R.L. HL-A antigens in myasthenia gravis. *Lancet I*:240–243, 1974.
Fu, S.M., Kunkel, H.C., Brusman, H.P., Allen, F.H., and Fotino, M. Evidence for linkage between HL-A histocompatibility genes and those involved in the synthesis of the second component of complement. *J. Exp. Med. 140*:1108, 1974.
Fu, S.M., Stern, R., Kunkel, H.G., Dupont, B., Hansen, J.A., Day, N.K., Good, R.A., Jersild, C., and Fotino, M. Mixed lymphocyte culture determinants and C_2 deficiency: LD-7a associated with C2 deficiency in four families. *J. Exp. Med. 142*:495–506, 1975.
Gebhard, R.L., Katz, S.J., Marks, J., Shuster, S., Trapani, R.J., Rogentine, G.N., and Strober, W. HL-A antigen type and small intestinal disease in dermatitis herpetiformis. *Lancet II*:760–763, 1973.
Gibofsky, A., Jaffe, E.A., Fotino, M., and Becker, C.G. The identification of HL-A antigens on fresh and cultured human endothelial cells. *J. Immunol. 115*:730–733, 1975.
Giles, C.M., Gedde-Dahl, T., Jr., Robson, E.B., Thorsby, E., Olaisen, B., Arnason, A., Kissmeyer-Nielsen, F., and Schreuder, I. Rg^a (Rodgers) and the HLA region: Linkage and associations. *Tissue Antigens 8*:143–149, 1976.
Giphart, M.J., Doyer, E., Wisse, E., and Bruning, J.W. Quantitative aspects of HL-A2 antigenic surface determinants studied with radiolabelled antibodies. *Histocompatibility Testing 1975*, pp. 739–746, F. Kissmeyer-Nielsen, ed., Munksgaard, Copenhagen, 1975b.
Goldstein, S., and Singal, D.P. Loss of reactivity of HL-A antigens in clonal populations of cultured human fibroblasts during aging in vitro. *Exp. Cell Res. 75*:278–282, 1972.
Goodfellow, P.N., Jones, E.A., Heyningen, V. van, Solomon, E., Bobrow, M., Miggiano, V., and Bodmer, W.F. The β_2-microglobulin gene is on chromosome 15 and not in the HL-A region. *Nature 254*:267–268, 1975.
Gorer, P.A. The antigenic basis of tumour transplantation. *J. Pathol. Bacteriol. 47*:231–252, 1938.
Gorer, P.A. The antigenic structure of tumors. *Adv. Immunol. 1*:345–393, 1961.
Gosset, T., Walford, R.L., Smith, G.S., Robins, A., and Ferrara, G.B. The Merrit alloantigenic system of human lymphocytes. *Histocompatibility Testing 1975*, pp. 687–691, F. Kissmeyer-Nielsen, ed., Munksgaard, Copenhagen, 1975.
Goulmy, E., Termijtelen, A., Bradley, B.A., and Rood, J.J. van HLA restriction of non HLA-A, B, C and D cell mediated lympholysis (CML). *Tissue Antigens, 8*, No. 5:317–326, 1976.
Granditsch, G., Ludwig, H., Polymenidis, Z., and Wick, G. Coeliac disease and HL-A 8. *Lancet II*:908, 1973.
Grey, H.M., Kubo, R.T., Colon, S.M., Poulik, M.D., Cresswell, P., Springer, T., Turner, N., and Strominger, J.L. The small subunit of HL-A antigens is β_2-microglobulin. *J. Exp. Med. 138*:1608–1612, 1973.
Grosse-Wilde, H., Netzel, B., Mempel, W., Ruppelt, W., Brehm, G., Bertrams, J., Ewald, R., Lenhard, V., Rittner, Ch., Scholz, S., and Albert, E.D. Immunogenetics of LD determinants in man. *Histocompatibility Testing 1975*, pp. 526–532. Published by Munksgaard, Copenhagen, Denmark.
Grumet, F.C., Payne, R.O., Konishi, J., and Kriss, J. HL-A antigens as markers for disease susceptibility and autoimmunity in Graves' disease. *J. Clin. Endocrinol. Metab. 39*:1115–1119, 1974.
Hämmerling, U., Aoki, T., Harven, E. de, Boyse, E.A., and Old, J.L. Use of hybrid antibody with anti-G and anti-ferritin specificities in locating cell surface antigens by electron microscopy. *J. Exp. Med. 128*:1461–1473, 1968.
Halim, A., Abbasi, K., and Festenstein, H. The expression of the HL-A antigens on human spermatozoa. *Tissue Antigens 4*:1–6, 1974.
Halim, K., and Festenstein, H. HLA-D on sperms. *Lancet II*: 1255–1256, 1975.
Hardy, P.A., Ling, N.R., and Knight, S.C. Exceptional lymphocyte stimulating capacity of cells from lymphoid cell lines. *Nature 223*:511–512, 1969.

Harms, K., Granditsch, G., Rossipal, E., Ludwig, H., Polymenidis, Z., Scholz, S., Wank, R., and Albert, E. D. In: *Coeliac Disease,* (W. Tu, J. M. Hekkergs, and A. S. Pena, eds.) pp. 215–228. H. E. Stenfert Kroese, Leiden, 1974.

Harris, R. Leukaemia antigens and immunity in man. *Nature (London) 241*:95–100, 1973.

Harris, R., and Zervas, J. D. Reticulocyte HL-A antigens. *Nature 221*: 1062–1063, 1969.

Haughton, G. Extraction of H-2 antigens from mouse tumor cells. *Transplantation 2*:251–260, 1964.

Hauptmann, G., Sasportes, M., Tongio, M. M., Mayer, S., and Dausset, J. The localization of the Bf locus within the MHS region on chromosome no. 6. *Tissue Antigens 7*:52–54, 1976.

Haynes, W. D. D., Jones, J. V., and Cumming, J. C. O. HL-A antigens on circulating platelets: ultrastructural demonstration. *Transplantation 18*:81–86, 1974.

Heinrich, D., Müller-Eckhart, C., and Czitron, A. Elution of HL-A specific antibodies from platelets. *Vox Sang. 27*:310–321, 1974.

Helenius, A., and Simmons, K. The Binding of detergents to lipophilic and hydrophilic proteins. *J. Biol. Chem. 247*:3656–3661, 1972.

Hilgert, I., Kandutsch, A. A., Cherry, M., and Snell, G. D. Fractionation of murine H-2 antigens with the use of detergents. *Transplantation 8*:451–461, 1969.

Hirschberg, H., Evensen, S. A., Henriksen, T., and Thorsby, E. Stimulation of human lymphocytes by allogeneic endothelial cells in vitro. *Tissue Antigens 4*:257–261, 1974.

Hirschberg, H., Kaakinen, A., and Thorsby, E. Presence of HLA-D determinants on human macrophages. *Nature 263*:63–64, 1976.

Hirschberg, H., and Thorsby, E. Lymphocyte activating alloantigens on human epidermal cells. *Tissue Antigens 6*:183–194, 1975.

Hirschfeld, J. Serologic codes: interpretation of immunogenetic systems. *Science 148*:968–971, 1965.

Hooff, J. P. van, Schippers, H. M. A., Hendriks, G. F. J., and Rood, J. J. van Influence of possible HL-A haploidentity on renal-graft survival in Eurotransplant. *Lancet I*:1130–1132, 1974.

Hooff, J. P. van, Steen, G. J. van der, Schippers, H. M. A., and Rood, J. J. van Efficacy of HL-A matching in Eurotransplant. *Lancet II*: 1385–1388, 1972.

Hunter, M.J., and Cummerford, S.L. Pressure homogenization of mammalian tissue. *Biochim. Biophys. Acta 47*:580–586, 1961.

Ivanyi, P., and Dausset, J. Allo-antigens and antigenic factors of human leukocytes. An hypothesis. *Vox sang. 11*:3, 1966.

Jacot-Guillarmod, H., Buzzi, G., Carbonara, A. O., Cone, R., and Ceppellini, R. Shedding of HL-A antigens and antibodies from lymphocyte surface.*Histocompatibility Testing 1975,* pp. 753–760, F. Kissmeyer-Nielsen, ed., Munksgaard, Copenhagen, 1975.

Jersild, C., Ammitzbøll, T., Clausen, J., and Fog, T. Association between HL-A antigens and measles antibody in multiple sclerosis. *Lancet I*:151, 1973a

Jersild, C., Dupont, B., Fog, T., Hansen, G. S., Nielsen, L. S., Thomsen, M., and Svejgaard, A. Histocompatibility-linked immune response determinants in multiple sclerosis. *Transplant. Proc. 5*, No. 4:1791–1796, 1973c.

Jersild, C., Fog, T., Hansen, G. S., Thomsen, M., Svejgaard, A., and Dupont, B. Histocompatibility determinants in multiple sclerosis, with special reference to clinical course. *Lancet II*:1221–1225, 1973b.

Jersild, C., Svejgaard, A., and Fog, T. HL-A antigens and multiple sclerosis. *Lancet I*:1240, 1972.

Johnson, M., Hattler, B., Alexander, K., and Carrier, C. Effect of granulocyte concentration of mixed lymphocyte culture. *Fed. Proc. 30*:1514 (Abstract), 1971.

Joint Report of the Fourth International Histocompatibility Workshop. *Histocompatibility Testing 1970,* pp. 2–47, (P. I. Terasaki, ed.), Munksgaard, Copenhagen, 19 .

Joint Report of the Fifth International Histocompatibility Workshop. *Histocompatibility Testing 1972,* p. 619, Munksgaard, Kopenhagen, 1973.

Joint Report from the Sixth International Histocompatibility Workshop Conference. II. Typing for HLA-D (LD-1 or MLC) determinants. *Histocompatibility Testing 1975,* pp. 414–458, Munksgaard, Copenhagen, 1976.

Jongsma, A., Someren, H. van, Westerveld, A., Hagemeijor, A., and Pearson, P. Localization of genes on human chromosomes using human-Chinese hamster somatic cell hybrids. Assignment of PGM_3 to chromosome C6 and regional mapping of the PGD, PGM_1 and Pep-C genes on chromosome A1. *Humangenetik 20*:195, 1973.

Kachru, R.B., and Mittal, K.K. Serological detection of HL-A antigens in human mammary secretion. *Histocompatibility Testing 1975*, pp. 404–413, F. Kissmeyer-Nielsen, ed., Munksgaard, Copenhagen, 1975.

Kahan, B.D., Pellegrino, M.A., Papermaster, B.W., and Reisfeld, R.A. Quantitative serologic parameters of purified HL-A antigens. *Transplant. Proc. 3*:227–230, 1971.

Kahan, D.B., and Reisfeld, R.A. Chemical markers of transplantation individuality solubilized with sonic energy. *Bacteriol. Rev. 35*:59–85, 1971.

Kahan, B.D., Reisfeld, R.A., Pellegrino, M.A., Curtoni, E.S., Mattiuz, P.L., and Ceppellini, R. Water soluble human transplantation antigens. *Proc. Natl. Acad. Sci. 61*:897–903, 1968.

Kandutsch, A.A. Intracellular distribution and extraction of tumor homograft enhancing antigens. *Cancer Res. 20*:264–268, 1960.

Kandutsch, A.A., and Reiner-Wenck, U. Studies on a substance that promotes tumor homograft survival (the 'enhancing substance'). Its distribution and some properties. *J. Exp. Med. 105*:125–139, 1957.

Kandutsch, A.A., and Stimpling, T.H. Partial purification of tissue isoantigens from mouse sarcoma. *Transplantation 1*:201–216, 1963.

Katagiri, M., Tanigaki, N., Kreitzer, V.P., and Pressman, D. Common antigenic structures of HL-A antigens. III. An HL-A common antigenic marker closely associated with HL-A alloantigenic activity and detected by use of rabbit anti-rhesus monkey cell membrane antibodies. *Immunology 27*:487–500, 1974.

Kerek, G., and Afzelius, B.A. The HL-A antigens on human spermatozoa. *Int. J. Fertil. 17*:120–126, 1972.

Keuning, J.J., Peña, A.S., Leeuwen, A. van, Hooff, J.P. van, Rood, J.J. van. HLA-DW3 associated with coeliac disease. *Lancet I*:506–508, 1976.

Kissmeyer-Nielsen, F., Jensen, K.B., Ferrara, G.B., Kjerbye, K.E., and Svejgaard, A. HL-A phenotypes in Hodgkin's disease. Preliminary report. *Transplant. Proc. 3*, No. 3:1287, 1971.

Kissmeyer-Nielsen, F., and Kjerbye, K.E. The human HL-A locus. Antibodies and antigens belonging to the LA- and 4-series. *Bull. Eur. Soc. Hum. Genet. 1*:58–63, 1967a.

Kissmeyer-Nielsen, F., and Kjerbye, K.E. Lymphocytotoxic microtechnique. Purification of lymphocytes by flotation. *Histocompatibility Testing 1967*, pp. 381–383, E.S. Curtoni, P.L. Mattiuz, and R.M. Tosi, eds., Munksgaard, Copenhagen, 1967b.

Kissmeyer-Nielsen, F., Svejgaard, A., Ahrons, S., and Nielsen, L.S. Crossing-over within the HL-A system. *Nature (Lond.) 224*:75, 1969.

Kissmeyer-Nielsen, F., Staub-Nielsen, L., Sandiberg, L., Svejgaard, A., and Thorsby, E. The HL-A system in relation to human transplantations. *Histocompatibility Testing 1970*, pp. 105–135, P.I. Terasaki, ed., Munksgaard, Copenhagen, 1970.

Koch, C.R., Frederiks, E., Eijsvoogel, V.P., and Rood, J.J. van. Mixed-lymphocyte-culture and skin-graft data in unrelated HL-A identical individuals. *Lancet II*:1334–1336, 1971.

Koch, C., Hooff, J.P. van, Leeuwen, A. van, Tweel, J. van den, Frederiks, E., Steen, G. van den, Schippers, H.M.A., and Rood, J.J. van. The relative importance of matching for the MLC versus the HL-A loci in organ transplantation. *Histocompatibility Testing 1972*, pp. 521–524, J. Dausset and J. Colombani, eds., Munksgaard, Copenhagen, 1973.

Kömpf, J., and Bissbort, S. Population genetics of red cell glyoxalase I (E.C.: 4.4.1.5). *Humangenetik 28*:175–176, 1975.

Kömpf, J., Bissbort, S., Gussman, S., and Ritter, H. Polymorphism of red cell glyoxalase I (E.C.: 4.4.1.5). A new genetic marker in man. *Humangenetic 27*:141–143, 1975a.

Kömpf, J., Bissbort, S., and Ritter, H. Red cell glyoxalase I (E.C.: 4.4.1.5): Formal genetics and linkage relations. *Humangenetik 28*:249–251, 1975b.

Kömpf, J., Bissbort, S., and Schunter, F. Confirmation of linkage between the loci for HL-A and glyoxalase I. *Hum. Genet. 32*:197–198, 1976.

Kourilsky, F.M., Silvestre, D., Levy, J.P., Dausset, J., Niccolai, M.G., and Senik, A. Immunoferritin studies of the distribution of HL-A antigens on human blood cells. *J. Immunol. 106*:454–466, 1971.

Kourilsky, F.M., Silvestre, D., Neauport-Sautes, C., Loosfelt, Y., and Dausset, J. Antibody-induced redistribution of HL-A antigens at the cell surface. *Eur. J. Immunol. 2*:249–257, 1972.

Kristensen, T., and Grunnet, N. Cell mediated lympholysis in man. Evidence of a separate CML locus within the major histocompatibility complex and an approach to CML typing. *Histocompatibility Testing 1975*, pp. 835–844, Munksgaard, Copenhagen, 1976.

Lamm, L.U., Friedrich, U., Petersen, G.B., Jørgensen, J., Nielsen, J., Therkelsen, A.J., and Kissmeyer-Nielsen, F. Assignment of the major histocompatibility complex to chromosome no. 6 in a family with a pericentric inversion. *Hum. Hered. 24*:273–284, 1974.

Lamm, L.U., Jørgensen, F., and Kissmeyer-Nielsen, F. Bf maps between HLA-A and D loci. *Tissue Antigens 7*:122–124, 1976.

Lamm, L.U., Kissmeyer-Nielsen, F., Svejgaard, A., Brunn Petersen, G., Thorsby, E., Mayr, W., and Høgman, C. On the orientation of the HL-A region and the PGM_3 locus in the chromosome. *Tissue Antigens 2*:205–214, 1972.

Lamm, L.U., Svejgaard, E., and Kissmeyer-Nielsen, F. PGM_3: HL-A is another linkage in man. *Nature (London) 231*:109–111, 1971.

Lamm, L.U., Thorsen, I.-L., Petersen, G.B., Jørgensen, J., Henningsen, K., Bech, B., and Kissmeyer-Nielsen, F. Data on the HL-A linkage group. *Ann. hum. Genet. 38*:383–390, 1975.

Leeuwen, A. van, Schuit, H.R.E., and Rood, J.J. van. Typing for MLC (LD). I. The selection of non stimulator cells by MLC inhibition test using SD identical stimulator cells (MISIS) and fluorescence antibodies studies. *Transpl. Proc. 3*:1539–1542, 1973.

Legrand, L., and Dausset, J. Serological evidence of the existence of several antigenic determinants (or factors) on the HL-A gene products. *Histocompatibility Testing 1972*, pp. 441–453, J. Dausset and J. Colombani, eds., Munksgaard, Copenhagen, 1973.

Legrand, L., and Dausset, J. Immunogenetics of a new lymphocyte system. *Transpl. Proc. 7*:5–8, 1975a.

Legrand, L., and Dausset, J. A second lymphocyte system (Ly-Li). *Histocompatibility Testing 1975b*, pp. 665–670, F. Kissmeyer-Nielsen, ed., Munksgaard, Copenhagen, 1975b.

Levis, W.R., and Miller, A.E. Leukocyte/skin cultures as a measure of histocompatibility in man. *Lancet II*:357–360, 1972.

Levy, J.A., Virolainer, M., and Defendi, V. Human lymphoid lines from lymph node and spleen. *Cancer 22*:517–524, 1968.

Lewis, C.M., Pegrum, G.D., and Evans, C.A. Intracellular location of specific antibodies reacting with human lymphocytes. *Nature (London) 247*:463–465, 1974.

Lightbody, J., Bernoco, Miggiano, V.C., and Ceppellini, R. Cell mediated lympholysis in man after sensitization of effector lymphocytes through mixed leukocyte cultures. *G. Bact. Virol. Immunol. 64*:243–254, 1971.

Löw, B., Messeter, S., Mansson, S., and Lindholm, T. Crossing-over between the SD-2 (FOUR) and SD-3 (AJ) loci of the human major histocompatibility chromosomal region. *Tissue Antigens 4*:405, 1974.

Lohrman, H.P., Novikons, L., and Graw, R.G. Stimulatory capacity of human B and T lymphocytes in mixed lymphocyte culture. *Nature 250*:144–146, 1974.

Loke, Y.N., Josey, V.C., and Borland, R. HL-A antigens on human trophoblast cells. *Nature 232*:403–405, 1971.

Loor, F., Forni, L., and Pernis, B. The dynamic state of the lymphocyte membrane factors affecting the distribution and turnover of surface immunoglobulins. *Eur. J. Immunol. 2*:203–212, 1972.

Ludwig, H., Polymenidis, Z., Granditsch, G., and Wick, G. HL-A1 and HL-A8 bei kindlicher Coeliakie. *Z. Immunitaetsforsch., Exp. Klin. Immunol. 146*:158, 1973.

Mackay, I.R., and Morris, P.J. Association of autoimmune active chronic hepatitis with HL-A1, 8. *Lancet 2*:793, 1972.

Mann, D.L. The effect of enzyme inhibitors on the solubilization of HL-A antigens with 3 M KCL. *Transplantation 14*:398–401, 1972a.

Mann, D.L. Comparison of HL-A alloantigens solubilized by papain and TIS. *Transplantation*

Antigens, pp. 287–298, B.D. Kahan and R.A. Reisfeld, eds., Academic Press, New York-London, 1972b.

Mann, D.L., Fahey, J.F., and Nathenson, S.G. Molecular comparisons of papain solubilized H-2 and HL-A alloantigens. *Histocompatibility Testing 1970,* pp. 461–468, P.I. Terasaki, ed., Munksgaard, Copenhagen, 1971.

Mann, D.L., Rogentine, G.N., Fahey, J.L., and Nathenson, S.G. Molecular heterogeneity of human lymphoid (HL-A) alloantigens. *Science 163*:1460–1462, 1969a.

Mann, D.L., Rogentine, G.N., Fahey, J.L., and Nathenson, S.G. Human lymphocyte membrane (HL-A) alloantigens: isolation, purification and properties. *J. Immunol. 103*:282–292, 1969b.

Manson, L.A. Extraction of membranous transplantation antigens by pressure homogenization. *Transplantation Antigens,* pp. 227–235, B.D. Kahan and R.A. Reisfeld, eds., Academic Press, New York-London, 1972.

Mapstone, R., and Woodrow, J.C. Acute anterior uveitis and HL-A27. *Lancet I*:681–682, 1974.

Marchalonis, J.J., Cone, R.E., and Sauter, V. Enzymatic iodination. A probe for accessible surface proteins of normal and neoplastic lymphocytes. *Biochem. J. 124*:921–931, 1971.

Marshall, W.H., Rigo, S.J., and Melman, S. Lymphocyte transformation and mitosis in vitro initiated by homologous macrophages. *Lancet I*:730–732, 1966.

Mattiuz, P.L., Ihde, D., Piazza, A., Ceppellini, R., and Bodmer, W.F. New approaches to population genetic and segregation analysis of the HL-A System. *Histocompatibility Testing 1970,* p. 193, P.I. Terasaki, ed., Munksgaard, Copenhagen, 1970.

Mawas, C., Christen, Y., Legrand, L., and Dausset, J. Cell-mediated cytotoxicity toward human lymphocytes: Comparison between in vivo immunisation and in vitro sensitization. *Transplant. Proc. 5*:1691–1695, 1973a.

Mawas, C., Sasportes, C., Christen, Y., Bernard, A., Dausset, J., Alter, B.J., and Bach, M.L. Cell mediated lympholysis (CML) in the absence of LD2 mixed lymphocyte reaction and CML in the presence of SD1–SD2 identity in two HL-A genotyped families. *Transplant. Proc. 5*:1683–1689, 1973b.

Mayr, W.R. Molekulare Assoziation des β_2-Mikroglobulins mit serologisch definierbaren Merkmalen an der Lymphozytenoberfläche. *Z. Immunitätsforschung 148*:92–96, 1974.

Mayr, R.W. The SD-3 locus of the HLA system with special reference to T5. *Histocompatibility Testing 1975,* pp. 330–335, F. Kissmeyer-Nielsen, ed., Munksgaard, Copenhagen, 1975.

Mayr, W.R., Bernoco, D., DeMarchi, M., and Ceppellini, R. Genetic analysis and biological properties of products of the third SD (AJ) locus of the HL-A region. *Transplant. Proc. 5*:1581–1593, 1973.

Mayr, W.R., Bissbort, S., and Kömpf, J. Confirmation of the linkage HLA/PGM_3. *Humangenetik 28*:173–174, 1975.

Mayr, W.R., Mayr, D., Kömpf, J., Bissbort, S., and Ritter, H. Possible linkage of HL-A and GLO. *Humangenetik 31*:241–242, 1976.

McCune, J.M., Humphreys, R.E., Yocum, R.R., and Strominger, J.L. Enhanced representation of HL-A antigens on human lymphocytes after mitogenesis induced by phytemagglutinin or Epstein-Barr virus. *Proc. Natl. Acad. Sci. 72*:3206–3209, 1975.

McDonald, W.C., Dobbins, W.O., and Rubin, C.E. Studies of the familial nature of celiac sprue using biopsy of the small intestine. *New Engl. J. Med. 272*:448–456, 1965.

McKenzie, I.F.C., and Morris, P.J. Leukocyte antigens in renal transplantation. II. HL-A and ABO antigens on kidney cells in culture. *Histocompatibility Antigens 1970,* pp. 309–318, P.I. Terasaki, ed., Munksgaard, Copenhagen, 1971.

McNeish, A.S., Nelson, R., and Mackintosh, P. HL-A1 and 8 in childhood coeliac disease. *Lancet I*:668, 1973.

Meera Khan, P., Volkers, W.S., Doppert, B.A., Bijnen, A.B., Schreuder, I., and Rood, J.J. van. The locus for glyoxalase I (*GLO*) is between *HLA-A* and PGM_3 on chromosome 6 of man. In: Proceedings of the Third International Conference on Human Gene Mapping. Baltimore (1975). *Birth Defects: Original Article Series* (The National Foundation, New York) (in press, 1976)

Melief, C.J.M., Hart, M. van der, Engelfriet, C.P., and Loghem, J.J. van. Immune adherence of leukocytes and fibroblasts derived from skin sensitized by cytotoxic leukocyte isoantibodies and complement, to the surface of indicator cells. *Vox Sang. 12*:374–389, 1967.

Mempel, W., Albert, E., and Burger, A. Further evidence for a Separate MLC-Locus. *Tissue Antigens 2*:250–254, 1972.
Mempel, W., Grosse-Wilde, H., Albert, E., and Thierfelder, S. Atypical MLC reactions in HL-A typed related and unrelated pairs. *Transplant. Proc. 5*:401–408, 1973a.
Mempel, W., Grosse-Wilde, H., Baumann, P., Netzel, B., Steinbauer-Rosenthal, I., Scholz, S., Bertrams, J., and Albert, E.D. Population genetics of the MLC response: Typing for MLC determinants using homozygous and heterozygous reference cells. *Transplant. Proc. 5*:1529–1534, 1973b.
Metzgar, R.S., Flanagan, J.F., and Mendes, N.F. Serological studies of extracted human tissue isoantigens. *Histocompatibility Testing 1967,* pp. 307–313, E.S. Curtoni, P.L. Mattine, and R.M. Tosi, eds., Munksgaard, Copenhagen, 1967.
Mickelson, E.M., Petersons, J.S., Flournoy, N., Clift, R.A., and Thomas, E.D. An estimate of the recombination frequency between the B locus and the D locus within the major histocompatibility complex. *Tissue Antigens 8*:247–252, 1976.
Mickey, M.R., Terasaki, P.I., Kreisler, M., Albert, E.D., and Sengar, D.P.S. Analysis of histocompatibility data from 1000 kidney transplants. *Tissue Antigens 1*:57–67, 1971.
Middleton, J., Crookston, M.C., Falk, J.A., Robson, E.M., Cook, P.J.L., Batchelor, J.R., Bodmer, J., Ferrara, G.B., Festenstein, H., Harris, R., Kissmeyer-Nielsen, F., Lawler, S.D., Sachs, J.A., and Wolf, E. Linkage of Chido and HL-A. *Tissue Antigens 4*:366–373, 1974.
Miggiano, V.C., Nabholz, M., and Bodmer, W.F. Detection of HL-A antigens and other antigens on fibroblast micro-monolayers using a fluorochromatic cytotoxic assay. *Histocompatibility Testing 1970,* pp. 623–630, P.I. Terasaki, ed., Munksgaard, Copenhagen, 1971.
Mittal, K.K. Human histocompatibility (HL-A) antigens in semen and their role in reproduction. *Sterility and Fertility 26*:704–710, 1975.
Mittal, K.K., Mickey, M.R., Singal, D.P., and Terasaki, P.I. Serotyping for homotransplantation. XVIII. Refinement of microdroplet lymphocyte cytotoxicity test. *Transplantation 6*:913–927, 1968.
Mittal, K.K., Mickey, M.R., and Terasaki, P.I. Cross reactive antibodies in "duospecific" anti-HL-A antisera. *Int. Symp. Standardisation HL-A Reagents, Copenhagen, Symp. Ser. Immunobiol. Standard 18*:165–170, 1972a.
Mittal, K.K., and Terasaki, P.I. Cross-reactivity in the HL-A system. *Tissue Antigens 2*:94–104, 1972b.
Miyajima, T., Hirata, A.A., and Terasaki, P.I. Escape from sensitization to HL-A antibodies. *Tissue Antigens 2*:64–73, 1972.
Miyakawa, Y., Tanigaki, N., Kreiter, V.P., Moore, G.E., and Pressman, D. Characterization of soluble substances in the plasma carrying HL-A alloantigenic activity and HL-A common antigenic activity. *Transplantation 15*:312–319, 1973a.
Miyakawa, Y., Tanigaki, N., Yogi, Y., and Pressman, D. An efficient method for isolation of HL-A antigens from hematopoietic cell lines. *J. Immunol. 107*:394–401, 1971a.
Miyakawa, Y., Tanigaki, N., Yagi, Y., and Pressman, D. Human transplantation antigens: isolation and radioimmunoassay. *Proc. Soc. Exp. Biol. (N.Y.) 136*:899–902, 1971b.
Miyakawa, Y., Tanigaki, N., Yagi, Y., and Pressman, D. Determination of human histocompatibility antigens in the peripheral blood by radioimmunoassay. *Transplantation 13*:481–485, 1972.
Miyakawa, Y., Tanigaki, N., Yogi, Y., and Pressman, D. Common antigenic structures of HL-A antigens. I. Antigenic determinants recognizable by rabbits on papain solubilized HL-A molecular fragments. *Immunology 24*:67–76, 1973b.
Moore, G.E., Gerner, R., and Franklin, H. Culture of normal human leukocytes. *J. Amer. Med. Assoc. 199*:519–524, 1967.
Moraes, J.R., and Stastny, P. Allo-antibodies to endothelial cell antigens. *Histocompatibility Testing 1975,* pp. 391–397, F. Kissmeyer-Nielsen, ed., Munksgaard, Copenhagen, 1975.
Morris, P.J., and Forbes, J.F. HL-A and Hodgkin's disease. *Transplant. Proc. III,* No. 3: 12, 75, 1971.
Morris, R., Metzger, A.L., Bluestone, R., and Terasaki, P.I. HL-A-W27—A clue to the diagnosis and pathogenesis of Reiter's syndrome. *New Engl. J. Med. 290*:554, 1974.
Morton, J.A., Pickels, M.M., and Sutton, L. The correlation between the Bg^a bloodgroup with

the HL-47 leukocyte group: determination of antigenic sites on red cells and leukocytes. *Vox Sang.* *17*:536–547, 1969.

Morton, J. A., Pickels, M. M., Sutton, L., and Skov, F. Identification of further antigens on red cells and lymphocytes. *Vox Sang.* *21*:141–153, 1971.

Mowbray, J. F., Hoffbrand, A. V., Holborow, E. J., Seah, P. P., and Fry, L. Circulating immune complexes in dermatitis herpetiformis. *Lancet I*:400–401, 1973.

Mueller-Eckhardt, C., Heinrich, D., and Rothenberg, V. Frequency and complexity of cross-reactive HL-A antibodies. Elution studies with platelets. *Int. Symp. Standardisation HL-A reagents, Ser. Immunobiol. Standard 18*:171–178, 1972.

Naito, S., Namerow, N., Mickey, M. R., and Terasaki, P. I. Multiple sclerosis: association with HL-A3. *Tissue Antigens 2*:1–4, 1972.

Nakamuro, K., Tanigaki, N., Kreiter, V. P., and Pressman, D. Common antigenic structure of HL-A antigens. IV. HL-A common portion fragment isolated from spent culture medium of human lymphoid cell lines. *Immunology 27*:1127–1139, 1974.

Nakamuro, K., Tanigaki, N., and Pressman, D. Multiple common properties of human β_2-microglobulin and the common portion fragment derived from HL-A antigen molecule. *Proc. Natl. Acad. Sci. 70*:2863–2867, 1973.

Nakamuro, K., Tanigaki, N., and Pressman, D. Isolation of HLA 33,000 dalton fragments carrying high HL-A alloantigenic activity. *Transplantation 19*:431–437, 1975.

Nathenson, S. G., and Davies, D. A. L. Solubilization and partial purification of mouse histocompatibility antigens from a membraneous lipoprotein fraction. *Proc. Natl. Acad. Sci. 56*:676–681, 1966.

Nathenson, S. G., and Shimada, A. Papain solubilization of mouse H-2 isoantigens: an improved method of wide applicability. *Transplantation 6*:662–664, 1968.

Neauport-Sautes, C., Bismuth, A., Kourilsky, F. M., and Manuel, Y. Relationship between HL-A antigens and β_2-microglobulin as studied by immunofluorescence on the lymphocyte membrane. *J. Exp. Med. 139*:957–968, 1974.

Neauport-Sautes, C., Silvestre, D., Kourilsky, F. M., and Dausset, J. Independence of HL-A antigens from the first and second locus at the cell surface. *Histocompatibility Testing 1972*, pp. 539–544, J. Dausset and J. Colombani, eds., Munksgaard, Copenhagen, 1973.

Nerup, J., Platz, P., Andersen, O. O., Christy, M., Lyngsøe, J., Poulsen, J. E., Ryder, L. P., Nielsen, L. S., Thomsen, W., and Sveygaard, A. HL-A antigens and diabetes mellitus. *Lancet II*:864–866, 1974.

Netzel, B., Grosse-Wilde, H., Rittner, Ch., Pretorius, A. M. G., Scholz, S., and Albert, E. D. HL-A/MLC recombination frequency and LD typing in HL-A/MLC/Bf/PGM3 recombinant families. *Histocompatibility Testing 1975*, pp. 955–959, Munksgaard, Copenhagen, 1976.

Netzel, B., Mempel, W., Albert, E.D., Baumann, P., and Grosse-Wilde, H. LD typing with lymphoblastoid cell lines. *Immunogenetics 2*:205–210, 1975.

Nilsson, K., Evrin, P. E., and Welsh, K. I. Production of β_2-microglobulin by normal and malignant human cell lines and peripheral lymphocytes. *Transplant. Rev. 21*:53–84, 1974.

Nordhagen, R., and Orjasaeter, H. Association between HL-A and red cell antigens. An autoanalyzer study. *Vox Sang. 26*:97–106, 1974.

Östberg, L., Linbloom, J. B., and Peterson, P. A. Subunit structure of HL-A antigens on cell surfaces. *Nature 249*:463–465, 1974.

Oh, S. K., Pellegrino, M. A., Ferrone, S., Sevier, E. D., and Reisfeld, R. A. Soluble HL-A antigens in serum. I. Isolation and purification. *Eur. J. Immunol. 5*:161–166, 1975.

Oh, S. K., Pellegrino, M. A., and Reisfeld, R. A. Hypertonic salt extraction of HL-A antigens: assessment of protease activity. *Proc. Soc. Exp. Biol. Med. 145*:1272–1277, 1974.

Olaisen, B., Teisberg, P., Gedde-Dahl, T., Jr., and Thorsby, E. The *Bf* locus in the HLA region of chromosome 6: Linkage and association studies. *Humangenetik 30*:291–296, 1975.

Opelz, G., Mickey, M., and Terasaki, P. I. HL-A and kidney transplants: reexamination. *Transplantation 17*:371–382, 1974.

Opelz, G., Sengar, D. P. S., and Mickey, M. R. Effect of blood transfusions on subsequent kidney transplant. *Transplant. Proc. 5*:253–259, 1973.

Opelz, G., and Terasaki, P.I. The role of the HL-A system in kidney transplants. *Transplant. Proc. 4*:No. 4:433–438, 1972.

Opelz, G., Mickey, M.R., and Terasaki, P.I. Identification of unresponsive kidney transplant recipients. *Lancet I*: 868–871, 1972.

Opelz, G., and Terasaki, P.I. Prolongation effect of blood transfusions on kidney graft survival. *Transplantation*, in press 1976.

Ott, J., Hecht, F., Linder, D., Lovrien, E.W., and Kaiser-McCaw, B. Human centromere mapping using teratoma data. *Third International Workshops on Human Gene Mapping*. In press 1975.

Papermaster, V.N., Papermaster, B.W., and Moore, G.E. Histocompatibility antigens of human lymphocytes in long term culture. *Fed. Proc. 28*: 379 (Abstract), 1969.

Papermaster, B.W., Papermaster, V.M., Reisfeld, R.A., Pellegrino, M.A., Ferrone, S., Kahan, B.D., Terasaki, P.I., Takasugi, M., and Albert, E.D. Characterization and isolation of HL-A antigens from continuous cultured human lymphocyte cell lines: A report of current progress. *Cellular Antigens*, pp. 186–199, A. Nowotny, ed., Springer-Verlag, Heidelberg-New York, 1972.

Parham, P., Humphreys, R.E., Turner, M.J., and Strominger, J.L. Heterogeneity of HLA antigen preparations is due to variable sialic acid content. *Proc. Natl. Acad. Sci. 71*: 3998–4001, 1974.

Parham, P., Terhorst, C., Herrmann, H., Humphreys, R.E., Waterfield, M.D., and Strominger, J.L. Immunological and chemical purity of papain-solubilized HL-A antigens. *Proc. Natl. Acad. Sci. 72*: 1594–1598, 1975.

Patel, R. Cytotoxic reactions of lymphocytes of blood, lymph node and thoracic duct origin with monospecific anti-HL-A antisera. *Transplantation 11*: 348–351, 1971.

Patel, R., and Terasaki, P.I. Significance of the positive cross match test in kidney transplantation. *New Engl. J. Med. 280*: 735, 1969.

Pellegrino, M.A., Ferrone, S., Natali, P.G., Pellegrino, A., and Reisfeld, R.A. Expression of HL-A antigens in synchronized cultures of human lymphocytes. *J. Immunol. 108*: 573–576, 1972.

Pellegrino, M.A., Ferrone, S., and Pellegrino, A. A simple micro-absorption technique for HL-A typing. *Proc. Soc. Exp. Biol. Med. 139*: 484–488, 1971.

Pellegrino, M.A., Ferrone, S., Pellegrino, A., Oh, S., and Reisfeld, R.A. Evaluation of two sources of soluble HL-A antigens: platelets and serum. *Eur. J. Immunol. 4*: 250–255, 1974.

Pellegrino, M.A., Ferrone, S., Pellegrino, A., and Reisfeld, R.A. A critical evaluation of the serologic assay for soluble HL-A alloantigens. *Symp. Ser. Immunobiol. Stand. 18*: 209–217, 1973.

Pellegrino, M.A., Pellegrino, A., and Kahan, B.D. HL-A antigens of human fetal cells. *Transplantation 10*: 425–430, 1970.

Persijn, G.G., Hooff, J.P. van, Kalff, M.W., and Rood, J.J. van. The effect of blood transfusions and HLA matching on renal transplantation in the Netherlands. *Transpl. Proc.* in press 1977.

Peterson, P.A., Cunningham, B.A., Berggard, I., and Edelman, G.M. β_2-microglobulin—a free immunoglobulin domain. *Proc. Natl. Acad. Sci. 69*: 1697–1701, 1972.

Peterson, P.A., Rask, L., and Lindblom, J.B. Highly purified papain-solubilized HL-A antigens contain β_2-microglobulin. *Proc. Natl. Acad. Sci. 71*: 35–40, 1974.

Petris, S. de, and Raff, M.C. Normal distribution, patching, and capping of lymphocyte surface immunoglobulin studied by electron microscopy. *Nature New Biol. 241*: 257–259, 1973.

Piazza, A. Haplotypes and linkage disequilibria from the three-locus phenotypes. *Histocompatibility Testing 1975*, pp. 923–927, F. Kissmeyer-Nielsen, ed., Munksgaard, Copenhagen, 1975.

Piazza, A., Mattiuz, P.L., and Ceppellini, R. Assortimento per gli apoltipi del sistense HL-A come possible mechanismo de selezione gametica ozigotica. *Haematologica 54*: 703–720, 1969.

Pierres, M., Fradelizi, D., Neauport-Sautes, C., and Dausset, J. Third HL-A segregant series: Genetic analysis and molecular independence on the lymphocyte surface. *Tissue Antigens 5*: 266–279, 1975.

Platz, P., Ryder, L., Staub Nielsen, L., Svejgaard, A., Thomsen, M., Nerup, J., and Christy, M. HL-A and idiopathic Addison's disease. *Lancet II*: 289, 1974.

Poulik, M.D., Bernoco, M., Bernoco, D., and Ceppellini, R. Aggregation of HL-A antigens at the lymphocyte surface induced by antiserum to β_2-microglobulin. *Science 182*: 1352–1355, 1973.

Poulik, M. D., Ferrone, S., Pellegrino, M. A., Sevier, D. E., Oh, S. K., and Reisfeld, R. A. Association of HL-A antigens and β_2-microglobulin: concepts and questions. *Transplant. Rev. 21*:106–125, 1974.

Poulik, M. D., and Motwani, N. Demonstration of a β_2-microglobulin on membrane of B lymphocytes. *Clin. Res. 20*:795 (Abstract), 1972.

Pretorius, A. M. G., Scholz, S., Kuntz, B., and Albert, E. D. Investigations of the red cell glyoxalase (GLO) in recombinant families. *Eur. J. Immunol. 6*, No. 10:759–761, 1976.

Preud'homme, J. L., Neauporte-Sautes, C., Piat, S., Silvestre, D., and Kourilsky, F. M. Independence of HL-A antigens and immunoglobulin determinants on the surface of human lymphoid cells. *Eur. J. Immunol. 2*:297–300, 1972.

Race, R. R., and Sanger, R. *Blood groups in man*; 6th ed. Blackwell, Oxford, 1975.

Rachelewski, G.S., Terasaki, P.I., Katz, R., and Stiehm, E.R. Increased prevalence of W27 in juvenile rheumatoid arthritis. *New Engl. J. Med. 290*:892–893, 1974.

Ragab, A. H., and Cowan, D. H. Separation of cells involved in the mixed leukocyte culture by velocity sedimentation. *Cell. Immunol. 7*:336–340, 1973.

Rapaport, F. T., Dausset, J., Converse, J. M., and Lawrence, H. S. Effect of freezing and storage upon the biological activity of transplantation antigens isolated from human blood leucocytes. *Histocompatibility Testing 1967*, pp. 315–320, E. S. Curtoni, P. L. Mattiuz, and R. M. Tosi, eds., Munksgaard, Copenhagen, 1967.

Rask, L., Österberg, L., Lindblom, B., Rernstedt, Y., and Peterson, P. A. The subunit structure of transplantation antigens. *Transplant. Rev. 21*:85–105, 1974.

Raum, D., Glass, D., Carpenter, C.B., Alper, Ch.A., and Schur, P.H. The chromosomal order of genes controlling the major histocompatibility complex, properdin factor B, and deficiency of the second component of complement. *J. Clin. Invest. 58*:1240–1248, 1976.

Reekers, P., McShine, R. L., Boon, J. M., and Kunst, V. A. J. M. HL-A antigens on erythrocytes. *Histocompatibility Testing 1975*, pp. 398–403, F. Kissmeyer-Nielsen, ed., Munksgaard, Copenhagen, 1975.

Reisfeld, R. A., Allison, J. P., Ferrone, S., Pellegrino, M. A., and Poulik, M. D. HLA antigens in serum and urine: Isolation and characterization and immunogenic properties. *Transplant. Proc. 8*:173–176, 1976.

Reisfeld, R. A., and Kahan, B. D. Transplantation antigens. *Adv. Immunol. 12*:117–200, 1970.

Reisfeld, R. A., and Kahan, B. D. Extraction and purification of soluble histocompatibility antigens. *Transplant. Rev. 6*:81–112, 1971.

Reisfeld, R. A., Pellegrino, M. A., and Ferrone, S. The immunologic and molecular profiles of HLA antigens isolated from urine. *J. Immunol. 118*:264–269, 1977.

Reisfeld, R. A., Pellegrino, M. A., Ferrone, S., and Kahan, B. D. Chemical and molecular nature of HL-A antigens. *Transplant. Proc. 5*:447–449, 1973.

Reisfeld, R. A., Pellegrino, M. A., and Kahan, B. D. Salt extraction of soluble HL-A antigens. *Science 172*:1134–1136, 1971 a.

Reisfeld, R. A., Pellegrino, M., Papermaster, B. W., and Kahan, B. D. HL-A antigens from a continuous lymphoid cell line derived from a normal donor. I. Solubilization and serologic characterization. *J. Immunol. 104*:560–565, 1970.

Reisfeld, R. A., Pellegrino, M., Papermaster, B. W., and Kahan, B. D. Serologic characterization of soluble HL-A antigens from continuous lymphoid cell lines derived from normal donors. *Histocompatibility Testing 1970*, pp. 455–460, P. I. Terasaki, ed., Munksgaard, Copenhagen, 1971 b.

Reisfeld, R. A., Sevier, E. D., Pellegrino, M. A., Ferrone, S., and Poulik, M. D. Association of HL-A antigens and β_2-microglobulin at the cellular and molecular level. *Immunogenetics 2*:183–197, 1975.

Rittner, Ch., Grosse-Wilde, H., Rittner, B., Netzel, B., Scholz, S., Lorenz, H., and Albert, E. D. Linkage group HL-A-MLC-Bf (properdin factor B). The site of the Bf locus at the immunogenetic linkage group on chromosome 6. *Humangenetik. 27*:173–183, 1975.

Rittner, C. H., Hauptmann, G., Grosshans, F., and Mayr, S. Linkage between HLA-A (major histocompatibility complex) and genes controlling the synthesis of the fourth component of complement. *Histocompatibility Testing 1975*, pp. 945–954, Munksgaard, Copenhagen, 1976.

Rodbard, D., and Chrambach, A. Estimation of molecular radius, free mobility, and valence using polyacrylamide gel electrophoresis. *Anal. Biochem. 40*:95–134, 1971.

Rogentine, G.N., and Gerber, P. HL-A antigens of human lymphoid cells in long term tissue culture. *Transplantation 8*:28–37, 1969.

Rogentine, G.N., and Gerber, P. Qualitative and quantitative comparisons of HL-A antigens on different lymphoid cell types from individuals. *Histocompatibility Testing 1970*, pp. 333–338, P.I. Terasaki, ed., Munksgaard, Copenhagen, 1971.

Rood, J.J. van. Leukocyte Grouping. A Method and Its Application. *Thesis, Leyden*. Drukkeris Pasmans, Dan Haag, 1962.

Rood, J.J. van. A proposal for international cooperation in organ transplantation: Eurotransplant. *Histocompatibility Testing 1967*, pp. 451–452, E.S. Curtoni, P.L. Mattiuz, and M.R. Tosi, eds., Munksgaard, Copenhagen, 1967.

Rood, J.J. van. LD-SD interaction *in vivo* and the allograft reaction. *Transplant. Proc. 5*, No. 4:1747–1750, 1973.

Rood, J.J. van, and Leeuwen, A. van. HL-A and the group five system in Hodgkin's disease. *Transplant. Proc. 3*:1283–1286, 1971.

Rood, J.J. van, and Leeuwen, A. van. Major and minor histocompatibility systems in man and their importance in bone marrow transplantation. *Transplant. Proc. VIII*, No. 3:429–436, 1976.

Rood, J.J. van, Leeuwen, A. van, Keuning, J.J., and Bussé van Oud, Alblas, A. The serological recognition of the human MLC determinants using a modified cytotoxicity technique. *Tissue antigens 5*:73–79, 1975b.

Rood, J.J. van, Leeuwen, A. van, Koch, C.T., and Frederiks, E. HL-A inhibiting activity in serum. *Histocompatibility Testing 1970*, pp. 483–487, P.I. Terasaki, ed., Munksgaard, Copenhagen, 1971.

Rood, J.J. van, Leeuwen, A. van, Parlevliet, J., Terijtelen, A., and Keuning, J.J. LD typing by serology. IV. Description of a new locus with three alleles. *Histocompatibility Testing 1975*, pp. 629–636, F. Kissmeyer-Nielsen, ed., Munksgaard, Copenhagen, 1975a.

Rood, J.J. van, Leeuwen, A. van, and Ploem, J.S. Simultaneous detection of two cell populations by two colour fluorescence and application to the recognition of B cell (Ia like) determinants. *Nature 262*:795–796, 1976

Rood, J.J. van, Leeuwen, A. van, and Santen, M.C.T. Anti-HL-A2 inhibitor in normal serum. *Nature 226*:366–367, 1970.

Rood, J.J. van, Leeuwen, A. van, Termijtelen, A., and Keuning, J.J. B-cell antibodies, Ia-like determinants, and their relation to MLC determinants in man. *Transplant. Rev. 30*:122–139, 1976b.

Ruddle, F.H., and Giblett, E.R. Report of the committee on the genetic constitution of autosomes other than chromosomes 1 and 2. *Birth Defects: Original Article Series*. Vol. XI, No. 3, The National Foundation, 1975. S. Karger, Basel-München-Paris-London-New York-Sydney 1975.

Russell, Th.J., Schultes, L.M., and Kuban, D.J. Histocompatibility (HL-A) antigens associated with psoriasis. *New Engl. J. Med. 287*:738–740, 1973.

Ryder, L.P., and Svejgaard, A. Associations between HLA and disease. *Report from the HLA and Disease Registry of Copenhagen, 1976*. Published by the authors, 1976.

Sachs, D.H., Cullen, S.E., and David, C.S. *Ir*-associated murine alloantigens. Serological and chemical definition of Ia specificities associated with the *H-2*^{b} haplotype. *Transplantation 19*:388–393, 1975a.

Sachs, D.H., David, C.S., Shreffler, D.C., Nathenson, S.G., and McDevitt, H.O. Ia antigens, proceedings of a workshop. *Immunogenetics 2*:301–312, 1975b.

Sandberg, L., Thorsby, E., Kissmeyer-Nielsen, F., and Lindholm, A. Evidence of a third sublocus within the HL-A chromosomal region. *Histocompatibility Testing 1970*, pp. 165–170, P.I. Terasaki, ed., Munksgaard, Copenhagen, 1970.

Sanderson, A.R. Cytotoxic reactions of mouse isoantisera: Preliminary considerations. *Brit. J. Exp. Pathol. 45*:398–408, 1964.

Sanderson, A.R. HL-A substances from human spleen. *Nature 220*:192–195, 1968.

Sanderson, A.R., and Batchelor, J.R. Transplantation antigens from human spleens. *Nature 219*:184–186, 1968.

Sanderson, A. R., Cresswell, P., and Welsh, K. I. Involvement of carbohydrate in the immunochemical determinant area of HL-A substances. *Nature New Biol. 230*:8–12, 1971.
Sanderson, A. R., and Welsh, K. I. Purification and structural studies of alloantigen determinants solubilized with papain. *Transplantation Antigens*, pp. 273–285, B. D. Kahan and R. A. Reisfeld, eds., Academic Press, New York, 1972.
Sanderson, A. R., and Welsh, K. I. Properties of histocompatibility (HL-A) determinants. I. Site density of antigens of the two segregant series on peripheral human lymphocytes. *Transplantation 17*:281–289, 1974.
Sasportes, M., Dehay, C., and Fellous, M. Variations of the expression of HL-A antigens on human diploid fibroblasts in vitro. *Nature 233*:332–334, 1971.
Schellekens, P. Th. A., and Eijsvoogel, V. P. Lymphocyte transformation in vitro. III. Mechanism of stimulation in the mixed lymphocyte culture. *Clin. Exp. Immunol. 7*:229–239, 1970.
Schlessinger, M., and Amos, D. B. Effect of neuraminidase on serological properties of murine lymphoid cells. *Transplant. Proc. 3*:895–897, 1971.
Schoefinius, H. H., Braun-Falco, O., Scholz, S., Steinbauer-Rosenthal, I., Wank, R., and Albert, E. D. Histokompatibilitätsantigene (HL-A) bei Psoriasis. *Deut. Med. Wochschr. 99*:440–444, 1974.
Scholz, S., Schattenkirchner, M., Harms, K., Steinbauer-Rosenthal, I., and Albert, E. D. Family studies in HL-A associated diseases. *Z. Immunitaetsforsch., Exp. Klin. Immunol. 148*:387–388, 1975.
Scholz, S., Schoefinius, H., Steinbauer-Rosenthal, I., Wank, R., Albert, E., and Braun-Falco, O. Association between HL-A antigen and psoriasis vulgaris. *Z. Immunitaetsforsch. 147*:4 (abstr.), 1974.
Schlosstein, I., Terasaki, P.J., Bluestone, R., and Pearson, C.M. High association of an HL-A antigen, W27, with ankylosing spondylitis. *New Engl. J. Med. 288*:704–706, 1973.
Schultz, J. S., and Shreffler, D. C. Studies on the serum fraction containing soluble inhibitors of anti-HL-A sera. *Transplantation 13*:186–188, 1972.
Schwartz, B. D., Kato, K., Cullen, S. E., and Nathenson, S. G. H-2 histocompatibility alloantigens. Some biochemical properties of the molecules solubilized by NP-40 detergent. *Biochemistry 12*:2157–2164, 1973.
Seamen, M.J., Bemson, R., Jones, M.N., Morton, J.A., and Pickles, M.M. The reaction of the Bennet Goodspeed group of antibodies tested with the autoanalyzer. *Brit. J. Haemat. 13*:464–473, 1967.
Seigler, H. F., Kremer, W. B., Metzgar, R. S., Ward, F. E., Taung, A. T., and Amos, D. B. HL-A antigenic loss in malignant transformation. *J. Natl. Cancer Inst. 46*:577–583, 1971.
Seigler, H. F., and Metzgar, R. S. Embryonic development of human transplantation antigens. *Transplantation 2*:478–486, 1970.
Shechy, M. J., Sondel, P. M., Bach, M. L., Wank, R., and Bach, F. H. HLA-LD (lymphocyte-defined) typing: a rapid assay with primed lymphocytes. *Science 188*:1308, 1975.
Shimada, A., and Nathenson, S. G. Murine histocompatibility-2 (H-2) alloantigens. Purification and some chemical properties of soluble products from H-2^b and H-2^d genotypes released by peptin digestion of membrane fractions. *Biochemistry 8*:4028–4062, 1969.
Shiner, M., and Shmerling, D. H. The immunopathology of coeliac disease. *Digestion 5*:77, 1972.
Silvestre, D., Kourilsky, F. M., Niccolai, M. G., and Levy, J. P. Presence of HL-A antigens on human reticulocytes as demonstrated by electron microscopy. *Nature 228*:67–68, 1970.
Singal, D. P., Berry, R., and Naipaul, N. HL-A inhibiting activity in human seminal plasma. *Nature New Biol. 233*:61–62, 1971.
Singer, S. J., and Nicolson, G. L. The fluid mosaic model of the structure of cell membranes. *Science 175*:720–731, 1972.
Smithies, O., and Poulik, M. D. Initiation of protein synthesis at an unusual position in an immunoglobulin gene. *Science 175*:187–189, 1972.
Snary, D., Goodfellow, P., Bodmer, W.F., and Crumpton, M.J. Evidence against a dimeric structure for membrane bound HLA antigens. *Nature 258*:240–242, 1975.
Snary, D., Goodfellow, P., Hayman, M. J., Bodmer, W. F., and Crumpton, M. J. Subcellular separation and molecular nature of human histocompatibility antigens (HL-A). *Nature 247*:457–461, 1974.

Snell, G. D. Methods for the study of histocompatibility genes. *J. Genetics 49*:87–108, 1948.
Snell, G. D. The genetics of transplantation. *J. Nat. Cancer Inst. 14*:691–700, 1953.
Solheim, B. G., Bratlie, A., Sandberg, L., Staub-Nielsen, L., and Thorsby, E. Further evidence of a third HL-A locus. *Tissue Antigens 3*:439–453, 1973.
Solheim, B. G., Bratlie, A., Winther, N., and Thorsby, E. LD-typing with antisera by planned immunization. *Histocompatibility Testing 1975,* pp. 713–718, F. Kissmeyer-Nielsen, ed., Munksgaard, Copenhagen, 1975.
Solheim, B. G., and Thorsby, E. β_2-microglobulin. Part of the HL-A molecule in the cell membrane. *Tissue Antigen 4*:83–94, 1974.
Someren, H. von, Westerveld, A., Hagemeijer, A., Mees, J. R., and Meera Khan, P. Human antigen and enzyme markers in man-Chinese hamster somatic cell hybrids. Evidence for synteny between the HL-A, PGM_3, ME_1, and IPO-B loci. *Proc. Nat. Acad. Sci. U.S.A. 71*:962, 1974.
Sondel, P. M., and Bach, F. H. Recognitive specificity of human cytotoxic T lymphocytes. II. The non-recognition of antigens controlled outside the major histocompatibility complex. *Tissue Antigens 7*:173–180, 1976.
Springer, T. A., and Strominger, J. L. Detergent-soluble HLA antigens contain a hydrophilic region at the COOH-terminus and a penultimate hydrophobic region. *Proc. Natl. Acad. Sci. 73*:2481–2485, 1976.
Springer, T. A., Strominger, J. L., and Mann, D. L. Partial purification of detergent soluble HL-A antigen and its cleavage by papain. *Proc. Natl. Acad. Sci. 71*:1539–1543, 1974.
Steinbauer-Rosenthal, I., Schattenkirchner, M., Schürer, W., Wank, R., Scholz, S., Schiessl, B., Brandenburg, H., and Albert, E. D. HL-A 27 in patients with ankylosing spondylitis (AS). *Z. Immunitaetsforsch., Exp. Klin. Immunol. 147*:6 (abstr.), 1974.
Stokes, P. L., Asquith, P., Holmes, G. K. T., Mackintosh, P., and Cooke, W. T. Histocompatibility antigens associated with adult coeliac disease. *Lancet II*:162, 1972.
Strominger, J. L., Cresswell, P., Grey, H., Humphreys, R. E., Mann, D., McCune, J., Parham, P., Robb, R., Sanderson, A.R., Springer, T.A., Terhorst, C., and Turner, M.J. The immunoglobulin-like structure of human histocompatibility antigens. *Transplant. Rev. 21*:126–143, 1974.
Suciu-Foca, N., Hansen, J. A., Dupont, B., Rubinstein, P., Fµ, S. M., Yunis, E., Mickelson, F., Thomas, D. L., Fotino, M., Whitsett, C., Jersild, C., Kunkel, H. G., Good, R. A., Dausset, J., and Reemtsma, K. Families with recombinations on the major histocompatibility complex (MHC) Unusual MLC reactions and LD typing. *Histocompatibility Testing 1975,* pp. 937–940, Munksgaard, Copenhagen, 1976.
Svejgaard, A., Bratlie, A., Hedin, P. J., Høgman, C., Jersild, C., Kissmeyer-Nielsen, F., Lindblom, B., Lindholm, A., Løw, B., Messeter, L., Møller, E., Sandberg, L., Staub-Nielsen, L., and Thorsby, E. The recombination fraction of the HL-A system. *Tissue Antigens 1*:81–88, 1971 b.
Svejgaard, A., Jersild, C., Staub-Nielsen, L., and Bødmer, W. F. HL-A antigens and disease statistical and genetical consideration. *Tissue Antigens 4,* No. 2:95–105, 1974a.
Svejgaard, A., and Kissmeyer-Nielsen, F. Cross-reactive human HL-A isoantibodies. *Nature (London) 219*:868–869, 1968.
Svejgaard, A.: Synergistic action of HL-A isoantibodies. *Nature (London) 222*:94–95, 1969.
Svejgaard, A., Kissmeyer-Nielsen, F., and Thorsby, E. HL-A typing of platelets. *Histocompatibility Testing 1970,* pp. 153–164, P. I. Terasaki, ed., Munksgaard, Copenhagen, 1971 a.
Svejgaard, A., Kjerbye, K. E., and Kissmeyer-Nielsen, F. The sensitivity of some of the methods used in leukocyte and platelet grouping. *Histocompatibility Testing 1967,* pp. 385–387, R. S. Curtoni, P. L. Mattiuz, and R. M. Tosi, eds., Munksgaard, Copenhagen, 1967.
Svejgaard, A., Staub-Nielsen, L., Svejgaard, E., Kissmeyer-Nielsen, F., Hjortshøj, A., and Zachariae, H. HL-A in psoriasis vulgaris and in pustular psoriasis – population and family studies. *Brit. J. Dermatol. 91*:145, 1974b.
Tanigaki, N., Katagiri, M., Nakamuro, K., Kreiter, V. P., and Pressman, D. Common antigenic structures of HL-A antigens. II. Small fragments derived from papain-solubilized HL-A antigen molecule. *Immunology 26*:155–168, 1974b.
Tanigaki, N., Miyakawa, Y., Yagi, Y., and Pressman, D. HL-A antigens from hematopoietic cell lines: molecular size and electrophoretic mobility. *J. Immunol. 107*:402–408, 1971.
Tanigaki, N., Miyakawa, Y., Yagi, Y., and Pressman, D. Radioiodinated soluble HL-A antigens:

HL-A alloantigenic characterization and use in the radioimmuneassay. *J. Immunol. Meth. 3*:109–126, 1973b.
Tanigaki, N., Nakamuro, K., Appella, E., Poulik, M.D., and Pressman, D. Identity of the HL-A common portion fragment and human β_2-microglobulin. *Biochem. Biophys. Res. Comm. 55*:1234–1239, 1973a.
Tanigaki, N., Nakamuro, K., Natori, T., Kreiter, V.P., and Pressman, D. Common antigenic structures of HL-A antigen molecules. V. An antigenic determinant characteristic of a 33,000 dalton fragment of HL-A antigen molecules. *Transplantation 18*:74–78, 1974a.
Tanigaki, N., Nakamuro, K., Natori, T., Minowada, J., and Pressman, D. Structure of HL-A antigens. The structural components of papain-solubilized HL-A antigen molecules. *Transplant. Proc. 7*:195–199, 1975.
Taylor, R.B., Duffus, W.P.H., Raff, M.C., and Petris, S.de. Redistribution and pinocytosis of lymphocyte surface immunoglobulin molecules induced by anti-immunoglobulin antibody. *Nature New Biol. 233*:225–229, 1971.
Teisberg, P., Olaisen, B., Gedde-Dahl, T., Jr., and Thorsby, E. On the localization of the *Gb* locus within the *MHS* region of chromosome No. 6. *Tissue Antigens 5*:257–261, 1975.
Terasaki, P.I., Kreisler, M., and Mickey, M.R. Presensitization and Kidney Transplant Failure. *Postgrad. Med. J. 47*:98–100, 1971.
Terasaki, P.I., and McClelland, J.D. Microdroplet assay of human serum cytotoxins. *Nature (London) 206*:998, 1964.
Terasaki, P.I., Opelz, G., Park, M.S., and Mickey, M.R. Four new B lymphocyte specificities. *Histocompatibility Testing 1975*, pp. 657–664, F. Kissmeyer-Nielsen, ed., Munksgaard, Copenhagen, 1975.
Terasaki, P.I., Thrasher, D.I., and Hauber, T.H. Serotyping for homotransplantation XIII. Immediate kidney transplantation rejection and associated preformed antibodies. *Advance in Transplantation*, pp. 225–229, Munksgaard, Copenhagen, 1967.
Terhorst, C., Parham, P., Mann, D.L., and Strominger, J.L. Structure of HLA antigens: Amino-acid and carbohydrate compositions and NH_2-terminal sequence of four antigen preparations. *Proc. Natl. Acad. Sci. 73*:910–914, 1976.
Thieme, T.R., Raley, R.A., and Fahey, J.L. Demonstration of molecular individuality of HL-A antigens. *J. Immunol. 113*:323–328, 1974.
Thomas, E.D., Storb, R., Clift, R., Fefer, A., Johnson, F.L., Neiman, P.E., Lerner, K.G., Glucksburg, H., and Buckner, C.D. Bone marrow transplantation. *New Engl. J. Med. 292*:832, 1975.
Thorsby, E. HL-A antigens on human granulocytes studied with cytotoxic isoantisera obtained by skin grafting. *Scand. J. Haematol. 6*:119–127, 1969.
Thorsby, E., Hirschberg, H., and Helgesen, A. A second locus determining human MLC response: Separate lymphocyte populations recognize the products of each different MLC-locus allele in allogeneic combinations. *Transplant. Proc. 5*:1523–1528, 1973.
Thorsby, E., and Kissmeyer-Nielsen, F. Lymphocytotoxic antisera of limited isospecificity after skin grafting in man. *Vox Sang. 14*:417, 1968.
Thorsby, E., and Lie, S. Antigens on human fibroblasts demonstrated with HL-A antisera and anti-human lymphocyte sera. *Vox Sang. 15*:44–53, 1968.
Ting, A., Mickey, M.R., and Terasaki, P.I. B lymphocyte alloantigens in Caucasians. *J. Exp. Med.*, in press 1976.
Turner, M.J., Cresswell, P., Parham, P., Strominger, J.L., Mann, D.L., and Sanderson, A.R. Purification of papain-solubilized histocompatibility antigens from a cultured human lymphoblastoid line, RPMI 4265. *J. Biol. Chem. 250*:4512–4519, 1975.
Turner, M.J., Strominger, J.L., and Sanderson, A.R. Enzymic removal and re-expression of a histocompatibility antigen, HL-A2, at the surface of human peripheral lymphocytes. *Proc. Natl. Acad. Sci. 69*:200–202, 1972.
Tweel, J.G. van den, Blussé van Oud Alblas, A., Keuning, J.J., Goulmy, E., Termijtelen, A., Bach, M.L., and Rood, J.J. van. Typing for MLC (LD). I. Lymphocytes from cousin-marriage offspring as typing cells. *Transplant. Proc. 5*:1535, 1973.
Uhlenbruck, G., Voigtmann, R., Salfner, B., Bube, F.W., and Seibel, E. Comparison of different cell types for the solubilization of HL-A substances. *Symp. Ser. Immunobiol. Stand. 18*:205–208, 1973.

Walford, R.L., Smith, G.S., and Waters, H. Histocompatibility systems and disease states with particular reference to cancer. *Transplant. Rev.* *7*:78–111, 1971.

Wank, R., Harms, K., Scholz, S., Steinbauer-Rosenthal, I., Brandenburg, H., Schiessl, B., and Albert, E. A study of HL-A antigens in 50 families of patients with coeliac disease. *Z. Immunitaetsforsch., Exp. Klin. Immunol.* *147*:147 (abstr.), 1974.

Weitkamp, L.R. Linkage of GLO with HLA and Bf. effect of population and sex on recombination frequency. *Tissue Antigens* *7*:273–279, 1976.

Weitkamp, L.R., and Guttormsen, S.A. Genetic linkage of a locus for erythrocyte glyoxalase (GLO) with HLA and Bf. In: Proceedings of the Third International Conference on Human Gene Mapping, Baltimore (1975). *Birth Defects: Original Article Series* (The National Foundation, New York) (in press, 1976).

Wernet, P., Jersild, C., Cunningham-Rundless, C., and Svejgaard, A. Dynamic and molecular characteristics of HL-A and HL-B (Ia-type) antigens on the surface of human lymphoid cells. *Histocompatibility Testing 1975*, pp. 735–738, F. Kissmeyer-Nielsen, ed., Munksgaard, Copenhagen, 1975.

Wernet, P., and Kunkel, H.G. Immunochemical aspects of Ia type B cell membrane specificities (HL-B) as candidates for a human MLC stimulator antigen system; molecular heterogeneity and distinction from the Fc receptor. *Histocompatibility Testing 1975*, pp. 731–734, F. Kissmeyer-Nielsen, ed., Munksgaard, Copenhagen, 1975.

White, A.G., Barnetson, R.St.C., Da Costa, J.A., and McClelland, D.B.L. HL-A and disordered immunity. *Lancet I*:108, 1973a.

White, A.G., Barnetson, R.St.C., Da Costa, J.A.G., and McClelland, D.B.L. The incidence of HL-A antigens in dermatitis herpetiformis. *Brit. J. Dermatol.* *89*:133–136, 1973b.

White, S.H., Newcomer, V.D., Mickey, M.R., and Terasaki, P.I. Disturbance of HL-A antigen frequency in psoriasis. *New Engl. J. Med.* *287*:740, 1972.

WHO-Terminology Report in *Histocompatibility Testing 1975*, pp. 5–11, Munksgaard, Copenhagen, 1976.

Wigzell, H. Quantitative titrations of mouse H-2 antibodies using Cr^{51}-labelled target cells. *Transplantation* *3*:423–431, 1965.

Wilson, L.A., and Amos, D.B. Subcellular localization of HL-A antigens. *Tissue Antigens* *2*:105–111, 1972.

Wilson, L.A., Amos, D.B., and Boyle, W. The subcellular location of antigens. *Cellular Antigens*, pp. 263–277, A. Nowotny, ed., Springer-Verlag, Heidelberg-New York, 1972.

Winchester, R.J., Dupont, B., Wernet, P., Fu, S.M., Hansen, J.A., Laursen, N., and Kunkel, H.G. Studies on HL-B, a system of non-HL-A alloantigens selectively expressed on B lymphocytes and its relation to DL determinants. *Histocompatibility Testing 1975*, pp. 651–656, F. Kissmeyer-Nielsen, ed., Munksgaard, Copenhagen, 1975b.

Winchester, R.J., Fu, S.M., Wernet, P., Kunkel, H.G., Dupont, B., and Jersild, C. Recognition by pregnancy serums of non-HL-A alloantigens selectively expressed on B lymphocytes. *J. Exp. Med.* *141*:924–929, 1975a.

Woolf, B. On estimating the relation between blood group and disease. *Ann. hum. Genet.* *19*:251–253 (1955).

Yasuda, N., and Kimura, M. A Gene-counting method of maximum likelihood for estimating gene frequencies in ABO and ABO-like Systems. *Ann. Hum. Genet. London 31*, 409:409–421, 1968.

Yunis, E.J., and Amos, D.B. Three closely linked genetic systems relevant to transplantation. *Proc. nat. Acad. Sci. (Wash.)* *68*:3031–3035, 1971.

Zachariae, H., Hjortshøj, A., and Kissmeyer-Nielsen, F. Reiter's disease and HL-A27. *Lancet II*:565–566, 1973.

Zervas, J.D., Delamore, L.W., and Israels, M.C.O. Leucocyte phenotypes in Hodgkin's disease. *Lancet II*:634, 1970.

Chapter 2

The Major Histocompatibility System of Subhuman Primate Species

H. BALNER *

1. Introduction

The major histocompatibility system (MHS) has been elaborately studied in only two subhuman primate species: the rhesus monkey (*Macaca mulatta*) and, to a much lesser extent, the chimpanzee (*Pan troglodytes*). Current information on the MHS of those two species will be reviewed rather extensively. The knowledge of tissue antigens of other primate species (except man, of course) is still rudimentary and does not yet warrant an elaborate discussion. Table 2.1 provides some information regarding the taxonomic rank of the various primates to be discussed.

We shall be dealing with aspects of serology, histocompatibility, immune responses, and genetic mapping of the MHS in primates, in that order. RhL-A, the major histocompatibility system of the rhesus monkey, will first be reviewed in some detail. ChL-A, the MHS of the chimpanzee, for which there is far less information, will be discussed separately. A third section of this chapter will deal with the fragmentary data available for tissue antigens of other primate species. Finally, similarities and cross-reactions between MHS determinants of various primate species, including man, will be discussed in the last section.

It should be realized that new data in three of the areas to be reviewed (MHS of rhesus, MHS of chimpanzees, and interspecies serology) are accumulating so rapidly that any manuscript must be somewhat obsolete by the time it appears in print. But the same holds true for the MHS information relating to mouse, man, dog, and other species. Thus, a quick overview of the state of affairs for subhuman primates in mid-1976 might be useful in providing a reference point for the future.

A further issue for the introduction may be the problem of MHS nomenclature. At the conclusion of the recent histocompatibility workshop in Aarhus (Kissmeyer-Nielsen et al., 1975), a new WHO-sponsored nomenclature was proposed for the human MHS. The conventional and convenient subdivision of the human *HLA* complex into serologically defined (SD) loci, MLC or lymphocyte defined (LD) loci etc., is to be abandoned. Instead, established loci will be designated as HLA-A, B, C, etc. (in rank order of discovery), whereas allelic determinants of each locus will be given numerical

* Staff member of the biology division of EURATOM. This publication is contribution number 959 of the Euratom Biology Division.

Table 2.1. Traditional Classification of Primate Genera

Suborder	Infraorder	Superfamily	Family	Subfamily	Genus	"Common" Designation
Prosimii	Tupaiiformes				*Tupaia*	
					Urogale	
	Lemuriformes				*Lemur*	
	Tarsiiformes				*Tarsius*	
	Lorisiformes			Lorisinae	*Loris*	
					Nycticebus	
					Arctocebus	
					Perodicticus	
				Galaginae	*Galago*	
Anthropoidea	Platyrrhini		Callithricidae		*Saguinus*	
			Cebidae		*Aotus*	
					Callicebus	
					Ateles	
					Saimiri	
					etc.	
	Catarrhini	Cercopithecoidea		Cercopithecinae	*Cercopithecus*	
					Cercocebus	
					Theropithecus	
					Macaca	Rhesus monkey, etc.
					Papio	Baboon
					Erythrocebus	
				Colobinae	*Colobus*	
					Presb. nasalis	
					Pygathrix	
		Hominoidea	Hylobatidae		*Hylobates sp.*	Gibbon
			Pongidae		*Pongo*	Orangutan
					Gorilla	
					Pan	Chimpanzee
			Hominidae		*Homo*	Man

designations: A_1, A_2, A_3, etc. Obviously, investigators dealing with the MHS of animals should eventually adopt a similar nomenclature.[1] However, because the rather extensive literature on the MHS of rhesus monkeys and

[1] By the end of 1976, the primate tissue typers had indeed reached agreement to adopt the new nomenclature (RhLA-A, RhLA-B, etc.).

chimpanzees has hitherto employed a conventional nomenclature, a sudden switch to the Aarhus proposals might be confusing. In this chapter, therefore, the conventional nomenclature will be used; the new internatnternational terminology may be used in future publications.

2. RhL-A, MHS of Rhesus Monkeys

2.1 Detection of Tissue Alloantigens

2.1.1 Serological Methods

Conventional Serologically Defined Antigens. The rhesus monkey was the first outbred animal species in which a MHS with separate, closely linked SD loci was established (Balner et al. 1971b; Gabb et al. 1972; Rogentine et al. 1971). Chronologically, the serological definition of the SD antigens of rhesus monkeys closely followed that of the SD antigens of the human HLA complex. In the context of this review, the SD antigens of RhL-A and the reagents defining them must be described in a cursory fashion; details on production, selection, and absorptions of the antibodies, etc., can be found in the literature.

In the earliest period (1964–1967), reagents were raised by cross-immunization of unrelated, unselected individuals (Balner et al. 1965b, 1967a; Bogden and Gray 1967). The usual immunization method was an exchange of skin grafts (which provided graft-survival data), followed by reate.c. or i.c. injections of blood or lymphocytes from the same donor. The initial technique for detecting specificities on leukocytes was agglutination. However, this was soon replaced by the more reliable lymphocytotoxicity and complement fixation techniques (Colombani et al. 1967; Kissmeyer-Nielsen and Kjerbye 1967; Mittal et al. 1968). The first reagents produced by the two principal teams of investigators (Rijswijk, Holland, and Bethesda, Maryland, USA) were mostly multispecific and required absorptions to "narrow" the specificity of the antibodies. The number of identified "broad" specificities steadily increased and the quality of reagents improved when it became possible to cross-immunize individuals that already shared identifiable broad specificities. In the meantime, pedigreed rhesus families had been raised in Rijswijk as well as Bethesda; the cross-immunization of selected sibs and half-sibs then led to the production of numerous oligo- and monospecific reagents. By 1970, the Rijswijk investigators were able to define several SD specificities; population and family studies led to the establishment of the RhL-A system as the MHS of rhesus monkeys (Balner et al. 1971b, 1971c) with probably two linked, segregating series of alleles controlling the SD antigens (see also Section 2.5).

At that point, the systematic production of alloantisera was begun. This was aimed at defining the still missing antigens of each segregant series. Eventually, testing was done exclusively with a one-step microcytotoxicity

Table 2.2. Phenotype Distribution of 25 Serologically Defined (SD) Antigens of the Two Segregant Series of RhL-A (testing for goodness of fit to Hardy-Weinberg equilibrium)

First Segregant Series

Gene freq.	Phenotypes		Obs.	Exp.
0.155	**9**	6	18	13.8
		10	5	10.3
		5	4	2.7
		1	2	2.0
		3	3	2.0
		19	7	7.3
		21	0	0.3
		23	7	5.2
		27	0	0.5
		22	6	3.4
		28	1	3.2
		33	2	2.0
		Null	11	12.5
0.195	**6**	10	12	13.0
		5	4	3.3
		1	0	2.6
		3	1	2.6
		19	3	9.1
		21	0	0.4
		23	3	6.5
		27	0	0.6
		22	3	4.3
		28	5	4.0
		33	7	2.6
		Null	22	17.5
0.146	**10**	5	3	2.4
		1	4	1.9
		3	1	1.9
		19	8	6.8
		21	0	0.3
		23	7	4.9
		27	2	0.4
		22	2	3.2
		28	3	3.0
		33	1	1.9
		Null	13	11.5
0.038	**5**	1	1	0.5
		3	0	0.5
		19	2	1.8
		21	0	0.1
		23	2	1.3
		27	0	0.1
		22	0	0.8
		28	0	0.8
		33	0	0.5
		Null	1	2.0
0.029	**1**	3	1	0.4
		19	0	1.3
		21	0	0.1
		23	2	1.0
		27	0	0.1
		22	0	0.6
		28	1	0.6
		33	1	0.4
		Null	1	1.5
0.030	**3**	19	3	1.3
		21	0	0.1
		23	3	1.0
		27	0	0.1
		22	0	0.6
		28	0	0.6
		33	0	0.4
		Null	1	1.5
0.103	**19**	21	1	0.2
		23	3	3.4
		27	0	0.3
		22	1	2.3
		28	3	2.1
		33	1	1.3
		Null	11	7.0
0.004	**21**	23	0	0.1
		27	0	0.0
		22	1	0.1
		28	0	0.1
		33	0	0.1
		Null	0	0.2
0.073	**23**	27	1	0.2
		22	2	1.6
		28	2	1.5
		33	0	1.0
		Null	1	4.5
0.007	**27**	22	0	0.1
		28	0	0.1
		33	0	0.1
		Null	0	0.3
0.048	**22**	28	1	1.0
		33	0	0.6
		Null	5	2.7
0.045	**28**	33	0	0.6
		Null	4	2.5
0.029	**33**	Null	1	1.5
0.099	Null	Null	1	2.3
Totals			228	228.0

$\chi^2 = 87.67$; $p = 0.22$ (78 D.F.)

Analysis of typing results obtained with the lymphocytes of 228 unrelated rhesus monkeys.

Table 2.2 (continued)

Second Segregant Series

Gene freq.	Phenotypes		Obs.	Exp.
0.110	**11**	13	2	3.7
		2	1	1.8
		14	3	1.4
		18	1	3.5
		25	2	1.5
		20	1	0.8
		26	14	12.2
		17	5	3.4
		24	3	4.9
		29	3	2.9
		31	0	0.7
		Null	12	10.5
0.074	**13**	2	0	1.2
		14	0	1.0
		18	2	2.3
		25	1	1.0
		20	1	0.5
		26	8	8.2
		17	2	2.3
		24	5	3.3
		29	2	2.0
		31	0	0.4
		Null	9	6.5
0.036	**2**	14	0	0.5
		18	2	1.1
		25	0	0.5
		20	1	0.3
		26	4	4.0
		17	1	1.1
		24	1	1.6
		29	0	1.0
		31	1	0.2
		Null	5	2.9
0.029	**14**	18	1	0.9
		25	0	0.4
		20	0	0.2
		26	7	3.2
		17	0	0.9
		24	2	1.3
		29	0	0.8
		31	0	0.2
		Null	0	2.2
0.069	**18**	25	1	1.0
		20	1	0.5
		26	3	7.7
		17	2	2.1
		24	6	3.1
		29	3	1.8
		31	0	0.4
		Null	8	6.0
0.031	**25**	20	0	0.2
		26	5	3.4
		17	3	1.0
		24	0	1.4
		29	0	0.8
		31	1	0.2
		Null	1	2.4
0.015	**20**	26	1	1.7
		17	0	0.5
		24	2	0.7
		29	0	0.4
		31	0	0.1
		Null	0	1.1
0.244	**26**	17	5	7.5
		24	8	10.8
		29	8	6.5
		31	2	1.5
		Null	32	30.8
0.068	**17**	24	3	3.0
		29	3	1.8
		31	1	0.4
		Null	5	5.8
0.097	**24**	29	2	2.6
		31	0	0.6
		Null	10	9.1
0.059	**29**	31	0	0.4
		Null	5	5.0
0.013	**31**	Null	1	1.0
0.155	Null	Null	4	5.5
totals			228	228.0

$\chi^2 = 61.97$; $p = 0.62$ (66 D.F.)

Analysis of typing results obtained with the lymphocytes of 228 unrelated rhesus monkeys.

assay on gradient-separated blood lymphocytes (Böyum 1968; Kissmeyer-Nielsen and Kjerbye 1967). Reagents of reasonable specificity were regularly exchanged between the few teams working in the field. Thus, the number of well-defined antigens increased by two or three per year. At the time of this writing, the Dutch team can identify some 25 conventional SD antigens, with about 10 percent blanks (undetected gene products) in each series. Table 2.2 shows the phenotype distribution in 228 unrelated monkeys of the 25 SD antigens identifiable by the Dutch team in 1975; there was clearly a good fit between observed and expected phenotypes (if Hardy-Weinberg equilibrium is assumed).

Confirmation of the existence of the two linked SD loci of RhL-A came from the National Institutes of Health (NIH) group in Bethesda. Rogentine et al. reported on the serology of five SD antigens. Three of these seemed to be alleles of one genetic locus, the other two possibly of a closely linked second locus (Rogentine et al. 1971). The first Primate histocompatibility workshop (Rijswijk 1971) established that the Rijswijk antigens 6, 9, and 10 of the first SD series corresponded to antigens 2, 1, and 5 of the NIH group (Balner et al. 1972a). The excellent correlations between the reactivity patterns of Rijswijk (BA) and Bethesda (RO) sera defining those three specificities when tested against cells from 87 unrelated rhesus monkeys are shown in Table 2.3. Further similarities among Rijswijk, Bethesda, and Birmingham reagents were established in 1973 during the second Primate workshop in Atlanta (Neefe et al. 1975a). A continued exchange of reagents among the various laboratories has since led to reasonable agreement on the definition of the majority of SD antigens of RhL-A. Table 2.4 presents the local designations of the "homologous" antigens of the first and second SD series of RhL-A. It can be seen that the majority of the antigens are independently recognized by at least two laboratories. Linkage disequilibrium (unexpectedly strong associations of antigens determined by two closely linked loci) between antigens of the first and second SD series of RhL-A has been observed by the Dutch as well as the Bethesda group (Neefe et al. 1975b; van Vreeswijk et al. 1976). Table 2.5 depicts the majority of the rhesus families analyzed. Positively demonstrable recombination between alleles of the SD_1 and SD_2 loci occurred only once[2] namely in child 00 of family ♂600 – ♀426. If all informative offspring available at Rijswijk are considered, including numerous offspring not depicted in Table 2.5 and those resulting from "inbreeding", the recombination frequency between the two SD loci can be estimated to be 0.29 percent, namely one recombinant out of 200 paternal and none out of 143 maternal haplotypes (van Vreeswijk et al. 1976; incidentally, other groups of investigators have not described any SD recombinants). The estimated recombination frequency between the two SD loci of RhL-A is therefore in the same order of magnitude as the frequency reported for the LA and Four loci of HLA (about 0.5 percent).

[2] Offspring ED of family ♂ 599 ×♀498 and CL of family ♂ 599 ×♀1115 were at one time considered as potential SD recombinants (Balner et al. 1973b). Results of recent absorption studies made those assumptions untenable.

Table 2.3. The Serological Definition of Three RhL-A Antigens in 1971

RhL-A6

Freq. pos.	Serum number and name	215	216	260	271	259	110
0.379	215 BA902.1	–					
0.414	216 BA1285.1	0.930	–				
0.391	260 BA1157.2	0.879	0.810	–			
0.416	271 RO966-E	0.893	0.920	0.814	–		
0.253	259 BA1171.3	0.835	0.777	0.815	0.766	–	
0.552	110 RO631-F	0.701	0.663	0.560	0.706	0.588	–

RhL-A9

Freq. pos.	Serum number and name	16	14	210	269	47	208	209	158
0.356	16 BA42A	–							
0.345	14 BA41E	0.975	–						
0.379	210 BA954.1	0.929	0.906	–					
0.390	269 RO403-F	0.920	0.894	0.836	–				
0.405	47 RO446-F	0.877	0.853	0.826	0.972	–			
0.402	208 RO309-F	0.858	0.835	0.832	0.893	0.828	–		
0.402	209 RO405-F	0.837	0.814	0.810	0.761	0.723	0.739	–	
0.414	158 BR2167-1805	0.775	0.748	0.802	0.840	0.770	0.745	0.801	–

RhL-A10

Freq. pos.	Serum number and name	233	234	235	236
0.287	233 RO303-F	–			
0.345	234 BA1121 XI	0.875			
0.322	235 BA1262.1	0.759	0.743	–	
0.299	236 BACF.2	0.862	0.741	0.679	–

Correlation coefficients between cytotoxic reactivity patterns of rhesus alloantisera defining antigens RhL-A6, -9, and -10 on lymphocytes from 87 unrelated rhesus monkeys (First International Workshop, Rijswijk, 1971).
Symbols BA, RO, and BR preceding the numerical designation of individual sera indicate their origin in the laboratories of Balner (Rijswijk), Rogentine (Bethesda), and Barnes (Birmingham). For further details, see Balner et al., 1972a.

Cross-reactivity between antigens of either segregant series of RhL-A has been observed. It has been described, in detail, for antigens 2 and 14 by the Rijswijk investigators (Balner et al. 1973b). Interestingly, antigen 14 strongly cross-reacted with antigen 2, but antigen 2 did not cross-react with antigen 14. (14+ 2– cells removed all reactivity from anti-2 sera but 2+ 14–

Table 2.4. Serologically Defined (SD) Antigens of the RhL-A Complex of Rhesus Monkeys (corresponding specificities recognized by the three principal teams, 1971–1975)

	Rijswijk workshop, 1971			Atlanta workshop, 1973			Serum exchange, 1975		
	Rijswijk	Bethesda	Birmingham	Rijswijk	Bethesda	Birmingham	Rijswijk	Bethesda	Birmingham
First segregant series				1			1		No participation
				3	16		3	16	
				5			5	414H	
	6	2		6	2		6	2	
	9	1		9	1	370	9	1	
	10	5		10	5		10	5	
	(12)	B2621		19	10	1867.37	19	10	
				21			21		
				r22			22		
				23	17		23	17	
				27			27		
				DS*	(18)		28	B4005, B2762^{II}	
							33	114H, 605H	
							Blank		
Second segregant series		2		2			2		No participation
		11		11	7	362.2	11	7	
		13		13	6	366.17	13	6	
		14		14			14		
				r17			17	443H	
				18			18	148.I	
				r20			20		
				r24			24	414H	
				r25			25	B3710^{II}	
				26	15		26	15	
					19			19	
					22			22	
							29	B3178^{II}	
							31		
							r32		
							Blank		

In anticipation of a new international nomenclature, only local designations are presented. The symbol r preceding some of the Rijswijk antigens indicates that alloantisera from a single animal define that (provisional) specificity. Gene frequencies for the 1975 Rijswijk antigens are presented in Table 2.2.

cells did not remove cytotoxic reactivity from anti-14 sera). A few other cases of probable cross-reactivity between SD antigens, mostly of the second series, have been reported more recently (van Vreeswijk et al. 1976).

A search for antigens of a third SD series (as an analogue of the human AJ or HLA-C locus) is in progress in Rijswijk as well as Bethesda. Unequivocal evidence for the existence of a third series of conventional SD antigens in rhesus monkeys was not available when this review was written.

The tissue distribution of RhL-A (SD) antigens has not been investigated systematically. Absorption studies demonstrated the presence of the antigens on leukocytes and platelets as well as spleen cells. In view of the similar organization of RhL-A and its human, canine, and murine analogues, one can assume that the tissue distribution of SD antigens of RhL-A will be similar to that observed for those of HLA, H-2, etc. Thus, nearly all nucleated cells of rhesus monkeys are likely to carry RhL-A (SD) antigens, probably with some quantitative variations for various organs and tissues.

Antigens with Restricted Tissue Distribution (Ia-Like Specificities). The first reports on murine Ia antigens[3] (David et al. 1973; Götze et al. 1973; Hauptfeld et al. 1973; Sachs and Cone 1973) were published in 1973. These serologically defined antigens are most readily detectable on B lymphocytes, and appear not to be carried by platelets. They are controlled by the I or Ir region of the H-2 system and seem to be relevant to histocompatibility (Klein 1975). A relation between Ia antigens and MLC-stimulator (MLC-s or LD) determinants has been proposed but not proved (Meo et al. 1975).

These developments, and reports on human alloantibodies possibly identifying LD or MLC-s determinants on lymphocytes (van Leeuwen et al. 1972; van Rood et al. 1975), led the Rijswijk investigators to initiate a systematic search for "non-SD" sera in rhesus monkeys. The aim was the serological identification of LD or MLC-s antigens or, alternatively, the detection of the equivalent of the murine Ia antigens. Among the methods tried were the cross-immunization of RhL-A identical siblings which stimulate in MLC (SD/LD recombinants) as well as mutual immunization of unrelated SD "full-house"[4] identical monkeys. The latter approach led to the production of several antisera that showed minimal complement-dependent cytotoxicity with conventional lymphocyte suspensions (mostly T-cells), but strong reactions with B-cell-enriched suspensions. In 1974, several promising reagents were provisionally analyzed (Balner and van Vreeswijk 1975). The reagents recognized a few specificities coded by the RhL-A region and were primarily carried by B lymphocytes, not by platelets. In a provisional population study, no positive association was found with reactivity patterns obtained with the available LD typing cells[5] (see Section 3.1.2). In view of these findings as well as the demonstration of immunocytological characteristics reminiscent of those of murine Ia antigens (Zaalberg et al. 1976), the specificities were tentatively designated as "Ia-like". Using the same method of immunization, the Rijswijk team subsequently raised 36 additional sera that seemed to recognize B cell alloantigens of similar characteristics. Results of a first population and family study performed with the available reagents (Balner et al. 1976; Roger et al. 1976), permitted the provisional conclusion that eleven new cell surface alloantigens of rhesus monkeys have been identified. They

[3] "Immune-region associated" antigens; see Chapter 7.

[4] Carrying four identifiable antigens of the two SD series of RhL-A.

[5] When proof-reading this chapter in December 1976, evidence for strong associations with B-cell or Ia-like antigens was available.

Table 2.5. Genotyping of Rhesus Monkey Families According to RhL-A (SD) Antigens

Parents and Offspring		SD Genotypes			Parents and Offspring		SD Genotypes			Parents and Offspring		SD Genotypes			Parents and Offspring		SD Genotypes		
♂381	ab	10	17/–	29	†♂598	ab	6	13/(19	17)	♂599	ab	1	–/10	13	♂600	ab	6	24/10	2
♀ 584	cd	6	14/ 6	11	*♀ 834	cd	28	2/–	–	*♀ 581	cd	9	11/ 1	26	♀ 597	cd	6	–/ 9	11
V	bd	–	29/ 6	11	UU	bc	19	17/28	2	G	bc	10	13/ 9	11	AB	bc	10	2/ 6	–
GO	bd	–	29/ 6	11	BD	bc	19	17/28	2	GG	bc	10	13/ 9	11	BF	bc	10	2/ 6	–
JJ	bc	–	29/ 6	14	EK	bc	19	17/28	2	DV	bc	10	13/ 9	11	CG	ad	6	24/ 9	11
AV	bc	–	29/ 6	14	CS	ad	6	13/–	–	AG	ac	1	–/ 9	11	HO	ad	6	24/ 9	11
BU	bc	–	29/ 6	14						CF	ac	1	–/ 9	11	DW	ac	6	24/ 6	–
CZ	bc	–	29/ 6	14											IW	bd	10	2/ 9	11
♀ 432	cd	5	26/21	14	*♀ 730	cd	10	13/33	11	*♀ 498	cd	19	11/10	18	♀ 669	cd	9	–/22	18
N	ac	10	17/ 5	26	FF	bd	19	17/33	11	NN	ac	1	–/19	11	AC	ad	6	24/22	18
FN	ac	10	17/ 5	26	ZZ	bc	19	17/10	13	AQ	ac	1	–/19	11	BI	ad	6	24/22	18
AK	bd	–	29/21	14	BT	ac	6	13/10	13	ED	ad	1	–/10	18	CR	ad	6	24/22	18
GM	bd	–	29/21	14	DA	ad	6	13/33	11	GU	bd	10	13/10	18	EL	bc	10	2/ 9	–
CP	ad	10	17/21	14											FS	bc	10	2/ 9	–
♀ 494	cd	3	14/ 5	14	♀ 832	cd	19	14/22	18	*♀ 590	cd	9	11/ 6	32	♀ 603	cd	21	–/ 3	11
L	ac	10	17/ 3	14	AD	bd	19	17/22	18	CV	bd	10	13/ 6	32	T	bd	10	2/ 3	11
CY	ac	10	17/ 3	14	BM	ad	6	13/22	18	GD	bd	10	13/ 6	32	DF	bd	10	2/ 3	11
AM	ad	10	17/ 5	14	CN	ac	6	13/19	14	EI	ad	1	–/ 6	32	FO	bd	10	2/ 3	11
AA	bd	–	29/ 5	14	DS	bc	19	17/19	14	HG	ac	1	–/ 9	11	GY	bc	10	2/21	–
															LF	bc	10	2/21	–
*♀ 852	cd	23	–/22	24	†♀ 589	cd	(–	17)/ 6	13	*♀ 1115	cd	19	18/21	24	♀ Y	cd	–	29/23	–
AH	ac	10	17/23	–	AE	ad	6	13/ 6	13	CL	ac	1	–/19	18	FA	ad	6	24/23	–
DN	ac	10	17/23	–	Z	ac	6	13/–	17	GZ	ac	1	–/19	18	HS	ad	6	24/23	–
EV	ad	10	17/22	24	BP	bc	19	17/–	17	EF	bd	10	13/21	24	HB	ac	6	24/–	29
BL	bd	–	29/22	24	FL	bd	19	17/ 6	13						MY	ac	6	24/–	29
															GC	bd	10	2/23	–
†♀ 594	cd	(6	?)/(9	18)	*♀ 728	cd	10	–/ 6	14	*♀ 493	cd	9	11/10	11	♀ 429	cd	10	26/27	?
BJ	bd	–	29/ 9	18	KK	ad	6	13/ 6	14	AX	bc	10	13/ 9	11	XX	bc	10	2/10	26
FU	bd	–	29/ 9	18	AS	bd	19	17/ 6	14	CK	bc	10	13/ 9	11	BG	ac	6	24/10	26
YY	ad	10	17/ 9	18	EP	ac	6	13/10	–	DM	bc	10	13/ 9	11					
*♀ 324	cd	9	20/10	25	*♀ 306	cd	6	11/ 6	29	*♀ 926	cd	23	–/19	25	♀ 1113	cd	19	24/19	26
CU	bc	–	29/ 9	20	SS	bc	19	17/ 6	11	DC	bc	10	13/23	–	FH	bc	10	2/19	24
EM	ac	10	17/ 9	20	BK	ac	6	13/ 6	11	FJ	ac	1	–/23	–	GN	bd	10	2/19	26
*♀ 1480	cd	9	26/19	11	*♀ 1114	cd	9	25/–	13	*♀ 1470	cd	10	26/ 9	26	♀ 2504	cd	9	26/ 9	25
EH	bd	–	29/19	11	EU	ac	6	13/ 9	25	FW	ac	1	–/10	26	IU	bc	10	2/ 9	26
GJ	ad	10	17/19	11											LJ	ad	6	24/ 9	25
*♀ 1472	cd	19	14/27	11						*♀ 1644	cd	10	–/19	11	♀ 426	cd	6	13/10	?
EQ	ac	10	17/19	14						HA	ac	1	–/10	–	EE	ac	6	24/ 6	13
															OO	a/bc	6	2/ 6	13
										*♀ 307	cd	1	–/19	26					
										EC	ac	1	–/ 1	–					

Parents and Offspring		SD	Genotypes	
♂1435	ab	9	13/10	26
♀ 1422	cd	19	29/19	–
FX	ac	9	13/19	29
JM	ac	9	13/19	29
HP	ad	9	13/19	–
MH	ad	9	13/19	–
GV	bc	10	26/19	29
♀ 1425	cd	6	26/ –	20
HQ	ac	9	13/ 6	26
JC	ac	9	13/ 6	26
ER	bc	10	26/ 6	26
GB	bd	10	26/ –	20
♀ 923	cd	22	? / –	26
FT	ad	9	13/ –	26
EJ	bd	10	26/ –	26
GX	bc	10	26/22	?
♀ T	cd	10	2/ 3	11
GQ	bc	10	26/10	2
IB	ac	9	13/10	2
HL	ad	9	13/ 3	11
♀ 1478	cd	6	26/ 6	11
HT	bc	10	26/ 6	26
MP	ad	9	13/ 6	11
♀ 1427	cd	6	11/ 9	?
GH	bc	10	26/ 6	11
HM	bc	10	26/ 6	11
♀ 1423	cd	19	26/ 5	17
EO	ac	9	13/19	26
HF	ad	9	13/ 5	17
♀ 1008	cd	10	13/27	26
IR	ac	9	13/10	13
LT	ac	9	13/10	13
♀ 2325	cd	23	26/ 9	17
IY	ac	9	13/23	26
LI	bd	10	26/ 9	17
♀ 2518	cd	6	11/ 6	25
IX	bc	10	26/ 6	11
MV	bd	10	26/ 6	25

Parents and Offspring		SD	Genotypes	
♂600	ab	6	24/10	2
♀852		23	–/22	24
IJ	bd	10	2/22	24
♀ 324		9	20/10	25
KG	bc	10	2/ 9	20
♂1033	ab	6	11/19	11
♀ 1480		9	26/19	11
JE	bc	19	11/ 9	26
♀ 1472		19	14/27	11
JB	ad	6	11/27	11

Parents and Offspring		SD	Genotypes	
♂600	ab	6	24/10	2
♀ 834		28	2/ –	–
IQ	bc	10	2/28	2
♀728		10	–/ 6	14
KI	ac	6	24/10	–
♂1033	ab	6	11/19	11
♀ 1114		9	25/ –	13
HR	ac	6	11/ 9	25
KO	ad	6	11/–	13
♂2315	ab	9	17/19	24
♀ 730		10	13/33	11
HU	ad	9	17/33	11
KX	ad	9	17/33	11
♀ 306		6	11/ 6	29
IP	ad	9	17/ 6	29
ML	bc	19	24/ 6	11

Parents and Offspring		SD	Genotypes	
♂600	ab	6	24/10	2
♀307		1	–/19	26
S	bd	10	2/19	26
♂2315	ab	9	17/19	24
♀ 1115		19	18/21	24
HY	bd	19	24/21	24
LO	bc	19	24/19	18
♀ 1470		10	26/ 9	26
IN	bd	19	24/ 9	26
♀1644		10	–/19	11
IL	ac	9	17/10	–
KP	bc	19	24/10	–
♂1435	ab	9	13/10	26
♀ 581		9	11/ 1	26
IA	ad	9	13/ 1	26
LQ	bd	10	26/ 1	26
♀ 498		19	11/10	18
HX	bc	10	26/19	11
MB	bc	10	26/19	11
♀ 590		9	11/ 6	32
HW	ad	9	13/ 6	32
MU	bc	10	26/ 9	11
♀ 493		9	11/10	11
HZ	bc	10	26/ 9	11
KU	bd	10	26/10	11
♀926		23	–/19	25
IC	bc	10	26/23	–
LB	bc	10	26/23	–

Parents are indicated by numerical designations, offsprings by capital letters; exceptions are mother Y (offspring of ♂381), and T (offspring of ♂600). Symbols a and b stand for paternal, c and d for maternal "haplotypes." Asterisks preceding the numbers of certain females indicate that they were mated also to different males. The results of such rematings are depicted in the second, third and fourth vertical columns on this page. The second column depicts the rematings of females originally belonging to the "harem" of male 381 (first column of opposite page), the third column those of harem 598 (second column of opposite page), the fourth and rightmost column those of harem 599 (third column of opposite page). Incidentally males 1033 and 2315 (shown on this page) have numerous other offspring which are not depicted in this table, but confirm the SD haplotypes presented here.
† = animal dead
( ) = haplotype deduced
? = homozygosity cannot be excluded

are controlled by the major histocompatibility complex but are distinct from the conventional serological defined (SD) antigens of RhL-A. As mentioned before the new specificities were termed "Ia-like" because of serological, immunocytological and other characteristics reminiscent of Ia antigens of the mouse. A formal genetic analysis led to the postulation of two segregant series, controlling eight of the eleven new specificities. Strong linkage disequilibria with SD antigens and genetic mapping on the basis of segregation studies in recombinant offspring in the families, placed at least one of the two loci in the vicinity of the SD_1 locus of RhL-A, in the region of the major MLC or LD_1 locus. For this and other reasons, the new B-cell alloantigens of rhesus monkeys are believed to be similar to or associated with the stimulator antigens of LD_1.

Further relationships among the SD, LD, and Ia-like antigens, including the mapping positions of the genes controlling them as well as their possible relevance to histocompatibility, are discussed below.

2.1.2 Cellular Methods

As described in more detail elsewhere in this volume, the mixed lymphocyte culture (MLC) has become an indispensible cellular technique to determine important antigens of the MHS. Bach and Amos first demonstrated that lymphocytes from HLA identical human siblings do not show mutual stimulation in culture, whereas other cell combinations do (Bach and Amos 1967). Thus, MLC reactivity in man is controlled by the HLA system. Subsequently, it was shown that a "major" MLC or LD_1 locus is situated outside the SD region of HL-A and that its determinants may be important for histocompatibility (Eijsvoogel et al. 1972b; Hamburger et al. 1971; Koch et al. 1971; Yunis and Amos 1971). Attempts have been made to define the human MLC-s or LD_1 determinants by direct serological methods (van Leeuwen et al. 1973; van Rood et al. 1975); there is suggestive, but as yet no unequivocal evidence that this can be achieved.

MLC work in rhesus monkeys started in 1970 when the Rijswijk investigators established a major MLR or LD_1 locus within the RhL-A system (Appelman and Balner 1972). This locus was separable from the two SD loci as shown by three unequivocal LD/SD recombinants (Balner and Toth 1973). MCL data for one pair of sibs, one of which was a recombinant between SD_1 and SD_2, suggested that the LD_1 locus might be situated on the side of the first SD series. Unfortunately, no other informative SD recombinants have since become available to confirm this assumption. Further studies by the Dutch group indicated that the LD_1 locus is moderately polymorphic and that one, possibly several "minor" LD loci linked to RhL-A must be assumed (Balner 1973). Independent studies by the Bethesda team also provided evidence for the existence of one major and at least one minor RhL-A-linked LD locus (Neefe et al. 1973).

An important refinement in recognizing LD determinants was introduced by Mempel et al. (1973): Human cells homozygous for an LD_1 determinant do not stimulate heterozygous cells carrying the same LD determinant. This principle of cellular LD-typing has since been adopted by those studying the MHC of man, dog, and monkey. In man and dogs, it has led to the establishment of several "alleles" of the LD_1 locus (Grosse-Wilde et al. 1975; Keunig et al. 1975; and appropriate chapters of this volume). For rhesus monkeys, the number of available LD typing cells is limited, but steadily increasing. Preliminary studies by the Dutch group with about a dozen LD typing cells (five of which are consanguinous) and by the Bethesda group (Neefe et al. 1976), suggest the existence of an allelic system of LD_1 determinants, also for the rhesus monkey. Close associations between LD_1 determinants and identifiable Ia-like antigens of RhL-A have been established (Balner and van Es, unpublished observations).

Because defining LD antigens with typing cells remains an intricate time-consuming method, vigorous efforts have been made to find means of defining LD_1 antigens by more direct techniques. A serological method has been mentioned above. Another promising approach is the so-called primed lymphocyte test, or PLT, recently described by F. H. Bach and colleagues (Sheehy et al. 1975). This method is currently applied by the Dutch group also to rhesus monkeys.

2.1.3 Relations Among SD, LD, and Ia-Like Antigens

Few studies have been made to characterize the tissue antigens of rhesus monkeys and to differentiate among them. Chemical characterization, the most reliable method, is discussed briefly in the next section. Here, a few empirical methods will be described that may shed light on the characteristics of cell surface antigens and their possible relationships.

Co-capping Experiments: Alloantisera against HLA and/or H-2 antigens will, under certain conditions, cause aggregation and redistribution of cell surface antigens and the formation of patches and/or polar caps on lymphocytes (Kourilsky et al. 1972; Taylor et al. 1971; Unanue et al. 1972). As a rule, antigens of different molecular structure will not "co-cap"; i.e., the other type of antigen will still be demonstrable on the cell surface if appropriate antisera and immunofluorescent techniques are applied. In rhesus monkeys, the Dutch investigators have recently found that antigens of the SD_1 and SD_2 series of RhL-A (both co-capping with β_2-microglobulin) do not co-cap with each other. Furthermore, an Ia-like antigen did not co-cap with SD_1 or SD_2 antigens or with β_2-microglobulin (Zaalberg et al. 1976), a finding that provides provisional evidence that, as in the mouse (Unanue et al. 1974), SD and Ia-like antigens are structurally distinct.

Immune precipitation: Precipitation of detergent-solubilized cellular antigens with specific alloantisera allows the differentiation of various types of antigens and an estimation of their respective molecular weights (Wernet and Kunkel 1973). In pilot experiments with rhesus monkey cells and sera, B. Tank was able to establish biochemical differences between antigens precipitated with anti-SD sera and those precipitated with an anti-Ia serum *(personal communication)*.

Inhibition of Mixed lymphocyte reactivity: Specific inhibition of MLR by various types of alloantisera (anti-SD, anti-LD, or anti-Ia) has been regarded as evidence that the various antigens are, if not identical or cross-reacting, at least located in the vicinity of each other on the cell surface (Ceppellini 1971). The Dutch investigators, working with rhesus monkeys, found that anti-SD sera specifically inhibit stimulator cells in MLC (Balner and Toth 1973); certain anti-Ia sera also specifically inhibit stimulator cells under similar conditions. However, they do not consider these findings as evidence for similarity between LD determinants and SD or Ia antigens; steric hindrance or other mechanisms could also explain the phenomenon.

Cell-mediated lympholysis (CML)—role of various antigens: CML is considered by some as an *in vitro* model of events occurring during graft recognition and rejection *in vivo*. Schematically, the principle of CML is stimulation of lymphocytes A by lymphocytes B in an MLC and a subsequent measurement of the destruction of PHA-transformed isotope-labeled lymphoblasts (of type B, C, D, etc.) by the triggered A cells (Lightbody et al. 1971). A popular theory holds that LD differences are essential for triggering, whereas SD differences are required as specific targets for the kill (Eijsvoogel et al. 1972a). This theory has not consistantly been supported by experimental data (Bach and Balner 1975), but CML remains an attractive tool for studying the trigger and effector phases of cellular immune responses. Pilot experiments by the Dutch group in rhesus monkeys have confirmed the requirement of LD disparity for the "triggering" of killer cells and SD differences to serve as targets. However, the exact role of SD_1, SD_2, Ia-like, and LD_1 determinants in the various stages of CML has not yet been determined.

2.2 Biochemistry

The biochemical characterisation of tissue antigens of subhuman primates has been somewhat neglected. In man and the mouse, papain digestion of the cell membranes followed by chromatography or detergent solubilization of membranes combined with immune precipitation of antigens by means of alloantisera are the most widely practised methods. By the use of these techniques, human and murine SD antigens have been fairly well characterised as glycoproteins with molecular weights of around 40,000 daltons that are closely associated with β_2-microglobulin molecules of about 10,000 daltons.

Of the subhuman primates, only antigens of rhesus monkeys, baboons, and chimps (see below) have been studied to some extent. Rogentine et al. subjected rhesus spleen cells to papain digestion according to the method of Mann et al. (1969) and Rogentine et al. (1972), and obtained water-soluble alloantigens. The product was checked for serologic specificity by inhibition of the lymphocytotoxic activity of appropriate alloantisera. Amino acid analysis of acrylamide gel fractions of these RhL-A (SD) antigens revealed striking qualitative similarities (but also quantitative differences) to the amino acid spectrum of SD antigens of mouse and man. However, an estimate of the molecular weight of an SD antigen of RhL-A was not reported. Clearly, much biochemical work remains to be done, particularly now that various types of cell surface antigens (SD, LD, Ia-like) can be identified in rhesus monkeys by various immunological methods. Using immunoprecipitation techniques, the Dutch investigators recently established that SD and Ia-like antigens of rhesus monkeys, are biochemically very similar to those of mouse and man (see also 2.1.3).

2.3 Histocompatibility

Direct proof that products of a genetic region are particularly important for histocompatibility can be obtained by intrafamily transplantations. A genetic system such as HLA or RhL-A consists of numerous, closely linked loci or systems. In families, such a chromosomal region is normally passed to each offspring as a unit or haplotype. The paternal contributions are traditionally called haplotypes a and b, the maternal ones c and d. The four types of offspring can thus share two parental haplotypes (genotypic identity), one haplotype, or none. If the gene products of a complex are of particular relevance to histocompatibility, grafts exchanged between genotypically identical sibs show a significantly prolonged survival as compared to non-identical controls. This simple approach has been followed by investigators studying the MHS of several species. It has become evident that all species studied so far have a genetic system with an overriding influence on allograft survival. These complexes are called "MHS," and their most convenient markers are the described SD antigens, the MLC-s or LD antigens and, more recently, the products of the immune response region, I or Ir.

The purpose of this section is to summarize the data currently available regarding the relevance of the RhL-A region to histocompatibility.

2.3.1 Transplantation in Related Rhesus Monkeys

As soon as the number of identifiable leukocyte "groups" was sufficient for reliable SD haplotyping of pedigreed monkeys, skin grafts were exchanged between full sibs of the rhesus families available in Rijswijk. The results showed that skin grafts exchanged between genotypically identical pairs had significantly longer survival times (14.3 ± 0.6 days) than appropriate controls (8.7 ± 0.2). This was a strong indication that the available SD markers were controlled by the rhesus monkeys' MHS. That assumption has since been confirmed in several ways; in analogy with HLA, the system was called RhL-A (Balner et al. 1971b).

In view of the scarcity of pedigreed rhesus families, transplantation experiments of a potentially terminal nature have been performed mostly with unrelated rhesus monkeys (see below). Certain pilot experiments with related animals have been performed by the Dutch group, however. When lethally irradiated monkeys were given bone marrow from RhL-A-identical siblings, the severity of the usually lethal graft-versus-host (GvH) disease was significantly reduced (U. W. Schaefer, *personal communication*). Such experiments are being continued on a modest scale; they might eventually provide an answer to the important clinical question of why a large proportion of patients treated with bone marrow from HLA-identical (MLC-negative) siblings still succumb to lethal GvH disease (Thomas et al. 1975). The experimental use of related rhesus monkeys for organ grafting seems unnecessary, because the available clinical data show that the fate of kidney grafts from MHS-identical human siblings is superior to that of grafts in any other host/donor combination (except monozygotic twins).

2.3.2 Transplantation in Unrelated Rhesus Monkeys

Although matching related individuals for MHS products is relatively easy (the offspring normally inherit the entire MHS region), selecting compatible unrelated host/donor combinations is a more complicated procedure. It entails separate matching for SD-, LD-, Ia-like, or other MHS determinants.[6] In view of its potential importance for clinical transplantation, matching of unrelated monkeys has been vigorously pursued in several laboratories. Currently available data are presented below; however, it should be realized that the data given may have only transient value because the precision of typing and matching for any category of antigens is improving year by year.

Transplantation of Skin. Historically, experiments with preimmunized rhesus monkeys provided the first evidence that serologically defined antigens on leukocytes are relevant for skin graft survival (Balner et al. 1965a). However, actual matching of host/donor combinations for SD products of RhL-A was started only after a reasonable number of antigens could be serologically identified. Early results, obtained with matching for two or three SD antigens, only suggested a positive influence of matching on skin allograft survival (Balner et al. 1972b). More reliable results could not be expected until the majority of the SD antigens were identifiable several years later. In 1974, the Rijswijk investigators demonstrated that full-house identity for RhL-A (SD) antigens definitely leads to prolongation of skin allograft survival in monkeys. Somewhat unexpectedly, MLC reactivity of the recipients against the graft donors did not seem to influence graft survival (Balner and van Vreeswijk 1975). Table 2.6, which summarizes the results obtained by the Dutch group during 1974/75, confirms the outcome of the previous experiments—namely, that matching for SD antigens leads to prolonged skin allograft survival and that antidonor MLC reactivity seems to be of minor importance. The 41 SD-identical host-donor combinations listed in Table 2.6 were retrospectively typed for the presence of Ia-like specificities (see p. 87). Although it is too early to draw conclusions, it is noteworthy that, in the

[6] Possible influences of a disparity for blood group systems are not the subject of this review and have been discussed elsewhere (Stone 1975). Up to now none of the known red cell systems of rhesus monkeys have been shown to be closely linked to the MHS.

Table 2.6. Influence of Matching for SD Antigens and MLC Reactivity on Skin Allograft Survival in Rhesus Monkeys

RhL-A (SD)	MLC[a] $R \rightarrow D_x$	Number of Comb. (n)	Mean Graft Survival in Days (S.D.)	Significance
Identical[b]	Positive[c]	33	12.0 (1.8)	$p<0.001$
	Negative[d]	8	11.6 (1.0)	
Not identical	Positive	19	9.7 (0.9)	
	Negative	8	10.2 (1.1)	$0.05>p>0.02$

[a] MLC activity of recipient lymphocytes against irradiated donor cells; "negative" combinations include a few that reacted very weakly (2–3× autologous counts).
[b] "Full-house" identical combinations, sharing four RhL-A (SD) antigens.
[c] Excluding one combination with a graft survival of 35 days; if that combination is included, the mean survival becomes 12.9 days (S.D. 4.3).
[d] Including four related animals that share one parental haplotype.

three combinations where the donor did not show detectable incompatibilities for Ia-like antigens, skin graft survival times were 13, 13, and 14.5 days, clearly above the average of 12 days.

Transplantation of Organs. Matching for RhL-A (SD) antigens in kidney grafting was first attempted by the Dutch group in the early 1970s (Dicke et al. 1971; Marquet et al. 1972). Those studies failed to show a positive effect of matching, possibly because "phenotypic identity" between host and donor was never complete (the pairs shared two or three SD antigens, never four). More favorable results of SD matching for kidney allograft survival in rhesus monkeys have not appeared in the literature so far. In the meantime, the number of identifiable RhL-A (SD) antigens has sharply increased (Table 2.4), and an elaborate program of prospective matching for kidney transplantation was carried out at the Rijswijk center. Current results indicate that host/donor matching for four conventional SD antigens (full-house identity) does not prolong the survival time of kidney allografts as was the case for skin allografts. However, in such SD identical combinations, MLR-non-reactivity of host- against donor-lymphocytes (prior to transplantation), had led to modest but significant prolongation of kidney allograft survival in unrelated monkeys (van Es et al. 1976).

Ortho- and heterotopic cardiac as well as hepatic transplantations have also been performed in rhesus monkeys. However, optimal techniques and methods of immunosuppression rather than matching for MHS products were the main points of interest in those studies. To our knowledge, realistic MHS matching has not yet been applied in this area of research in monkeys.

Transplantation of Bone Marrow. For many years, rhesus monkeys have served as the optimal model to study graft versus host disease (GvH disease) in irradiated bone marrow-treated individuals. The first attempts to mitigate the fulminating GvH disease in monkeys by matching unrelated host-donor combinations for RhL-A antigens were made in the early 1970s. Although some of the results seemed encouraging (Neefe et al. 1974), solid evidence for a beneficial influence of SD or LD matching in marrow transplantation has not yet been obtained. This could be due to the limited knowledge of the MHS determinants at the time of those studies. The currently available methods for typing and matching for products of the MHS in rhesus monkeys have led to a renewed interest in this important field of research. Hence, investigations are in progress in Rijswijk and Bethesda to determine the influence of matching for SD, LD, or Ia-like antigens on GvH disease in this primate species.

2.4 MHC-Linked Immune Responses

The reasons for studying the genetics of the immune response are discussed at length elsewhere in this volume. In the mouse, the species most extensively studied, the majority of the known immune response genes map within the MHS, in the so-called I region of the H-2 system (McDevitt and Benacerraf 1969). Other genes of the I region control the Ia antigens, have a major influence on MLC and GvH reactivity, and on the interaction between T- and B-lymphocytes (Bach et al. 1972b; Klein 1975). Most important, Ir genes may play a significant role in susceptibility to diseases and oncogenic viruses (Benacerraf and Dorf 1974; Lilly 1965; McDevitt and Benacerraf, 1969).

Interest in the genetics of the immune response of the rhesus monkey stems from the phylogenetic closeness of the monkey to man and the extensive knowledge of the RhL-A system already available. In initial experiments, the Dutch investigators, in collaboration with McDevitt's group, studied the humoral response to the synthetic polypeptide (TG)AL, the antigen initially used to identify the Ir-1 locus of mice (McDevitt and Benacerraf, 1969). Preliminary results from studies in a few rhesus families suggested that the responder status was inherited together with a particular RhL-A haplotype (Balner 1973). Data on cellular reactivity such as skin reactions and *in vitro* lymphocyte responses to the antigen were inconclusive.

In close collaboration with Dorf and Benacerraf, the immune response studies were continued by the Dutch investigators, using GA and DNP-GL as antigens (linear copolymers of L-glutamic acid and L-alanine or L-lysine, the latter conjugated to dinitrophenyl). In unrelated monkeys, it appeared that strong humoral responses and measurable delayed-type skin reactions could be elicited in some of the animals, whereas others were low responders or nonresponders. There was no correlation between responder status to GA or GL and any of the RhL-A (SD) antigens (reagents identifying Ia-like antigens and LD-typing cells were not yet available). A subsequent segregation analysis of data for 21 rhesus families (sired by three different males) demonstrated that the capacity to respond to GA and DNP-GL was also controlled by genes located in the RhL-A system (Dorf et al. 1974, 1975). Table 2.7 presents the humoral anti-GA responses of members of harem 598.

Table 2.7. Humoral Response of Related Rhesus Monkeys to the Antigen GA

Parents and Offspring[a]	RhL-A Genotype[b]	Antibody Response (ABC-33)[c]
♂ 598	a B	†
♀ 589	c d	†
Z	a c	0.1
BP	B c	1023
FL	B d	300
♀ 832	C d	81
AD	B d	148
BM	a d	26
DS	B C	170
♀ 834	c d	41
UU	B c	4410
BD	B c	>9000
EK	B c	<0.1 ←
CS	a d	47
♀ 434	c d	†
K	B c	>9000
♀ 728	c D	462
KK	a D	2801
AS	B D	>9000
EP	a c	0.2
♀ 306	c D	118
SS	B c	3484
BK	a c	5.7
♀ 833	c d	<0.1
CT	a c	<0.1
♀1114	c d	6.6
EU	a c	
♀1355	c d	†
EG	B c	3056

[a] Parents are indicated with numerical symbols; offspring with letters.
[b] Paternal RhL-A haplotypes are indicated with a or b (a single father for all offspring); maternal haplotypes with c and d (different for each family). Capital letters indicate haplotypes controlling responsiveness to GA (copolymer of glutamic acid and alanine).
[c] Antigen binding capacity for undiluted serum expressed as picomoles of ligand bound per milliliter of serum. GA humoral responses are based on primary sera taken 3 weeks after initial immunizations; sera taken 7 days after boosting confirmed these data.
† Indicates that animal has died. Assignment of "reactive" RhL-A haplotype is based on data obtained from the other parents and offspring. Arrow indicates proposed recombinant for the Ir-GA gene.
Modified from Table VII in Dorf et al. 1975.

Because the GA response "segregated" with RhL-A haplotypes in all informative families (including those not shown in Table 2.7), the aberrant negative reaction of offspring EK (Table 2.7, ♀834) was regarded as provisional evidence for recombination between a proposed Ir-GA gene and the

Table 2.8 Humoral Response to DNP-GL in a Rhesus Family with Two LD/SD Recombinant Offspring

Parents and Offspring	RhL-A Genotype	Antibody Response to DNP-GL	Site of Proposed Recombination (↓)
♂381	A b	+	
♀584	c d	–	
JJ	b c	–	
AV	b c	–	
BU	b c	–	↓
CZ	A b c	–	LD_1-IrGL-SD-Bf
V	b d	–	↓
GO	A b d	+	LD_1-IrGL-SD-Bf

Symbols a, b, c, and d stand for paternal (a, b) and maternal (c, d) haplotypes. The capital A indicates that all offspring of "harem ♂381" with haplotype a were responders to DNP-GL. Offspring CZ and GO inherited the LD_1 determinants of paternal haplotype a but the SD genes of haplotype b. Consequently, the Ir-GL gene may be located between the LD_1 locus and the SD region of RhL-A. (DNP-GL is a copolymer of glutamic acid and lysine, coupled to dinotrophenol.) The symbols used in the extreme right column are explained in the text and in Figure 1. Modified from Table 3 in Dorf et al. 1974.

LD-SD region of RhL-A (see also Section 2.5). Data for responses to DNP-GL in another pedigree (♂381) provided interesting information on the probable location of a proposed Ir-GL gene in the RhL-A system. Three offspring of male 381 had been shown to be recombinants between the LD and SD region of RhL-A (Balner and Toth 1973). In two of those, the response to DNP-GL segregated with the LD part of the haplotype; in the third case, with the SD part. Table 2.8 schematically depicts the data for one of those families (♂381/♀584). The results tentatively localize the Ir-GL gene between the LD and SD regions of RhL-A (Balner et al. 1973a; Dorf et al. 1974).

Immune response studies in rhesus monkeys are being continued by the Rijswijk workers (in collaboration with others[7]) using the synthetic polypeptides (TG)AL and (PheG)ProL and certain purified ragweed extracts as antigens. Preliminary results indicate that responses to some of the latter antigens are not controlled by the RhL-A region.

2.5 Genetic Organization of the RhL-A System

Certain aspects of the genetic organization or the "mapping" of the RhL-A system have already been discussed in the preceding sections of this chapter. In this section, Figure 2.1 will be used as a guideline to summarize the developments of the past few years that have led to the tentative mapping of a number of loci in the RhL-A system.

[7] For (TG)AL and (PheG)ProL with E. Mozes of the Weizmann Institute, Israel. For ragweed antigens with D. Marsh of Johns Hopkins, Baltimore, Md., USA.

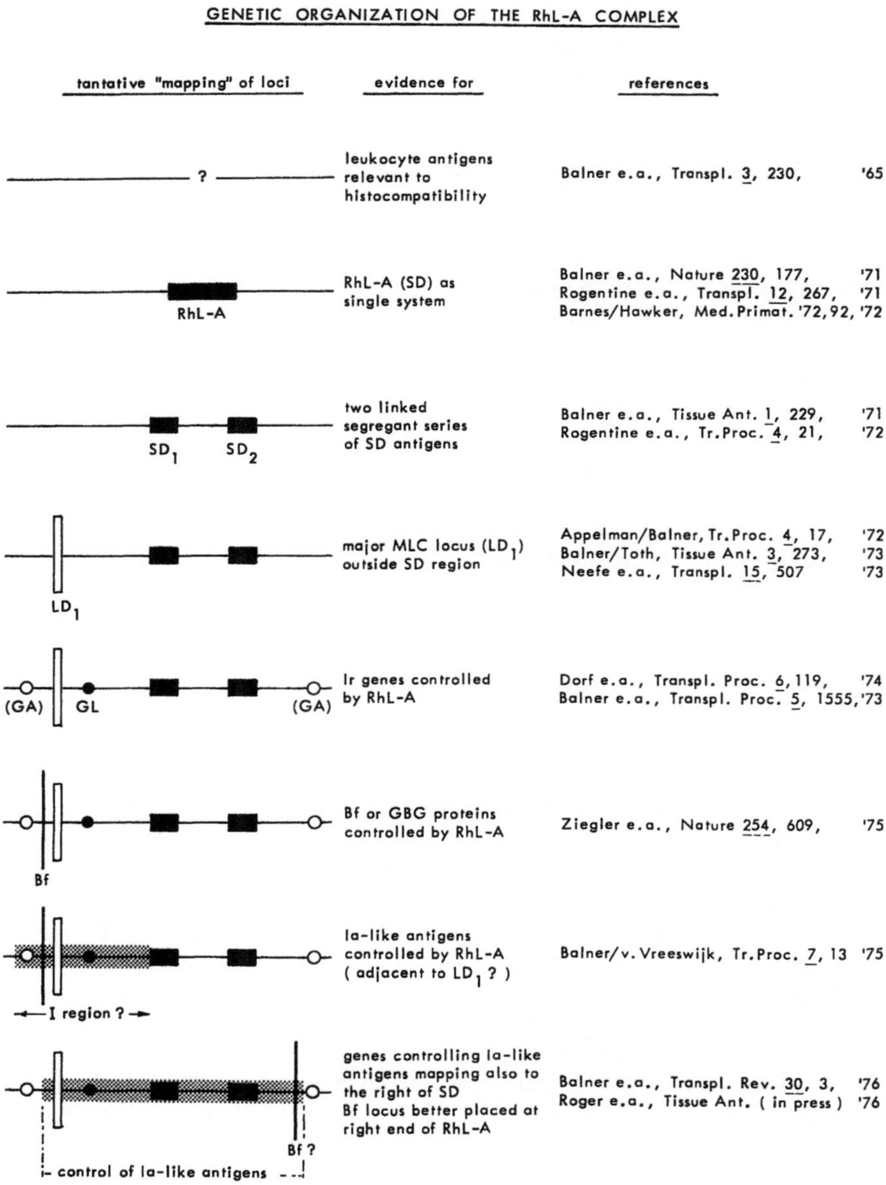

Fig. 2.1. Genetic organization of the RhL-A system

Around 1970, evidence was obtained that a number of fairly well-defined SD antigens of rhesus monkeys are probably controlled by genes of a single system. The methods used for antigen identification and for data analysis in related and unrelated animals were similar to those used for the study of HLA in man. Haplotyping of families and intersib skin-grafting experiments by the Rijswijk team proved the relevance of the system to histocompatibility and led to its name, RhL-A (Balner et al. 1971b). Evidence that the antigens were controlled by two segregant series was not yet available.

Approximately a year later, the Dutch and American investigators independently demonstrated control of the identifiable SD antigens by two closely linked loci (Balner et al. 1971c; Gabb et al. 1972; Rogentine et al. 1972). The number of definable antigens was still small, but it increased rapidly in the following years. The first Primate histocompatibility workshop (Rijswijk 1971) led to international acceptance of RhL-A as the MHS of rhesus monkeys and to agreement on the serological definition of certain antigens (Balner et al. 1972a).

The next step was the identification of a major MLC locus in the RhL-A complex. Again, the Rijswijk and Bethesda investigators independently and more or less simultaneously established the existence of a major MLC locus (LD_1 or Lad_1) closely linked to the SD region and one or more minor loci probably controlled by the same chromosomal segment (Balner and Toth 1973; Neefe et al. 1973). Data obtained with cells from several recombinant offspring in the Rijswijk rhesus colony placed the LD_1 system outside the SD region of RhL-A. However, its location *vis-à-vis* the two SD loci (adjacent to SD_1 or to SD_2) could not be firmly established, because only a single SD_1/SD_2 recombinant with an appropriate sibling (sharing the other parental haplotype) was available. Thus, the exact location of LD_1 versus SD_1 and SD_2 remains to be determined, although recent evidence for the mapping position of various genes and loci within RhL-A, supports the original assumption of LD_1 lying adjacent to SD_1 (Balner et al. 1976).

In the early 1970s, interest in the genetics of the immune response was greatly stimulated by the discovery of possible associations between HLA antigens and disease susceptibility in man (Möller 1975). These observations, plus the previous elegant work on the genetics of the immune response and disease susceptibility in mice (Lilly 1965) and the discovery of MHS-linked Ir genes in guinea pigs (Benacerraf and McDevitt 1972; Polák et al. 1968), prompted similar work in rhesus monkeys. Collaborations ensued between the Dutch workers and those who had established histocompatibility-linked Ir genes in rodents and guinea pigs. In 1973, preliminary evidence was obtained that suggested that MHC-linked genes also control the humoral response to the synthetic polypeptide (TG)AL in the rhesus monkey (Balner et al. 1973a). Lack of informative data precluded the actual mapping of a proposed (TG)AL gene within the RhL-A system. Shortly thereafter, an Ir gene controlling the humoral response to the copolymer GL (conjugated to DNP) was found to be located in the RhL-A system, probably between the LD_1 locus and the SD region (Dorf et al. 1974). The same authors proposed the existence of another MHC-linked Ir gene of rhesus monkeys, the Ir-GA gene, which was tentatively located outside the LD-SD region of RhL-A, either to its left or right (Dorf et al. 1975; see also Section 2.4 and Table 2.7).

Table 2.9. Genotyping for Serologically Defined (SD) Antigens of RhL-A and Properdin Factor B (Bf) Genes in Rhesus Monkey Families

Parents and Offspring	SD[a] Haplotype	Bf Type	Parents and Offspring	SD Haplotype	Bf Type	Parents and Offspring	SD Haplotype	Bf Type	Parents and Offspring	SD Haplotype	Bf Type
♂381	ab	SS	♂598[b]	ab	(SIF)	♂599	ab	FS	♂600	ab	SF
♀584	cd	SS	♀834	cd	FS	♀581	cd	FF	♀669	cd	SS
V	bd	SS	UU	bc	FF	G	bc	SF	AC	ad	SS
JJ	bc	SS	BD	bc	FF	GG	bc	SF	BI	ad	SS
AV	bc	SS	CS	ad	S1S	AG	ac	FF	CR	ad	SS
BU	bc	SS	EK	bc	FF	CF	ac	FF	EL	bc	FS
CZ	bc	SS				DV	bc	SF	FS	bc	FS
♀432	cd	G1F	♀730	cd	SG1	♀1115	cd	SS1	♀603	cd	FS
N	ac	SG1	FF	bd	FG1	CL	a/bc	FS	T	bd	FS
AK	bd	SF	BT	ac	S1S	EF	bd	SS1	DF	bd	FS
CP	ad	SF	DA	ad	S1G1	GZ	ac	FS	FO	bd	FS
FN	ac	SG1							GY	bc	FF
♀852	cd	FS	♀832	cd	FS	♀498	cd	SF	♀597	cd	FF
AH	ac	SF	AD	bd	FS	NN	ac	FS	AB	bc	FF
BL	bd	SS	BM	ad	S1S	AQ	ac	FS	BF	bc	FF
DN	ac	SF	CN	ac	S1F	ED	a/bd	FF	CG	ad	SF
EV	ad	SS	DS	bc	FS←				DW	ac	SF
♀594[b]	cd	(.S)	♀589[b]	cd	(SS1)	♀590	cd	SS	♀429	cd	G1F
YY	ad	SS	Z	ac	S1S	CV	bd	SS	XX	bc	FG1
BJ	bd	SS	AE	ad	S1S1	EI	ad	FS	BG	ac	SG1
FU	bd	SS	BP	bc	FS	GD	bd	SS			
						HG	ac	FS			
♀494	cd	SF	♀728	cd	G1S	♀493	cd	G1F			
L	ac	SS	KK	ad	S1S	AX	bc	SF←			
AA	bd	SF	AS	bd	FS	CK	bc	SG1			
AM	ad	SF	EP	ac	S1G1	DM	bc	SG1			
CY	ac	SS									
♀324	cd	S1S1	♀306	cd	FS	♀926	cd	SS			
CU	bc	SS1	SS	bc	FF	DC	bc	SS			
EM	ac	SS1	BK	ac	S1F	FJ	ac	FS			

[a] By convention, a and b are paternal, c and d maternal haplotypes; for details see Balner 1973.
[b] Animal is dead; ( ) Bf type "deduced," when possible. Arrows indicate suggested recombinants for the Bf locus. Recent absorption studies reduce the likelihood that offspring CL and ED (of families 599/1115 and 599/498, respectively) are "conventional" SD recombinants; their SD haplotypes are therefore most probably a/c and a/d (see also Table 2.5).
From Ziegler et al. 1975a.

In 1974, it was found that the human properdin factor B (Bf) of the "alternative complement pathway" is polymorphic and controlled by a locus in the HLA system (Allen 1974). Shortly thereafter, Ziegler et al. described a similar B factor (Bf) polymorphism for rhesus monkeys (Ziegler et al. 1975b). This led to a collaborative study with the Dutch workers to investigate possible linkage of Bf with RhL-A. An elaborate family study (Table 2.9) soon provided evidence that the Bf locus of rhesus monkeys is part of the RhL-A system (Ziegler et al. 1975a). It was tentatively mapped outside and to the left of the LD-SD region of RhL-A. However, more recent mapping of the RhL-A system (in connection with the identification of numerous Ia-like specificities, see below and p. 87) tends to place the Bf locus to the right of the SD region rather than to the left[8] (Balner et al. 1976; Roger et al. 1976).

Interesting new information regarding the mapping of RhL-A comes from the study of the Ia-like antigens. For reasons discussed in Section 2.1, those specificities are provisionally regarded as the monkey's analogues of the murine Ia antigens. Pilot studies in rhesus families, conducted in 1974, suggested control of some of the Ia-like antigens by the RhL-A system and data obtained with one particular reagent placed the gene controlling that specificity in the vicinity of the LD_1 locus (Balner and van Vreeswijk 1975). Subsequent studies in 1975 led to the identification of several new Ia-like specificities, the majority of which are controlled by loci firmly linked to RhL-A. However, the most recent data obtained in rhesus families (including six offspring with recombinations among SD, LD, Ir, or Bf genes) expand the region of RhL-A in which the genes controlling Ia-like specificities could be located. In fact, haplotyping of more than 16 families and a population study of 118 unrelated animals permitted the postulation of at least one allelic series, controlling several Ia-like specificities (hatched area of the RhL-A model at the bottom of Figure 2.1). Detailed information is presented elsewhere (Balner et al. 1976; Roger et al. 1976).

3. ChL-A, the MHS of Chimpanzees

As mentioned in Section 1, the tissue antigens of chimpanzees have been investigated far less extensively than those of man, the rhesus monkey, and several other species. Consequently, the existance of two linked loci controlling serologically defined antigens of chimpanzees has been described only recently (Balner et al. 1974b), and evidence that these SD antigens are the markers of the chimp's major histocompatibility system (ChL-A) is still tenuous. In view of the limited number of unrelated animals available and an even greater scarcity of captive chimp families, the identification of further SD antigens and other gene products of the ChL-A system is expected to take much time. Yet a vivid interest in ChL-A and its products continues,

[8] Data available at the time of proofreading (Dec. '76) support the original assumption that the Bf locus is situated to the left of the SD region.

and the study of the MHS of man's closest relative is being pursued. In this section, the current knowledge of the chimpanzee's "own" tissue alloantigens will be summarized; in the last section, similarities between the MHS products of several primate species, including man and the chimpanzee, will be discussed. There are only two teams of investigators actively involved in the study of ChL-A: one originating at Duke University, Durham, North Carolina, USA (Metzgar, Dorf, Seigler, and Ward), the other at the Primate Center TNO and at Leiden University in Holland (Balner, van Vreeswijk, D'Amaro, van Rood, van Leeuwen, with Gabb [Adelaide, Australia] as consultant for genetics). Because there is relatively little information regarding the biochemistry of ChL-A products,[9] and because no data are available on ChL-A-linked immune response genes, those subjects will not be considered further in this section.

3.1 Detection of Tissue Alloantigens

3.1.1 Serological Methods

Shulman performed the first alloimmunizations of chimpanzees in 1964. Of 18 animals immunized with platelets and leukocytes, only one formed demonstrable alloantibodies. This serum, which did not react with human cells (the original aim of the experiment), was not analyzed further (Shulman et al. 1965). During the past decade, the Duke and the Dutch investigators have made dermined efforts to identify the SD antigens of the chimpanzee's MHS. Chronologically, this era can be divided into three "periods." In the first six or seven years, both teams produced sera by random alloimmunizations. Those sera identified the initial groups or "broad" chimpanzee specificities. The second period began around 1972, after the first Primate Workshop in Rijswijk (Balner et al. 1972a). Based on matching of host/donor combinations according to the then-identifiable leukocyte groups, the Dutch began to produce antisera of narrower specificity. Those efforts led to the identification of a dozen "short" antigens and the postulation of two closely linked segregant series controlling these SD antigens (Balner et al. 1974a, 1974b). The third period has only just began (1975): Serum producers and unrelated immunizing donors are matched more accurately for all identifiable SD antigens, and related chimpanzees (sibs and half-sibs) are used for the production of antisera.

The methods used for alloimmunizations, for testing the reagents against lymphocytes, and for data analysis were essentially the same as those used for man and rhesus monkeys. The leukoagglutination test was rapidly replaced by the more reproducible microlymphocytotoxicity test, and conven-

---

[9] ChL-A specificities can be extracted from the cell membrane using the same techniques as those employed for the solubilization of human HLA antigens; the soluble products of human and chimpanzee origin have similar molecular characteristics on Sephadex gels (Dorf et al. 1970).

tional absorptions (with platelets and/or leukocytes) were done to improve the quality of the sera and test the degree of specificity.

The first period of chimpanzee typing began in the mid-1960s. In 1967 the Dutch described the reactivity patterns of their first five chimp alloantisera; when tested on a small panel of chimp and human leukocytes, these sera seemed to detect HLA-related antigens (4a, 4b, 7c; see below) on human as well as chimp cells (Balner et al. 1967c). In 1969 and 1970, the same investigators described the first "broad" chimpanzee specificities: Five groups of alloantisera gave similar reactivity patterns when tested against cells of 46 unrelated chimpanzees. According to absorption studies, three groups detected chimpanzee alloantigens defined by operationally monospecific sera, the other two groups of sera detected 4a- and 4b-like specificities (Balner et al. 1970). In 1971, the Dutch screened 198 unrelated chimpanzees with 27 selected alloantisera. This study suggested the existence of eight leukocyte groups, several of which turned out to be antigens of the current ChL-A (SD) system. Statistical relationships among those eight early groups were consistent with control by a single genetic system (Balner et al. 1971a). Simultaneously and independently, the Duke investigators described seven broad chimpanzee groups based on the testing of 47 cell samples with 53 chimp sera (Dorf and Metzgar 1970a). They had also raised chimp sera that were able to identify antigens 4a and 4b on chimp and human cells. This initial period of chimp typing was concluded by comparing the reactivity patterns of the available sera during the first primate workshop in 1971 (Balner et al. 1972c; Metzgar et al. 1972a). Fifty-five of the sera were used to define 14 provisional chimpanzee groups, which were given ChW (chimp workshop) designations. Table 2.10 shows the resulting similarities among the groups defined by the Dutch and the Americans; about 50 percent of the chimp groups were recognized by both teams. The proposed similarities with HLA-like antigens are also shown in the table (see also below). The associations of reactivity patterns of the sera defining the various ChW groups can be found in the joint report of the first workshop (Balner et al. 1972a).

The second period of chimpanzee typing was characterized by the production of alloantibodies after a more meaningful selection of donors for alloimmunization (matched according to all identifiable groups) and by the use of optimal dilutions of existing oligospecific sera. Table 2.11 gives the phenotype distribution in 60 unrelated chimpanzees of 11 "narrow" specificities of the two proposed segregant series of ChL-A (Balner et al. 1974a). It can be seen that only antigens 111 and 106 of the "first period" (ChW-111 and ChW-106 of Table 2.9) remained as candidate antigens of the first and second segregant series, respectively. Evidence for linkage between the proposed loci of ChL-A was obtained in a family study carried out during the second Primate workshop (Atlanta 1973). Figure 2.2 shows a small part of the pedigree studied. It is apparent that haplotype 111–117 was passed from Soda to Franz and to Dena and subsequently to the great-grandchild Stanford (for details, see Balner et al. 1974b). The reason that the described antigens are believed to be the SD markers of the chimpanzee's MHS are given below.

Table 2.10. Leukocyte Specificities of Chimpanzees: Relation Between Workshop and Previous Nomenclature

Workshop Nomenclature	Original Rijswijk/Leiden Nomenclature	Original Duke Nomenclature	Similarities with Human Antigens	
			Firm	Vague
ChW4	1	I, II	4a	HLA-A11
ChW6	4	III	4b	
ChW11	8		HLA-A11	
ChW101		VIII		
ChW102	2	VI		
ChW103	5			
ChW104	6	I		
ChW105	3	IV		7cAA
ChW106	3 (short)			7cAA
ChW107	4 (short)			4b
ChW108	8 (short)		HLA-A11	
ChW109				
ChW110		VII		4b
ChW111	7 (short)			

For detailed explanation of symbols, etc., see "Joint Report of the First International Primate Workshop," Rijswijk, 1971 (Balner et al. 1972a).

The third period of chimpanzee typing has now been started by the Dutch investigators. The availability of more than 20 chimpanzees born at the Rijswijk center between 1970 and 1976 now permits the mutual immunization of several sibs and half-sibs sharing one ChL-A haplotype. Moreover, the increased possibilities of selecting immunizing donors among unrelated animals also permits the production of typing reagents of higher specificity and better quality. Results already available suggest that some of the group-specific sera described in 1974 show subdivisions similar to the "splits" observed for human typing reagents defining certain HLA antigens. Preliminary absorption, population, and family studies with the new chimp alloantisera have led to the identification of six or more new SD antigens. Provisional results obtained with the new reagents permit a more reliable identification of several of the previously established SD antigens (although a few of those tentative "older" antigens may have to be abandoned as biological entities). An elaborate serological analysis (absorptions, etc.) and a world-wide population and family study using these new reagents, is in progress.

At the time of this writing, no data are available on which to assume the existence of a third SD series of CHL-A; Ia-like alloantigens have also not yet been identified in chimpanzees.

3.1.2 Cellular Methods

Mixed lymphocyte cultures between chimpanzee cells (or chimpanzee cells cultured with human cells; see below) have been performed since 1970 (Bach

Table 2.11. Phenotype Distribution of 11 Specificities in Two Proposed Segregant Series of ChL-A (60 Unrelated Chimpanzees)

First Series

Gene frequency	Group 1	Group 2	Observed	Expected
0.1810	108	112	1	1.32
		113	6	3.74
		111	2	2.09
		Null	11	12.61
0.0608	112	113	0	1.25
		111	1	0.70
		Null	5	3.80
0.1720	113	111	2	1.98
		Null	11	11.89
0.0961	111	Null	6	6.21
0.4901	Null	Null	15	14.41
			60	60.00
	$\chi_5^2=2.59$	$0.8>p>0.7$		

Second Series

Gene frequency	Group 1	Group 2	Observed	Expected
0.0508	115	116	0	0.26[b]
		117	2	0.42[b]
		118	1	0.80[b]
		119	0	0.21[c]
		120	1	0.26[c]
		106	0	0.71[c]
		Null	2	3.29
0.0427	116	117	0	0.35[d]
		118	1	0.67[d]
		119	0	0.17[e]
		120	1	0.22[e]
		106	0	0.59[e]
		Null	3	2.74
0.0688	117	118	2	1.09
		119	0	0.28[e]
		120	0	0.35[f]
		106	0	0.96[f]
		Null	4	4.53
0.1316	118	119	1	0.54[g]
		120	0	0.67[g]
		106	3	1.83
		Null	7	9.15
0.0341	119	120	0	0.17[h]
		106	0	0.47[h]
		Null	3	2.17
0.0423	120	106	1	0.59[h]
		Null	2	2.72
0.1159	106	Null	9	7.95
0.5138	Null	Null	17	15.84
			60	60.00
	$\chi_9^2=6.37$	$0.8>p>0.7$		

This analysis is based on the data for 60 unrelated chimpanzees (the Rijswijk colony). Specificity 114 of the first series was not analyzed, for reasons explained in Balner et al. 1974b. The gene frequencies were determined by the gene-counting method of maximum likelihood; a, b, c, etc., indicate that classes so labeled have been pooled in calculating χ^2. From Balner et al. 1974b.

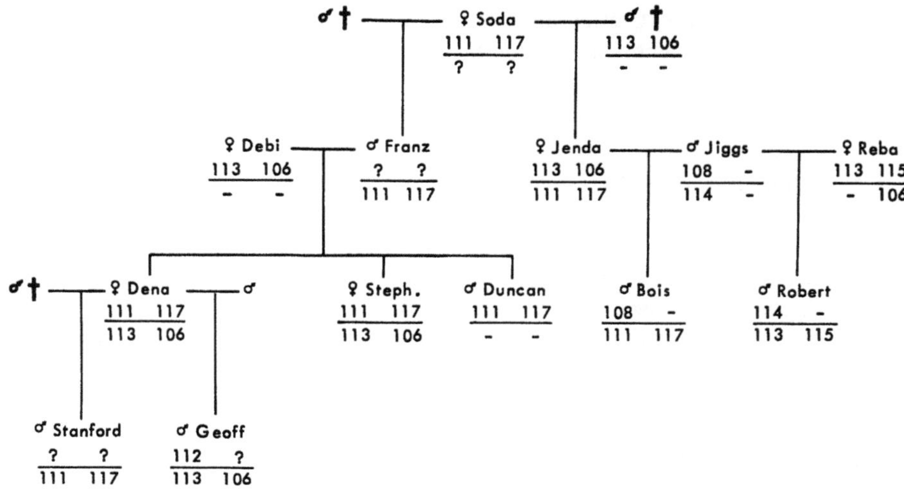

Fig. 2.2. Provisional genotyping of a chimpanzee pedigree for serologically defined specificities of the proposed ChL-A system (part of the colony at the Yerkes Primate Center, Atlanta, Ga., USA). Symbols 108, 111, 112, 113, 114 are specificities of the first; 106, 115, and 117 of the second segregant series of ChL-A (other known antigens are not represented on these cells). Paternal and maternal "haplotypes" above and below horizontal lines, respectively. The deduction of some of the haplotypes, including those of deceased animals, is based on data for the complete pedigree published elsewhere (Balner et al. 1974b). A dash indicates that assumed specificity is serologically still unidentified. A question mark means that homozygosity for the corresponding specificity cannot be excluded

et al. 1972a). As in other species, cultures of cells from unrelated, unmatched individuals virtually always show stimulation[10]. Apparently, the number of unrelated chimpanzees available at any laboratory is too small to find the odd MLC-negative combination, and the selection of SD full-house identical combinations (10 percent of which may be MLC-negative in man or rhesus monkey) has not been possible up to now.

To establish a major MLC locus linked to ChL-A, MLC studies with cells from members of chimpanzee families are required: If sibs genotypically identical for ChL-A do not show stimulation in MLC, while any other combination does, this would permit the assumption of a ChL-A-linked LD_1 locus in chimpanzees. Moreover, the hypothesis of ChL-A as the MHS of chimpanzees would be further supported (although not proved) by such a finding. In 1973, Seigler and colleagues at Duke University had access to a sufficient number of chimpanzee siblings to test the hypothesis. They performed classical MLC studies in the chimpanzee families available at

[10] Techniques used and levels of stimulation observed in chimp MLC's are similar to those described for man, rhesus monkey and other species. Certain interesting anomalies, like the rather frequent occurrence of high thymidine incorporation when lymphocytes from some of the chimpanzees are cultured alone ("autologous" cultures without allogeneic cells or mitogens), are to be published shortly (A. A. van Es, *in preparation*).

the Yerkes Primate Center and reported that genotypically identical sibs did not stimulate, whereas nonidentical sibs did (Seigler et al. 1974).

Preliminary results of LD typing of chimpanzee lymphocytes with human homozygous LD-typing cells are discussed in the last section of this chapter.

3.2 Histocompatibility

The limited number of chimpanzees in research laboratories, their preciousness and the technical problems of working with such large primates are the reasons for the scarcity of data regarding allograft survival in chimpanzees. If we consider the rather provisional character of SD typing in chimps and the virtual absence of other matching procedures, it will be understood why proving the relevance of the proposed ChL-A system to histocompatibility has been impossible. Yet some circumstantial evidence that the described SD antigens may be the markers of the chimp's MHS has become available. Table 2.12 shows that the survival times of skin grafts exchanged between two pairs of chimps sharing one or two ChL-A haplotypes are distinctly longer than those observed for grafts exchanged between unmatched, unrelated individuals. Although the number of combinations is small, the difference in mean survival time is significant. This limited information on skin allograft survival obtained in a few related and unrelated chimps of the Rijswijk center, might be regarded as provisional evidence that the identifiable SD antigens are controlled by the chimpanzee's major histocompatibility system, ChL-A.

In other laboratories, chimpanzees have also been used on a limited scale for renal, hepatic, and/or cardiac allografting. However, the results of those experiments are not relevant to the current discussion, because meaningful typing and/or matching of the unrelated chimpanzees was not performed and immunosuppression was applied in most instances.

Table 2.12. Survival of Skin Allografts in Chimpanzees

	Unrelated Animals ($n=24$)	Sibs and Half-sibs Sharing One or Two ChL-A Haplotypes ($n=4$)
Individual survival times of grafts (in days)	10, 10, 10, 10, 10, 10, 10, 10	15
	11, 11, 11, 11, 11	16
	12, 12, 12, 12, 12, 12, 12	17
	13, 13, 13	19
	14	
Mean (±S.D.)	11.3 (±1.20)	16.8 (±1.71)
Significance	$p<0.001$	

All animals were unimmunized before skin grafting; they received two grafts from each donor and no immunosuppression. Techniques and methods for evaluating graft survival have been described (Balner et al. 1965a).

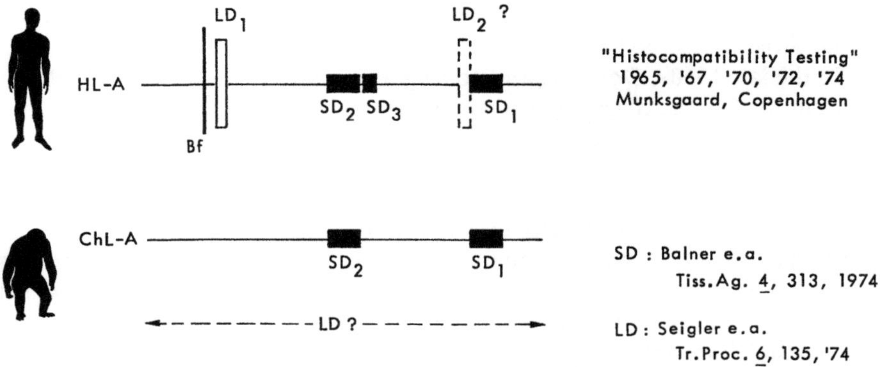

Fig. 2.3. Current state of genetic mapping of the proposed ChL-A system and comparison with the human HLA system

3.3 Genetic Organization of the ChL-A System

Although the working hypothesis of ChL-A as the major histocompatibility system of chimpanzees was proposed some years ago (Balner et al. 1971a), meaningful genetic mapping of the ChL-A region has not been possible so far. Figure 2.3 demonstrates the paucity of information available for the ChL-A system compared to that for HLA (the now obsolete, original nomenclature is used). The reasons for placing the SD_1 and SD_2 loci of ChL-A "in parallel" with the human LA and Four series, respectively, is detailed in the reference given in Figure 2.3 and is discussed briefly in the last section of this review, dealing with interspecies similarities. The existence of a major MLC or LD_1 locus within the ChL-A system can be safely predicted. However, as indicated earlier, the available experimental data do not yet permit the definite incorporation of an LD_1 locus into the ChL-A system, nor to determine its mapping position. Data for other genetic markers, in particular those that are MHS-linked in related species such as man or rhesus monkey (Ir, Ia, Bf, enzymes, etc.), are not yet available for chimpanzees.

4. Tissue Antigens of Other Subhuman Primates

4.1 Baboons

Three subgenera of baboons (*Papio ursinus, P. cynophalus,* and *P. anubis*) have been widely used in biomedical research, including transplantation (Dubernard et al. 1971; Murphy and Brede 1972; Myburgh et al. 1971). Concerted efforts by two teams[11] have led to the identification of a few

[11] Downing and colleagues in Durban, South Africa, and A. D. Barnes and colleagues in Birmingham, U.K.

leukocyte groups of baboons, but a major histocompatibility system of either of the three mentioned baboon species has not yet been established.

In the late 1960s, Downing and colleagues began the production of alloantisera in the South-African *P. ursinus* (Downing et al. 1972). Sixteen baboons were immunized with skin and leukocytes from unselected donors. Fifteen of the sera showed interesting reactivity patterns when tested against lymphocytes of 45 baboons (cytotoxicity). A chi-square analysis revealed positive associations among the reactivity patterns of some of the sera; they were "grouped" together but not analyzed further. Subsequently, these groups of sera were used to match six pairs of baboons for alloimmunization which led to the production of antibodies of narrower specificity (Downing et al. 1974). The characteristics of those reagents are currently being investigated by absorptions as well as by population and family studies (H. J. Downing, *personal communication*). Recently, Downing has also applied parent-offspring immunizations and raised several interesting additional sera. Provisional data obtained with those sera indicate that they may identify SD antigens controlled by separate loci. However, it is not yet possible to state that the antigens are controlled by a single genetic region, nor is there published evidence that they are serological markers of the baboon's MHS.

Barnes and colleagues from Birmingham studied the tissue antigens of the two other commonly used baboon species, *P. anubis* and *P. cynocephalus*, both imported from Kenya. Initially, the selection of donors for immunization was made by typing the animals with RhL-A, HLA, and various other types of antisera (Barnes and Hawker 1972); in this manner four interesting sera were produced, two by alloimmunization (cyno/cyno), the other by cross-immunization (cyno/anubis). These sera, as well as those produced by Downing in *P. ursinus*, were tested against a small panel of lymphocytes from *P. cynocephalus* and *P. anubis*. Limited absorption studies suggested that two of the Birmingham sera were oligospecific. However, no similarities were found between the reactivity patterns of the Birmingham and Durban alloantisera (Ford et al. 1974).

In summary, the MHS of the principal baboon species of central and southern Africa have not yet been established; however, investigations to reach that goal are in progress. Certain similarities between the tissue antigens of *P. cynocephalus* and those of rhesus monkeys (RhL-A) are discussed below (see Section 5.2).

4.2 Other Primate Species

Crab-eating monkeys (*Macaca irus*) and stumptail macaques (*M. arctoides*) are used extensively in various kinds of biomedical research. Nevertheless, little attention has been paid to the study of their tissue antigens. The Dutch investigators are currently raising stumptail alloantisera that are likely to identify the conventional SD antigens of that species. Although predictable, there is as yet no proof that the antigens currently being identified by that team, are the SD markers of the stumptail monkey's MHS. On the other hand, there is fairly solid evidence that several of the RhL-A antigens (or antigens very similar to them) are also present on lymphocytes of stumptail macaques and that these SD antigens are probably controlled by two closely linked series of alleles (see Section 5.2).

The study of tissue antigens of several widely used species of New World monkeys has been conspicuously neglected. Limited data on MLC reactivity in one or two common marmoset species are available (N. Gengozian and G. Mahouy, *personal communication*), but serious attempts to identify the marmosets' tissue antigens by serological means have not been reported.

In summary, the tissue antigens of primate species other than man, the chimpanzee, and the rhesus monkey have not been thoroughly investigated. At the Rijswijk center, work is in progress to identify the serological markers of the stumptail macaque's MHS.

5. Similarities Among Tissue Antigens of Various Primate Species

One way of studying the evolutionary development of the mammalian MHS is to look for similarities among the products of that important chromosomal region. This can be done, for instance, by testing cells from one species with alloantisera produced in another. Before discussing the various methods employed in interspecies typing of primates, the terminology used in this last section should be briefly explained.

The MHS of any species is best defined by intraspecies typing with alloantisera; the latter are obtained by immunization with tissue from individuals of the same genus (human-antihuman, chimp-antichimp, etc.). Interspecies typing is the expression used for the testing of alloantisera from one species against the cells of another. Such studies include interspecies absorptions and elutions as well as the retesting of the absorbed and/or eluted reagents against the cells of both species involved.

The expression "interspecies" is used for the typing between closely related species (e.g., human sera tested against chimp cells) as well as for the testing between remotely related species (e.g., rhesus sera tested against human cells). However, a distinction is made with regard to the method of producing the antibodies; sera produced by immunizing animals with antigens from a closely related species are called *cross-immune* (e.g., chimp-antihuman), sera produced by immunization with tissue from a remotely related species are termed *heteroimmune* (e.g., rabbit-antihuman). Tissue antigens of primates have also been investigated with cross-immune and heteroimmune antisera. But those studies contributed little to the detection of similarities among tissue antigens of the various primate species and will therefore not be reviewed. On the other hand, the availability of excellent alloantisera defining the MHS products of man, the chimpanzee, and the rhesus monkey offered an attractive way of studying similarities among the antigens of those species. The results of such studies also provide leads on the evolutionary development of the MHC. However, as we shall see below, there can be pitfalls and technical difficulties in interspecies typing,[12] and conclusions about antigenic similarities among species should therefore be drawn with great caution.

5.1 Similarities Between Alloantigens of Man and Chimpanzee

5.1.1 Human Alloantisera Tested with Chimpanzee Cells

Shulman first tested human alloantisera against chimpanzee cells in 1964. Although he failed to show polymorphism on chimpanzee cells, he was able to fractionate the multispecific human sera by absorption with chimp platelets (Shulman et al. 1965). Thus, he could demonstrate indirectly that chimpanzees may carry tissue antigens similar to those of man.

In 1966, the investigators at Duke University detected polymorphism on chimp leukocytes, using human alloantisera of undefined specificity. Unfortunately, absorption studies were not performed and conclusions regarding the similarity of tissue antigens of chimp and man could not be drawn (Metzgar and Zmijewski 1966). Shortly thereafter, the Dutch team was able to report the "probable presence" of eight defined human alloantigens on chimpanzee cells (Balner et al. 1967b). The antigens in question were the broad human specificities identifiable in the mid-1960s and the techniques used were leukocyte agglutination and absorptions.

These early encouraging results prompted both teams of investigators to continue the work on a larger scale and with more sophisticated techniques. By 1970, many monospecific HLA antisera, more reliable testing procedures, and numerous interesting chimp alloantisera had become available. Thus, it soon became possible to predict, with some confidence, which of the "HLA-like" antigens were likely to be carried by chimpanzees. The criteria used to determine this "likelihood" are depicted schematically in Table 2.13. A summary of the data available in the early and mid-1970s is presented in Table 2.14. The left part of the table shows the results obtained by typing chimp cells with human sera, employing various techniques (sometimes including absorptions to corroborate the results of direct typing). Space limitations prevent a detailed description of the serological data that have been published in numerous reports by the American (Dorf and Metzgar et al. 1970a, 1970b; Metzgar et al. 1972b) and the Dutch investigators (Balner et al. 1971a; van Leeuwen et al. 1972; van Rood et al. 1972) between 1967 and 1972. Suffice it to say that there was fair agreement between results obtained independently by both teams. Moreover, if the presence of an HLA-like antigen on chimp cells was considered "probable" at any particular

[12] One of the complications is the occasional presence in the test sera of preformed, heterophile antibodies, in some species combinations. However, such interfering antibodies can be easily removed by absorption with red cells of the primate species to be tested (Dorf and Haber 1972).

Table 2.13. Criteria for Assuming the Presence of HLA-like Antigens on Chimpanzee Cells

Serological Conditions That Apply		Likelihood That HLA-like Antigen Is Present on Chimp Cells
1. A single HLA serum shows polymorphism, using one technique		Unlikely
2. Several HLA sera show concordant typing results	using one technique	Unlikely
	using several techniques	Possible
3. HLA reactivity removed by absorption with chimp cells (retesting on human cells)		Probable
4. "Meaningful" results obtained in absorption and elution studies using cells and sera of both species (see text for explanation)		Very likely
5. Alloimmunization of chimpanzees yields antibody of same HLA specificity in man		Very likely

time, this was nearly always confirmed in subsequent studies using better reagents and more refined techniques. A summary of the serological results obtained during the most recent human histocompatibility workshop (Aarhus 1975) is depicted graphically in Figure 2.4.

5.1.2 Chimpanzee Alloantisera Tested with Human Cells

The logical counterpart of the described work with human alloantisera and chimpanzee cells is the testing of human cells with chimp alloantisera. As indicated above, the Dutch investigators produced chimp alloantisera with defined specificity against human cells in 1966 (Balner et al. 1967c). The identified specificities were the broad or supertypic 4a, 4b, and 7c. In the following years, all newly produced chimp alloantisera[13] were screened against panels of selected human cells (using various techniques) and the number of chimp sera with "interesting" reactivity patterns against human cells increased steadily. By 1971, a respectable number of "HLA-like" antigens could be identified on human cells with chimp alloantisera. Once again, the serological data cannot be presented in the context of this review, and the reader is referred to the ample literature for details (Balner et al. 1970; Dorf and Metzgar 1970a; Metzgar et al. 1972b; van Rood et al. 1972). However, the reactivity of several chimpanzee alloantisera showing particularly high correlations with HLA sera (when both were tested against human cells) is shown in Table 2.15. A summary of the serological results available by 1975 is presented in Table 2.14 (second broad column). It can be seen that chimp alloantisera can define at least three antigens of the first as well as the second series of HLA (A1, A11, A29, and Bw15, Bw17, Bw22,

[13] These sera were produced by both teams in the framework of identifying the ChL-A system, see Section 3.1

Table 2.14. HLA Related Specificities Detected with Human and Chimpanzee Alloantisera Tested Against Chimpanzee and Human Cells, Respectively

HLA Antigens		Human Alloantisera Tested with Chimpanzee Cells: Early Data (1966–1971) Duke Team	Early Data (1966–1971) Dutch Team	Recent Data – Workshop Sera: Evian, 1972 Duke Team	Evian, 1972 Dutch Team	Aarhus, 1975 Dutch Team	Chimpanzee Alloantisera Tested with Human Cells: Early Data (1966–1971) Duke Team	Early Data (1966–1971) Dutch Team	Recent Data (1975) Dutch Team	Conclusions: HLA-like Antigens Present or Possibly ( ) Present on Chimp Cells	ChL-A Antigens Possibly Related to the "Shared" HLA Antigens	
	1	(1*)	1*	1	1	1		1	1	1	112	
	2											
	3	(3*)		(3)		3		(3)	(3)	(3)		
	9 {W23								(9)			
	9 {W24											
First	10 {W25											
series	10 {W26	(10)	(10)	(10)					(10)	(10)		First
of HLA	11	11*	11*	11	11	11	11	11	11	11	W108	series of
(LA,	19 {29		29		29	29			29	29	W111	ChL-A
HLA-A)	19 {W30											
	19 {W31					W31						
	19 {W32					W32	W32			(W32)		
	W33											
	28	(28)	(28*)	(28)	(28)		(28)			(28)	(113)	
	W34											
	(MO) W36					W36						

		5											
		7	(7*)	(7*)	(7)					(7)	(7)	(W106)	
		8	(8)										
		12	(12)	(12)	(12)					(12)			
		13	(13)	(13)	(13)								
		14		(14)									
Second		18											
series		27		27*		27	27				(27)		Second
of HLA	(W5)	W35											series of
(Four,	(W10)	W40											ChL-A
HLA-B)		W15		W15*	W15	W15	W15		W15	W15	W15	115	
		W16											
		W17		W17*	W17	W17	W17	(W17)	(W17)	W17	W17	119	
		W22		W22*		W22	W22		W22	W22	W22	W106	
	(TY)	W37				W37				W37			
	(W161)	W38				38							
	(Sab)	W41											
	(MWA)	W42					W42						
		4a	4a*	4a*	4a	4a		4a	4a	4a	4a	4a	
"Super-		4b	4b	4b*	4b	4b		4b	4b	4b	4b	4b	
typic"		6a		(6a)									
specifi-		7a		(7a)									
cities		7b		(7b)									
		7c*		7c*					7c				

The HLA nomenclature in the extreme left column shows the older designations as well as the "splits" agreed upon at the 6th human histocompatibility workshop (Aarhus, 1975).

In the body of the table, asterisks indicate that the proposed presence of an antigen is based also on absorptions with cells of the other species. Brackets indicate that the serological evidence for the sharing of the antigen is tenuous. For detailed information see references in the text.

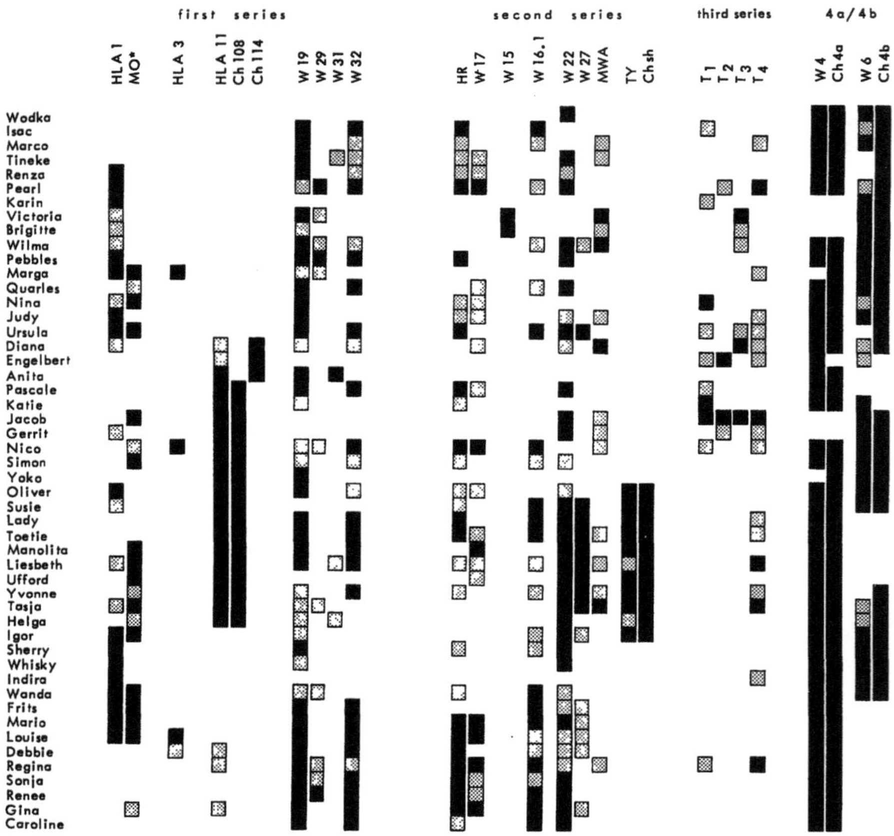

Fig. 2.4. Serological interspecies typing between man and chimpanzee (lymphocytotoxicity). Results of typing 50 chimpanzees with 137 human workshop sera (1975), the "Leiden HLA serum set," and several groups of chimpanzee alloantisera (Ch 108, Ch 114, Ch 4a, Ch 4b, and Ch-sh). Solid squares ■ = strongly positive reactions with majority of sera defining a group; stippled squares ▣ = weakly positive; negative reactions are left blank. (From Schreuder et al. 1975)

respectively). If the rules of Table 2.13 are adhered to, it appears that these are the six "HLA-like" antigens that are most probably carried by chimpanzees (extreme right columns of Table 2.14; compare also Bodmer et al. 1972). Another good candidate might be the new HLA antigen TY or W37: As can be seen in Figure 2.4, one particular chimp alloantiserum (Ch-Sh) showed an identical reactivity pattern with human TY sera when both types of sera were tested against chimpanzee lymphocytes. However, this chimp alloantiserum has not yet been screened against human cells.

How similar are the tissue antigens that, according to the serological data reviewed above, are shared by chimpanzee and man? Biochemical characterization of individual antigens of either species has not reached the degree of sophistication to provide the answer. On the other hand, meticulous ab-

Table 2.15. Chimpanzee Alloantisera Tested with Human Cells

Chimpanzee Alloantisera (and ChL-A Groups)	Human Alloantisera Against	2×2 Associations of Reactivity Patterns			
		+/+	+/−	−/+	−/−
Ti_5 (W108)	HLA-A11	15	1	0	174
An_{23} (115)[a]	W15	22	1	1	120
El_{14} (W106)	W22	7	2	0	49
Sera W4 (4a)	4a	58	1	0	23
Sera W6 (4b)	4b	68	0	1	13

[a] Complement fixation on human platelets; all other sera tested by lymphocytotoxicity.

sorption and elution studies can be very useful in this respect. Employing those techniques, Dorf et al. were able to show a striking similarity (but also distinct differences) between the human HLA-A11 antigen and its chimpanzee counterpart ChW 108 (Dorf et al. 1972). Unfortunately, similar experiments have not yet been performed with sera identifying any of the other antigens that seem to be shared by man and chimpanzee.

5.1.3 Chimpanzee and Human Alloantisera Tested with Cells from Other Primate Species

Chimp alloantisera have been used to "type" small numbers of unrelated gorillas and orangutans. Although the three species involved belong to the same taxonomic family (Pongidae, see Table 2.1), the chimp sera that define ChL-A antigens in chimpanzees and show interesting patterns in man, never reacted concordantly[14] in either gorillas or orangutans (Metzgar et al. 1972a). The serological data obtained by the American as well as the Dutch investigators are not interpretable, also because systematic absorption studies have never been done. An interesting observation made by both teams was that most gorillas reacted strongly with anti-4a sera but hardly ever with anti-4b sera, whereas orangutans virtually never reacted with anti-4a sera and nearly always with anti-4b sera.

Reactivity patterns of chimpanzee alloantisera tested against cells from rhesus monkeys and stumptail macaques have been obtained and analyzed. It is interesting that these lower primates also seem to carry 4a- and 4b-like specificities (Bright and Balner 1976) and that the distribution of those broad human antigens (unlike in gorillas and orangutans) is similar to that seen in man and chimpanzee (see below).

Human alloantisera produced equally uninteresting results when tested with small panels of gorilla and orangutan cells (Seigler et al. 1972). The Duke investigators speculated that an antigen similar to HLA-B12 might be present in orangs and one similar to HLA-B7 on gorilla cells. This was assumed on the basis of rather concordant typing results with groups of

[14] Lack of concordance means that not all sera identifying a particular alloantigen react positively or negatively against a cell of the other species.

antisera but never corroborated by absorption studies. In conclusion, it is peculiar that chimpanzee and human alloantisera (which show highly interesting cross-reactivity with each other) should produce such uninterpretable results when tested with cells from gorillas and orangutans. In fact, these data can be regarded as suggestive evidence that the latter species share few (if any) SD antigens with man and chimpanzee.

Human alloantisera were also tested against cell panels from rhesus monkeys and stumptail macaques (lymphocytotoxicity). Reactivity patterns were similar to those observed with chimp alloantisera; few of the sera showed distinct patterns of cytotoxicity, and none of the groups of sera defining a particular HLA antigen showed a concordant pattern with monkey cells. However, as was the case with chimp alloantisera, the monkey cells did react with the anti-4a and/or the anti-4b sera, albeit less avidly than with analogous chimp-alloantisera. The presence of 4a- and 4b-like antigens on rhesus monkey cells had already been postulated by the Dutch team in 1967; this was done on the basis of absorption studies using human antisera and rhesus monkey leukocytes (Balner et al. 1967c). Recent elaborate serological studies, including meticulous absorptions, confirmed and expanded the early observations that macaques carry antigens similar to 4a and 4b of man and the chimpanzee (Bright and Balner 1976). Unlike in gorillas and orangutans (see above), the phenotypic distribution of those antigens in lower monkeys is as follows: Virtually all rhesus or stumptail macaques tested carry either 4a or 4b, or both. The tracing of those supertypic antigens down the evolutionary ladder to the lower Old World monkeys revives the early speculations by the Dutch investigators (Balner et al. 1971a; van Rood et al. 1972) that 4a and 4b may well be the "basic substance" from which the important tissue antigens of primates evolved.

Finally, some investigators (Murphy et al. 1969) have described the reactivity of human alloantisera with baboon lymphocytes (*P. ursinus*). In 1971, Cohen et al. (1970) reported on interesting polymorphic reactivity patterns of numerous HLA sera; however, absorptions were not performed, so the data remain basically uninterpretable.

5.1.4 Cellular Methods

In view of the observed similarities between the serologically defined antigens of the human and chimpanzee MHS, it seemed worthwhile to look for similarities in other products of that chromosomal region. Mixed lymphocyte cultures between chimpanzee and man had been performed in the early 1970s (Bach et al. 1972a); the degree of stimulation obtained in such interspecies MLCs was very similar to that obtained in MLCs performed with human or chimpanzee cells only. Interesting as this may be, it provided no information regarding the possible similarities between the LD antigens of man and the chimpanzee. The recent availability of reliable human LD-typing cells (discussed elsewhere in this volume), prompted the Dutch team to test their chimpanzees against the panel of human LD-typing cells available at

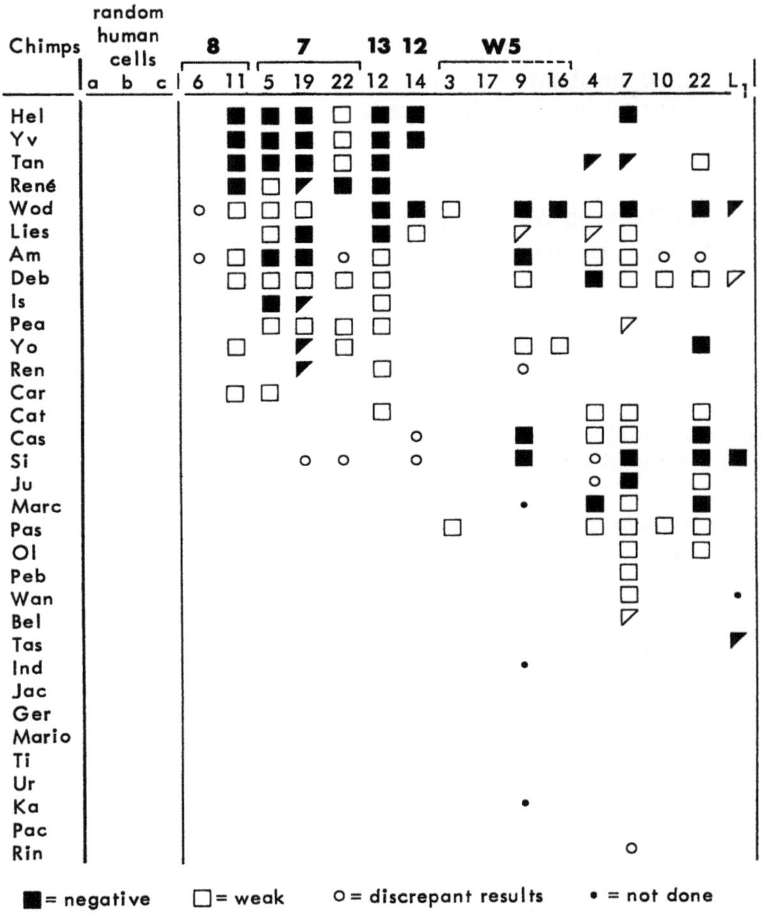

Fig. 2.5. Provisional "LD typing" of chimpanzees with human lymphocytes. Results of testing lymphocytes from 30 chimpanzees with human LD-typing cells in unilateral mixed cultures. Triangular symbols indicate that tests were performed only once (in all other instances they were done at least twice, on different days). Results are based on stimulation index. The HLA associations of groups of LD-typing cells (with the same specificity in man) are indicated in bold type at the top

the Leiden blood bank (Keunig et al. 1975; van Rood et al. 1976). Preliminary results of that study are schematically depicted in Figure 2.5. It can be seen that certain chimpanzee cell samples were not stimulated by the human typing cells in unilateral MLCs (solid black squares in Figure 2.5). Because chimp cells are always stimulated by "normal" human cells (not homozygous for LD determinants), this would suggest that some of the chimpanzees' LD determinants may be similar to those of man. However, the observed reactivity patterns with typing cells of each LD specificity are not strictly concordant[15], which suggests cross-reactivities rather than close similarities between the LD determinants of man and chimpanzee. The actual relationship will not be clarified until larger numbers of reliable human typing cells become available for testing with chimp cells.

5.2 Similarities Between Alloantigens of Rhesus Monkeys and Those of Other Primate Species

The interesting results obtained by interspecies typing between chimpanzee and man prompted the Dutch investigators to extend the studies to some of the "lower" Old World primates. The optimal reagents to use were obviously the monospecific alloantisera defining the RhL-A antigens of rhesus monkeys (see Section 1). The Southeast Asian stumptail macaques (*Macaca arctoides*) and a Central African baboon species (*Papio cynocephalus*) were primarily investigated. Serological interspecies reactivities among rhesus monkeys (RhL-A), chimpanzees (ChL-A), and humans (HLA) were also studied, but only in a rather cursory fashion.

The experimental protocols used in interspecies typing among the lower primates were basically the same as those used for typing between man and chimpanzee. They were direct serological testing of RhL-A sera against gradient-separated lymphocytes from the other species (cytotoxicity) as well as conventional absorptions performed with the second species' cells. Platelets from five positively and one or two negatively reacting cells were usually used for absorption (4×10^8 platelets/0.1 ml serum). Subsequently absorbed sera were retested on the cells of rhesus monkeys as well as those of the other species. Conclusions about the "sharing" (or similarity) of tissue antigens between the two species were drawn from the outcome of such testing, as indicated below.

Initial experiments by the Dutch team were performed in the late 1960s when only a few of the "short" RhL-A antigens had been identified. It could be shown that cells from stumptail macaques gave "polymorphic" patterns with the majority of the rhesus sera, sometimes showing "concordant" positive results with all sera defining a particular specificity. Although absorption studies were not performed at the time, the simple typing results suggested the sharing of several antigens between rhesus and stumptail monkeys (Dersjant et al. 1972). The conclusions were confirmed and extended by more detailed studies in the early 1970s; by that time, 20 RhL-A antigens of rhesus monkeys were fairly well defined. The upper part of Table 2.16, involving nearly a 100 unrelated and 50 related stumptail monkeys at the Rijswijk center, summarizes the results of those studies. It can be seen that only five RhL-A antigens were deemed "identical"; one was considered "similar" and the others were dissimilar or totally absent on cells of stumptail

[15] Human cells usually react similarly positive or negative with all typing cells of a particular LD specificity (Keunig et al. 1975).

Table 2.16. Presence of RhL-A-like Antigens on Cells from Stumptail Macaques and Baboons (Conclusions Based on Lymphocytotoxicity Tests and Absorptions)

	Rhesus Alloantisera Tested with			
	Stumptail Lymphocytes (*M. arctoides*)		Baboon Lymphocytes (*P. cynocephalus*)	
	First Series of RhL-A	Second Series of RhL-A	First Series of RhL-A	Second Series of RhL-A
"Identical" antigen	6 9 19	11 14	1 6 19	2 11
"Similar" antigen	1		5	
Reactivity negative or uninterpretable	Other RhL-A antigens		Other RhL-A antigens	

For explanation see text. Studies were performed between 1971 and 1973; no information is available for RhL-A antigens identified after 1973.

macaques. The criterion for identity was that all sera defining a group reacted "concordantly" positive or negative with stumptail cells and that, after absorption with any positive stumptail cell, reactivity against positive rhesus *and* stumptail cells was removed. If absorption removed reactivity only against the positive stumptail cells (but not the rhesus cells), the corresponding antigen was considered "similar." The distribution of the identical and similar RhL-A antigens in stumptail macaques seemed compatible with the hypothesis that RhL-A-like antigens present on stumptail cells may also be controlled by one genetic region. In fact, recent interspecies typing of the members of stumptail families at Rijswijk with all currently available rhesus alloantisera, increased the number of RhL-A-like antigens carried by stumptail lymphocytes and suggested that they are controlled by two closely linked SD series, also in the stumptail macaque. Because too few stumptail alloantisera are available at this time, it is not yet possible to test the proposed similarities from the "opposite serological direction"—i.e., testing rhesus lymphocytes with stumptail alloantisera that define the stumptail's own SD antigens controlled by the MHS (see Section 5.1).

On a somewhat smaller scale[16], rhesus alloantisera were tested against baboon cells (*P. cynocephalus*) (E. K. Toth, *unpublished data*). The methods used were nearly identical to those described above and a summary of the results is given in the right part of Table 2.15. Again, the data obtained in unrelated animals and baboon families were compatible with control of the "shared" antigens by a single genetic system, probably similar to RhL-A. However, in this species, the amount of data was insufficient to draw conclusions about the control of the RhL-A-like antigens by two distinct SD loci.

[16] Collaboration of the Rijswijk Primate Center and the Southwest Foundation for Research and Education, San Antonio, Texas, USA.

As indicated above (Section 4.1), a fair number of baboon alloantisera have recently been raised and it would be interesting to test the same colony of baboons with those reagents. Unfortunately, those sera were not yet available at the time of the described interspecies typing.

The sharing of SD antigens between rhesus monkeys and stumptail macaques is not at all surprising. The two species originate in adjacent areas of Southeast Asia and their size, outward appearance, etc., are similar. The apparent sharing of as many SD antigens between rhesus monkeys and baboons came as a bit of a surprise, because the region of origin as well as the animals' appearance are totally dissimilar. The finding that several of the RhL-A antigens (6, 19 and 11) are present in all three species investigated, is rather interesting. If these cross-reacting or "similar" antigens are found also in other lower primate species (as has been the case for the human 4a/4b specificities, see above), the rather wide global distribution and evolutionary "persistance" of these MHS products might have biological significance.

We can be brief about the interspecies typing between rhesus monkeys on the one hand and the two higher primate species, man and chimpanzee, on the other. The work performed by the Dutch team can be summarized as follows. When rhesus alloantisera were tested against panels of human and chimpanzee cells, none of the groups of sera defining RhL-A antigens showed concordant results, although many individual sera displayed polymorphic patterns (clearcut positive and negative reactions in cytotoxicity testing). These results are not interpretable until thorough computer analyses of reactivity patterns and selected absorption studies will have been done. Nevertheless, it was interesting to observe that the RhL-A sera that showed a particular reactivity pattern against chimp cells (only negative, only positive, or clearcut polymorphic reactions) usually displayed a very similar reactivity pattern when tested against human cells. On the other hand, when these same sera were tested against small panels of orangutan lymphocytes, the reactivity patterns were erratic, with no resemblance whatsoever to the patterns observed in chimp and man.[17]

Finally, in the reverse situation, the testing of rhesus monkey cells with human and chimpanzee alloantisera, similar uninterpretable reactivity patterns were obtained. Only sera with anti-4a or anti-4b reactivity showed an interesting polymorphism, which has already been discussed in detail (Section 5.1.3).

Acknowledgments. We thank Miss G. A. Bauer and Miss D. v. d. Velden for the patient typing and retyping of the lengthy manuscript and the many tables. Mr. J. de Kler is thanked for the preparation of the illustrations and Dr. A. Ford for making linguistic corrections in the original manuscript.

[17] When testing RhL-A sera against dog cells and cells from some 20 mouse strains, the results were also erratic and uninterpretable. In those combinations, however, preexistent heteroantibodies may interfere more strongly than in interprimate typing.

References

Allen, F. H., Jr. Linkage of HL-A and G.B.G. *Vox. Sang. 27*:382–384, 1974.

Appelman, A. W. M., and Balner, H. Mixed leukocyte cultures in rhesus monkeys. *Transplant. Proc. 4*:17–20, 1972.

Bach, F. H., and Amos, D. B. Major histocompatibility locus in man. *Science 156*:1506–1508, 1967.

Bach, F. H., and Balner, H. The role of LD and SD determinants in MLC (mixed lymphocyte cultures) and CML (cell-mediated lympholysis). *Transplant. Proc. 7*:877–878, 1975.

Bach, F. H., Engstrom, M. A., Bach, M. L., and Sell, K. W. Histocompatibility matching. VII. Mixed leukocyte cultures between chimpanzee and man. *Transplant. Proc. 4*:97–105, 1972a.

Bach, F. H., Widmer, M. B., Bach, M. L., and Klein, J. Serological defined and lymphocyte defined components of the major histocompatibility complex in the mouse. *J. Exp. Med. 136*:1430–1444, 1972b.

Balner, H. Current knowledge of the histocompatibility complex of rhesus monkeys (a brief review). *Transplant. Rev. 15*:50–61, 1973.

Balner, H., D'Amaro, J., and Visser, T. P. Tissue typing of chimpanzees. I. Evidence for two allelic series of leukocyte antigens. *Transplant. Proc. 6*:141–149, 1974a.

Balner, H., et al. Joint report of first histocompatibility workshop on Primates. *Transplant. Proc. 4*:141–147, 1972a.

Balner, H., Dersjant, H., van Leeuwen, A., and van Rood, J. J. Identification of two major leukocyte antigens of rhesus monkeys and their relation to histocompatibility. *In* E. S. Curtoni, P L. Mattiuz, and R. M. Tosi (eds.), *Histocompatibility Testing*, pp. 267–276, Munksgaard, Copenhagen, 1967a.

Balner, H., Dersjant, H., and van Rood, J. J. A method to relate leukocyte antigens and transplantation antigens in monkeys. *Transplantation 3*:230–234, 1965a.

Balner, H., Dersjant, H., and van Rood, J. J. Leukoagglutinating iso-antibodies in rhesus monkeys. *Transplantation 3*:402–422, 1965b.

Balner, H., Dersjant, H., van Vreeswijk, W., and Gabb, B. W. Tissue typing of rhesus monkeys: Application in transplantation research. *Transplant. Proc. 4*:3–9, 1972b.

Balner, H., Dorf, M. E., de Groot, M. L., and Benacerraf, B. The histocompatibility complex of rhesus monkeys. III. Evidence for a major MLR locus and histocompatibility-linked Ir genes. *Transplant. Proc. 5*:1555–1560, 1973a.

Balner, H., Gabb, B. W., D'Amaro, J., van Vreeswijk, W., and Visser, T. P. Evidence for two linked loci controlling the serologically defined leukocyte antigens of chimpanzees (ChL-A). *Tissue Antigens 4*:313–328, 1974b.

Balner, H., Gabb, B. W., Dersjant, H., van Vreeswijk, W., van Leeuwen, A., and van Rood, J. J. Heterologous antisera for human histocompatibility testing. *Transplant. Proc. 3*:1088–1098, 1971a.

Balner, H., Gabb, B. W., Dersjant, H., van Vreeswijk, W., and van Rood, J. J. Major histocompatibility locus of rhesus monkeys. *Nature 230*:177–180, 1971b.

Balner, H., Gabb, B. W., Toth, E. K., Dersjant, H., and van Vreeswijk, W. The histocompatibility complex of rhesus monkeys. I. Serology and genetics of the RhL-A system. *Tissue Antigens 3*:257–272, 1973b.

Balner, H., van Leeuwen, A., Dersjant, H., and van Rood, J. J. Chimpanzee iso-antisera in relation to human leukocyte antigens. *In* E. S. Curtoni, P. L. Mattiuz, and R. M. Tosi (eds.), *Histocompatibility Testing*, pp. 257–265, Munksgaard, Copenhagen, 1967b.

Balner, H., van Leeuwen, A., Dersjant, H., and van Rood, J. J. Defined leukocyte antigens of chimpanzees. Use of chimpanzee isoantisera for leukocyte typing in man. *Transplantation 5*:624–642, 1967c.

Balner, H., van Leeuwen, A., van Vreeswijk, W., Dersjant, H., and van Rood, J. J. Leukocyte antigens of rhesus monkeys (RhL-A) and chimpanzees (ChL-A); similarities with the human HL-A system. *Tissue Antigens 1*:229–238, 1971c.

Balner, H., van Leeuwen, A., van Vreeswijk, W., Dersjant, H., and van Rood, J. J. Leukocyte antigens of chimpanzees and their relation to human HL-A antigens. *Transplant. Proc. 2*:454–462, 1970.

Balner, H., and Toth, E. K. The histocompatibility complex of rhesus monkeys. II. A major locus controlling reactivity in mixed lymphocyte cultures. *Tissue Antigens 3*:273–290, 1973.

Balner, H., and van Vreeswijk, W. The major histocompatibility complex of rhesus monkeys (RhL-A). V. Attempts at serological identification of MLR determinants and postulation of an I region in the RhL-A complex. *Transplant. Proc. 7*:13–20, 1975.

Balner, H., van Vreeswijk, W., Dersjant, H., D'Amaro, J., van Leeuwen, A., and van Rood, J. J. Leukocyte antigens of chimpanzees (ChL-A). *Transplant. Proc. 4*:43–48, 1972c.

Balner, H., van Vreeswijk, W., de Groot, M. L., and D'Amaro, J. The major histocompatibility complex of rhesus monkeys. IV. Serological identification of several new antigens of both series of RhL-A. *Transplant. Proc. 6*:111–117, 1974c.

Balner, H., van Vreeswijk, W., and Roger, J. H. Ia-like antigens of rhesus monkeys; current state of serology and genetics. *Transpl. Rev. 30*:3–17, 1976.

Barnes, A. D., and Hawker, R. J. Leukocyte antigens in baboons: A preliminary to tissue typing for organ grafting. *Transplant. Proc. 4*:37–42, 1972a.

Barnes, A. D., and Hawker, R. J. The production of leukocyte typing sera in monkeys and babbons. *Med. Primatol.* 92–99, 1972b.

Benacerraf, B., and Dorf, M.E. Genetic control of specific immune respònses. *In* L. Brent and J. Holborow (eds.), *Progress in Immunology* II, Vol. 2, pp. 181–190, North-Holland Publishing Co., Amsterdam, 1974.

Benacerraf, B., and McDevitt, H. O. Histocompatibility-linked immune response genes; A new class of genes that controls the formation of specific immune responses has been identified. *Science 175*:273–278, 1972.

Bodmer, W. Population studies. I. General Introduction. *In* J. Dausset and J. Colombani (eds.), *Histocompatibility Testing* 1972, pp. 622–667, Munksgaard, Copenhagen, 1972.

Bogden, A. E., and Gray, J. H. Report SAM-TR-67-14, USAF School of Aerospace Medicine, Brooks Air Force Base, Texas, 1967.

Böyum, A. Separation of leukocytes from blood and bone marrow. *Scand. J. Clin. Lab. Invest. 21*:97, 1968, suppl. 97.

Bright, S., and Balner, H. The antigens 4a and 4b in rhesus monkeys and stumptailed macaques. *Tissue Antigens 8*:261–271, 1976.

Ceppellini, R. Old and new facts and speculations about transplantation antigens of man. *In* B. Amos (ed.), *Progress in Immunology,* pp. 973–1025, Academic Press, New York and London, 1971.

Cohen, E., Gregory, S., Dozier, A., Groenewald, J. H., and Murphy, J. P. Human type erythrocyte A-B-0 groups and leukocyte antigens of *Papio ursinus,* South Africa. *Med. Primatol. 148–152, 1970.*

Colombani, J., Colombani, M., Benajam, A., and Dausset, J. Leukocyte and platelet antigens defined by platelet complement fixation test (Antigens 1, 5, 6, 11, and 14). *In* E.S. Curtoni, P. L. Mattiuz, and R. M. Tosi (eds.), *Histocompatibility Testing* 1967, pp. 413–417, Munksgaard, Copenhagen, 1967.

David, C. S., Shreffler, D. C., and Frelinger, J. A. New lymphocyte antigen system (LNA) controlled by the Ir region of the mouse H-2 complex. *Proc. Natl. Acad. Sci.* (USA) *70*:2509–2514, 1973.

Dersjant, H., van Vreeswijk, W., and Balner, H. Cross-specific tissue typing between rhesus monkeys and chimpanzees. *Transplant. Proc. 4*:93–96, 1972.

Dicke, H. W., Marquet, R. L., Heystek, G. A., and Balner, H. Effect of immunosuppressive treatment and leukocyte antigen matching on kidney allografts in rhesus monkeys. *Transplant. Proc. 3*:484–487, 1971.

Dorf, M. E., Balner, H., and Benacerraf, B. Mapping of the immune response genes in the major histocompatibility complex of the rhesus monkeys. *J. Exp. Med. 142*:673–693, 1975.

Dorf, M. E., Balner, H., de Groot, M. L., and Benacerraf, B. Histocompatibility-linked immune response genes in the rhesus monkey. *Transplant. Proc. 6*:119–123, 1974.

Dorf, M. E., Boyle, W., and Metzgar, R. S. Serological analysis of soluble chimpanzee histocompatibility antigens. *Fed. Proc. 29*:507, 1970.

Dorf, M. E., and Haber, J. A. Leukocyte antigens of primates. *Primates in Med. 6*:67–114, 1972.

Dorf, M. E., and Metzgar, R. S. Serological relationship of human, chimpanzee and gorilla lymphocyte antigens. *In* P. E. Terasaki (ed.), *Histocompatibility Testing* 1970, pp. 287–296, Munksgaard, Copenhagen, 1970a.

Dorf, M. E., and Metzgar, R. S. The distribution of human HL-A antigens in chimpanzees and gorillas, *Med. Primatol.* 12–23, 1970b.

Dorf, M.E., Toth, E.K., and Balner, H. Cross-reactions of HL-A antibodies. V. Relationships between the human HL-A and chimpanzee ChW-11 specificities. *Tissue Antigens 2*:461–472, 1972.

Downing, H. J., Brain, P., Hammond, M. G., Vos, G. H., and Webb, G. R. Leukocyte antigens of baboons. *Transplant. Proc. 4*:33–36, 1972.

Downing, H. J., Burgess, B. J., Vos, G. H., Burgers, L. E., and Webb, G. R. Transplantation antigens in the chacma baboon papio ursinus kerr. *Transplant. Proc. 4*:169–172, 1974.

Dubernard, J. M., et al. Renal skin and xenografts from baboons to macaques: Effect of antilymphocyte globulins. *Transplant. Proc. 3*:545–550, 1971.

Es, A. A. van, Marquet, R. L., Vreeswijk, W. van, and Balner, H. The influence of matching for RhL-A (SD) antigens and of mixed lymphocyte reactivity on allograft survival in unrelated rhesus monkeys *Transpl. Proc.* (in press), 1976.

Eijsvoogel, V. P., et al. Position of a locus determining mixed lymphocyte reaction (MLR), distinct from the known HL-A loci, and its relation to cell-mediated lympholysis (CML). *In* J. Dausset and J. Colombani (eds.), *Histocompatibility Testing* 1972, pp. 501–508, Munksgaard, Copenhagen, 1972a.

Eijsvoogel, V. P., Koning, L., de Groot, M. L., Huismans, L., van Rood, J. J., van Leeuwen, A., and du Toit, E. D. Mixed lymphocyte culture and HL-A. *Transplant. Proc. 4*:199–204, 1972b.

Ford, C. H. J., King, L. M., and Barnes, A. D. Further studies of tissue typing sera in baboons. *Transplant. Proc. 6*:151–155, 1974.

Gabb, B. W., Piazza, A., D'Amaro, J., and Balner, H. Genetics of RhL-A system of rhesus monkeys. *Transplant. Proc. 4*:11–16, 1972.

Götze, D., Reisfeld, R. A., and Klein, J. Serologic evidence for antigens controlled by the Ir region in mice. *J. Exp. Med. 138*:1003–1008, 1973.

Grosse-Wilde, H., Vriesendorp, H. M., Netzel, B., Mempel, W., Kolb, H. J., Wank, R., Thierfelder, S., and Albert, E. D. Immunogenetics of seven LD alleles of the DL-A complex in Mongresls Beagles and Labradors. *Transplant. Proc. 7*:159–164, 1975.

Hamburger, J., Crosnier, J., Descamps, B., and Rowinski, D. The value of present methods used for the selection of organ donors. *Transplant. Proc. 3*:260–267, 1971.

Hauptfeld, V., Klein, D., and Klein, J. Serological identification of an Ir-region product. *Science 18*:167–169, 1973.

Keunig, J. J., Termijtelen, A., Blussé van Oud Alblas, A., van den Tweel, J. G., Schreuder, I., and van Rood, J. J. Typing for MLC (LD). *Transplant. Proc. 7*:35–39, 1975.

Kissmeyer-Nielsen, F., and Kjerbye, K. E. Lymphocyte micro-technique purification of lymphocytes by flotation. *In* E. S. Curtoni, P. L. Mattiuz, and R. M. Tosi (eds.), *Histocompatibility Testing* 1967, pp. 381–383, Munksgaard, Copenhagen, 1967.

Kissmeyer-Nielsen, F., Svejgaard, A., and Thorsby, E. (eds.). *Histocompatibility Testing* 1975, Munksgaard, Copenhagen, 1975.

Klein, J. *Biology of the Mouse Histocompatibility-2 Complex: Principles of Immunogenetics Applied to a Single System*. Springer Verlag, Berlin, 1975.

Koch, C. T., Frederiks, E., Eijsvoogel, V. P., and van Rood, J. J. Mixed-lymphocyte-culture and skin-graft data in unrelated HL-A identical individuals. *Lancet II*:1334–1336, 1971.

Kourilsky, F. M., Silvestre, D., Neauport-Sautes, C., Loosfelt, Y., and Dausset, J. J. Antibody-induced redistribution of HL-A antigens at the cell surface. *Eur. J. Immunol. 2*:249–257, 1972.

van Leeuwen, A., et al. Study of the HL-A system in a colony of chimpanzees. *In* J. Dausset and J. Colombani (eds.), *Histocompatibility Testing* 1972, pp. 49–53, Munksgaard, Copenhagen, 1972.

van Leeuwen, A., Schuit, H. R. E., and van Rood, J. J. Typing for MLC (LD). I. The selection of nonstimulator cells by MLC inhibition tests using SD-identical stimulator cells (MISIS) and fluorescence antibody studies. *Transplant. Proc. 5*:1539–1542, 1973.

Lightbody, J. J., Bernoco, D., Miggiano, V. C., and Ceppellini, R. Cell mediated lympholysis in man after sensitization of effector lymphocytes through mixed leukocyte cultures. *G. Batt. Virol. 14*:243–254, 1971.

Lilly, F. The histocompatibility-2 locus and susceptibility to tumor induction. *Natl. Cancer Inst. Monogr. 22*:631–641, 1965.

Mann, D. L., Rogentine, G. N., Jr., Fahey, J. L., and Nathenson, S. G. Human lymphocyte membrane (HL-A) alloantigens: Isolation, purification and properties. *J. Immunol. 103*:282–292, 1969.

Marquet, R. L., Heystek, G. A., and van Bekkum, D. W. Heterotopic heart and kidney transplantation in rhesus monkeys. *Med. Primatol. 2*:125–133, 1972.

McDevitt, H. O., and Benacerraf, B. Genetic control of specific immune responses. *Adv. Immunol. 11*:31–74, 1969.

Mempel, W., Grosse-Wilde, H., Baumann, P., Netzel, B., Steinbauer-Rosenthal, I., Scholz, S., Bertrams, J., and Albert, E. D. Population genetics of the MLC response: Typing for MLC determinants using homozygous and heterozygous reference cells. *Transplant. Proc. 5*:1529–1534, 1973.

Metzgar, R.S., Seigler, H. F., Ward, F. E., Hill, E. D., and Mohanakumar, T. Characterization of chimpanzee leukocyte alloantisera. *Transplant. Proc. 4*:49–54, 1972a.

Metzgar, R. S., Ward, F. E., and Seigler, H. F. Study of the HL-A system in chimpanzees. *In* J. Dausset and J. Colombani (eds.), *Histocompatibility Testing* 1972, pp. 55–61, Munksgaard, Copenhagen, 1972b.

Metzgar, R. S., and Zmijewski, C. M. Species distribution of human tissue isoantigens. I. Detection of human tissue isoantigens in chimpanzees. *Transplantation 4*:84–93, 1966.

Mittal, K. K., Mickey, M. R., Singal, D. P., and Terasaki, P. I. Serotyping for homotransplantation. XVIII. Refinement of microdroplet lymphocyte cytotoxicity test. *Transplantation 6*:913–917, 1968.

Meo, T., David, C. S., Rijnbeek, A. M., Nabholz, M., Miggiano, V. C., and Shreffler, D. C. Inhibition of mouse MLR by anti-Ia sera. *Transplant. Proc. 7*:127–129, 1975.

Möller, G. (ed.). HL-A and disease. *Transplant. Rev. 22*, 1975.

Murphy, G.P., et al. Correlation of tissue typing tests in baboon renal allotransplants. *J. Surg. Res. 9*:19–28, 1969.

Murphy, G. P. and Brede, H. D. Baboon allotransplantation. *Primates in Med. 7*:44–54, 1972.

Myburgh, J. A., Smith, J. A., Mieny, C. J., and Mason, J. A. Hepatic allotransplantation in the baboon. III. The effects of immunosuppression and administration of donor-specific antigen after transplantation. *Transplantation 12*:202–210, 1971.

Neefe, J. R., Jr., Balner, H., Barnes, A. D., Ford, C., Rogentine, G. N., Jr., van Vreeswijk, W., and Ward, F. E. Progress in rhesus histocompatibility typing resulting from the second international nonhuman primate histocompatibility workshop (1973). *Tissue Antigens 6*:77–79, 1975a.

Neefe, J. R., Ellis, E.B., and Rogentine, G. N. Rhesus lymphocyte alloantigens. III. Identification of new antigens. *Tissue Antigens 6*:195–204, 1975b.

Neefe, J. R., Merritt, C. B., Darrow, C. C., and Rogentine, G. N. Beneficial influence of limited histocompatibility of bone marrow grafted to unrelated rhesus monkeys preconditioned with X-ray and ALS. *Transplant. Proc. 6*:125–128, 1974.

Neefe, J. R., Maurer, B., and Sachs, D. H. Definition of eighteen SD antigens and two LD antigens of the RhL-A monkey major histocompatibility complex. *Transpl. Proc.* (in press), 1976.

Neefe, J. R., Vaal, L., Darrow, C. C. I. I., and Rogentine, G. N., Jr. Mixed lymphocyte reactivity in rhesus sibships. *Transplantation 15*:507–510, 1973.

Polák, L., Barnes, J. M., and Turk, J. L. The genetic control of contact sensitization to inorganic metal compounds in guinea-pigs. *Immunology 14*:707–711, 1968.

Rogentine, G. N., Merritt, C. B., Vaal, L. A., Ellis, E. B., and Darrow, C. C. I. I. Rhesus lymphocyte alloantigens. II. Serologic genetic and chemical characteristics. *Transplant. Proc. 4*:21–24, 1972.

Rogentine, G. N., Vaal, L., Ellis, E. B., and Darrow, C. C. I. I. Rhesus lymphocyte alloantigens. I. Identification of a major alloantigen system. *Transplantation 12*:267–270, 1971.

Roger, J. H., van Vreeswijk, W., Dorf, M. E., and Balner, H. The major histocompatibility complex of Rhesus monkey. VI. Serology and Genetics of Ia-like antigens. *Tissue Antigens* 67–86, 1976.

van Rood, J. J., van Leeuwen, A., and Balner, H. HL-A and ChL-A: Similarities and differences. *Transplant. Proc. 4*:55–62, 1972.

van Rood, J. J., van Leeuwen, A., Keunig, J. J., and Blussé van Oud Alblas, A. The serological recognition of the human MLC determinants using a modified cytotoxicity technique. *Tissue Antigens 5*:73–79, 1975.

van Rood, J. J., van Leeuwen, A., Parlevliet, J., Termijtelen, A., and Keunig, J. J. LD typing and serology. IV. Description of the major locus with 3 alleles. *In* F. Kissmeyer-Nielsen, A. Svejgaard, and E. Thorsby (eds.), *Histocompatibility Testing*, pp. 629–636, Munksgaard, Copenhagen, 1976.

Sachs, D. H. and Cone, J. L. A mouse B-cell alloantigen determined by gene(s) linked to the major histocompatibility complex. *J. Exp. Med. 138*:1289–1304, 1973.

Schreuder, I., van Leeuwen, A., and Balner, H. A further study on the detection of HL-A-like antigens in a colony of chimpanzees. *In* F. Kissmeyer-Nielsen, A. Svejgaard, and E. Thorsby (eds.), *Histocompatibility Testing* 1975, pp. 130–135, Munksgaard, Copenhagen, 1975.

Seigler, H. F., Metzgar, R.S., Ward, F.E., and Reid, D.M. Reactions of human HL-A sera with orang-utan and gorilla lymphocytes. *Transplant. Proc. 4*:83–86, 1972.

Seigler, H. F., Ward, F. E., Metzgar, R. S., Stulting, S. M., Phaup, M. B., and Adams, B. J. Mixed lymphocyte culture responses in chimpanzee families. *Transplant. Proc. 6*:135–139, 1974.

Sheehy, M. J., Sondel, P. M., Bach, M. L., Wank, R., and Bach, F. H. HL-A LD (lymphocyte defined) typing: A rapid assay with primed lymphocytes. *Science 188*:1308–1310, 1975.

Shulman, N. R., Moor-Jankowski, J., and Hiller, M. C. Platelet and leukocyte isoantigens common to man and other animals. *In* H. Balner, F. J. Cleton, and J. G. Eernisse (eds.), *Histocompatibility Testing* 1965, pp. 113–123, Munksgaard, Copenhagen, 1965.

Stone, W. H. Immunogenetic studies of rhesus. 1975. The Rhesus monkey, II. (G.H. Bourne ed.). Academic Press.

Taylor, R. B., et al. Redistribution and pinocytosis of lymphocyte surface immunoglobulin molecules induced by anti-immunoglobulin antibody. *Nature New Biol. 233*:225–229, 1971.

Thomas, E. D., et al. Bone marrow transplantation. *N. Engl. J. Med. 292,* part 1 and 2:832–843 and 895–902, 1975.

Unanue, E. R., Dorf, M. E., David, C. S., and Benacerraf, B. The presence of I region-associated antigens on B cells in molecules distinct from Ig and H-2K and H-2D. *Proc. Natl. Acad. Sci.* (USA) *71*:5014–5016, 1974.

Unanue, E. R., Perkins, W.D., and Karnovsky, M. J. Ligand-induced movement of lymphocyte membrane macromolecules. I. Analysis by immunofluorescence and ultrastructural radioantography. *J. Exp. Med. 136*:855–906, 1972.

van Vreeswijk, W., Roger, J. H., D'Amaro, J., and Balner, H. The major histocompatibility complex of rhesus monkeys, Rhl-A. VII. Identification of five new serologically defined antigens. *Tissue Antigens* (in press, July 1976).

Wernet, P. and Kunkel, H. G. Demonstration of specific T-lymphocyte membrane antigens associated with antibodies inhibiting the mixed leukocyte culture in man. *Transplant. Proc. 5*:1875–1881, 1973.

Yunis, E. J. and Amos, D. B. HL-A mixed leukocyte reaction (MLR) and hypersensitivity delayed reaction (HDR). Three closely linked genetic systems relevant to transplantation. *Proc. Natl. Acad. Sci.* (USA) *68*:3031–3035, 1971.

Zaalberg, P. B., Fasbender, M. J., and Balner, H. "Ia-like" antigens of rhesus monkeys are distinct from conventional RhL-A antigens, β microglobulin, and immunoglobulin. *Immunogenetics 3*:499–505, 1976.

Ziegler, J. B., Alper, Ch. A., and Balner, H. Properdin factor B and histocompatibility loci linked in the rhesus monkey. *Nature 254*:609–611, 1975a.

Ziegler, J.B., Watson, L., and Alper, Ch.A. Genetic polymorphism of properdin factor B in the rhesus: Evidence for single subunit structure in primates. *J. Immunol. 114*:1649–1653, 1975b.

Chapter 3

The Major Histocompatibility System of the Dog

H. M. VRIESENDORP, H. GROSSE-WILDE, and M. E. DORF

1. Introduction

1.1 The Dog as an Experimental Model

Dogs are frequently used as experimental animals in transplantation research. For ethical and economical reasons this use should be limited to those experimental protocols in which members of the canine species will provide the best answers to the questions that an investigator wants to answer. This will be the case when transplantation surgeons require an experimental subject of a size and temperament that allows major operations and intensive postoperative care. Dogs may also be useful when new biological concepts, after their development in inbred murine strains, need further definition and clarification in an outbred preclinical animal model. In such an animal model histocompatibility systems should be amenable for analysis for a proper evaluation of the results obtained and an extrapolation to the treatment of human patients. Because of this and because of other advantageous properties of dogs, such as large family size and relatively short gestation and generation times (63 and 360 days, respectively), histocompatibility has been studied in this species.

The degree to which the dog can be considered a realistic model for subsequent human studies is often questioned. It is generally believed that all dogs (and, in particular, dog breeds) are inbred to some degree. This implies the absence of an important experimental group in dogs, i.e., unrelated outbred donor-recipient pairs. This issue was recently discussed elsewhere (Joint Report Second International Workship on Canine Immunogenetics 1976) where it was shown that truly unrelated, outbred dogs can be found, even within breeds, when appropriate genetic studies are done. Therefore dogs can be considered as suitable preclinical animal model when the required genetic information is obtained. The most important genetic information in this regard is histocompatibility. In this chapter the current state of knowledge of dog histocompatibility will be described.

1.2 Short History of Dog Histocompatibility Studies

In 1964 the first studies on dog alloantisera that aimed at a definition of histocompatibility structures (Puza et al. 1964; Rubinstein and Ferrebee 1964;

Kasakura et al. 1964; Altman and Simonsen 1964) were reported. Later Epstein and co-workers (1968) demonstrated that matching related donor-recipient pairs for dog leukocyte specificities prolonged bone marrow graft survival. In 1971 it was shown by Vriesendorp et al. that one chromosomal area was involved in the genetic control of most of the dog leukocyte specificities recognized at that time and that genetic information on the same chromosome had a major influence on the survival of skin, small intestine, and heart allografts. The abbreviation DLA was introduced in which, in analogy to the human HLA system, D stands for dog, L for leukocyte, and A for the fact that this complex chromosomal area carries major histocompatibility information and that it is the first genetic region to be discovered that control leukocyte antigens.

As in other mammals, reactivity in mixed leukocyte cultures (MLCs) of dogs appeared to be under genetic control of one chromosomal area (Templeton and Thomas 1971). Later this locus (or loci) was found to be located within the DLA system (Templeton et al. 1973; van der Does et al. 1973).

International cooperation in the larger field of canine immunogenetics, including histocompatibility genetics, was begun informally in 1972, and since then more or less formally by the organization of workshops. Two have been held so far, one in Rotterdam, the Netherlands, in 1972, and one in Portland, Oregon, USA, in 1974. A third one is in the planning stage for 1978 in Munich, Germany. These occasions have provided excellent opportunities for the comparison of reagents and techniques, nomenclature decisions, and the planning of future research efforts. This fruitful international cooperation is gratefully acknowledged here, because many of the data reported have been generated directly or indirectly by these joint efforts.

2. DLA Genetics

2.1 Nomenclature

In 1974 a nomenclature subcommittee was established for dog histocompatibility determinants by the International Union of Immunological Societies. Its activities have been synchronized to the international workshops on canine immunogenetics. This committee adheres to a nomenclature policy as formulated by Swisher (1963) for biomedical notation systems and to a maximum resemblance to human HLA nomenclature decisions when applicable.

The latest nomenclature decisions have been included in the Joint Report of the Second International Workshop on Canine Immunogenetics (1976). The dog major histocompatibility system has been designated DLA. Loci within this complex are numbered with consecutive letters starting with A. Alleles receive the prefix DLA followed by a dash and the letter of their locus, followed by their allele number. DLA alleles are numbered from 1 on in sequence of their discovery. However, an earlier nomenclature decision was left intact in which numbers were given to alleles of the different segregant series. Therefore the series DLA-A, DLA-B, and DLA-C shows gaps in the allele numbers. A provisional nomenclature is given to genetic variation within the major histocompatibility system that is less well defined, or that has not been allocated to a locus yet. Here the first letter of the investigator's name or home town is used, followed by a number for serologically defined antigens. For lymphocyte-defined alleles the prefix DLA and a number from 50 on are utilized.

In this chapter the following subdivisions within the DLA complex have been used for loci and their alleles and gene products: SD when they are *s*erologically *d*efined by microlymphocytotoxicity techniques (Section 2.2); LD when they are *l*ymphocyte *d*efined by mixed lymphocyte cultures (Section 2.3); Ir when they are defined by the presence or absence of a specific humoral *i*mmune *r*esponse (Section 2.4); and R when they are involved in the *r*esistance against allogeneic bone marrow grafts (Section 2.5).

2.2 Serologically Defined Antigens

2.2.1 Methodology (see Table 3.1)

Test. Limited experience was obtained with complement-fixation methods (Gluckman and Vriesendorp, *unpublished observations*), probably indicating that complement-fixing antibodies do exist that recognize dog thrombocyte antigens that are similar to dog leukocyte serologically defined (SD) antigens. In general, however, two different modifications of a microlymphocytotoxicity technique have been in use:

1. A one-stage test (Kissmeyer-Nielsen and Kjerbye 1967; Vriesendorp 1973) in which cells, antiserum, and complement are allowed to interact from the very start of the incubation period of 30 min at 37° C
2. A two-stage test (Terasaki and McCelland 1964; Albert et al. 1973b), which is performed at room temperature and in which cells and antiserum are incubated for 30 min, followed by a second incubation period with complement.

In agreement with human experience (Ahrons and Kissmeyer-Nielsen 1973), the two-stage test was found to be more sensitive (Smid Mercx et al. 1975; Saison and Vriesendorp, *unpublished observations*). In the past most of the dog typing sera have been raised in immunization schedules in which a one-stage test was used as the test procedure (Vriesendorp et al. 1971, 1972, 1973). The majority of one-stage sera (though not all) do show extra reactions in a two-stage testing procedure. Most of these reactions occur in so-called cross-reactive groups (Smid Mercx et al. 1975) (see Section 2.2.3). A convenient two-stage testing procedure that will accommodate one-stage sera must still be developed. In this way the more numerous one-stage sera of good specificity could be used in the more practical two-stage testing technique. In both one- and two-stage testing in dogs, lower reproducibility rates (i.e., 85 to 90 percent) have been reported than those commonly found

Table 3.1. Methodology of Dog SD Typing

Microcytotoxicity test	
	1. One-stage
	2. Two-stage
	3. Modified two-stage (not yet operational)
Serum production	
	1. Organ allograft
	2. Injections of leukocytes
	3. Pregnancy sera
	4. Injections of spleen acetone powder

in man (95 to 99 percent). This makes it necessary to type each dog on at least two different occasions. The results analyzed in this chapter, with the exception of the data reported in Section 2.6.2, were obtained by typing dogs on at least two different days using a one-stage microcytotoxicity test.

Sera Production. The four different immunization methods that have been used to produce dog allolymphocytotoxins are listed in Table 3.1. When organs or leukocytes are grafted for the purpose of inducing specific antisera (Table 3.1, methods 1 and 2), preselected, unrelated donor-recipient pairs with only one antigen difference should be used. If this cannot be achieved, one haplotype-different littermates or parent-child combinations are excellent alternatives. Sera should be harvested as soon as a strong positive cross-match is found with donor lymphocytes. Extended immunization procedures carry the risk of spoiling the specificity of the antisera raised (Vriesendorp et al. 1971; van der Does et al. 1973). Several organ allografts (method 1) have been shown to give rise to the development of dog allocytotoxins. Skin allografts are easy to perform, and their fate can be easily followed by visual inspection. Obviously, no information on the interesting parameter of graft survival is obtained when method 2 (leukocyte injections) is used, although excellent reagents can be produced (van der Does et al. 1973). Sera of female dogs in the postpartum period (method 3) can be a good source of typing reagents, because cross-placental immunization of the mother by the fetus does occur in dogs (Vriesendorp et al. 1971, 1973). This method will be attractive in a large kennel, where good breeding records are kept and blood samples of sires can be obtained for screening and specificity determination. In one stage testing a low percentage (± 15 percent) of postpartum sera were found to be useful typing sera (Vriesendorp et al. 1973). A much higher (± 40 percent) percentage was observed in two-stage testing (Vriesendorp and Visser, *unpublished observations*). The fourth method shown in Table 3.1 is in development by Zweibaum and co-workers (Léon et al. 1975a). The use of spleen acetone powders as immunogenic material for xenogeneic or allogeneic hosts and as absorption material for further refinement of the produced antisera seems to hold great promise for the production of large quantities of excellent tissue-typing reagents (Léon et al. 1975b).

2.2.2 Sera Analysis

The analysis of dog sera has followed the example set by van Rood in 1962 for human leukocyte serology by the application of a computerized approach (Vriesendorp et al. 1972; Joint Report First International Workshop on Canine Immunogenetics 1973). Computer programs were used to cluster sera with common reactivity patterns on the basis of a statistical analysis of their results in a population of unrelated animals. In Table 3.2 the data are given for the best known clusters of dog alloantisera from a previously unpublished analysis of 1973. The presence or absence of a group was determined by looking at the reactivity patterns of all sera in a cluster. Only when the "leading" serum of a cluster and some or all of the other sera within the same cluster were positive with the lymphocytes of an individual was an antigen marked as present. These clusters are presumed to recognize *one* leukocyte antigen or group per cluster, because (1) the groups have low phenotype frequencies; (2) predictions of population genetics for monofactorial groups are met (see Section 2.2.3); (3) some absorption studies were performed in which 0.1 ml of antiserum was absorbed

Table 3.2. Correlations Among Dog Alloantisera with Similar Reactivity Patterns ($n=100$)

SD Group	Sera	R^a		
1	D 0322			
	B 27	50		
	D 1198	50	50	
2	14022			
	B 191	60		
	D 1216	67	60	
3	B 0297			
	B 156	54		
	B 622	47	34	
4	D 121			
	1	88		
	D 544	66	71	
	14009	81	77	54
5	Ca 22			
	14011	52		
	D 173	62	57	
	B 120	63	71	69
6	14021			
	B 609	45		
	3894	46	48	
	S 13	40	44	43
7	D 1228			
	D 595	61		
	14016	40	44	
8	14014			
	B 30	63		
9	14020			
	14019	88		
	D 168	66	64	
10	B 604			
	3896	43		
	B 26.2	53	57	
	14018	74	47	46
11	14017			
	Ca 34	73		
	1302	48	47	
12	D 1185			
	D 2298	79		
13	3897			
	3895	52		
	14022	44	40	

[a] $R=\sqrt{(\chi^2/n)}\times 100$, where n is the number of individuals tested, and χ^2 is the value with Yates' correction of the two-by-two contingency table of the results of the two sera.

Table 3.3. Relationships Among DLA SD Antigens

DLA-A — χ^2 of Independence with Yates' Correction[a]

	1	2	3	7	8	9
1						
2	0.0					
3	0.0	−0.3				
7	0.0	0.0	−0.3			
8	0.0	0.0	−2.9	0.0		
9	0.0	−0.1	−2.3	−1.0	−0.6	
10	−0.1	0.0	0.0	0.2	0.0	−2.9

DLA-A — χ^2 of allelism

	1	2	3	7	8	9
2	0.0					
3	0.0	0.0				
7	0.0	0.0	1.1			
8	0.0	0.0	1.0	0.0		
9	0.0	0.0	0.0	0.2	0.8	
10	0.1	0.0	3.9 (hatched)	5.0 (hatched)	0.8	1.1

DLA-A
$n = 100$ unrelated dogs of different breeds

DLA-B — χ^2 of Independence with Yates' Correction[a]

	4	5	6
4			
5	−9.6		
6	−0.6	1.0	
13	0.1	0.0	−0.2

DLA-B — χ^2 of allelism

	4	5	6
5	1.8		
6	0.2	0.0	
13	5.8 (hatched)	5.9 (hatched)	0.0

DLA-B
$n = 100$ unrelated dogs of different breeds

DLA-C — χ^2 of Independence with Yates' Correction[a]

	12	R 15
11		
12	−4.0	
R 15	−0.3	−8.4

DLA-C — χ^2 of allelism

	11	12
12	0.1	
R 15	0.8	2.8

DLA-C
$n = 70$ unrelated dogs of different breeds

The hatched areas show exceptions to expectations and are further discussed in Section 2.2.3.
[a] A negative sign is given to a χ^2 value from a two-by-two comparison where $ad < bc$; a, b, c, and d being, respectively, the + +, + −, − +, and − − results of the two sera.

with 10^8 peripheral leukocytes. Data compatible with "operational" monospecificity of the reagents were obtained for DLA-A1, DLA-A10, DLA-B4 (Vriesendorp, *unpublished observations*), and DLA-A8 (Saison and Doble 1975). When low numbers of unrelated individuals are tested, the interrelationships among the different SD antigens can be looked at most efficiently by applying two χ^2 tests, one assuming independence and one assuming allelic relationships between pairs of antigens (Andresen et al. 1963). Such data are shown in Table 3.3, where the antigens are arranged in three series of multiple alleles, indicated as DLA-A, DLA-B, and DLA-C. One new antigen, R 15 (recognized by five newly produced antisera), has been added to the antigens of Table 3.2. Antigens are arranged in one series when low or negative χ^2 values of independence and low (<3.8) χ^2 values of allelism are found between them. The three series of allelic specificities given in Table 3.3 conform to this rule with a minimum of exceptions, which are hatched in the table, and which will be discussed in Section 2.2.3. The working hypothesis as shown here, that at least three different SD loci exist within the DLA complex, is in accordance with other data obtained in families and populations of unrelated individuals (see Section 2.2.3).

The tissue distribution of the DLA SD antigens is largely unknown. They are present on lymphocytes and thrombocytes from the peripheral blood and have so far not been found on erythrocytes in direct serological tests or by absorptions (Bull and Vriesendorp, *unpublished observations*). Suggestive indirekt evidence for the presence of SD antigens in skin, small bowel, pancreas, and heart tissues has been obtained. Recipients of allografts of these tissues produced good SD reagents during and after rejection (Vriesendorp et al. 1971; Westbroek et al. 1972).

2.2.3 Genetics

Population Data. In Table 3.4 the gene frequencies are given for the currently known DLA SD antigens in unrelated dogs. The formula $GF = 1-(1-PF)^{1/2}$ is used, in which GF and PF stand for gene and population frequency, respectively. Antigen P 17 (Joint Report Second International Workshop on Canine Immunogenetics 1976) is shown in parentheses because sera recognizing this antigen were not available in the studies analyzed here. The gene frequency of P 17 is the one computed from the second international workshop material. The total number of individuals tested to reach the estimates of gene frequencies in Table 3.5 is 115 for DLA-A antigens and 70 for DLA-B and C antigens.

In Figure 3.1 the distribution of the antigens is given. No triplets are found in any series. Hardy-Weinberg equilibrium appears to be present in

Table 3.4. Gene Frequencies of Currently Known DLA SD Antigens

DLA-A		DLA-B		DLA-C	
1	0.013	4	0.163	11	0.172
2	0.058	5	0.163	12	0.130
3	0.296	6	0.106	R 15	0.146
7	0.106	13	0.122	BL	0.552
8	0.026	R 16	0.024[a]		
9	0.115	BL	0.422		
10	0.110				
BL	0.276	(P17	0.147)		
Number of unrelated individuals tested:					
115		70		70	

[a] New, still provisionally defined, specificity.

Table 3.5. Haplotypes of DLA SD Antigens Found in Family Studies

DLA-A Antigens	DLA-B Antigen					
	4	5	6	13	R 16	Blank
1	+	+	+	+	−	+[11]
2	+	+[11]	+	+	−	+
3	+	+	−	+	−	+[11 12 R 15]
7	+	+	−	+	+	+[12]
8	−	−	−	+	+	+[R 15]
9	+[12]	+	+[12]	+	−	+[12]
10	+	+	+	−	−	+[R 15]
Blank	+	+[R 15]	−	+	+	+[11 12 R 15]

DLA-C antigens are indicated in the area of the DLA-A, DLA-B haplotype with which they were found to segregate.

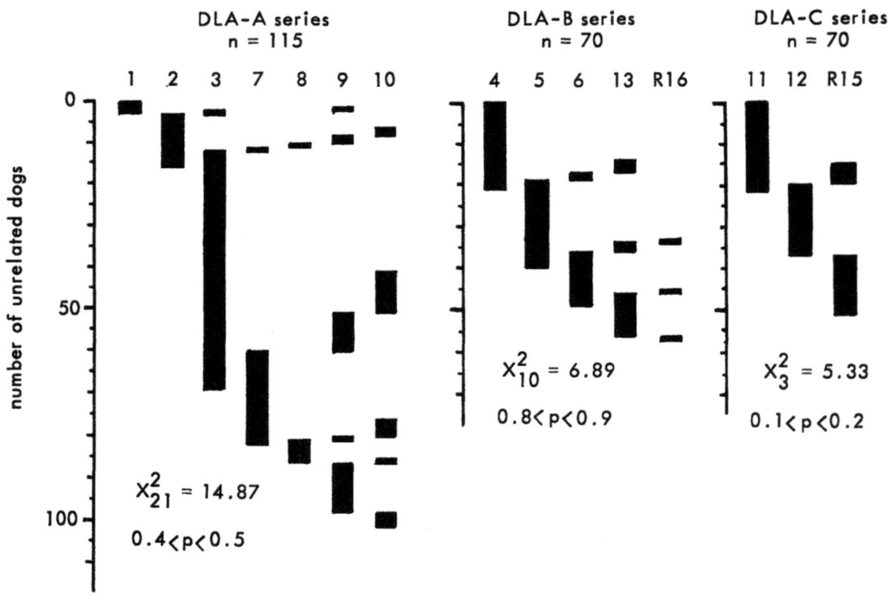

Fig. 3.1. Distribution of DLA-SD antigens in unrelated animals. Results are rearranged in each series for optimal visualization

the DLA-A and B series and to be less convincing in the DLA-C series. Previously (Vriesendorp et al. 1973), DL 11 and DL 12 (now DLA-C11 and DLA-C12) were reported as belonging to the second DLA SD series (now DLA-B). This was caused by the assumption that these antigens were recognized by extra antibodies in DLA-A2 and DLA-A9 sera, respectively. New immunizations and absorptions have shown that this is not the case and that the association in reactivity patterns between DLA-A9 and DLA-C12 and between DLA-A2 and DLA-C11 is caused by the linkage disequilibrium

Table 3.6. Common Combinations of DLA Antigens

I (Family Data)

DLA-A Antigen	DLA-B Antigen	Percent Expected $\times 10^{-3}$	Percent Found $\times 10^{-3}$	Δ $\times 10^{-3}$	Ratio[a] Found/Exp.
10	4	11	24	13	2.2
2	5	16	77	61	4.8
9	6	34	130	96	3.8
10	6	15	30	15	2.0
7	13	25	95	70	3.8
8	13	11	36	25	3.3
3		55	124	69	2.3

II (Data of Unrelated Individuals)

DLA-C Antigen	DLA-A Antigen				
11	2	17	113	96	6.7
11	3	70	145	75	2.1
11	8	10	32	22	3.2
12	9	41	226	185	4.5
R 15	3	75	194	119	2.6
R 15	7	35	97	62	2.8

DLA-C Antigen	DLA-B Antigen				
11	5	56	128	77	2.3
12	4	42	114	72	2.7
12	6	28	86	58	3.1
12	13	32	86	54	2.7
R 15	5	48	143	91	3.0

[a] Only those Δ are listed that have a ratio found/exp. of 2.0 or higher.

present between these pairs of antigens (see Table 3.6 and section on linkage disequilibrium).

Family Data. Dog families were studied for the segregation of individual SD antigens and the construction of haplotypes of SD antigens of different series. SD antigens appear to segregate according to expectations for a simple mendelian factor (Vriesendorp et al. 1971, 1972). In Table 3.5 is given a list of the haplotypes that have been identified so far. Because of the overrepresentation of beagles and labrador retrievers in this material, exact frequencies of haplotypes cannot be given. Linkage disequilibrium between antigens of different series does occur in dog breeds and in mongrel dogs, which causes some haplotypes to be more frequent than others. Frequent beagle haplotypes are 1, 13, –; 2, 4, 11; 2, 5, 11; 3, –, 11; 7, –, –; 9,

4, 12; and 9, 6, 12. In labrador retrievers, 2, 13, 11; 9, 5, 12; and 9, 6, 12 are often found. In mongrel dogs, 3, –, R 15; 3, –, 11; 8, 13, –; 9, 6, 12; 10, 4, –; and 10, 6, – are frequently occurring haplotypes (see also Table 3.6 and section on linkage disequilibrium).

Each of the four different DLA haplotypes within a family appears to have an equal chance of being present in a given offspring. This can be illustrated by the observation that SD, LD homozygotes in test matings occur not more or less frequent than would be expected. In eight litters, consisting of a total of 57 pups, 21 SD and LD homozygotes were found, whereas 19.25 were expected. This observation also argues against a pronounced selective advantage or disadvantage for the presence of major histocompatibility differences between mother and offspring.

The absence of doublets in the more than 100 family studies performed so far (i.e., antigens that are presumed to be controlled by alleles never segregated *en bloc*) supports the present hypothesis of the existence of three SD series and the allocation of the particular antigens to them. Recombination within the DLA complex will be discussed in Section 2.7.

Linkage Disequilibrium. The term *linkage disequilibrium* is used to describe the nonrandom association between alleles of different series. In families, positive linkage disequilibrium between alleles will cause a certain haplotype to be more frequent than the product of the gene frequencies of each of the alleles in such a haplotype. In unrelated individuals, it will lead to positive associations between antigens of different series. Several explanations can be offered for the existence of this phenomenon (Cavalli Sforza and Bodmer 1970). Suggestive evidence for selective forces, favoring some human SD histocompatibility antigen combinations above others and thus as an explanation for the linkage disequilibrium between them, have been found (Bodmer 1973). In Table 3.6 the dog SD antigen pairs with the highest linkage disequilibrium are shown. These are expressed in a value for the parameter of linkage disequilibrium or delta (Δ), computed according to Mattiuz et al. (1970), and in a ratio of the found and expected frequency of a given antigen combination. DLA-C antigens appear to show their highest delta values mainly with DLA-A antigens. This and the previously noted associations 2–11 and 9–12 could be an argument for a closer relationship between the loci DLA-C and DLA-A than between the loci DLA-C and DLA-B (see Section 2.7). The deltas found in dogs are considerably higher than the ones in primates (e.g., Joint Report Fourth Human Histocompatibility Workshop 1970; Albert et al. 1973a; and for subhuman primates see Chapter 2 in this volume). The same tendency is observed for delta values between dog LD and SD antigens (van den Tweel et al. 1974; Grosse-Wilde et al. 1974, 1975). A likely explanation for the high delta values in dogs is a founder or bottleneck effect (Vriesendorp 1973). Dog history has probably known periods and/or areas in which only a limited number of animals was available for further propagation. The DLA haplotypes of such animals will be overrepresented in subsequent generations. Such a mechanism will not necessarily lead to inbreeding and loss of genetic variation. However, besides this presumed bottleneck effect other mechanisms (such as, perhaps, natural selection) will in all probability have contributed to the high delta values found in dogs (Grosse-Wilde et al. 1975a). It is important to note that the presence of a high degree of linkage disequilibrium entails a danger in the analysis of donor selection studies for organ transplantation. An investigator might be misled to assume that alleles that he has determined have a histocompatibility effect. In fact, however, the real histocompatibility alleles are of another locus on the same chromosome and linkage disequilibrium exists between the recognized "pseudo" histocompatibility alleles and unrecognized "real" histocompatibility alleles. The effects of different loci within the major histocompatibility system (MHS) will be more difficult to separate in the dog, where a high linkage disequilibrium exists, than in other outbred species where this is not the case. Higher linkage disequilibrium parameters do, however, have a practical advantage for experimental studies, in that it is easier to obtain unrelated donor recipient pairs that are matched for one, two or more systems of the MHS.

Cross-Reactivity. Because of space limitations only the final decision on the presence of an antigen is given in Figure 3.1, not the results of individual sera. Sera recognizing DLA-A3 or -7 or -10 frequently have extra reactions with cells of animals carrying one of these three antigens. Similar results have been obtained with anti DLA-B5 and DLA-B13 sera. A third specificity (not included in this review, because of its imperfect recognition) is also recognized by some of the "long" DLA-B5 sera and in all probability belongs to the DLA-B series. In a new series of immunizations, again antibodies were raised with activity against cells carrying any of the three antigens DLA-A3, -A7 or, -A10 or any of the antigens DLA-B5, -B13, extra antigen of the B series, although only one of the three antigens was present in the donor and absent in the recipient. Thus, these two groups of antigens have been proposed as being cross-reactive (Joint Report First International Workshop on Canine Immunogenetics 1973), although formal absorption studies are lacking. These "cross-reactions" can also be offered as an explanation for the hatched aberrant results in Table 3.3. The too high values of the χ^2 of allelism for the antigen pairs 3–7, 3–10, and 4–13 and 5–13 are in all probability caused by an imperfect recognition of groups 10 and 13 in the analysis of the 1973 data, where too many extra reactions of the not completely specific antisera are scored as proper 10 or 13 reactions. This will cause positive associations between allelic antigens that crossreact. Since 1973, short sera for 10, 5, and 13 have become available, as can also be seen from the good fit for Hardy-Weinberg equilibrium in the more recent data reported in this chapter, in contrast to earlier reports (Joint Report First and Second Workshop on Canine Immunogenetics 1973, and 1976).

Besides P 17, three other new groups have been found, R 18, 19, and 20, which will be reported in full when their analysis has been completed.

2.3 Lymphocyte-Defined Antigens

Dog lymphocytes isolated from peripheral blood or other sources and cocultivated for several days in an allogeneic mixture (*m*ixed *l*ymphocyte *c*ulture = MLC) are able to undergo blastogenesis and mitosis. This *in vitro* stimulation is, as in other mammalian species, an immunological specific reaction based on inherited differences in membrane structures of the participants in the mixture, which can presently not be defined by antisera and can therefore be labeled as lymphocyte defined (LD).

2.3.1 Methodology

MLC Culture System. Several authors have described successful culture methods for the dog MLC test (Templeton and Thomas 1971; van der Does et al. 1973; Gluckman et al. 1973; Grosse-Wilde et al. 1973; Goldman et al. 1975a). The most widely used technique is a microculture system in flat or round bottom Microtiter plates first described for human MLC testing by Hartzman and co-workers in 1971. The separation of lymphocytes from defribinated or heparinized blood is done mainly by gradient centrifugation (Ficoll/Isopaque, etc.). Because in the case of heparinized blood the contamination with granulocytes is sometimes rather high, some authors prefer to separate lymphocytes from buffy coat cells diluted with culture medium (Grosse-Wilde, *unpublished observations;* Gluckman et al. 1973). The following media are reported to give sufficient support for the growth of dog lymphocytes in the MLC test: MB752/1, RPMI1640, and MEM-S buffered with $NaHCO_3$ or Hepes. As in the majority of other mammalian cell cultures, 10 to 20 percent serum or plasma is needed. The use of serum-free medium (Click et al. 1972) has not been successful in dogs so far (Grosse-Wilde, *unpublished observations*). DNA synthesis in the stimulating cell population can be blocked in order to obtain one-way MLC tests by mitomycin-C treatment or X-irradiation with approximately 2500 rad. Dog lymphocytes can be cultured successfully in quantities of 1×10^5 stimulating cells and 1×10^5 responding cells. Higher ratios (2:1; 4:1) of stimulating and responding cells give rise to equal or higher MLC reactivity, whereas lower ratios (1:2; 1:4) result in less positive or even negative MLCs (Bijnen, *personal communication*). ^{3}H- or ^{14}C-thymidine are generally used as nucleoacid precursors. Harvesting of the MLCs and further processing for liquid scintillation counting can be done by techniques already described for human or murine MLC tests (Hartzman et al. 1972). The peak of a positive MLC response measured by radioactive-labeled thymidine incorporation is usually observed between day 6 and 7 of culture.

The possibility of cryopreserving LD-typing cells in Microtiter plates has been described recently for dogs (Netzel et al. 1975). The application of this technique will facilitate further studies with LD-typing cells (see Section 2.3.2), in view of the growing number of different LD-typing cells recognized in the dog.

2.3.2 Definition of LD-Typing Cells

Normal MLC tests between unrelated and related individuals can only discriminate between identity or disparity for the MLC determinants carried by the individuals under study. An important step forward has been the use of MLC homozygous cells in one-way MLC tests as reference for the presence of a particular LD specificity. The principles behind the definition of MLC homozygous cell are described in the chapter on human histocompatibility, and can similarly be applied to the dog (Grosse-Wilde et al. 1973). Table 3.7 gives an example for the definition of an LD homozygous dog

Table 3.7. Definition of LD-Homozygous Dog by Family MLC Study

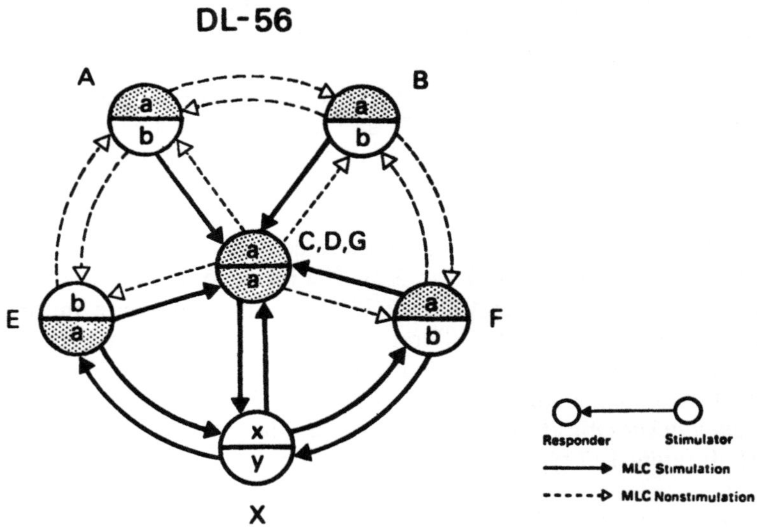

HMV102 010774

	DL-A	Am	Bm	Cm	Dm	Em	Fm	Gm	Xm
A	1-13/3-12	851	901	534	956	256	385	572	68 546
B	1-13/3-12	557	255	397	394	652	341	138	45 976
C	1-13/1-13	24 792	12 252	496	819	18 503	14 165	836	19 807
D	1-13/1-13	58 466	44 712	716	843	17 707	40 433	573	34 361
E	1-13/3-12	747	620	473	565	872	641	437	69 227
F	1-13/3-12	298	556	120	208	454	114	345	85 581
G	1-13/1-13	81 485	40 456	984	892	24 752	91 822	492	82 209
X	3-12/9-6	33 097	98 356	65 108	82 801	30 011	71 184	48 099	207

cpm from quadruplicates

A Dog No 07 Father
B 08 Mother (possible Littermates)
C L16 Child 1 Ref Dog DL-56
D L17 Child 2 Ref Dog DL-56
E L18 Child 3
F L19 Child 4
G L20 Child 5 Ref Dog DL-56
X D8 unrelated Control

Table 3.8. Well Known DLA LD Specificities

LD type:		Frequently associated SD type		Origin:
	50		2-4	Munich, Germany
	51		2-5	Munich, Germany
	52		9-6	Munich, Germany
	53		3-12	Munich, Germany
	54		10-5	Rijswijk, Netherlands
	55		3-bl	Rijswijk, Netherlands
	56		1-13	Munich, Germany
	57		8-13	Paris, France
	58		9-4	Rijswijk, Netherlands

by a family study: Sire and dame in this case DLA-SD genotypically identical littermates (DLA-A1-B13/A3-C12). The SD typing in the offspring revealed that L16, L17, and L20 are homozygous for SD antigens DLA-A1-B13, and L18 and L19 are heterozygous and SD identical to their parents. The MLC reactions indicate that L16, L17, and L20 are LD homozygous as well, because they do not stimulate any of the family members with the DLA-A1-B13 haplotype whereas they are stimulated by their heterozygous family members. A substantial number of additional homozygotes have been detected, and subsequent cross-testing of these cells has so far revealed up to nine different LD-typing cells (Table 3.8). The results of these cross-testing experiments were interpreted as follows: If LD homozygotes are mutually MLC positive, they should carry different LD determinants. More recently, several groups have reported additional LD-homozygous dogs (Gluckman et al. 1975; Goldmann et al. 1975; Bijnen, *personal communication*; Storb, *personal communication*). It is expected that in the near future a battery of up to 15 different LD typing cells will be available.

Definition of LD-Typing Response. LD-typing cells, found in MLC family studies, require further characterization in unrelated individuals. LD-homozygous cells are useful in population studies only if differences in a MLC response against the typing cell can be demonstrated between individuals with and without the LD allele. In order to demonstrate the discriminative power of a particular LD-typing cell, the raw CPM (*c*ounts *p*er *m*inute) obtained in each experiment can be recalculated in so-called stabilized relative responses (RRstab.), as described by Thomsen and co-workers in 1975 for HLA-D typing. Figures 3.2 and 3.3 contain the histograms of such responses for the seven longest known LD specificities (DLA 50 through 56). The histograms of DLA 51, 52, 53, 55, and 56 show a clear bimodal distribution with an incision approximately at the 35 percent RRstab. level. This indicates that these typing cells distinguish very well between individuals positive or negative for the determinant under study. DLA 50 and 54 have a less optimal discriminatory power. The last histogram in Figure 3.3 summarizes LD-typing results obtained with these seven specificities. As can be seen from the bimodal distribution curve, a relative small percentage (13 percent) of the overall

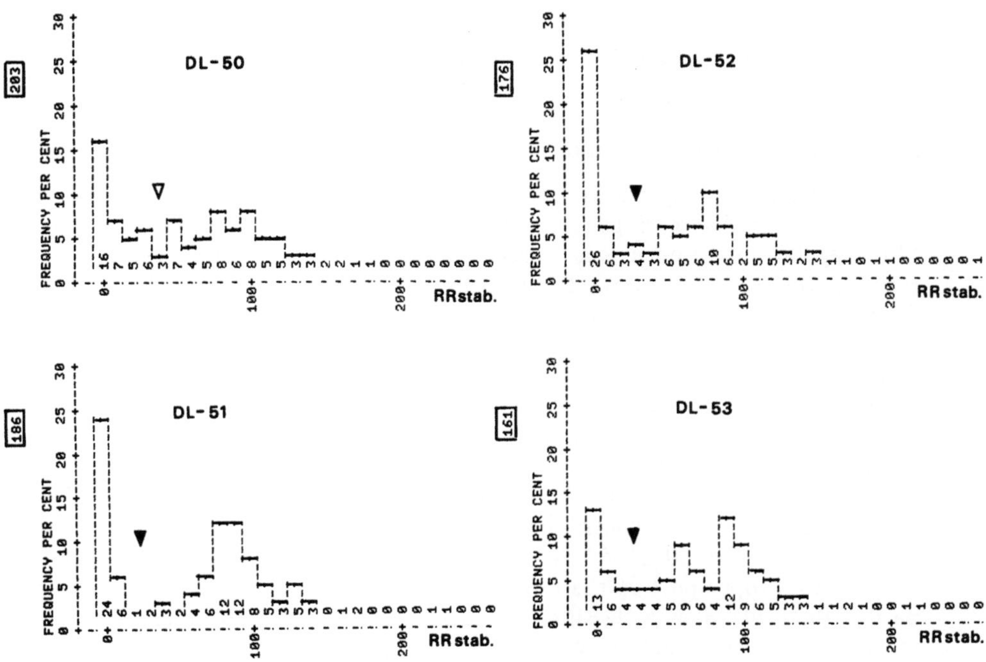

Fig. 3.2. Stabilized relative responses to DLA LD-typing cells, I

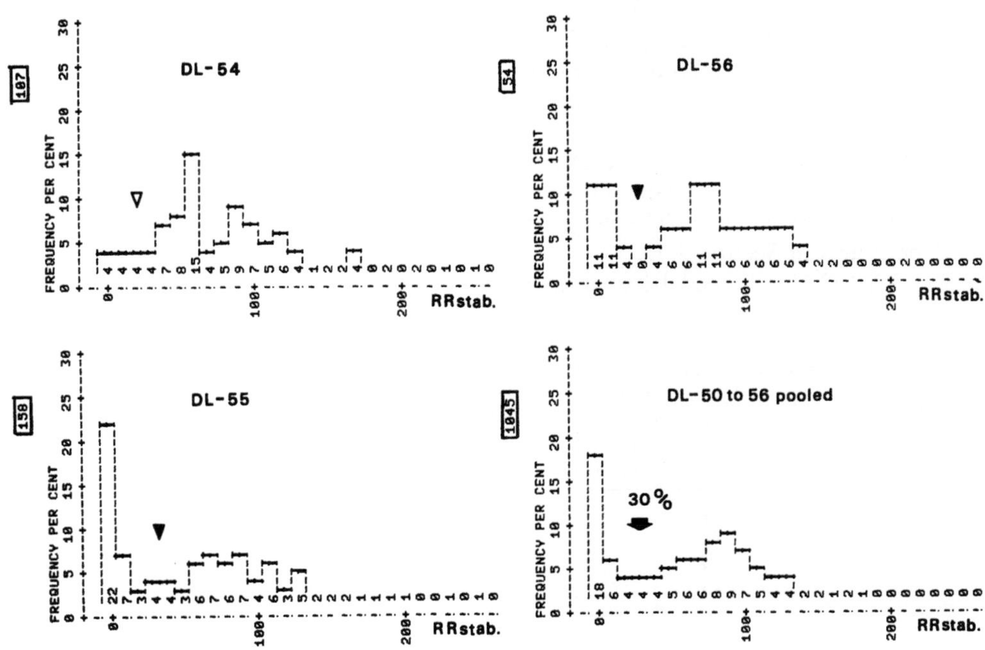

Fig. 3.3. Stabilized relative responses to DLA LD-typing cells, II

typing data fall in the critical range between 20 and 50 percent RRstab. in dogs, in contrast to earlier observations in humans (Grosse-Wilde et al. 1975b).

2.3.3 Genetics of LD Determinants

Family Studies. Family segregation studies were performed in a beagle colony with 50 informative matings for the traits DLA 50, 51, 52, 53, 56 (Table 3.9). No irregular inheritance was observed because the offspring were found positive only for LD specificities also present in the parents. Although the family material is rather small (especially for DLA 52 and 56), the distribution of positive and negative haplotypes does not appear to differ significantly from the expected 1:1 ratio. LD identity between two individuals is assumed when they are not stimulated by the same LD-typing cells. In contrast to serological typing, this can be checked *in vitro* by doing a direct MLC test. An example is given in Table 3.10. The SD and LD genotype of the parents (56-1-13/53-3-12 × 51-2-5/50-2-4) was already established by previous studies. The MLC reactions between the littermates 1 through 6 and toward the LD-typing cells DL 50, 51, 53, 56 together with the SD genotypes are depicted as RRstab. (upper part of the table) and plotted in a histogram. The lower part of the table gives a classification analogue to serological interpretations in plus and minus reaction, where a plus represents a MLC reaction below 35 percent RRstab. and a minus above 35 percent RRstab. The LD typing in this offspring reveals that child 1 and 3 and child 4 and 5, LD-type identical (DLA 51 and 50 and DLA 50 and 53, respectively). These typing results are confirmed by the fact that both pairs are indeed MLC identical as proved by intrafamiliar MLC testing, whereas all the other combinations are MLC different as predicted by LD typing.

In addition, this family gives an example that the genes coding for LD determinants are linked to those coding for the SD antigens because serologically identical littermates (1 and 3, 4 and 5) also typed identical with the MLC reference cells. The crossing-over frequency between LD and SD can be found in Section 2.7.

MLCs performed between *unrelated* individuals that are not stimulated

Table 3.9. Segregation Analysis of Five DLA LD Specificities

LD Type	Parents (+ /–)×(– /–) (– /–)×(+ /–)	Offspring (+ /–)	(– /–)	Ratio (+ /–):(– /–)
50	11	30	23	1.3
51	16	35	47	0.7
52	3	8	14	0.6
53	14	36	33	1.1
56	6	17	23	0.7
Total	50	126	140	0.9

Table 3.10. LD Typing and LD Identity in a Family

HMV263 210475

SD - Type	1m	2m	3m	4m	5m	6m	50	51	53	56
1 1-13/2-5		78	7	95	80	103	52	12	147	10
2 1-13/2-4	102		100	132	107	114	7	72	59	10
3 1-13/2-5	14	105		111	182	117	100	10	94	12
4 3-12/2-5	92	106	92		18	71	94	22	6	143
5 3-12/2-5	62	160	88	19		98	152	6	4	82
6 3-12/2-4	143	51	120	65	80		9	129	3	75

% R R stab.

F : DLA 56-1-13/53-3-12

M: 51-2-5/50-2-4

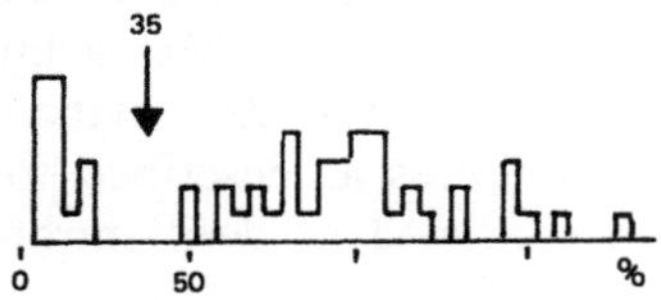

LD - Type	1m	2m	3m	4m	5m	6m	50	51	53	56
1 56/51		-	+	-	-	-	-	+	-	+
2 56/50	-		-	-	-	-	+	-	-	+
3 56/51	+	-		-	-	-	-	+	-	+
4 53/51	-	-	-		+	-	-	+	+	-
5 53/51	-	-	-	+		-	-	+	+	-
6 53/50	-	-	-	-	-		+	-	+	-

Class. + = < 35 % R R stab.
- = > 35 % R R stab.

by the same two LD-typing cells are frequently positive (Bijnen, *personal communication*). This suggests the existence of more than one locus in the genetic control of MLC reactivity, which would be in accordance with the observed inheritance *en bloc* of two different LD determinants by Grosse-Wilde et al. in 1975. The total number of different LD loci within the DLA system cannot be given as yet. The data collected so far suggest that at least two exist. DLA 50, 51, 52, and 55 are in all probability alleles from a different locus than DLA 53 and 54 (Grosse-Wilde et al. 1975). These two loci are in this chapter provisionally called DLA-D and DLA-E. However, international agreement on this notation has not yet been reached. For DLA 56 through 58, not enough data are available to decide whether they belong to one of these loci. The possible practical complications of more loci in the control of MLC reactivity, as far as the use of LD-homozygote reference cells is concerned, will have to be determined in further studies. Suffice it here to state that some cells might be "more homozygous" than others. The low-grade stimulation of some cells by the LD-typing cells might be explained by the influence of a second MLC system, for which the reference cells are not homozygous or for which there is no similarity between responder and typing cell. Cells that are homozygous for more than one LD determinant will more often show a lack of stimulation with random individuals than cells that are homozygous for only one LD determinant. This phenomenon could lead to "splits" in the currently known LD alleles.

2.4 Immune Response Genes

2.4.1 Methodology

A preliminary study of immune response (Ir) genes in dogs has been performed in which three random linear copolymers of amino acids have been used for immunizations. Copolymers of L-glutamic acid with L-alanine (GA), L-lysine (GL), or L-tyrosine (GT) were synthezised to order by Pilot Chemicals, Inc., Watertown, Massachusetts, USA. DNP-GL was prepared as described by Benacerraf and Levine (1962). Animals were immunized using the same procedures as described for rhesus monkeys (Dorf et al. 1975a). In brief, it consisted of deep intramuscular injections of a total of 100 µg of GA and 50 µg of DNP-GL, each in the two hind legs and both in complete Freund adjuvant. Skin tests were done 3 weeks later intradermally in 0.1 ml injections doses of 10 and 50 µg for each. After a minimum resting period of 7 weeks after the skin tests, a new immunization schedule was started with a dose of 100 µg of GT for the first injection and following subsequently the same procedures as outlined for GA and GL. Serum samples were collected on days 0, 21, and 28 of the immunization procedure and stored at −20° C until assayed. A Farr assay (Katz et al. 1970; Dorf et al. 1973) was used to measure the antibody response of immunized animals. A rabbit antidog immunoglobulin serum or ammonium sulfate was used to precipitate antigen antibody complexes. Results are compared to results with the serum of day 0 and expressed as +, ±, or − according to the percentage of antigen binding at a 1/5 serum dilution, being ≧40, between 10 and 40 or ≦10, respectively.

2.4.2 Genetics

Unrelated Dogs. Table 3.11 gives the results of immunizations performed in limited numbers of unrelated dogs. In this study it was observed that the immune responses among the dogs tested were rather weak in comparison to the humoral responses observed in guinea pigs (Bluestein et al. 1971) and rhesus monkeys (Dorf et al. 1975) to these same antigens. The ability

Table 3.11. Immunization with Copolymers of Amino Acids in Unrelated Dogs

Antigen[a]	Number of Animals with a Humoral Immune Response of Type			Gene Frequency[b] of Immune Response Gene
	−	±	+	
GA	5	1	19	0.53
GL	2	1	15	0.67
GT	20	1	4	0.11

[a] For abbreviations see text.

[b] Computed assuming ± response to be positive, with the formula $GF=1-(1-PF)^{1/2}$, where GF and PF are gene and population frequency, respectively.

Table 3.12. Family Studies of Immune Response Against GA in Dog Families

Family	Parents	Litter	DLA[a]	GA Response
1	♂		AB	Not tested
	♀		CD	–
		1	BC	+
		2	AD	–
		3	AD	–
2	♂		AB	Not tested
	♀		CD	–
		1	BD	–
		2	BC	–
		3	AD	+
		4	AD	+
3	♂		AB	Not tested
	♀		CD	Not tested
		1	AD	±
		2	BC	±
		3	BC	±
		4	BC	±
		5	AC	+
		6	AC	+
		7	BD	–

[a] The ABCD notation is used here, in which each parental DLA haplotype is indicated by a letter.

of an animal to produce antibodies against a certain antigen appeared to be polymorphic for all three antigens tested; i.e., responders and nonresponders have been found. The occurrence of equivocal responders (indicated as ±) is disturbing and makes a genetic analysis less reliable. This problem of responders in the dog has not been solved so far. In mice studies it appeared that the magnitude of a specific immune response is influenced by many different loci (Biozzi et al. 1971; Dorf et al. 1973). One might assume that products of equivalent loci in dogs sometimes have a negative influence on the expression of the Ir genes studied. In the present analysis weak responses were scored as positive.

Family Data. GA: Three informative segregation patterns were observed for this antigen (Table 3.12). In six additional families with a total of 43 siblings, GA responses were monomorphic. Only positive (30) or weak responses (13) were found. The three segregation patterns observed are in accordance with DLA inheritance. Only two of the six parents were available for testing.

GT: In four families (17 siblings in all), no antibodies against GT were found in parents or offspring. In two families (13 siblings in all), one isolated positive offspring was found. One of them appeared to have antibodies in the preimmune serum of day 0. The other positive animal remains unexplained. It could be an example of a requirement for two complementing

Table 3.13. Family Studies of Immune Response Against GT in Dog Families

Family	Parents	Offspring	DLA[a]	GT Response
1	♂		AB	−
	♀		CD	+
		1	BC	−
		2	AC	+
		3	BD	−
		4	AC	+
		5	AD	+
		6	AD	+
2[b]	♂		AB	+
	♀		CD	−
		1	AD	−
		2	A/BC	+
		3	A/BC	−
		4	AD	−
3	♂		AB	Not tested
	♀		CD	Not tested
		1	AD	−
		2	AD	−
		3[c]	BC	−
		4	BC	+
		5	BC	±
		6	BC	±

[a] The ABCD notation is used here, in which each parental DLA haplotype is indicated by a letter.
[b] Serological and MLC results of family 2 were reported by van den Tweel et al. (*J. Exp. Med.* *140*:825–836, 1974): they showed that offspring 2 obtained DLA-D and DLA-A specificities from the B haplotype and DLA-B antigens from the A haplotype. Offspring 3 inherited the DLA-D specificity from the A haplotype and the DLA-A and B specificities from the B haplotype. This localizes the Ir-GT response outside DLA-A.
[c] This animal was LD and SD identical with sibs 4, 5, and 6. The discrepancy in GT response indicates a recombination between the DLA-D and the Ir-GT loci and localizes Ir-GT to the left of DLA-D (see also family 2 in this table and Figure 5).

IrGT response genes for a positive response as described in mice by Dorf et al. 1975b. The three remaining informative families, i.e., those with positive and negative responders within a litter, are given in Table 3.13. The data suggest an *en bloc* inheritance of the GT response and DLA haplotypes. In families 2 and 3 exceptions occur, which could be explained by crossing-over. This matter is discussed in more detail in Section 2.7.

GL: Only one family of the nine was informative for GL inheritance; in all the others only responders were found. One nonresponder animal was found among seven littermates. It was the only animal in this litter receiving a paternal B and a maternal D DLA haplotype.

The conclusion of these preliminary data is that results of immunizations in dogs for the detection of Ir genes have given suggestive information about (1) the presence of these genes in this species, and (2) linkage between Ir genes and the DLA complex. The major problem that remains to be solved by further experimentation is the definition of conditions in which the difference in antibody response between responders and nonresponders is wider.

2.5 Allogeneic Resistance (R)

Soon after the discovery of the protection that injected bone marrow (BM) cells can offer against radiation-induced death, it was observed that the number of cells needed to achieve this purpose was among other things dependent on the donor of the injected BM cells. An animal that received a lethal dose of total body irradiation (TBI) needed more BM cells to survive from an allogeneic donor than from an isologous or autologous one (van Bekkum and Vos 1957). Similar results were reported for dogs (Thomas et al. 1959).

2.5.1 Methodology

In 1971 Cudkowicz and Bennett demonstrated, in studies of this phenomenon in mice, that the resistance (R) against allogeneic BM cells after a lethal dose of TBI was a genetically determined property and effectuated by the recipient. The genetic control of R appeared to be located within the major histocompatibility system of this species. Subsequent studies of this group led to the concept that macrophages play an important role in allogeneic resistance (Lotzová and Cudkowicz 1974). A reliable *in vitro* assay for R is not yet available in mice (Vriesendorp et al. 1976). The only way to demonstrate unequivocally the presence of R is *in vivo*. This is illustrated by the data obtained in dogs given in Figure 3.4. Three different treatment schedules were applied to dogs after a supralethal dose of TBI. Variations were noted in the changes of the peripheral leukocyte levels in the different experimental groups. In dogs that received 4×10^8 BM cells/kg body weight of a DLA-identical donor, a gradual recovery to normal counts (around day 30) was found. In contrast, after a similar number of BM cells of a DLA-not identical donor, only a temporary elevation in leukocyte counts occurred. Animals died subsequently from the complications of BM aplasia. Animals without BM treatment underwent the same fate, but did not show this temporary rise in peripheral leukocytes. Similar patterns were seen in thrombocyte and reticulocyte levels in the three experimental groups. The absence of a lasting take of the injected BM cells in the animals that died was verified by histological examinations showing the absence of graft-versus-host (GvH) reactions and no regeneration of hemopoietic tissues. The injection of silica particles after TBI appeared to abrogate R in dogs (Vriesendorp 1975b), which indicates that in dogs also macrophages might play a role in allogeneic resistance.

2.5.2 Genetics

In dogs the DLA system appeared to be of importance in the genetic control of R (Vriesendorp et al. 1975a, 1975b, 1975c). This is shown by the data

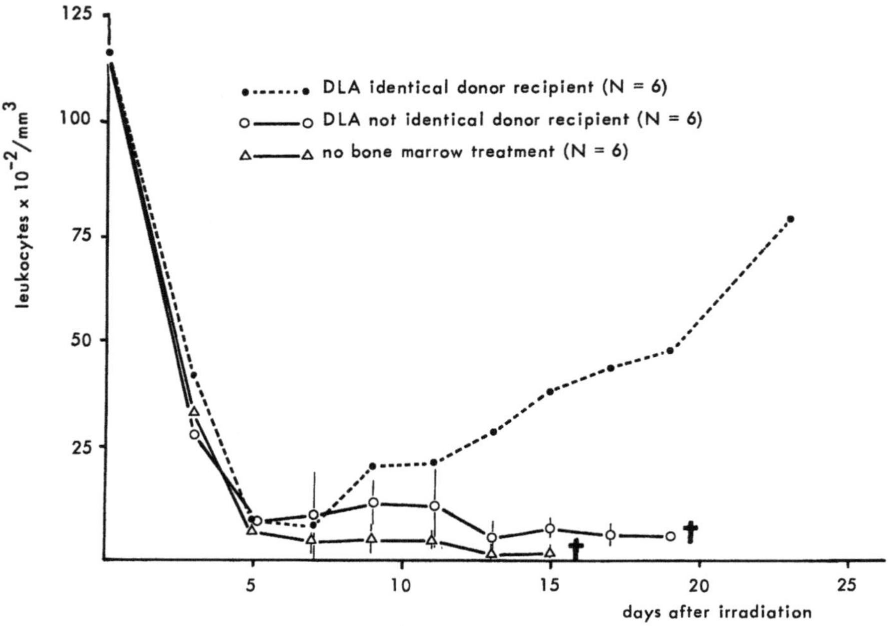

Fig. 3.4. Peripheral leukocyte levels in irradiated dogs with and without bone marrow treatment. 4×10^8 BM/kg body weight were given 24 hr after a total body irradiation of 750 or 800 rad

in Figure 3.4 and Table 3.14. The experimental protocol for the transplantation of BM cells has been similar in all animals, i.e. conditioning with 750 rad of TBI with X-rays, followed by the i.v. injection of 4×10^8 BM cells/kg body weight 24 hr later. Experimental groups 1 and 2 in Table 3.14 show that R is controlled on the same chromosome as on which the DLA complex is located. Results in experimental group 4 from Table 3.14 suggest that neither LD nor DLA-A nor DLA-B genes control R in dogs, because two examples of persisting takes were found in a group of 11 animals that were LD and/or SD different. This concept has been confirmed in additional unrelated donor-recipient pairs where a negative MLC, or a combined DLA-A, B and C identity, between donor and recipient, was not sufficient to secure a lasting BM take (Vriesendorp et al. 1975b, and unpublished observations).

The data in the third experimental group of Table 3.14 show that linkage disequilibrium must be present between SD and LD alleles on the one hand and R alleles on the other hand, because R was found to be absent in 8 out of 8 unrelated LD- and SD-identical donor-recipient pairs, in contrast to the 2 out of 11 in LD- and/or SD-mismatched pairs. In all probability, R control will be located between the LD and SD loci, because no example of R was found in 33 DLA-A-, SD-, and LD-identical donor-recipient pairs. BM grafts in DL-A recombinants that would allow a more precise mapping of the R region within the DLA complex have not yet been performed.

Table 3.14. Genetics of Take of Allogeneic Dog Bone Marrow

Exp. Group	DLA Differences Donor-Recipient[a]			Number of Recipients	Relationship of Donor and Recipient[b]	Proportion of Persisting Takes
	LD	DLA-B	DLA-A			
1	=	=	=	33	Sibs B→B	33/33
2	≠	≠	≠	4	Sibs B→B	0/4
3	=	=	=	8	Unr. B→B (2) Unr. M→B (6)	8/8
4	≠[c]	≠	≠	11	Unr. B→B (4) Unr. M→B (7)	1/4 1/7

[a] When SD groups were present in the donor and not in the recipient or when recipient lymphocytes were stimulated in MLC by donor cells, a ≠ sign is given. An = sign shows that this was not in fact the case.

[b] Breeds are given as B (beagle) or M (mongrel); unr. = unrelated.

[c] In the four B→B and in three of the seven M→B combinations, LD differences were not determined. The take in the M→B group occurred in a LD-incompatible combination.

2.6 Other Markers

2.6.1 PhosphoGlucoMutase 3

Phosphoglucomutase-3 (PGM-3) is a polymorphic leukocyte enzyme in men as well as in dogs (Meera Khan et al. 1973). In human families linkage between PGM-3 and HLA could be demonstrated in paternal segregation patterns. Similar results have been obtained in the First and Second International Workshops on Canine Immunogenetics (Meera Khan et al. 1976). In male segregation patterns a peak lod score of 3.033 was found at a recombination frequency of 10 percent. The lod score for female segregation patterns was negative. The fact that evidence for linkage can be found only in male segregation patterns is explained by the presence of higher recombination frequencies between PGM-3 and the major histocompatibility system in females. The exact location of the PGM-3 locus is unknown. If the situation in the dog is analogous to the one in man (Bijnen et al. 1976), one would anticipate it to be located outside DLA-D (see Section 2.7).

2.6.2 Immune Response-Associated Antigens (Ia) and Complement Markers

In several species immune response genes have been found to be linked to genes controlling antigens, which can be determined with antisera, but which in contrast to regular SD antigens show a preferential occurrence on B-lymphocytes, epidermal cells, macrophages, and sperm cells (Sachs et al. 1975; Balner and van Vreeswijk 1975). Such antigens have been labeled Ia (*I*mmune response genes *a*ssociated) antigens. An attempt has been made to define Ia antigens in dogs by exposing B-cell-enriched lymphocyte suspensions to postpartum sera. The percentage of B-cells in the cell suspensions was enhanced by separating the peripheral blood samples twice on ficoll isopaque gradients. Before the second gradient, the cells from the interphase of the first gradient were allowed to form rosettes with human O erythrocytes. Rosetting cells (approximately 50 percent and presumably T-lymphocytes) were spun down in the second gradient and cells of the second interphase were used for testing. A two-stage microcytotoxicity test with 50 postpartum sera was applied to "normal" lymphocyte samples and to "B-cell-enriched" lymphocyte samples. A small group of sera appeared to be positive only when tested with B-cells. The reactivity patterns of these sera were, however, identical with known SD antigens, and thrombocyte absorptions did remove the antibody activity. These data show that (1) the "B-cell" test employed is a more sensitive method for the measurement of anti-SD antibodies than the ordinary two-stage cytotoxicity test; (2) the postpartum sera investigated did not contain anti-Ia antibodies. These observations are in accordance with data obtained by Balner and van Vreeswijk in 1975 in rhesus monkeys. Further studies will have to be done to determine if Ia antigens can be defined in dogs.

Some genetically controlled polymorphisms of complement factors were found to be linked to the MHS in mice (Démant et al. 1973), men (Allen 1974; Fu et al. 1974), and rhesus monkeys (Ziegler et al. 1975). Recently polymorphism was found for a complement factor in dogs, in all probability C 3 (Rittner and Grosse-Wilde, *unpublished observations*). In preliminary family studies no linkage was found between this marker and DLA.

2.7 Genetic Organization of DLA System

The cluster of loci (SD, LD, Ir, R, PGM-3) that have been identified within the DLA region are known to be separate loci because alleles of these various loci show different distribution patterns in populations of unrelated, randomly selected animals. Separation by recombination events has been reported for DLA-B and DLA-A (recombination frequency ±0.7 percent; 95 percent confidence limits 0.1–2.2) (Vriesendorp et al. 1973), for DLA-A on the one hand and a MLC locus (DLA-D) on the other hand (van den Tweel et al. 1974; Joint Report Second International Workshop on Canine Immunogenetics 1976), and for the Ir-GT and DLA-D locus (see Section 2.4.2). A recent estimate of the crossing-over frequency between SD and LD was obtained in still unpublished studies of Bijnen and Vriesendorp, that is 0.71 percent (95 percent confidence limits 0.1–2.4). This estimate does not take into account that there is in all probability more than one LD locus in the DLA region.

The exact mapping of other loci within the DLA complex is not known. This is shown in Figure 3.5 by a question mark or by the remark that the locus is in the DLA area without giving an exact position of this locus. A question mark is given to those loci for which some indications exist about its possible whereabouts. This is the case for the PGM-3 locus, which

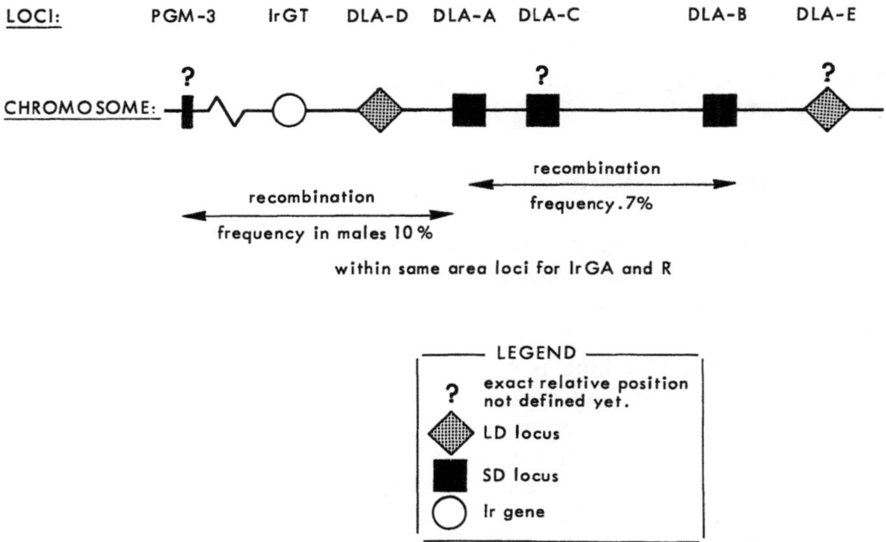

Fig. 3.5. Genetic organization of DLA complex. Recombinations were observed between DLA-A and DLA-D (van den Tweel et al., 1974), DLA-A and DLA-B (Vriesendorp et al., 1973), and DLA-D and Ir-GT (see Section 2.4.2, Table 3.13)

if the analogy with man is complete, should map to the left of DLA-D (Bijnen et al. 1976). High parameters for linkage disequilibrium between alleles suggest short distances between these loci. Because higher deltas were found between DLA-A and DLA-C alleles than between DLA-B and DLA-C alleles, this suggests that DLA-C is in all probability closer to the DLA-A locus than the DLA-B locus (see Section 2.2.3). In Section 2.3.3 are discussed the results that lead to the postulation of a provisional second LD locus (i.e., DLA-E). Grosse-Wilde et al. reported in 1975 that higher linkage disequilibrium parameters were found between DLA 50, 51, 52, 55, and DLA-B antigens than between DLA 50 to 55 and DLA-A antigens. This would locate the DLA-E locus close to DLA-B. Unpublished observations of Bijnen and Vriesendorp would place DLA-E outside the two SD loci to the right of DLA-B.

The data for locating the Ir-Ga and R loci within the DLA complex are given in Sections 2.4.2 and 2.5.2, respectively. For these markers more exact mapping data are not yet available.

3. Transplantation Biology of DLA

Studies of the DLA complex are not merely an excercise in genetics, but have as ultimate goal the definition of reliable methods of donor selection. In dogs donor selection for organ grafting and its effect on allograft survival has been studied in two experimental groups: (1) related and (2) unrelated donor-recipient pairs. As will be shown, effects of current donor selection procedures vary in these groups because of the still imperfect donor selection methods used.

3.1 Related Donor-Recipient Pairs

For various types of organs, donors have been selected from the recipient's family members by typing for SD antigens. A summary of the results obtained by the group in the laboratory for experimental surgery of the Erasmus University, Rotterdam, is given in Figure 3.6. For all organs a significant influence of DLA matching is observed. Similar data have been reported from the group working in Cooperstown in the United States for skin (Dausset et al. 1971), renal (Rapaport et al. 1970), heart (Rapaport et al. 1971), and liver allografts (Chandler et al. 1971). The same trend was observed in these data, in that the survival of skin grafts was less effected (MST 24.7 days) by donor selection and that kidney, heart, and liver allografts had a more extended survival of 27.3, 33.9, and 76.7 days, respectively. However, the absolute mean survival times for each organ are not comparable in the two different research groups. This might be due to differences in

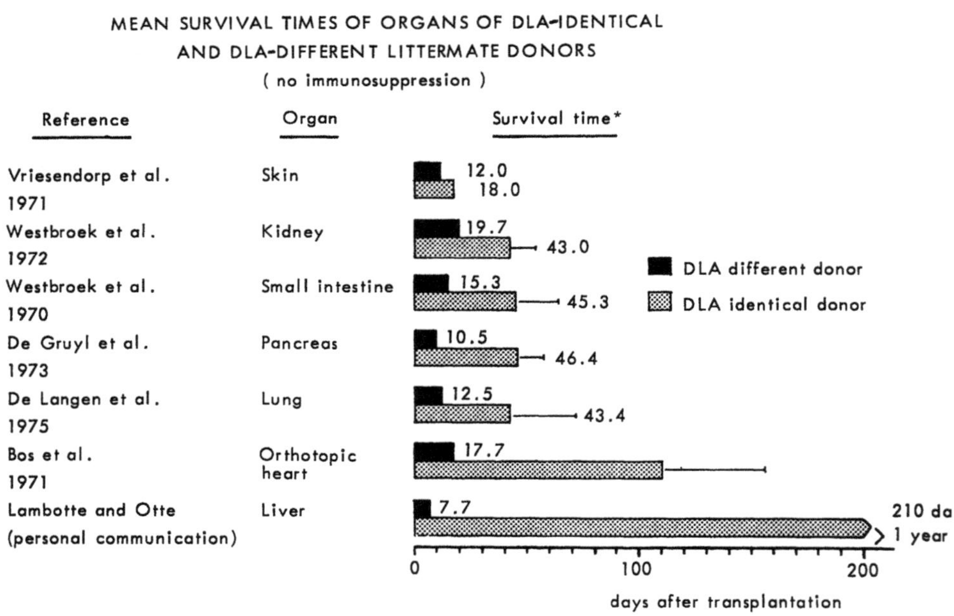

* One standard deviation of the mean is given. Each mean is computed from survival times of at least six different animals, with the exception of liver allografts where only two animals have been grafted.

Fig. 3.6. Mean survival times of organs of DLA-identical and DLA-different littermate donors

genetic background of the experimental animals, in operation procedures, in animal care, or in the tissue-typing reagents used. Variables that might induce differences in survival of grafts from different histological types, *within one laboratory,* include, among others: (1) intrinsic differences between vascular and avascular transplants, e.g., skin versus kidney; (2) differences in immunogenicity of the various organs; (3) a greater vulnerability of some organs to rejection (e.g. the conduction system of the heart [Dausset et al. 1971]; and (4) the use of third-party blood transfusions at the time of operation. It is clear from Figure 3.6 that the more complicated surgical procedures of heart and liver allografts are correlated with longer mean survivals of DLA-identical organs and a larger standard deviation of the mean survival times. The blood transfusions that are routinely needed for the recipients during such difficult surgical procedures might be of relevance here. Preliminary results of an ongoing analysis of the influence of blood transfusions are available and will be discussed in Section 3.3. With such a complicated phenomenon as graft survival and with a list of at least four variables, it is impossible to determine without further studies which one(s) is (are) determining the differences found in survival times of different organs. It is of interest to note that also in dogs liver allografts can survive for a very prolonged time without the use of immunosuppression. This would confirm that it is the organ and not the species that causes the reported prolonged liver allograft survival in pigs (Calne et al. 1967).

Bone marrow grafts differ from other organ allografts in that in the preparation ("conditioning") of the recipient, immunosuppressive procedures such as TBI have to be used to secure a take of the transplanted cells. Moreover, a successful graft is capable of killing its recipient by means of the so-called GvH reaction (van Bekkum and de Vries 1967). Early studies by Epstein and co-workers (1968, 1971) showed an important influence of matching for leukocyte specificities on host versus graft (HvG) as well as GvH reactions. A more detailed genetic analysis of GvH reactions in DLA-identical donor-recipient littermate pairs was made by Storb et al. (1973) and Vriesendorp et al. (1975b, 1975c). A pronounced effect of DLA matching on the incidence of GvH reactions was found in both studies. In DLA-identical pairs only approximately 50 percent of the animals showed signs of GvH, whereas in unrelated or DLA-mismatched sibling pairs this occurs in almost 100 percent. An extensive analysis of the influence of DLA matching on HvG reactions after TBI have been summarized in Section 2.5.

In addition to the effect of donor selection by DLA serology on graft survival, effects on histology and function of rejecting organs and on the efficacy of immunosuppression were found. Westbroek and co-workers (1972) noted that the functional abnormalities in rejecting DLA-identical and DLA-nonidentical kidneys were different. In short-surviving, DLA-different kidneys, biochemistry data of urine and serum indicated an overall ischemic kidney lesion. In longer-surviving, DLA-identical kidneys, a more selective tubulus dysfunction was found. In the same study the histology of graft rejection was compared to the donor-recipient relationship. More extensive histological studies were done by an evaluation of sequential biopsies of small intestine and heart allografts in tissue-typed dogs (Westbroek et al. 1971; Penn et al. 1976). In these studies DLA identity appeared to have an effect on both of the two most prominent signs of allograft rejection: (1) graft arteritis and (2) cellular infiltration of the graft. The cellular infiltration appeared later and was less aggressive in DLA-identical grafts. Sometimes it seemed even to disappear (Penn et al. 1976). The arteritis in DLA-identical grafts occurred for the first time around the third week after grafting, became gradually more intense, and was subsequently the final cause of allograft failure. A different sequence of events is found in DL-A-mismatched grafts where a fast and massive cellular infiltration is thought to be the major effector mechanism in the rejection process. The efficacy of some immunosuppressive regimens was found to be more pronounced in DLA-matched or partially-matched than in DLA-completely mismatched donor-recipient pairs (de Gruyl 1973; Storb et al. 1972).

3.2 Unrelated Donor-Recipient Pairs

Unrelated matched donor-recipient pairs have been tested in three different situations: (1) kidney allografts (Westbroek et al. 1975); (2) HvG reactions (Vriesendorp et al. 1975a, 1975b, 1975c); (3) GvH reactions (Storb et al. 1975; Kolb et al. 1975; Vriesendorp et al. 1975a). In all the cited reports the results indicated at best a marginal effect of LD and/or SD matching. The existence of additional loci within the DLA complex, which are different from the known LD and SD loci and which have an important histocompatibility effect, must therefore be postulated. In sibling donor-recipient pairs where DLA haplotypes inherit in the vast majority of cases without the occurrence of crossing-over, LD and SD typing can be used as "flags" to follow the inheritance of the more relevant histocompatibility structures in the same chromosomal area. In unrelated donor-recipient pairs the histocompatibility structures need to be identified, because a one-to-one relationship between LD or SD types and such structures does not hold. The marginal effects of LD or SD typing under these circumstances are at the moment best explained by the existence of linkage disequilibrium between LD and/or SD alleles on the one hand and additional histocompatibility alleles that must still be defined on the other hand.

3.3 Blood Transfusions and Graft Survival

In man, blood transfusions are the most frequently performed transplantations of allogeneic cells. The success rate of other transplants is influenced by preceding blood transfusions. Halasz et al. reported in 1964 a beneficial influence of small quantities of dog blood on the survival of subsequent renal allografts of the same donor. However, similar positive results did not appear in the literature after this initial report. Negative results were found by Storb and co-workers (1970, 1971) for canine bone marrow grafts. Transfusions of donor blood from a DLA-identical as well as a DLA-not identical donor lowered the percentage of successful takes of subsequent BM grafts. The same observation was made with blood transfusions of third parties. In kidney transplantation in dogs (Obertop et al. 1975; Bull and Vriesendorp, *unpublished observations*) an ultrashort graft survival was noted when after blood transfusions a positive cross-match was present between recipient's serum and donor's lymphocytes. No influence or even a prolonged graft survival was noted when this was not the case, notwithstanding the preceding immunization with donor blood (Obertop et al. 1975). A retrospective analysis of human kidney transplants (Opelz et al. 1973) showed that some but not all of the patients undergoing chronic haemodialysis developed antibodies against the allogeneic lymphocytes that were infused with the regularly required blood transfusions. This group of patients could thus be divided according to their humoral antibody response to blood transfusions as "responders" and "nonresponders." The survival of a subsequent kidney graft was found to be significantly better in nonresponder recipients. A beneficial influence of SD matching could be demonstrated in responder recipients. This lead to the formulation of the following working hypothesis: The immune response against infused allogeneic lymphocytes is controlled by the same genetically determined mechanisms in the host as the immune response against a transplanted kidney. Persons not reacting with antibody formation against transfused allogeneic lymphocytes would also not, or would but to a lesser degree, react against an allogeneic kidney. The dog is an ideal model for the testing of this hypothesis. In ongoing studies of this subject Bull and co-workers (*unpublished observations*) have found that after a number of transfusions of third parties in dog litters, responders and nonresponders were found. If this respondership is a simple Mendelian trait (which still remains to be demonstrated), then the results obtained indicate that this "response locus" is not linked to or correlated with DLA inheritance. The survival of a DLA-identical kidney from a sibling donor appeared not to be influenced by the responder status of the recipient, which is at variance with the earlier-mentioned human experience and argues against the hypothesis mentioned earlier. The survival of DLA mismatched kidneys was slightly better in nonresponders, when compared to responders. Most of the variables of blood transfusions and subsequent kidney grafting can be controlled and investigated in the dog model, which seems therefore to be optimally suited for further studies of this important subject.

4. Minor Histocompatibility Systems

The prolonged but limited survival as given in Figure 3.6 of DLA-identical allografts indicates that in the long run minor histocompatibility differences will cause graft rejection in dogs. Such systems are not amenable to analysis, however, because the tools with which to identify the different polymorphic structures controlled by these systems still need to be developed. Suggestive evidence for the presence of sex linked (Y as well as X) minor histocompatibility systems was recently obtained (Vriesendorp et al., *unpublished observations*).

The human ABO blood group system has been identified in the past as having some histocompatibility effect (Dausset and Rapaport 1966; Cepellini et al. 1969). An immunogenetic system in dogs with some similarities to the ABO system is the so-called canine secretory alloantigen system (CSA), which has been identified in a series of studies by Zweibaum and co-workers (e.g., Zweibaum et al. 1974). The equivalent system in the rabbit was shown to have a histocompatibility effect (Zweibaum and Bouhon 1973). In dogs CSA incompatibility did not appear to correlated with GvH reactions in DLA-identical donor-recipient pairs (Vriesendorp et al. 1975c). No further systematic studies of possible histocompatibility effects of CSA structures have been performed so far.

The occurrence of GvH in DLA-identical donor-recipient pairs (Storb et al. 1973; Vriesendorp et al. 1975c) is by definition under the control of minor histocompatibility systems. Suggestive evidence was found for a locus controlling GvH reactions on a chromosome that also codes for PGM-2 (Vriesendorp et al. 1975a, 1975c). Thus two similar linkage groups seem to be present in dogs: (1) PGM-2 and a minor GvH locus, and (2) PGM-3 and DLA. This could be an indication of duplication events in evolutionary history, which generated various histocompatibility systems from one common ancestor chromosomal area. Typing for the PGM-2-linked GvH locus by means of serological or other immunogenetical methods is not yet possible. A growing number of other genetic markers is being discovered in dogs (Joint Report Second International Workshop on Canine Immunogenetics 1976). The possibility that these systems have histocompatibility effects has not been tested so far.

5. Concluding Remarks

In the introduction to this chapter it was stated that the use of dogs in experimental medicine should be a deliberate decision and be limited to those protocols for which they are the optimal experimental animals. The amount of information available in dog histocompatibility at the present time, which was documented in the preceding paragraphs, is not yet complete, but allows for the use of dogs in a wide variety of "subclinical" experimental protocols. Although the procedures and reagents necessary to obtain the currently available genetic information in dogs are not cheap or easy to perform, it should be stressed here that this information is essential for a proper use of dogs in transplantation studies. The albeit laudable urge of many "dog" transplantation surgeons to simplify the preoperative analysis should not have as its consequence that no histocompatibility studies are done. The obtained results will be less easily interpreted or extrapolated to human conditions and therefore needlessly cruel to the experimental subjects when the relevant genetic tests are not performed. A growing group of internationally cooperating scientists (see Joint Reports Dog workshops) is eager to provide the necessary assistance in dog histocompatibility studies, because this will lead to a better use of dogs in the laboratory and a faster development of new histocompatibility concepts in this species. Recently two reference centers for dog histocompatibility have been established for this purpose by the International Committee for Laboratory Animals (ICLA 1975).

References

Ahrons, S., and Kissmeyer-Nielsen, F. HL-A typing: Influence of methodological variation. *Symp. Series Immunobiol. Std. 18*:85–88. Karger, Basel, 1973.

Albert, E.D., Mickey, M.R., Ting, A., and Terasaki, P.I. Deduction of 2140 HL-A haplotypes and segregation analysis in 535 families. *Transplant. Proc. 5*:215–221, 1973a.

Albert, E.D., Storb, R., Erickson, V.M., Graham, T., Parr, M., Templeton, J.W., Mickey, M.R., and Thomas, E.D. Serology and genetics of the DL-A system I. Establishment of specificities. *Tissue Antigens 3*:417–430, 1973b.

Allen, F.H. Linkage of HL-A and GBG. *Vox. Sang. 27*:382–000, 1974.

Altman, B., and Simonsen, M. Cytotoxic antibody and hemagglutinin in canine homotransplantation. *Ann. N.Y. Acad. Sci. 120*:28–34, 1964.

Andresen, E., Baker, L.N., and Rowe, K.E. The usefulness and limitation of two-by-two tables in distinguishing between allelism and non-allelism based on random population data. *Immunogenet. Letters 3*:15–20, 1963.

Balner, H., and van Vreeswijk, W. The major histocompatibility complex of rhesus monkeys (RHL-A) V—Attempts at serological identification of MLR determinants and postulation of a I region in the RhL-A complex. *Transplant. Proc. 7*:13–20, 1975.

Benacerraf, B., and Levine, B.B. Immunological specificity of the delayed and immediate hypersensitivity reactions. *J. Exp. Med. 115*:1023–1043, 1962.

Bijnen, A.B., Schreuder, I., Meera Khan, P., Allen, F.H., Giles, C.M., Los, W.R.T., Volkers, W.S., and van Rood, J.J. Linkage relationships of the loci of the major histocompatibility complex in families with a recombination in the HLA region. *J. Immunogenet., 3*:171–183, 1976.

Biozzi, G., Stiffel, C., Boutillier, Y., and Decreusefond, C. Genetic regulation of the function of antibody-producing cells. *In* B. Amos (ed.), *Progress in Immunology*; 1st Int. Congr. Immunol., pp. 529–545, Academic Press, New York, 1971.

Bluestein, H.G., Green, I., and Benacerraf, B. Specific immune response genes of the guinea pig. II. Relationship between the poly-L-lysine gene and the genes controlling immune responsiveness to copolymers of L-glutanic acid and L-alanine and L-glutanine acid and L-glutanic acid and L-tyrosine in random bred Hartley guinea pigs. *J. Exp. Med. 134*:471–481, 1971.

Bodmer, W.F. Population genetics of the HL-A system: Retrospect and prospect. *In* J. Dausset and J. Colombani (eds.), *Histocompatibility Testing*, pp. 611–619, Munksgaard, Copenhagen, 1973.

Bos, E., Meeter, K., Stibbe, J., Vriesendorp, H.M., Westbroek, D.L., de Vries, M.J., Nauta, J., and van Rood, J.J. Histocompatibility in orthotopic heart transplantation in dogs. *Transplant. Proc. 3*:155–156, 1971.

Calne, R.Y., White, H.J.O., Yoffa, D.E., Maginn, R.R., Binns, R.M., Samuel, J.R., and Molina, V.P. Observation of orthotopic liver transplantation in the pig. *Br. Med. J. 2*:478–480, 1967.

Cavalli Sforza, L.L., and Bodmer, W.F. *The Genetics of Human Populations.* W.H. Freeman, San Francisco, 1970.

Cepellini, R., Mattiuz, P.L., Scudeller, G., and Visetti, M. Experimental allotransplantation in man. II. The role of A_1, A_2 and B antigens. *Transplant. Proc. 1*:390–394, 1969.

Chandler, J.G., Villar, H., Lee, S., Williams, R.J., Nakagi, N.T., Ferrebee, J.W., and Orloff, M.J. The influence of histocompatibility matching according to lymphocyte types on orthotopic liver transplantation in dogs. *Surgery 71*:807–816, 1971.

Click, R.E., Benck, L., and Alter, B.J. Immune responses *in vitro*. I. Culture conditions for antibody synthesis. *Cell. Immunol. 3*:264–276, 1972.

Cudkowicz, G., and Bennett, M. Peculiar immunobiology of bone marrow allografts. I. Graft rejection by irradiated responder mice. *J. Exp. Med. 134*:83–102, 1971.

Dausset, J., and Rapaport, F.T. The role of blood group antigens in human histocompatibility. *Ann. N.Y. Acad. Sci. 129*:408–420, 1966.

Dausset, J., Rapaport, F.T., Cannon, F.D., and Ferrebee, J.W. Histocompatibility studies in a closely bred colony of dogs. III. Genetic definition of the DL-A system of canine histocompatibility, with particular reference to the comparative immunogenicity of the major transplantable organs. *J. Exp. Med. 134*:1222–1237, 1971.

de Gruyl, J., Westbroek, D.L., Dijkhuis, C.M., Vriesendorp, H.M., MacDicken, I., Elion-Gerritsen, W., Verschoor, L., Hulsmans, H.A.M., and Hörchner, P. Influence of DL-A matching, ALS and 24 hour preservation on isolated pancreas allograft survival. *Transplant. Proc. 3*:755–759, 1973.

de Langen, Z.J., de Jong, B., Eysink Smeets, M., Vriesendorp, H.M., Jeruzalem, Ch.R., and Wildevuur, Ch.R.H. Unmodified lung allograft survival related to the major histocompatibility complex in the dog. *In* J.P. Cachera (ed.), *Abstracts of the 10th Congress of the European Society for Experimental Surgery*, pp. 166, 1975.

Démant, P., Capková, J., Hinzová, E., and Vorácová, B. The role of the histocompatibility 2-linked Ss Slp region in the control of mouse complement. *Proc. Natl. Acad. Sci. (USA) 70*:863–864, 1973.

Dorf, M.E., Balner, H., and Benacerraf, B. Mapping of the immune response genes in the major histocompatibility complex of the rhesus monkey. *J. Exp. Med. 142*:673–693, 1975.

Dorf, M.E., Dunham, E.K., Johnson, J.P., and Benacerraf, B. Genetic control of the immune response. The effect of non H-2 linked genes on antibody production. *J. Immunol. 112*:1329–1336, 1973.

Dorf, M.E., Stimpfling, J.H., and Benacerraf, B. Requirements for two H-2 complex Ir genes for the immune response to the l-GLU, l-LYS-l-PHE terpolymer. *J. Exp. Med. 141*:1459–1463, 1975.

Epstein, R.B., Storb, R., Ragde, H., and Thomas, E.D. Cytotoxic antisera for bone marrow grafting in littermate dogs. *Transplantation 6*:45–58, 1968.

Epstein, R.B., Storb, R., and Thomas, E.D. Relation of canine histocompatibility testing to marrow grafting. *Transplant. Proc. 3*:161–164, 1971.

Fu, S.W., Kunkel, H.G., Brusman, H.P., Allen, F.P., Jr., and Fotino, M. Evidence for linkage between HL-A histocompatibility genes and those involved in the synthesis of the second component of complement. *J. Exp. Med. 140*:1108–1111, 1974.

Gluckman, E., Parr, M., Mickelson, E., Schroeder, M.L., and Storb, R. Mixed leucocyte cultures in dogs. A micro-technique, using gradient separated cells. *Transplantation 15*:642–645, 1973.

Gluckman, E., Schroeder, M.L., Storb, R., Goselink, H., Johnson, S., Graham, T.C., Pretorius, G., and Thomas, E.D. One-way nonstimulation of mixed leukocyte culture in dog families. *Transplantation 19*:36–42, 1975.

Goldman, S.F., and Flad, H.D. Histocompatibility testing in dogs. I. A semimicro mixed lymphocyte culture (MLC) technique for histocompatibility matching in dogs. *Tissue Antigens 5*:145–154, 1975.

Goldman, S.F., Krumbacher, K., Schnappauf, H., and Flad, H.D. Definition of MLC specificities in the dog. *Transplant. Proc. 7*:389–393, 1975.

Grosse-Wilde, H., Baumann, P., Netzel, B., Kolb, H.J., Wank, R., Mempel, W., and Albert, E.D. One way non stimulation in MLC related to DL-A homozygosity. *Transplant. Proc. 5*:1567–1571, 1973.

Grosse-Wilde, H., Vriesendorp, H.M., Wank, R., Mempel, W., Dechamps, B., Honauer, U.,

Baumann, P., Netzel, B., Kolb, H. J., and Albert, E. D. Identification of four MLC specificities in the dog. *Tissue Antigens 4*:229–237, 1974.

Grosse-Wilde, H., Netzel, B., Mempel, W., Ruppelt, W., Brehm, G., Bertrams, J., Ewald, R., Lenhard, V., Rittner, Ch., Scholz, S., and Albert, E. Immunogenetics of LD determinants in man. *In* F. Kissmeyer-Nielsen (ed.), *Histocompatibility Testing 1975*, pp. 526–532, 1975.

Grosse-Wilde, H., Vriesendorp, H. M., Netzel, B., Mempel, W., Kolb, H. J., Wank, R., and Albert, E. D. Immunogenetics of 7 LD alleles of the DLA complex in mongrels, beagles and labradors. *Transplant. Proc. 7* (Suppl. 1): 159–169, 1975.

Halasz, N. A., Orloff, M. J., and Hirose, F. Increased survival of renal homografts in dogs after injection of graft donor blood. *Transplantation 2*:453–458, 1964.

Hartzman, R. J., Bach, M. L., and Bach, F. H. Precipitation of radioactivity labeled samples: A semi-automatic multiple-sample-processor. *Cell Immunol. 4*:182–186, 1972.

Hartzman, R. J., Segall, M., Bach, M. L., and Bach, F. H. Histocompatibility matching. II. Miniaturization of the mixed lymphocyte culture test. *Transplantation 11*:268–273, 1971.

ICLA reference centers for histocompatibility testing in dogs. *ILAR News 19*:9, 1975.

Joint Report Fourth Human Histocompatibility Workshop. *Histocompatibility Testing*, Munksgaard, Copenhagen, 1970.

Joint Report First International Workshop on Canine Immunogenetics. *Tissue Antigens 3*:145–163, 1973.

Joint Report Second International Workshop on Canine Immunogenetics. *Transplant. Proc. 8*:289–314, 1976.

Kasakura, S., Thomas, E. D., and Ferrebee, J. W. Leukocytotoxic isoantibodies in the dog. *Transplantation 2*:274–280, 1964.

Katz, D. H., Paul, W. E., Goidl, E. A., and Benacerraf, B. Carrier function in anti-hapten immune responses. I. Enhancement of primary and secondary anti-hapten antibody responses by carrier preimmunization. *J. Exp. Med. 132*:261–282, 1970.

Kissmeyer-Nielsen, F., and Kjerbye, F. E. Lymphocytotoxic microtechnique. Purification of lymphocytes by flotation. *In* E. S. Curtoni, P. L. Mattiuz, and R. M. Tosi (eds.), *Histocompatibility Testing*, pp. 381–383, Munksgaard, Copenhagen, 1967.

Kolb, H. J., Rieder, I., Grosse-Wilde, H., Netzel, B., Mempel, W., Scholz, S., Albert, E. D., and Thierfelder, S. Canine marrow grafts in donor recipient combinations with one way non stimulation in the MLC. *Transplant. Proc. 7*:461–464, 1975.

Léon, S., Zweibaum, A., Vriesendorp, H. M., and Smid Mercx, B. H. J. Production of tissue typing reagents in rabbits immunized with dog-spleen dry acetone powder. *Transplant. Proc. 7*:379–382, 1975a.

Léon, S., Vriesendorp, H. M., Zweibaum, A., Fléché-Seban, C., and Chevalier, G. Application à l'étude sérologique du système majeur d'histocompatibilité du chien (DLA) des propriétés antigéniques et immunogènes de la poudre acétonique de rate. *C.R. Acad. Sci. (Paris), Series D—1653 281*:1653–1656, 1975b.

Lotzová, E., and Cudkowicz, G. Abrogation of resistance to bone marrow grafts by silica particles. Prevention of the silica effect by the macrophage stabilizer poly-2-vinylpyridine N-oxide. *J. Immunol. 113*:798–803, 1974.

Mattiuz, P. L., Ihde, D., Piazza, A., Ceppellini, R., and Bodmer, W. F. New approaches to the population genetic and segregation analysis of the HL-A system. *In* P. I. Terasaki (ed.), *Histocompatibility Testing*, pp. 193–205, Munksgaard, Copenhagen, 1970.

Meera Khan, P., Los, W. R. T., van der Does, J. A., and Epstein, R. B. Iso enzyme markers in dog blood cells. *Transplantation 15*:624–628, 1973.

Meera Khan, P., Vriesendorp, H. M., Saison, R., Volkers, W., Los, W. R. T., and Doppert, B. Homologies between the human and canine phosphoglucomutases. *Manuscript in preparation*, 1976.

Netzel, B., Grosse-Wilde, H., and Mempel, W. MLC reactions with dog lymphocytes frozen in microtiter plates. *Transplant. Proc. 7*:403–405, 1975.

Obertop, H., Jeekel, J., Vriesendorp, H. M., MacDicken, I., and Westbroek, D. L. The effect of donor blood on renal allograft survival in DL-A tissue typed beagle littermates. *Transplantation 20*:49–52, 1975.

Opelz, G., Sengar, D.P.S., Mickey, M.R., and Terasaki, P.I. The effect of blood transfusion on subsequent kidney transplants. *Transplant. Proc. 5*:253–259, 1973.

Penn, O.C.K.M., MacDicken, I., and Bos, T. Histopathology of rejection in DL-A identical canine cardiac allografts. *Transplantation 22*:313–322, 1976.

Puza, A., Rubinstein, P., Kasakura, S., Vlakovic, S., and Ferrebee, J.W. The production of isoantibodies in the dog by immunization with homologous tissue. *Transplantation 2*:722–733, 1964.

Rapaport, F.T., Boyd, A.D., Spencer, F.C., Lower, R.R., Dausset, J., Cannon, F.D., and Ferrebee, J.W. Histocompatibility studies in a closely bred colony of dogs. II. Influence of the DL-A system of canine histocompatibility upon the survival of cardiac allografts. *J. Exp. Med. 133*:260–274, 1971.

Rapaport, F.T., Hanaoka, T., Shimada, T., Cannon, F.D., and Ferrebee, J.W. Histocompatibility studies in a closely bred colony of dogs. I. Influence of leucocyte groups antigens upon renal allograft survival in the unmodified host. *J. Exp. Med. 131*:881–893, 1970.

Rubinstein, P., and Ferrebee, J.W. Efforts to differentiate iso hemagglutinins in the dog. *Transplantation 2*:734–741, 1964.

Sachs, D.H., Davis, C.S., Shreffler, D.C., Nathensen, S.G., and McDevitt, H.O. Meeting report Ir associated antigen. *Immunogenetics 2*:301–000, 1975.

Saison, R., and Doble, E. The reproducibility of reactions obtained with cytotoxic antisera directed against various DL-A specificities. *Transplant. Proc. 7*:353–360, 1975.

Smid Mercx, B.M.J., Duyzer-den Hartog, B., Visser, T.P., and Vriesendorp, H.M. Serological studies of canine histocompatibility antigens. *Transplant. Proc. 7*:361–364, 1975.

Storb, R., Epstein, R.B., Rudolph, R.H., and Thomas, E.D. The effects of prior transfusion on marrow grafts between histocompatible canine siblings. *J. Immunol. 195*:627–633, 1970.

Storb, R., Kolb, H.J., Graham, T.C., Leblond, R., Kolb, H., Lerner, K.G., and Thomas, E.D. Marrow grafts between histo-incompatible family members. *Rev. Eur. Etudes Clin. Biol. 17*:680–685, 1972.

Storb, R., Rudolph, R.H., Graham, T.C., and Thomas, E.D. The influence of transfusions from unrelated donors upon marrow grafts between histocompatible canine siblings. *J. Immunol. 107*:409–413, 1971.

Storb, R., Rudolph, R.H., Kolb, H.J., Graham, T.C., Mickelson, E., Erickson, V., Lerner, K.G., Kolb, H., and Thomas, E.D. Marrow grafts between DL-A matched canine littermates. *Transplantation 15*:92–100, 1973.

Storb, R., Weiden, P., Schroeder, M.L., and Graham, T.C. Marrow grafts between LD-hetero- and homozygous littermates. *Transplant. Proc. 7*:459–460, 1975.

Swisher, S.N. Bio medical notation systems. *JAMA 185*:21–26, 1963.

Templeton, J.W., Moseley, H.S., and Fletcher, W.S. Production of skin graft survival by MLC testing. *Tissue Antigens 3*:168–169, 1973.

Templeton, J.W., and Thomas, E.D. Evidence for a major histocompatibility locus in the dog. *Transplantation 11*:429–431, 1971.

Terasaki, P.I., and McClelland, J.D. Microdroplet assay of human serum cytotoxins. *Nature 219*:998–1000, 1964.

Thomas, E.D., Ashley, L.A., Lochte, H.L., Jaretzki, A., III, Sahler, O.D., and Ferrebee, J.W. Homografts of bone marrow in dogs after lethal total body irradiation. *Blood 14*:720–736, 1959.

Thomsen, M., Platz, P., Ortved Andersen, O., Christy, M., Lyngsøe, J., Nerup, I., Rasmussen, K., Ryder, L.P., Staub Nielsen, L., and Svejgaard, A. MLC typing in juvenile diabetes mellitus and idiopathic addison's disease. *Transplant. Rev. 22*:125–147, 1975.

van Bekkum, D.W., and de Vries, M.J. *Radiation Chimaeras*, Logos Press, Academic Press, London/New York, 1967.

van Bekkum, D.W., and Vos, O. Immunological aspects of homo- and heterologous bone marrow transplantation in irradiated animals. *J. Cell Comp. Physiol. 50*:139–156, 1957.

van den Tweel, J.G., Vriesendorp, H.M., Termytelen, A., Westbroek, D.L., Bach, M.C., and van Rood, J.J. Genetic aspects of canine mixed leucocyte cultures. *J. Exp. Med. 140*:825–836, 1974.

van der Does, J.A., van Rood, J.J., Walker, W., and Epstein, R.B. Consequent intrafamilial immunization for DL-A haplotyping in canines. *J. Exp. Med. 137*:494–503, 1973.

Vriesendorp, H.M. Major histocompatibility complex of the dog. Thesis, Erasmus University, Rotterdam; Bronder Offset, Rotterdam, 1973.

Vriesendorp, H.M., Bijnen, A.B., Zurcher, C., and van Bekkum, D.W. Donor selection and bone marrow transplantation in dogs. *In* F. Kissmeyer-Nielsen (ed.), *Histocompatibility Testing*, pp. 963–971, Munksgaard, Copenhagen, 1975a.

Vriesendorp, H.M., D'Amaro, J., van der Does, J.A., Westbroek, D.L., and Epstein, R.B. Analysis of the DL-A system in families and populations of healthy and diseased individuals. *Transplant. Proc. 5*:311–315, 1973.

Vriesendorp, H.M., Epstein, R.B., D'Amaro, J., Westbroek, D.L., and van Rood, J.J. Polymorphism of the DL-A system. *Transplantation 14*:299–307, 1972.

Vriesendorp, H.M., Löwenberg, B., Visser, T.P., Knaan, S., and van Bekkum, D.W. The influence of genetic resistance and silica particles on survival after bone marrow transplantation. *Transplant. Proc. 8*:483–489, 1976.

Vriesendorp, H.M., Rothengatter, C., Bos, E., Westbroek, D.L., and van Rood, J.J. The production and evaluation of dog allolymphocytotoxins for donor selection in transplantation experiments. *Transplantation 11*:440–445, 1971.

Vriesendorp, H.M., Zurcher, C., and van Bekkum, D.W. Engraftment of allogeneic dog bone marrow. *Transplant. Proc. 7*:465–468, 1975b.

Vriesendorp, H.M., Zurcher, C., Bull, R.W., Los, W.R.T., Meera Khan, P., van den Tweel, J.G., Zweibaum, A., and van Bekkum, D.W. Take and graft vs host reactions of allogeneic bone marrow in tissue typed dogs. *Transplant. Proc. 7* (Suppl. 1):849–853, 1975c.

Westbroek, D.L., Rothengatter, C., Vriesendorp, H.M., and van Rood, J.J. Histocompatibility and heterotopic segmental small bowel allograft survival in dogs. *Eur. Surg. Res. 2*:401–407, 1970.

Westbroek, D.L., Rothengatter, C., Vriesendorp, H.M., van Rood, J.J. Willighagen, R.G.J., and de Vries, M.J. Histocompatibility and allograft rejection in canine small bowel transplants. Evidence for the existence of a major histocompatibility locus in the dog. *Transplant. Proc. 3*:157–160, 1971.

Westbroek, D.L., Silberbusch, J., Vriesendorp, H.M., van Urk, H., Roemeling, H.W., Schönherr-Scholtes, Y., and de Vries, M.J. The influence of DL-A histocompatibility on the function and pathohistological changes in unmodified canine renal allografts. *Transplantation 14*:582–589, 1972.

Westbroek, D.L., Vriesendorp, H.M., van den Tweel, J.G., de Gruyl, J., and van Urk, H. Influence of SD and LD matching on kidney allograft survival in unrelated mongrel dogs. *Transplant. Proc. 7*:427–430, 1975.

Ziegler, J.B., Alper, C.A., and Balner, H. Properdin factor B and histocompatibility loci linked in the rhesus monkey. *Nature 254*:609–611, 1975.

Zweibaum, A., and Bouhou, E. Studies on digestive groups. II. Influence of the digestive group A system on skin allografts in rabbits. *Transplantation 15*:294–297, 1973.

Zweibaum, A., Oriol, R., Feingold, N., Dussaulx, E., Rousset, M., and Chevalier, G. Studies on canine secretory allo antigens (CSA). *Tissue Antigens 4*:115–129, 1974.

Chapter 4

4. The Major Histocompatibility System of Cattle, Pig, Rabbit, and Syrian Hamster

4.1 The Major Histocompatibility System of Cattle

P. IVANYI

4.1.1 Introduction

Cattle are an animal species in which histocompatibility research has barely begun. This contrasts with the fact that for blood and serum group systems cattle represent one of the most studied species. This work followed the possible association of polymorphic loci with different indices of production character. They are also used for precise genetic marking of breeding animals. It has become a routine procedure in countries with a highly developed organization of cattle breeding for animals that are to become the founders of the breeding and production herds to be held under control by genetic markers as provided by blood and serum groups (for references to the extensive literature on this topic, see X–XII European conferences on animal blood groups and biochemical polymorphism).

4.1.2 Blood Cell Chimerism, Immunological Tolerance, and Free Martinism in Cattle Twins

Cattle occupied an important role at the early stages of research of immunological tolerance to histocompatibility antigens. About 90 percent of dizygotic cattle twins are chimeras and have a mixture of two antigenically distinct kinds of erythrocytes. Erythrocyte mosaicism or chimerism is believed to arise from the *in utero* vascular anastomosis between dizygotic twins permitting an interchange of primordial erythropoietic cells and the persistence of mixed blood types in each twin. Consequently, members of a twin pair (or even a quintuplet) show identical blood types (Owen 1945; Owen et al. 1946). Anastomosis of the vessels of unlike-sex twins presumably allows for exchange of hormones, resulting in the free martin condition (Lillie 1916). Tissues that give rise to histocompatibility antigens are likewise exchanged, because dizygotic twins with erythrocyte mosaicism usually accept each others skin (Anderson et al. 1951). In contrast, the tissues that produce the J factor of cattle blood (Stormont 1949) and transferrins (Datta and Stone 1963) are not exchanged.

Erythrocyte mosaicism was used to study possible somatic cell mating. One chimeric twin was found whose blood contained, at three years of age, 10 percent of that of his co-twin. At eight years of age, three blood types were found, the two "parental" types, each representing 2 percent, and a "hybrid" type that represented 96 percent of the cell population. Stone et al. (1964) postulated that the hybrid cell type resulted from "mating" between the two hematopoietic tissues and that the hybrid type had a distinct selective advantage.

4.1.3 The Unknown MHS in Cattle

Of the total of about 12 blood group systems studied in cattle, the B system emerges as highly polymorphic. Because the MHS is the most polymorphic system hitherto known in every species, the B system might be a fair candidate for this role. More than 50 different B antigens have been described. Recombination events have been observed in a frequency of 0.2 to 0.3, indicating the involvement of a complex genetic region (Bouw and Fiorentini 1970; Sellei and Rendel 1970). However, data that might point to the role of the B system in histocompatibility are still missing.

The second prominent complex blood group system is the S system. The number of defined antigens in the S system is lower than that of the B system. However, the immunogenetic analysis was hampered by the peculiar serological complexity, which results in a rapid rising of subgroups (the phenomenon of antigen subdivision), in inclusions, and in extensive cross-reactions of the reagents employed (Grosclaude 1963, 1965). Naturally occurring isoantibodies of the S blood group system were reported by Stone and Miller (1961). These might correspond to the antibodies found by Iha et al. (1973) in 26 percent of multiparous cows. Thus with some degree of heuristics, the S blood group system might be predicted to represent the cattle MHS.

At least one indirect experimental approach points to this possibility. Borovská and Démant (1967) examined 30 typing sera against antigens of cattle blood group systems A, B, C, F, L, S, and Z for the presence of cytotoxic antibodies against lymph node cells. (The typing reagents were obtained from the laboratory of Dr. J. Matoušek, Liběchov.) Simultaneously, the erythrocytes of the unrelated 63 animals were examined with all sera for the presence of the erythrocyte antigens that they detected. All the sera examined were produced by alloimmunization by several injections of whole blood, and all were found to contain cytotoxic antibodies. However, a significant correlation between the erythrocyte antigen pattern and the cytotoxic reaction was found only for two anti-S sera (anti-S_2 and anti-U_1). These two sera also showed a highly significant positive correlation of their respective cytotoxic reactions. On the basis of these preliminary tests, the above-mentioned authors concluded: "if the premise is accepted that alloimmune cytotoxic antibodies appearing in the sera are directed against antigens of the main histocompatibility system of the given species, as has been proved in mice, man and rats (Iványi

1966), the results presented here indicate that the S system is probably the main histocompatibility system of cattle." Ostrand-Rosenberg and Stormont (1974) used a similar approach to the problem as did Borovská and Démant. Twenty-four reagents against erythrocyte blood groups of ten systems showed no apparent correlation with leukocyte antigens detected by the same sera using the microcytotoxicity tests. According to these authors this result is in contradiction to the report of Borovská and Démant. However, only 13 blood samples were tested, and the reaction pattern of two of the four anti-S system reagents (anti-S and anti-U_1) suggests a possible association of erythrocyte and leukocyte antigens for these particular specificities. These findings, according to our view, leave open the possibility that the S blood group system represents the bovine MHS. It is necessary to keep in mind that for MHS antigens the relation between erythrocyte and leukocyte presentation is rather complex (for illustration see the problem of HLA presentation on human red cells).

4.1.4 Cattle Alloimmune Sera Cross-Reacting with HLA Antigens

Another hint concerning the MHS might have come from the experiments of Iha et al. (1973). Alloimmune cattle sera obtained after immunization with whole blood, leukocytes, or from parous cows were tested by the microdroplet lymphocytotoxic assay on human peripheral lymphocytes. Several of these sera, even after absorption with human erythrocytes, exhibited discriminating cytotoxic activity with human cells. The cattle sera were tested on 50 human lymphocyte samples, and the 2×2 associations of the cattle sera activities with HLA antigens of the human cells were computed. Several significant positive associations were found, the most significant being that with HLA-A2, B12, 7, 27, and W35, as well as 4a (W4) and 4b (W6). Preliminary family studies and twin studies indicated, in accordance with population studies, that cattle alloimmune sera exhibit differential cytotoxicity on human lymphocytes depending on the HLA profile of the individual cells. These findings indicate that extensive serological cross-reactions exist between the human MHS (HLA) and the presumed MHS in cattle. The latter, however, remains undiscovered. Iha et al. (1973) did not refer to the specificities present in the alloimmune cattle sera (with regard to bovine alloantigens) that were tested on the human cells.

The same authors noticed that some anti-HLA sera reacted differentially on cattle lymphocytes. These results indicated that human lymphocytotoxic sera contain antibodies that cross-react with cattle lymphocyte antigens. However, there was no convincing evidence that these cross-reactions are correlated to known HLA specificities, nor did the activities of the human antisera on the cattle lymphocytes correlate with any of the known cattle erythrocyte antigen systems.

Rabbit antisera against the mouse H-2-linked Ss serum protein were tested for cross-reacting substances in cattle sera, but no positive reactions were found (Borovská et al. 1971).

Preliminary experiments can be found that aim to identify the cattle MHS with the help of alloimmune antilymphocyte cattle sera. However, these efforts have so far resulted only in preliminary methodological information (McGary 1969; McGary and Stone 1970; Millot 1966). Schmid and Otto (1970) refer briefly to the possibility of identifying three antigens by alloimmune antilymphocyte cattle sera (Mu-L/bov/1-3). Alloimmune sera from multiparous cows might be expected to represent a hopeful source of operationally monospecific antibodies. However, it is known that, in cattle, transplacental alloimmunization to blood group antigens is missing. Nevertheless, Iha et al. (1973) reported the presence of cytotoxic antibodies in the sera of multiparous cows.

4.2 The Major Histocompatibility System of Pig

P. Ivanyi

4.2.1 Introduction

The greater number of works on histocompatibility in pigs was initiated by the observation that liver allografts survive for a long period in surprisingly high proportions. It is still unclear whether this difference is due only to some peculiarities in immune responsiveness and/or tolerance induction or whether some degree of homogeneity in histocompatibility loci is also involved.

4.2.2 Blood Group Systems

About 15 blood group systems (labeled A to O) have been studied in the pig. Antigens of the A, E, and N systems were found to be present on leukocytes and other tissue cells by absorption tests (Hála 1967; Simon and Hojný 1970). For the A system this might constitute the analogous system to the human (and other species) ABO or ABO-like systems, including the lymphocytotoxic action of some anti-A sera (Simon and Hruban 1972). The representation of some E and G blood group system specificities was confirmed by the cytotoxic action of the respective antisera. Furthermore, a significant correlation was found for the reaction pattern in the hemagglutination test and the lymphocytotoxicity test for anti-E and anti-G sera. For an anti-Gb reagent (reaction frequency 56 percent) tested by both tests on 100 unrelated pigs, the correlation coefficient mounted to 0.92, i.e., almost perfect identity. Absorption experiments indicated the monospecificity of the serum. Similar results were obtained with anti-E sera. A cytotoxic anti-E serum correlated perfectly with the presence of Ea and El blood group antigens. Absorption experiments showed that the antibody cross-reacts with both Ea and E1 antigens (Hruban et al. 1972). Production of specific anti-E and anti-G hemagglutinins was observed after skin grafting (Saison and Ingram 1963; Hruban et al. 1974).

The findings of Hruban et al. (1974) strongly support the thesis that the E blood group system represents a minor histocompatibility system. This possibility is supported by the finding of E system antigens on lymphocytes and possibly on epidermal cells. The role of skin graft survival was directly tested when 29 siblings from inbred families (identical in MHS) were grafted by E-compatible or -incompatible skin grafts from siblings. The MST (31.5 versus 19.9, see also Table 4.1) differ at the $0.01 > p < 0.05$ level. Interestingly, in other species with well-defined MHS, we do not know about a comparable situation (i.e., serologically well-defined minor H systems), except possibly the role of the C blood group system in chicken. The E system seems to be the most complex blood group system in pigs, represented by a chromosomal segment including two or more loci of 2 centimorgans in length (Baker 1971).

Vaiman et al. (1970) found no indication for the identity of the pig MHS, the SL-A system (*vide infra*), with A, B, G, E. J. K blood group systems, and White et al. (1973) with A/O, E, I, K, L, M systems.

4.2.3 The MHS in Pig: SL-A (SD) or PL-A (LD)

4.2.3.1 Serological Studies

With the help of alloimmune cytotoxic sera obtained after skin grafting between related or unrelated pigs, groups of unrelated pigs and families were tested by the lymphocytotoxicity test. The reaction pattern of the sera was evaluated on cells from unrelated pigs ($N=487$) by correlation analysis (the mass x^2 method) and on families by segregation analysis. Correlation coefficients of two to three sera assigned to the individual antigens varied between 1.0 and 0.40 (mostly around 0.80). Absorption experiments showed the monospecificity of some sera, or at least operational monospecifity. Four antigens with codominant inheritance were defined and unequivocally assigned to one genetic system, designated SL-A. The antigens were designated SL-A1 (24 percent), SL-A2 (36 percent), SL-A3 (7 percent), and SL-A4 (15 percent) (Vaiman et al. 1971, 1972).

Leukocyte antigens with different designations (L1, Simon and Hruban 1971; Mu-Ly 1-3, Mu-Gr 1-23, Schmid and Otto 1971; Schmid and Cwik 1972) were also described. It is not known whether all belong to the SL-A system.

Alloimmune cytotoxic antilymphocyte sera can be absorbed by boar spermatozoa. This finding suggests that at least some lymphocyte antigens are shared by sperm cells (Jílek and Veselský 1972). The specificity of the sera were not specified.

Soluble inhibitor substances of heteroimmune and allommune lymphocytotoxic antibodies were found to be regularly present in serum of pigs (Schmid and Cwik 1972; Cwik and Schmid 1975). Their specificity was shown in only

Table 4.1. Survival Times of Different Pig Allografts

Organ or Tissue Grafted	Number of Transplants	Graft Survival or MST in Days	Donor-Recipient Relationship	Reference
1. Skin	41	6.8 ± 1.8	MHS-nonidentical siblings	White et al. 1973
2. Skin	100	9.7 ± 1.2	MHS-identical siblings	White et al. 1973
3. Skin	18	33.5 ± 2.6	Duroc breed siblings[a]	Baker and Andersen 1974
4. Skin	22	40.1 ± 4.1	Hampshire breed, siblings[a]	Baker and Andersen 1974
5. Skin	48	5.6 ± 1.1	MHS-incompatible siblings } outbred	Hruban et al. 1974
6. Skin	27	9.8 ± 2.3	MHS-compatible siblings } matings	Hruban et al. 1974
7. Skin	8	6.1 ± 1.0	MHS-incompatible siblings } semiinbred	Hruban et al. 1974
8. Skin	29	22.4 ± 7.8	MHS-compatible siblings } matings	Hruban et al. 1974
9. Skin	23	19.9 ± 5.8	E blood group-incompatible siblings[b]	Hruban et al. 1974
10. Skin	6	30.5 ± 12.5	E blood group-compatible siblings[b]	Hruban et al. 1974
11. Intestine	11	12.7 ± 48	MHS-incompatible siblings	Vaiman et al. 1972
12. Intestine	35	49.5 ± 2.1	MHS-identical siblings	Vaiman et al. 1972
13. Intestine	7	1/7 > 15	MHS-nonidentical siblings	Chomette et al. 1974
14. Intestine	21	10/27 > 15	MHS-identical siblings	Chomette et al. 1974
15. Kidney	1	< 16	MHS-nonidentical siblings	Bradley et al. 1972
16. Kidney	4	> 16	MHS-semiidentical siblings	Bradley et al. 1972
17. Kidney	4	> 76	MHS-identical siblings	Bradley et al. 1972
18. Kidney	12	11.5 ± 2.2	MHS-incompatible siblings	Vaiman et al. 1972
19. Kidney	12	109 ± 22.1	MHS-identical siblings	Vaiman et al. 1972
20. Kidney	12	18.8	MHS-semiidentical siblings	White et al. 1973
21. Kidney	16	84–490	MHS-identical siblings	White et al. 1973
22. Kidney	2	< 14	Unrelated	White et al. 1973
23. Kidney	8	< 30	MHS-nonidentical siblings	Chomette et al. 1974
24. Kidney	8	> 30	MHS-identical siblings	Chomette et al. 1974

[a] Matched for sex and blood groups of ten genetic loci.
[b] MHS-identical, partially inbred siblings.

one experiment, where an anti-SL-A3 serum was employed. Surprisingly, 84 of 112 pig sera were able specifically to inhibit anti-SL-A3, whereas the SL-A3 antigen was detectable on lymphocytes of only 14 of those animals. It is not clear whether these inhibitors are analogous to the HLA substances found in human sera by van Rood (see Chapter 1 on HLA) and/or significant for antigen-induced immunosuppression in connection with organ grafts, especially those of liver allografts in pigs (see below). More studies are needed to elucidate the biochemical nature and biological role of soluble inhibitor serum substances as well as comparative studies from other species.

Anti-SL-A sera were used to demonstrate independent movement of immunoglobulin and histocompatibility antigen on the lymphocyte membrane (Binns et al. 1972).

Buschman et al. (1975) described differences in the ability of pigs from different breeds to produce anti-DNK hapten antibodies. These differences correlated with the distribution of some leukocyte antigens whose classification was not clarified.

4.2.3.2 Mixed Lymphocyte Culture Studies

Mixed lymphocyte cultures (MLC) served well for the identification of the SL-A system when it was found that littermate piglets can be grouped in four groups on the basis of negative MLC. The MLC between individuals of the different groups were regularly positive (Viza et al. 1970; Vaiman et al. 1970a, 1970b). Mutual negative MLC ensured also prolonged graft survival (Vaiman et al. 1970a, 1970b), and later the MLC pattern was found to correlate perfectly with the segregation of serologically defined SL-A haplotypes in families (Vaiman et al. 1973). However, in one family of pigs genotyped for the SL-A system, a recombination was observed between the serologically defined antigens and MLC determinants. This suggests different but linked loci for SL-A antigens and MLC determinants. With the help of the observed SL-A recombinant haplotype, alloimmune sera were produced between sibs that differed only at the supposed MLC locus. The antibodies obtained were cytotoxic preferentially to B-lymphocytes. Thymocytes had very low absorbing capacity, and platelets had none. These findings led Vaiman et al. (1975) to suggest that the specificities detected correspond to the Ia antigens of the mouse H-2 system.

Two levels of positive response were described for MLC tests performed between siblings, dependent on the gene-dose effect. Indications were obtained that this difference may be important in renal allograft survival, because four grafts differing by two alleles were rejected before day 16 and four grafts differing by only one allele survived beyond day 37 (Table 4.1) (Bradley et al. 1972).

Bradley et al. (1974) compared the polymorphism of the serologically defined SL-A locus with that of the MLC-defined SL-A (PL-A) locus. Although unrelated serological identical individuals were found, several unrelated pigs shared the same MLC determinants. This finding led to the suggestion "that the number of MLR alleles might be relatively restricted in comparison to the number of alleles for serologically defined gene products." A similar conclusion was derived from experiments performed with homozygous SL-A cells. This approach also indicated the presence of common gene products between two completely different breeds of pigs (Large White and Landrace) (Bradley et al. 1973, 1974). However, two independent communications are at variance with this finding, claiming that negative MLC tests occur only between individuals of the same breed (Festenstein 1970; Parker et al. 1975).

4.2.3.3 Histocompatibility and Transplantation in Pigs

In spite of some interesting peculiarities concerning pig liver allografts, which will be discussed later, the role of the pig's MHS for allograft survival, as in other species, was clearly demonstrated (Table 4.1). The data can be summarized as follows:

1. Skin graft survival is in similar ranges as in other species and is influenced by MHS haplotype differences.
2. Kidney graft survival is very short in unrelated combinations. When grafted between siblings, a clearcut influence of MHS haplotype differences can be observed. However, MHS-identical sibs survive without immunosuppression for a relatively long period compared to other species. The role of MHS differences was shown also for intestine allografts.
3. The role of MHS differences is not clear in pig liver allograft survival and will be discussed separately in more detail.

4.2.3.4 Pig Liver Transplantation and the Role of Histocompatibility Genetics

Several authors have shown that the donor-recipient relationship in relation to the pig MHS, the SL-A system, is decisive for skin, kidney, and intestine graft survival (Table 4.1). This, however, does not hold for pig liver allografts. Approximately 80 percent of grafts performed even between unrelated individuals show a long-term survival. A number of experiments were initiated as a result of the original observations of Calne et al. (1967) and Riddell et al. (1967) on prolonged pig liver allograft survival. To a certain extent this holds also for other species (Calne et al. 1970; Calne 1971), but it seems that liver transplantation in pigs gives extraordinary good results. Several approaches were used to elucidate this phenomenon (Calne et al. 1969), but the explanation is still lacking. The situation is well characterized by Calne (1971):

> In pigs, the difference between the usual fierce rejection of skin, heart and kidney allografts compared with the often indefinite survival of liver grafts has been the main object of our study over the last three years. It was found that liver allografts specifically protected donor grafts of skin, heart and kidney, the protection of skin and heart being modest, whereas kidney grafts have been protected for as long as $2^1/_2$ years. Why allografts

of skin and heart have been less well protected than kidney has not been explained. Tissue specific antigens might be involved—alternatively a mild immune reaction may cause more damage to skin and heart than to kidney. Heterotopic liver allografts have protected donor kidney allografts from rejection within 24 hours after which time the liver has been removed and the kidney has continued to function for up to 8 months. Because this protective effect of a liver graft is donor-specific, it must involve transplantation antigens.

In connection with the aim of this book, we are interested in the possible genetic requirements of pig liver transplantation. All data points to the fact that the phenomenon of graft acceptance cannot be explained by an extraordinary and unexpected genetic homogeneity of pigs for histocompatibility antigens and particularly of the SL-A system. Even though the polymorphism of the SL-A system was hitherto studied only to a limited extent (see above), it was clearly shown that the donor-recipient relationship for the SL-A system greatly influences skin and other graft survival; however, this was not found to hold for liver grafts. Calne repeatedly pointed out that histocompatibility genetics may not play a major role in pig liver transplantation

It seems nevertheless very important to stress the question of whether the SL-A system has any influence on liver graft survival. No critical tests could be found in the literature. Tests that would compare the grafting results between pairs of genotyped (SL-A) siblings in sufficiently large series are missing. The relatively high number of tests that would resolve such a question emerge also behind the fact that technical and other nonimmunological reasons of graft failure are relatively more frequent for liver than for other organ grafts.

Recent data point to a most surprising finding, which might be highly relevant to the problem discussed. Bradley et al. (1974) showed that the polymorphism of the locus defined by mixed lymphocyte cultures is much more restricted than that of the serologically defined loci. MLC tests were found to be negative even between individuals of largely different breeds, such as Large White and Landrace. One of the allelic MLC products defined in domesticated pigs was found to be present even in European Wild Boar. Recent experiments of Parker et al. (1975) are at variance with these findings; these authors found only 13 percent of MLC tests to be negative in unrelated pigs. Negative MLC tests occurred only between individuals of the same breed (thus necessarily "related"), whereas none of the 109 tests performed between individuals of different breeds was negative. Older experiments of Festenstein (1970) were in the same line. If, nevertheless, the findings of Bradley et al. (1974) were confirmed, this might serve as a clue for the understanding of some peculiarities of organ grafting in pigs and might open new horizons not only for pig liver transplantation genetics but for the evaluation of the role of MHS in organ transplantation or transplantation immunology in general. Indirectly indicative of this possibility are some experiments performed with liver extracts in mice by Hilgert (1974). Successful liver grafts are known to prolong the survival of other grafts (skin, kidney). Analogously, liver extracts induce a state of specific tolerance to skin grafts in mice. However, this is valid only for donor-recipient mouse combinations that do not differ at the H-2K and H-2I regions, or shortly at the H-2K end. Clearly, more critical experiments with liver grafts performed between individuals carefully analyzed for mutual relation for the SL-A region are highly desirable. If the SL-A system has any role in pig liver transplantation, the favorable situation granted by other factors might serve as a potent tool for elucidation of some functional aspects of the pig MHS itself.

4.3 The Major Histocompatibility System of Rabbit

P. Ivanyi

4.3.1 Introduction

The rabbit has been used to discover the immunological nature of allotransplantation reaction (Medawar 1944, 1945). Medawar (1945) also pointed out that several histocompatibility systems must have been presumed to exist in this species; the minimal estimate was seven. This view was deduced from the finding that none of the 528 allografts exchanged between 201 rabbits survived more than 25 days, and that only 25 grafts survived more than 15 days. This material has represented up to now one of the greatest collections of graft exchange among unrelated individuals. In these early studies Medawar (1946) also pointed to the preferential presence of histocompatibility antigens on rabbit leukocytes and epidermal cells because of the inability to produce transplantation immunity by red cells alone.

4.3.2 Blood Groups and Histocompatibility

Studies of rabbit erythrocyte blood group systems as well as immunoglobulin allotypes represented an important source of knowledge for the study of alloantigenic differences. Of the six blood group systems studied (for review, see Cohen 1958 and Cohen and Tissot 1965), the most thoroughly described system was that given an independent designation from more than ten laboratories on the basis of actual rediscovery of the system. The first was probably Castle and Keeler (1933), who used two alloantibodies originally prepared by Levine and Landsteiner (1929). Their designation was anti-H_1 and anti-H_2 (without any meaning for histocompatibility). The problems of the nomenclature were discussed in detail by Cohen (1958, 1962), who also presented the tables of comparative terminology. In this section we shall use the designation adopted by Cohen, i.e., the Hg system. At least six specificities were detected in the Hg system, two of them being "interaction" antigens. Experimental work was performed by means of the Hg system on a large number of problems, including transfusion reactions produced by infusion of incompatible erythrocytes or high-titered alloantisera, active and passive induction of experimental hemolytic disease of the newborn, association of Hg blood groups with genetic regulation of alloantibody production, occurrence of interaction antigens, linkage and population genetics studies, transplacental transfer of antibodies, induction of immunological tolerance, the role of the Hg system in transplantation immunity (for references, see Cohen 1962; Cohen and Tissot 1965; Cohen et al. 1964; Iványi 1962, 1964, 1966; Iványi and Iványiová 1961; Iványi et al. 1959). This system was also suspected to present the rabbit MHS, but only slight differences in skin graft survival were reported. Skin grafts exchanged between rabbits of a closed colony genotyped for the Hg system indicated the influence of some incompatible combinations on first-set skin graft survival. Although Hg-compatible grafts had a mean survival time of 9.3 days, in three Hg-incompatible combinations referred to as strong differences (on the basis of the strength of the red cell antigen) graft survival was 6.1 to 6.4 days. In some other Hg-incompatible combinations (referred to as weak), graft survival was 8.4 to 9.1 days (Cohen et al. 1964). However, skin grafting among partially inbred rabbits genotyped for the Hg system (Fabian et al. 1963) and other experiments (Iványi 1962, 1964, 1966) showed conclusively that the Hg system was not the MHS of the rabbit. This was finally shown by the detection of the RL-A rabbit MHS system, which is not linked to the Hg system (*vide infra*).

The recognition of the Hg system as a minor histocompatibility system still remains open. However, apart from the above data (Cohen et al. 1964), there are few data that would support this possibility. The reasons for doubt are as follows: (1) Tolerance induction to skin grafts exchanged between newborn siblings did not depend on Hg blood groups; (2) very high titers (1:500) of haemagglutinins in the recipient did not influence the survival time of Hg-incompatible skin grafts, and anti-Hg antibodies had no cytotoxic effect on lymphocytes; (3) Hg antigens were not present, or were difficult to detect, on cells other than erythrocytes; (4) skin grafts between individuals of semiinbred populations survived for long periods even between Hg-incompatible animals; (5) immunization with pure suspensions of epidermal cells alone did not lead to anti-Hg hemagglutinin production (Iványi 1962, 1964, 1965, 1966; Fabian et al. 1963; Ivašková and Iványi 1966). However, a puzzling question arises when considering the fact, described primarily by Zotikov (1956) and confirmed by a number of other authors (cf. Iványi 1965; Matej 1968, 1969), that relatively strong anti-Hg hemagglutinins appear almost regularly after Hg-incompatible skin transplantation in rabbits. A simple explanation offers itself that these antibodies occur as a result of the presence of erythrocytes in the skin graft. This assumption is also supported by the finding that even as small a dose as 2×10^6 erythrocytes is sufficient to produce agglutinin formation in some rabbits (Iványi and Ujhelyiová 1958). This view could not be confirmed by Matej (1968), who concluded that much larger amounts of blood are needed for hemagglutinin production than traces of erythrocytes likely to be present in the transplant. Another assumption remains that the antigens of the Hg system are present in an unknown, concealed form even in epidermal cells and that their immunogenic capacity manifests itself only during immunization in the form of transplantation.

When the Hg blood group system is considered as a minor histocompatibility system, it may occupy a similar position in relation to the MHS as does the E blood group system in pigs and the C blood group system in chickens. In all these cases, a complex blood group system of a given species represents a minor histocompatibility system. Interestingly, there is no indication of a similar situation in man. However, it is not clear that it is not artificial to analogize the parallels from these species concerning the existence of a number of complex blood group loci in each species all of which may play some minor role in histocompatibility.

Rabbits can be typed as A(+) or A(−) according to the presence of a human A blood group-like substance in their body fluids and some tissues mainly in the mucose of the digestive tract (the so-called digestive groups). A(−) rabbits frequently have "natural" anti-human A erythrocyte agglutinins in their serum. Zweibaum and Bouhou (1973) tested the role of digestive group A on skin allografts. Four types of experiments indicate the role of A(+) as a histocompatibility factor: (1) of the four possible combinations given by A(+) and A(−) rabbits, skin grafts in A(−) recipients from A(+) donors were rejected in a significantly shorter time than in all other combinations (MST 5.5 versus 8.5 to 9.0, respectively). (2) In A(−) recipients receiving grafts from A(+) and A(−) donors at the same time, the A(+) grafts were regularly rejected earlier than the A(−) grafts. (3) In all nine A(−) recipients of first-set A(+) grafts, second-set grafts from A(+) donors behaved as white grafts. (4) "Hyperacute" rejection (on day 4 to 5) of first-set grafts was observed only in A(−) recipients receiving A(+) grafts. This situation strongly resembles the accelerated rejection of skin grafts in man from A donors to O recipients with two exceptions. First, in rabbits no correlation was found between the actual anti-A titer and the degree of skin graft survival, and second, in A(−) recipients the anti-A antibody titer remained unmodified after graft rejection.

4.3.3 The Rabbit MHS

4.3.3.1 Studies on Noninbred Strains

Serological Studies. Long before the discovery of the rabbit MHS, the occurrence of alloimmune lymphocytotoxic antibodies had been demonstrated after transplantation or injection of lymphoid cells (Terasaki et al. 1961; Kapitchnikov et al. 1962; Young et al. 1963; Govallo et al. 1964; Ivašková and Iványi 1966; Matej 1970a). The aim of these experiments was to clarify the tactical and methodological aspects of the approach, to ascertain the mutual role of antierythrocyte and antileukocyte antibodies, and to point to the specificity of cytotoxic antibodies. Although the kinetics of cytotoxic antibody production was followed in relation to different forms, doses, routes of injections, etc., the results are difficult to generalize, because they depend on the donor-recipient MHS relations. This point of view could not be followed in these pilot studies. The majority of experiments indicate that the production of cytotoxic antibodies is very efficient after skin graft transplantation followed by i.p. injections of lymphoid cells. It is important that these experiments showed the distinct nature of hemagglutinating and cytotoxic antibodies formed after skin transplantation (Ivašková and Iványi 1966; Matej 1970a). Ahrons and Lund (1972) showed that a correlation exists between lymphocytotoxic antibodies and the fate of kidney allografts in rabbits.

After the illustrative demonstration of leukocyte antigen identification of an extremely complex system in the outbred human population, a number of authors applied the same approach to rabbits. Series of antileukocyte antibodies were prepared and tested on panels of "unrelated" rabbits with subsequent analysis of the mutual reaction patterns of the sera employed. The outcome was the definition of several leukocyte antigens whose mutual relations indicated that they belonged to one genetic system. In the experiments of Black (1967), 26 alloimmune sera were tested by the cytotoxic test on the leukocytes of 52 unrelated rabbits. At least three groups of sera could be prepared for the definition of three leukocyte antigens. Démant (1968a, 1968b) tested 54 alloimmune sera on 101 unrelated rabbits. Thirty-eight sera exhibited significant associations, and seven groups of sera could be produced for the definition of seven leukocyte antigens. Matej (1970b, 1970c, 1973) tested 13 sera on 117 rabbits and defined three leukocyte antigens. He was also the first to propose the designation RL-A for the MHS in rabbits (Matej 1970c). Similarly, Ehlers and Ahrons (1971) defined 18 specificities by a corresponding number of antisera and proposed the designation RL-A. Simultaneously, all these authors demonstrated the role of the detected leukocyte antigens in allograft survival (see below).

Thus, little doubt remained that the approach that had been successfully applied to human outbred populations could be used for the detection of the rabbit MHS where more rapid progress was clearly hampered by the absence of well-defined, widely distributed homozygous inbred strains. The consequence of this situation was an unfortunate further fate of the works mentioned above, which evidently duplicated each other's efforts and thus led to subsequent rediscoveries of the rabbit MHS. This development is very similar to that encountered with research on rabbit blood group systems (see Cohen 1958, 1962). After conducting the published experiments (all in a more or less preliminary stage), the individual laboratories ceased further continuous work; thus, the important reference points that might have facilitated further progress are absent. Doubtless the reason behind these difficulties is the absence of widely represented reference inbred rabbit strains.

For the time being, the only laboratory performing continuous work along the same line seems to be that of Dr. C. Cohen at the Center of Genetics, University of Illinois, and it will be described here in more detail.

Twelve somewhat related rabbit lines used in this research came from an essentially closed colony; these 12 lines all descended from matings involving no more than 14 individuals at generation zero. In 1972, the coefficient of inbreeding ranged from 0.59 to 0.83 (Tissot and Cohen 1972). Twenty-five cytotoxic antisera were prepared after skin graft exchange among (1) partially inbred siblings (14 useful sera from 54 experiments), (2) rabbits from different lines (11 useful sera from 26 experiments), (3) or by lymphoid cell immunization between unrelated rabbits (one useful serum from five experiments). The sera obtained were tested on groups of rabbits from different inbred lines, individuals known to be homozygous for RL-A alleles, on segregating families, and on a randomely selected panel of 65 cells from a closed colony of 800 rabbits. The latter results were analyzed by the correlation coefficient that evaluated the mutual relationship of 18 antisera on a 2×2 table basis. The outcome of this work was the definition of seven RL-A alleles (RL-A^{a} to RL-A^{g}) and their distribution in ten inbred lines (inbred reference lines: Sh1, Sh3, Sh5, Sh6, Sh11, Sh13, FA1, FA2, FA5). Altogether, ten RL-A specificities were defined (designated R-1 to R-10) and their presentation on individual RL-A alleles described. This appears to represent the developmental stage of the RL-A chart (Table 4.2) analogous to that of the mouse H-2 or rat H-1 chart (Tissot and Cohen 1972).

It is obvious that the situation still did not approach the formal level of the mouse H-2 or rat H-1 system. Some of the inbred lines had a relatively low coefficient of inbreeding and included individuals heterozygous for the RL-A alleles. The individual RL-A antigenic specificities (R-1 to R-10) are not conclusively defined by the homozygous donor-recipient strains used for the reference serum production. The monospecificity of the individual sera were not conclusively tested by cross-absorption tests. Nevertheless, these data, if further elaborated and connected with the final establishment of homozygous highly inbred strains, might represent the basis of further rabbit histocompatibility immunogenetics.

Because some inbred strains were of common ancestry, their more detailed serological examination was of interest (Tissot and Cohen 1974). Three inbred strains, Sh5, Sh6, and Sh9, were examined by a battery of 43 independent

Table 4.2. The RL-A Chart

Allele	Typing Serum										Line
	R-1	R-2	R-3	R-4	R-5	R-6	R-7	R-8	R-9	R-10	
RL-A^{a}	+	+	−	+	−	−	+	+	−	+	Sh3, Sh13, Fa5, Fa1, Sh11
RL-A^{b}	+	+	+	+	+	−	+	+		−	Fa2, Fa5
RL-A^{c}	+	−	+	+	+	+	−	−	−	−	Sh9, Sh1, Sh6, Fa2, Fa1
RL-A^{d}	+	−	+	+	−	−	+	−	+	−	Sh6, Sh13
RL-A^{e}	−	−	+	+	−	+	−	+		−	Sh1
RL-A^{f}	+	−	+	−	+	+	−	−		−	Sh5
RL-A^{g}	−	−	+	+	−	+	+	+	−	−	Sh5

From Cohen and Tissot (1972).

alloimmune sera. The RL-A^g and RL-A^d alleles gave very similar reaction patterns, differing from each other by only one to three reactions. These very slight serological differences indicate that, if they had a common origin, there were opportunities for recombination or mutation within the RL-A locus.

The relative concentration of RL-A antigens 1 and 2 was studied by absorption tests (Matej 1970c). The highest levels of the antigens were found in the liver, spleen, and lungs, somewhat lower levels in the kidneys and the lowest levels in the myocardium and brain.

Simultaneous typing for RL-A alleles and blood group antigen E of the He blood group locus on rabbit families has shown that the He blood group locus and the RL-A locus are closely linked (Tissot and Cohen 1974). This observation should lead to a reconsideration of some aspects of hemagglutinin production after skin transplantation in rabbits.

Mixed Lymphocyte Culture Studies. On the basis of MLC tests in the RL-A genotyped rabbits, the close association of the rabbit major MLC locus with the RL-A locus was shown (Tissot and Cohen 1974). No critical recombinant was detected that gave conclusive proof of a closely linked but separate locus for the MLC determinants in addition to those serologically defined. However, the three serologically very slightly different alleles (which possibly evolved from a common ancestor by mutation or recombination) were mutually MLC nonstimulatory, indicating that they share the MLC locus determinant region(s) while differing in some parts of the serologically defined regions. This finding also indicates that the serologically defined and MLC determinants in the rabbit are genetically separable.

Immune Response Studies. Preliminary data indicate the linkage of RL-A with immune response genes (Ir). The results of immunization with human gamma globulin have shown that the RL-A^g allele is associated with the high response and the RL-A^f and RL-A^c alleles with the poor response to this immunogen. Strong antibody response behaved as a dominant trait. The difference between good and poor antibody producers was about tenfold. This finding might be significant for the selection of rabbits to produce potent antihuman globulin sera frequently used in immunohematological tests (e.g., the Coombs test).

4.3.3.2 Studies on Inbred Strains

The maintenance of inbred strains has proved to be decisive for successful progress of histocompatibility genetics in the mouse, rat, and chicken. This must also hold for further progress in rabbit work, however much it may contrast with the extreme time- and space-consuming requirements. Another difficulty in the rabbit is the inbreeding depression, which seems to be so sever that the lines frequently become extinct (Chai 1974). This might be possibly overcome in the future by transmitting the same RL-A alleles into different breeds and thus combining inbreeding with selection on a more heterogeneous genetic background. Another possibility might be the transfer by successive backcross matings of a series of RL-A alleles to an established highly inbred strain where inbreeding depression has already been overcome.

In addition to the Sh and FA inbred lines of Cohen (see above), the development of several inbred lines at the Jackson Laboratory was reported by Chai (1964, 1968, 1969, 1974) and used for genetic studies of histocompatibility in rabbits. It was shown that with increasing coefficient of inbreeding there is an increase in the proportion of long-term surviving skin grafts in contrast to a short survival of grafts exchanged between unrelated strains (e.g., the percentage survival of grafts exchanged within the strains was 21.6, 43.7, and 100 in generation 11-14, 15-17, and 18, respectively (Chai 1974). Similar results were obtained by Fabian et al. (1963) and Colberg and Dannenberg (1965). Inbred lines B and Y (F20) were used to estimate the number of segregating H loci. A Y female crossed with a B male at the twentieth generation of inbreeding produced the F_2 and F_3 generation. A total of 158 skin grafts were exchanged among these individuals and the frequency distribution of survival times was analyzed. The number of segregating loci was estimated to be 19.2 (with fiducial limits 16.4 to 24.7). Furthermore, the frequency distribution of graft survival time suggested that one locus was operating for rejection until day 21 to 23 and another for rejection until day 33 to 34. These two loci were designated RbH-1 and RbH-2. It was noticed that RbH-1 was probably the same as RL-A.

Thus, at least three notations appear for the rabbit MHS: RLC (Black 1967), RL-A (Matej 1970d; Ehlers and Ahrons 1971; Tissot and Cohen 1972), and RbH-1 (Chai 1974). RL-A is in the same line with HLA, SL-A, ChL-A, RhL-A, RbH-1 with H-2 in mice, and RtH-1 in rats.

4.3.3.3 Histocompatibility Testing in Rabbits and the Role of RL-A Antigens

In unrelated rabbits only Black (1967) could find by means of 26 alloimmune cytotoxic sera slight, but significant, differences for skin graft survival between compatible and incompatible pairs. Matej (1970d) and Cohen and Tissot (1974) found no difference between RL-A antigen-compatible or -incompatible combinations. However, in experiments of Matej (1970d), incompatible grafts were rejected more rapidly (3.2 to 5.0 versus 6.5 to 7.3 days) in preimmunized recipients. Cohen and Tissot (1974) were able to prove the role of RL-A antigens after 6-MP treatment (Table 4.3).

The probable role of RL-A antigens on corneal intralamellar transplantation was tested by 18 different cytotoxic alloimmune sera. Immune reactions (lymphocyte infiltration around the grafts) were observed only in RL-A-incompatible grafts. The lymphocyte infiltration of the grafts was more pronounced after presensitization with donor skin graft in incompatible combinations but absent after presensitization in compatible combinations. However, no details were given about the RL-A specificities involved (Ehlers and Ahrons 1971).

The major role of RL-A antigens in histocompatibility was conclusively shown on related rabbits.

Table 4.3. Skin Graft Survival in Rabbits

Recipients		Mean Graft Survival	
		Control	6-MP-Treated
RL-A mismatched and MLC-positive	Unrelated	7.3	9.3
	Noninbred siblings	8.0	8.5
	Inbred siblings[a]	8.3	9.6
RL-A mismatched and MLC negative	Unrelated	n.d.	9.4
RL-A identical and MLC negative	Unrelated	7.9	14.2
	Noninbred siblings	11.3	16.8
	Inbred siblings[a]	14.1	24.9

[a] Not more than 11F generations.
From Cohen and Tissot (1974).

Démant (1968a, 1968b) used 54 cytotoxic sera (which determined seven antigens) to test the role of serotyping on skin graft survival in newborn rabbits. It was known that tolerance induction to allogeneic skin grafts in newborn rabbits depended on the degree of donor-recipient relationship (Ványi and Iványiová 1961; Iványi 1964). Furthermore, prolonged survival of maternal as compared with paternal skin grafts in newborn rabbits indicated that maternal grafts enjoyed a certain degree of tolerance that tended to disappear rather rapidly after birth (Iványi and Démant 1965; Démant et al. 1966). The significant correlation found between serologically determined compatibility and prolonged graft survival indicated that antigenic differences between mother and fetus were one of the decisive factors in the induction of tolerance or immunity toward maternal antigens. The data obtained indicated that in the combinations with a small antigenic difference between mother and fetus tolerance was induced and the graft survival was prolonged, whereas in the combination with a great antigenic difference the fetus was sensitized and the graft survival was shortened (Démant 1968a, 1968b).

The role of RL-A antigens as part of the MHS was clearly shown by skin graft experiments performed between siblings. In the experiments of Matej (1970d), incompatible grafts were rejected on day 5 to 7, whereas compatible grafts were rejected on day 6 to 26 (with a MST for RL-A.1 of 15.44, for RL-A.2 of 12.25, and for RL-A.3 of 10.01 days, respectively). The experiments of Cohen and Tissot (1974) are summarized in Table 4.3. It is clear that RL-A identity ensures prolonged graft survival between siblings from noninbred as well as partially inbred parents and that this effect becomes much more apparent after 6-MP treatment. It should be noticed that in an exceptional combination of Sh6 line (RL-A^h) versus Sh9 (RL-A^c) line bearing serologically very similar but nevertheless distinct alleles (the two haplotypes can be traced to a probably common origin), 6-MP treatment had almost no effect on graft survival in spite of MLC negativity.

In summary, skin grafting experiments have shown that the RL-A system plays a decisive role in graft survival. In unrelated combinations the role of RL-A identity can be shown after presensitization or 6-MP treatment. In siblings (from noninbred or partially inbred families) the role of RL-A antigens is evident in untreated animals and becomes more apparent after 6-MP treatment. Negative MLC without serological RL-A identity is not sufficient to ascertain prolonged graft survival. Serologically identical, but MLC-positive, combinations have not yet been tested.

4.3.4 Rabbits Recognize H-2 and HLA Specificities

Several authors have shown that xenogeneic antisera raised in rabbits against insoluble or partly purified soluble membrane preparations of mouse or human lymphoid cells contain antibodies that recognize H-2 and/or HLA specificities or determinants inherited in association with them (for review, see Metzgar and Seigler 1972; Rapaport 1972; Ferrone and Pellegrino 1973). However, only a few of these experiments resulted in clear conclusions concerning the specificities involved. Billing and Terasaki (1974) were able to obtain monospecific anti-HLA-A9 rabbit sera after immunization with human serum HLA antigens. They presumed that the nondegraded nature of the serum antigen, compared to HLA antigens isolated from cells, was the reason for increased specificity of the rabbit antibody response. In similar experiments with extensively purified HLA antigens by papain solubilization from human lymphoblast-cultured cell lines, Robb et al. (1975) obtained high titered (1:190 to 1:1900) monospecific anti-HLA-A2 sera. Human cells possessing the HLA-A28 specificity (which is cross-reactive with HLA-A2) possessed an intermediate susceptibility to lysis. The sera contained in addition an anti-HLA activity that was not type-specific. Because purified beta$_2$-microglobulin reduced the titers of the serum by only 4 to 10 percent and without influence on its specificity, it was presumed that the second activity was directed toward a common determinant(s) on the 34.000-dalton HLA subunit.

All these data indicate that in rabbits mono- (or oligo-) specific anti-HLA sera can be produced by appropriate immunization procedures. Data are not yet available, however, that show how these findings correlate with the presence of rabbit histocompatibility products that cross-react with certain HLA and H-2 specificities.

Abeyounis and Milgrom (1969) have shown that rabbit alloimmune sera obtained after skin or kidney rejection have serological activity against murine L-cell fibroblasts. Different mouse strains, which share the H-2^k haplotype, were able to absorb anti-L cell activity; several H-2^b mouse strains had no absorbing capacity. One pair of congenic mouse strains, differing only by the H-2^k and H-2^b haplotypes, was included in these experiments. These findings have shown that alloimmune posttransplant rabbit sera contain antibodies that react on mouse cells with antigens controlled by H-2 or closely linked genes.

In a basically similar approach, alloimmune rabbit sera obtained after skin transplantation were found to exert cytotoxic activity against some human lymphocytes (Albert et al. 1969). When such sera were tested on human families, it appeared that the inheritance of human lymphocyte antigens detectable by eight rabbit sera might be governed by the HLA locus or a closely linked locus. This was supported by the finding that HLA genotyping was as possible with rabbit sera as on the basis of HLA typing and also that the rabbit sera always gave identical reaction patterns with lymphocytes of siblings who had HLA-identical antigens. However, attempts to correlate these serological reactions with particular HLA antigens have failed thus far. The specificity of the cytotoxic rabbit antibodies and their possible relation to RL-A antigens was not followed in any work.

All these data indicate that mono- (or oligo-) specific anti-HLA sera can be produced in rabbits by appropriate immunization procedures. Moreover, alloimmune rabbit sera cross-react with certain antigenic products of the HLA and H-2 genetical regions. The role of specific RL-A region products in these phenomena has not yet been ascertained.

4.4 The Major Histocompatibility System of Syrian Hamster

W.R. Duncan, J.W. Streilein, and P. Ivanyi

Early work with Syrian hamsters (*Mesocricetus auratus*) suggested that the members of this species are unlike other mammals in that they appear to be incapable of rejecting skin allografts acutely (Adams et al. 1958b; Schöne 1961; Skowron-Cendrzak and Spisak-Plonka 1958). However, subsequent studies by Billingham and Hildermann (1958), using animals from several closed colonies in England, demonstrated that some hamsters were capable of rejecting skin allografts in very prompt fashion, with survival time in the range of 9 to 11 days.

Evidence that various inbred strains of hamsters exhibit disparity at a major transplantation antigen locus was first obtained by Billingham et al. (1960). These workers studied F_2 hybrids derived from strains that acutely rejected reciprocal first-set skin grafts and found that allelic genes at only one to three different segregating loci determined the fate of skin allografts in hamsters. From the rejection patterns observed, it was suggested that at least one strong and one or two minor loci were operative in skin graft rejection. It was hypothesized that this surprisingly low number of H loci might be attributable to the limited gene pool from which all domesticated hamsters are thought to be derived; all Syrian hamsters in research today are the descendants of three littermates captured in Syria in 1930 (Adler 1948). More recently, a reevaluation of H loci in hamsters by Silvers et al. (1975) suggests that the paucity of such loci is more apparent than real and may be related to the inability of this species to reject full-size skin allografts when only minor histoincompatibility exists between the donor and the recipient; with the use of smaller grafts, these investigators obtained evidence for as many as ten different H loci in hamsters.

Recent studies by Duncan and Streilein (1976a) have shown that certain inbred strain combinations of hamsters give patterns of reciprocal skin graft rejection, mixed lymphocyte reactivity, and graft-versus-host reactivity, which suggests that hamsters possess a MHS equivalent. Genetic analysis utilizing segregent F_2 and backcross populations revealed that the allelic genes responsible for these traits are linked in a genetic region similar to the major histocompatibility complex found in other mammals; this linkage group in the hamster was designated Hm-1. However, among SGR, MLR, and GvHR, the linkage was not found to be as tight as would be expected for an MHS equivalent based on the murine and human models. Moreover, preliminary experiments have suggested that control of serum levels of complement (CH_{50}) and the immune response to bovine serum albumin are each under single, dominant gene control, but that the loci at which the alleles reside are not linked to Hm-1.

Further, Duncan and Streilein (1976b) have confirmed the results previously reported by Palm et al. (1967), i.e., that hamsters are unable to produce detectable hemagglutinating or cytotoxic alloantibodies specific for transplantation antigens. In addition, specific xenoantisera (rat, rabbit) were shown to be incapable of distinguishing between putative antigens dictated by different Hm-1 haplotypes. Other studies (Duncan and Streilein 1976c) revealed that hamsters were incapable of displaying strong cell-mediated cytotoxicity reactions to allogeneic targets but did develop minimal cytotoxicity to Ia-type determinants expressed only in T-lymphoblasts (not B-cell blasts or fibroblasts).

Thus, Syrian hamsters possess a genetic region similar in some aspects to the conventional mammalian MHS, but different in others. Current data suggest that all commercially available hamster strains are identical for the classical serologically detectable (SD) determinants but differ at regions of the MHS that code for lymphocyte-activating determinants (Lad), which are expressed only on T-cells and incite SGR, MLR, and GvHR.

References

Abeyounis, C.J., and Milgrom, F. Tissue isoantigens shared by rabbits and mice. *Transplant. Proc. 1*:556–559, 1969.

Adams, R.A., Patt, D.I., and Lutz, B.R. Long term persistence of skin homografts in untreated hamsters. *Transplant. Bull. 3*:41–42, 1956.

Adler, S. Origin of the golden hamster Cricetus auratus as a laboratory animal. *Nature (London) 162*:256–257, 1948.

Ahrons, S., and Lund, B. Renal transplantation in rabbits VIII. *Tissue Antigens 2*:112–122, 1972.

Albert, E., Kano, K., Abeiounis, C.J., and Milgrom, F. Detection of human lymphocyte isoantigens by rabbit homotransplantation sera. *Transplantation 8*:466–471, 1969.

Anderson, D., Billingham, R.E., Mapkin, G.H., and Medawar, P.B. The use of skin grafting to distinguish between monozygotic and dizygotic twins in cattle. *Heredity 5*:379–382, 1951.

Baker, L.N. A red cell system in pigs: Irregular genetic transmission. *Vox Sang. 21*:57–64, 1971.

Baker, L.N., and Andersen, E. Skin grafting in pigs: Evidence for a histocompatibility mechanism. *Transplantation 2*:118–119, 1974.

Billing, R.J., and Terasaki, P.I. Rabbit antisera to HL-A9 isolated from normal serum. *Transplantation 17*:231–234, 1974.

Billingham, R.E., and Hildemann, W.H. Studies on the immunological responses of hamsters to skin grafts. *Proc. R. Soc. Lond. (B) 149*:216–223, 1958.

Billingham, R.E., Sawchuck, G.H., and Silvers, W.K. Studies on the histocompatibility genes of the Syrian hamster. *Proc. Natl. Acad. Sci. (USA) 46*:1079–1090, 1960.

Binns, R.M., Symons, D.B.A., and White, D.J.G. Demonstration of the movement of histocompatibility antigen and immunoglobulin on the pig lymphocyte membrane by immunofluorescence. *J. Physiol. 226*:44, 1972.

Black, L. Histocompatibility testing in the rabbit. *Transplantation 5*:390–409, 1967.

Borovská, M., and Démant, P. Specificity of cytotoxic antibodies in typing sera against cattle blood group antigens. *Folia Biol. (Praha) 13*:473–475, 1967.

Borovská, M., Kořínek, J., Václavíková, I., and Démant, P. Ss protein: Search for cross-reacting substances in different species. *Folia Biol. (Praha) 17*:183–285, 1971.

Bouw, J., and Fiorentini, A. Structure of loci controlling complex blood group systems in cattle. *In XIth European Conference on Animal Blood Groups*, p. 109, W. Junk, The Hague, 1970.

Bradley, B.A., Edwards, J.M., Dunn, D.C., and Calne, R.Y. Quantitation of mixed lymphocyte reaction by gene dosage phenomenon. *Nature New Biol. 240*:54–56, 1972.

Bradley, B.A., Edwards, J.M., and White, D.J. Histocompatibility genotyping by the mixed lymphocyte reaction. *Tissue Antigens 3*:340–347, 1973.

Bradley, B.A., White, D.J., and Edwards, J.M. Restriction of polymorphisms defined by mixed lymphocyte reactions in the pig. *Tissue Antigens 4*:283–290, 1974.

Buschmann, H., Radzikowski, A., Kräusslich, H., Schmid, D.O., and Cwik, S. Untersuchungen über die Immunantwort gegenüber DNP-Hapten in mehreren Schweinerassen. *Zentralblatt Veterinaermed. 22*:155–161, 1975.

Calne, R.Y. Antigen induced immunosuppression for organ grafting. *Transplant. Proc. 3*:21–26, 1971.

Calne, R.Y., Davis, D.R., Pena, J.R., Balner, H., de Vries, M., Herbertson, B.H., Millard, P.R., Joysey, V.C., Seaman, M.J., Samuel, J.R., Stibbe, J., and Westbroek, D.L. Hepatic allografts and xenografts in primates. *Lancet i*:103–106, 1970.

Calne, R.Y., Sells, R.A., Pena, J.R., Davis, D.R., Millard, P.R., Herbertson, B.M., Binns, R.M., and Davies, D.A.L. Induction of immunological tolerance by porcine liver allografts. *Nature 223*:472, 1969.

Calne, R.Y., White, H.J.O., Yoffa, D.E., Binns, R.M., Maginn, R.R., Herbertson, R.M., Millard, P.R., Molina, V.P., and Davis, D.R.: Prolonged survival of liver transplants in the pig. *Br. Med. J. iv*: 645–648, 1967.

Castle, W.E., and Keeler, C.E. Blood group inheritance in the rabbit. *Proc. Natl. Acad. Sci. (USA) 19*:92–98, 1933.

Chai, C.K. Skin grafts between inbred rabbits. *Transplantation 2*:436–437, 1964.

Chai, C.K. The effect of inbreeding in rabbits. *Transplantation 6*:689–693, 1968.

Chai, C.K. The effect of inbreeding in rabbits: inbred lines, discrete characters, breeding performance and mortality. *J. Hered. 60*:64–70, 1969.

Chai, C.K. Genetic studies of histocompatibility in rabbits: identification of major and minor genes. *Immunogenetics 1*:126–132, 1974.

Chomette, G., Garnier, H., Vaiman, M., Auriol, M., and Hachimi, A.E.: System d'histocompatibilité S.L.A. et allotransplantations viscérales (intestin et rein) chez le porc. *Arch. Anat. Pathol. (Paris) 22*:17–23, 1974.

Cohen, C. On blood groups and confusion in the rabbit. *Transplant. Bull 5*:21–23, 1958.
Cohen, C. Blood groups in rabbits. *Ann. N.Y. Acad. Sci. 97*:26–36, 1962.
Cohen, C., DePalma, R.G., Colberg, J.E., Tissot, R.G., and Hubay, C.A. The relationship between blood groups and histocompatibility in the rabbit. *Ann. N.Y. Acad. Sci. 120*:356–361, 1964.
Cohen, C., and Tissot, R.G. Blood groups in the rabbit. Two additional isoantibodies and the red cell antigens they identify. *J. Immunol. 95*:148–155, 1965.
Cohen, C., and Tissot, R.C. The effect of the RL-A locus and the MLC locus on graft survival in the rabbit. *Transplantation 18*:150–154, 1974.
Colberg, J.E., and Dannenberg, A.M. An evaluation of inbred rabbit populations by skin homotransplantation. *Nature 207*:777–778, 1965.
Cwik, S., and Schmid, D.O. Immunogenetic properties of SL-A inhibitor substances in serum of pigs. *J. Immunogenet. 2*:27–30, 1975.
Datta, S.P., and Stone, W.H. Transferrins in cattle twins. *Proc. Soc. Exp. Biol. Med. 113*:756–759, 1963.
Démant, P. The role of serologically detected histocompatibility differences for the survival time of maternal skin grafts in newborn rabbits. *In* J. Dausset, J. Hamburger, and G. Mathé (eds.), *Advance in Transplantation*, pp. 325–329, Munksgaard, Copenhagen, 1968a.
Démant, P. Histocompatibility antigens in rabbits and their significance for the survival of maternal skin grafts in newborn rabbits. *Folia Biol. (Praha) 14*:9–20, 1968b.
Démant, P., Iványi, P., and Ivašková, E. Prolonged survival of maternal skin grafts in newborn rabbits. *Ann. N.Y. Acad. Sci. 129*:234–240, 1966.
Duncan, W.R., and Streilein, J.W. Definition and analysis of the major histocompatibility complex in Syrian hamsters. Ph. D. dissertation, Southwestern Medical School, Dallas, Texas, 1976a.
Duncan, W.R., and Streilein, J.W. The Major Histocompatibility Complex in Syrian Hamsters: Are 50 Determinants Present? Transplant. Proc. (in press), 1976b.
Duncan, W.R., and Streilein, J.W. Analysis of the major histocompatibility complex in Syrian hamster. III. Cellular and Humoral Immunity to Alloantigens J. Immunol. (in press), 1976c.
Ehlers, N., and Ahrons, S. The influence of histocompatibility upon the corneal immune reaction after intralamellar allotransplantation in rabbits. *Tissue Antigens 1:23–31, 1971.*
Fabian, G., Iványi, P., and Széky, P. Skin transplantation in partially inbred rabbits. *Folia Biol. (Praha) 9*:440–443, 1963.
Ferrone, S., and Pellegrino, M.A. HL-A antigens, antibody, and complement in the lymphocytotoxic reaction. *In* R.A. Reisfeld and W.J. Mandy (eds.), *Contemporary Topics in Molecular Immunology*, Vol. 2, pp. 185–236, Plenum Press, New York, 1973.
Festenstein, H. Discussion. *In* Strong and weak histocompatibility antigens. *Transplant. Rev. 3*:95–96, 1970.
Govallo, V.I., Konstantinova, U.T., and Kosobkova, V.F. Immunological reactions in homotransplantation of large and small skin grafts in rabbits. *Folia Biol. (Praha) 10*:117–123, 1964.
Grosclaude, F. Alleles du locus S de groupes sanguins des bovins. *Ann. Biol. Animal Biochem. Biophys. 3*:433–435, 1963.
Grosclaude, F. Studies on the S blood group system in French cattle breeds. *In* J. Matoušek (ed.), *Blood Groups of Animals Proceedings of the 9th European Animal Blood Group Conference*, p. 79, Czechslovak Academy of Science, Prague, 1965.
Grothaus, E.A., and Cohen, C. Isoantigens common to erythrocytes and other tissue cells in the rabbit. *Transplantation 11*:122–127, 1971.
Hála, K. Occurrence of erythrocyte antigens on cells from various tissues of the pig. *Folia Biol. (Praha) 13*:189–192, 1967.
Hilgert, I. Variation in the type of immune response to mouse histocompatibility antigens as the function of their form. *J. Immunogenet. 1*:153–207, 1974.
Hruban, V., Simon, M., and Hradecký, J. Alloantigens common to erythrocytes and leukocytes in pigs. *Anim. Blood Groups Biochem. Genet. 3*:157–161, 1972.
Hruban, V., Simon, M., and Hradecký, J. Histocompatibility studies in pigs from outbred and semi-inbred families. *Anim. Blood Groups Biochem. Genet. 5*:171–176, 1974.
Iha, T.H., Gerbrandt, G., Bodmer, W.F., McGary, D., and Stone, W.H. Crossreactions of

cattle lymphocytotoxic sera with HL-A and other human antigens. *Tissue Antigens 3*:291–302, 1973.

Ivânyi, P. Notes on the problem of the relationship of blood groups to transplantation of skin in rabbits. *Folia Biol. (Praha) 8*:322–327, 1962.

Ivânyi, P. Immunological tolerance on newborn rabbits. IV. Further studies on skin transplantation in newborn rabbits. *Folia Biol. (Praha) 10*:433–460, 1964.

Ivânyi, P. Relation of blood groups to transplantation antigens in rabbits. *In Blood Groups of Animals; Proceedings of the 9th European Animal Blood Group Conference 1964*, pp. 401–403, Czechoslovak Academy of Science, Prague, 1965.

Ivânyi, P. Blood groups and transplantation antigens. *Ann. Inst. Pasteur 110*:144–154, 1966.

Ivâny, P., and Démant, P. Prolonged survival of maternal skin grafts in newborn rabbits. *Folia Biol. (Praha) 11*:321–323, 1965.

Ivânyi, P., and Ivânyiovâ, D. Immunological tolerance in rabbits III. Succesful skin homotransplantation in newborn rabbits. *Folia Biol. (Praha) 7*:369–372, 1961.

Ivânyi, P., Tomâšková, M., and Ivânyi, J. Über die Bedeutung der Identifizierung der Blutgruppen bei Kaninchen für die Modellversuche in der Immunohämatologie. *Z. Immunitätsforschung 117*:134–146, 1959.

Ivânyi, P., and Ujhelyiovâ, M. Determination of the amount of blood group incompatible erythrocytes adequate for inducing isoimmune agglutinins in rabbits (in Slovak). *Bratisl. Lek. Listy 38*:93, 1958.

Ivašková, E., and Ivânyi, P. The study of allogeneic cytotoxic antibodies in partly inbred rabbits. *Folia Biol. (Praha) 12*:176–183, 1966.

Jílek, F., and Veselský, L. The occurrence of lymphocytes antigens on boar spermatodoa. *J. Reprod. Fertil. 31*:295–298, 1972.

Kapitchnikov, M. M., Ballantyne, D. L., and Stetson, C. A. Immunological reactions to skin homotransplantation in rabbits and rats. *Ann. N.Y. Acad. Sci. 99*:497–503, 1962.

Levine, P., and Landsteiner, K. On immune isoagglutinins in rabbits. *J. Immunol. 17*:559–565, 1929.

Lillie, F. R. The theory of the freemartin. *Science 43*:611–613, 1916.

Matej, H. Hemagglutinating antibodies after skin transplantation in rabbits. *Arch. Immunol. Ther. Exp. 16*:757–772, 1968.

Matej, H. Blood groups in rabbits detected by means of posttransplantation hemagglutinins. *Arch. Immunol. Ther. Exp. 17*:200–206, 1969.

Matej, H. Cytotoxic antibodies after skin allotransplantation in rabbits. *Arch. Immunol. Ther. Exp. 18*:29–41, 1970a.

Matej, H. Antigenic differentiation of rabbit lymphocytes. *Arch. Immunol. Ther. Exp. 18*:42–53, 1970b.

Matej, H. Further studies on antigenic differentiation of rabbit lymphocytes. *Arch. Immunol. Ther. Exp. 18*:173–184, 1970c.

Matej, H. Studies on histocompatibility in skin allotransplantation in rabbits. *Arch. Immunol. Ther. Exp. 18*:315–326, 1970d.

Matej, H. Transplantation antigens in rabbits. *In International Symposium on Standardization of HL-A Reagents, Copenhagen, 1972;* Symposium Series on Immunobiological Standards, vol. 18, pp. 246–250, Karger, Basel, 1973.

Matej, H., and Wieczorek, Z. Cytophilic and cytotoxic antibodies in sera of rabbits after allogeneic skin grafts. *Arch. Immunol. Ther. Exp. 23*:329–333, 1975.

McGary, D. R. *Immunology of cattle lymphocytes.* M.S. thesis, University of Wisconsin, Madison, 1969.

McGary, D. R., and Stone, W. H. Immunogenetic studies of cattle lymphocytes. *Fed. Proc. 29*:508, 1970.

Medawar, P. B. The behaviour and fate of skin autografts and skin homografts in rabbits. *J. Anat. 78*:176–199, 1944.

Medawar, P. B. A second study of the behaviour and fate of skin homografts in rabbits. *J. Anat. 79*:157–170, 1945.

Medawar, P. B. Immunity to homologous grafted skin. II. The relationship between the antigens of blood and skin. *Br. J. Exp. Pathol. 27*:15–24, 1946.

Metzgar, R.S., and Seigler, H.F. Species-distribution and evolutionary development of HL-A antigens. *In* B.D. Kahan and R.A. Reisfeld (eds.), *Transplantation Antigens*, pp. 209–224, Academic Press, New York, 1972.

Millot, P. Groupes thrombocytaires chez les bovins. *In Proceedings of the Xth European Conference on Animal Blood Groups*, p. 129, Inst. Nat. Rech. Agronom., Paris, 1966.

Ostrand-Rosenberg, S., and Stormont, C. Bovine leukocyte antigens. *Anim. Blood Groups Biochem. Genet. 5*:231–237, 1974.

Owen, R.D. Immunogenetic consequences of vascular anastomoses between bovine twins. *Science 102*:400–401, 1945.

Owen, R.D., Davis, H.P., and Morgan, R.F. Quintuplet calves and erythrocyte mosaicism. *J. Hered. 37*:291–297, 1946.

Palm, J.W., Silvers, W.K., and Billingham, R.E. The problem of histocompatibility in wild hamsters. *J. Hered. 58*:40–44, 1967.

Parker, J.R., Hickman, R., and Terblanche, J. Mixed lymphocyte culture studies in pigs which survive transplants without immunosuppression. *Transplantation 19*:276–279, 1975.

Rapaport, F.T. The biological significance of cross-reactions between histocompatibility antigens and antigens of bacterial and/or heterologous mammalian origin. *In* B.D. Kahan and R.A. Reisfeld (eds.), *Transplantation Antigens*, pp. 181–208, Academic Press, New York, 1972.

Riddell, A.G., Terblanche, J., Peacock, J.H., Tierris, E.J., and Hunt, A.C. Experimental liver homotransplantation in pigs. *In* J. Dausset, J. Hamburger, and G. Mathé (eds.), *Advances in Transplantation*, Munksgaard, Copenhagen, 1967.

Robb, R.J., Humphreys, R.E., Strominger, J.L., Fuller, T.C., and Mann, D.L. Rabbit anti-HL-A2 sera. *Transplantation 19*:445–447, 1975.

Saison, R., and Ingram, D.G. Production of specific haemagglutinins in pig after receiving skin homografts. *Nature 197*:296–297, 1963.

Schmid, D.O., and Cwik, S. Soluble leukocyte antigens in serum of pigs. *Tissue Antigens 2*:255–261, 1972.

Schmid, D.O., and Otto, F. Contribution to serology of lymphocytes in cattle and pigs. *In Proceedings of the XIIth European Conference on Animal Blood Groups*, p. 117, Akademiai Kiado, Budapest, 1970.

Schmid, D.O., and Otto, F. Zur Serologie der Granulozytenantigene beim Schwein. *Zentralblatt Veterinaermed. 18*:205–210, 1971.

Schöne, G. Transplantation und Genetik. *Beitr. Klin. Chir. 202*:129–159, 1961.

Sellei, J., and Rendel J. A probable crossing-over between two B-alleles of cattle blood groups. *In XIth European Conference on Animal Blood Groups*, p. 115, W. Junk, The Hague, 1970.

Silvers, W.K., Gasser, D.L., and Murphy, M.R. Number of histocompatibility loci in Syrian hamsters. *J. Immunol. 115*:1309–1311, 1975.

Simon, M., and Hojný, J. A study on lymphocyte antigens in pigs by means of anti-erythrocyte reagents. *In Proceedings of the XIIth European Conference on Animal Blood Groups*, pp. 369–374, Akademiai Kiado, Budapest, 1970.

Simon, M., and Hruban, V. Lymphocyte typing in pigs: Evidence for antigen L 1. *Anim. Blood Groups Biochem. Genet. 2*:95–100, 1971.

Simon, M., and Hruban, V. Cytotoxic action of pig anti-A erythrocyte antibodies. *Vox Sang. 13*:208–211, 1972.

Skowron-Cendrzak, A., and Spisak-Plonka, I. Skin homografts in the golden hamster. *Folia Biol. (Praha) 6*:187–189, 1958.

Stone, W.H., Friedman, J., and Fregin, A. Possible somatic cell mating in twin cattle with erythrocyte mosaicism. *Proc. Natl. Acad. Sci. (USA) 51*:1036–1044, 1964.

Stone, W.H., and Miller, W.J. Naturally occurring isoantibodies of the S blood group system in cattle. *J. Immunol. 86*:165–169, 1961.

Stormont, C. Acquisition of the J substance by the bovine erythrocytes. *Proc. Natl. Acad. Sci. (USA) 35*:232–234, 1949.

Terasaki, P.I., Bold, E.J., Cannon, J.A., and Longmire, W.P. Antibody response to homografts. VI. *In vitro* cytotoxins produced by skin homografts in rabbits. *Proc. Soc. Exp. Biol. Med. 106*:133–138, 1961.

Tissot, R. G., and Cohen, C. Histocompatibility in the rabbit. Identification of the major locus. *Tissue Antigens 2*:267–279, 1972.

Tissot, R. G., and Cohen, C. Histocompatibility in the rabbit. Linkage between RL-A, MLC and the He blood group locus. *Transplantation 18*:142–149, 1974.

Vaiman, M., Arnoux, A., Filleul, X., and Nizza, P. Le systême d'histocompatibilité SL-A du porc: Étude par la technique des cultures mixtes de leucocytes. *C.R. Acad. Sci. (Paris), Serie D. 271*:1724–1727, 1970a.

Vaiman, M., Garnier, H., Kunlin, A., Hay, J. M., Parc, R., Bacour, F., Fagniez, P. H., Villiers, P. A., Lecointre, J., Bara, M. F., and Nizza, P. The SL-A histocompatibility system in the Sus scrofa species. *Transplantation 14*:541–550, 1972.

Vaiman, M., Haag, J., Arnoux, A., and Nizza, P. The histocompatibility complex SL-A in the pig. Possible recombination between the regions governing MLR and serology respectively. *Tissue Antigens 3*:204–211, 1973.

Vaiman, M., Renard, C., La Fage, P., Ameteau, J., and Nizza, P. Evidence for a histocompatibility system in swine (SL-A). *Transplantation 10*:155–164, 1970b.

Vaiman, M., Renard, C., La Fage, P., Ameteau, J., and Nizza, P. Détermination d'un systéme d'histocompatitibilité chez le porc (Sus scrofa) le systéme SL-A. *Ann. Biol. Anim. Biochem. Biophys. 11*:41–54, 1971.

Vaiman, M., Renard, C., Ponceau, M., Lecointre, J., and Villiers, P. A. Alloantigénes sous la dépendance de la region SL-A controlant la reaction lymphocytaire mixte chez le porc. *C.R. Acad. Sci. (Paris) 280*:2809–2812, 1975.

Viza, D., Sugar, J. R., and Binns, R. M. Lymphocyte stimulation in pigs: Evidence for the existence of a single major histocompatibility locus, PL-A. *Nature 227*:949–950, 1970.

White, D. J. G., Bradley, B., Calne, R. Y., and Binns, R. M. The relationship of the histocompatibility locus in the pig to allograft survival. *Transplant. Proc. 5*:317–320, 1973.

Young, A. M., Hopkins, J. P., and Esparza, A. Humoral aspects of skin transplantation in the rabbit. *Am. J. Pathol. 43*:227–235, 1963.

Zotikov, E. A. Changes of immunological characters in rabbit sera after skin homotransplantation (in Russian). *Biull. Eksp. Biol. Med. 42*:58–62, 1956.

Zweibaum, A., and Bouhou, E. Studies on digestive groups. II. Influence of the digestive group A system on skin allografts in rabbits. *Transplantation 15*:294–297, 1973.

Chapter 5

The Major Histocompatibility System of the Guinea Pig

A. F. GECZY and A. L. DE WECK

1. Introduction

The investigation of guinea pig leukocyte antigens has lagged considerably behind the first documented reports of mouse (Gorer 1936) and human (Dausset 1958) leukocyte antigens. Although the guinea pig has been used extensively in a wide variety of immunological studies, particularly for investigations of genetic control of the immune response and its relationship to histocompatibility-linked immune response genes (McDevitt and Benacerraf 1969), until recently, relatively little effort has been invested into the serological and genetic aspects of the major histocompatibility system (MHS) in this species.

From data on the proportion of parental strain grafts surviving in F_2 and backcross animals from strain 2 and strain 13 guinea pigs and from the proportion of F_2 animals retaining both parental strain grafts, Bauer (1960) estimated that no less than six histocompatibility genes control the rejection of strain 2 grafts and no less than four genes the rejection of strain 13 grafts. Of course, these studies yield no information about whether products of these histocompatibility genes would all be represented on lymphocyte membranes. The presence of immunogenic histocompatibility antigens on leukocyte membranes was established by Walford et al. (1962), who detected antibodies to leukocyte antigens in strain 2 and strain 13 guinea pigs following skin homografts. Similarly, antibodies reacting with the lymphocytes of strain 2 or strain 13 animals have been obtained by immunization with lymphoid cells, lymphoid cell homogenates, or tumor cells (Kahan et al. 1969; Martin et al. 1970; Ellman et al. 1970).

However, because histocompatibility differences among the inbred strain 2 and strain 13 include more than one gene and gene product, such multispecific antisera give little information about the various histocompatibility antigens possessed by the particular species.

Apart from a single paper by Brummerstedt and Franks (1970) and two (de Weck et al. 1971; Sato and de Weck 1972) from our group, no reports have appeared on attempts to define the major histocompatibility system of the guinea pig by serological techniques. In 1972 Sato and de Weck identified four serologically defined leukocyte antigens (designated A, B, C, and D) by cross-immunizing with lymphoid cells of outbred animals originating from a closed colony of random-bred guinea pigs. The antigens B, C, and D were thought to be alleles of a single locus, and the term GPLA was proposed for these leukocyte alloantigens. Recent studies (Geczy et al. 1975a) have established that the specificity originally designated as A did not behave in allelic fashion with B, C, and D but appeared to be governed by another genetic region, which could be equivalent to the Ia region of the mouse H-2 complex (Shreffler and David 1975).

A number of studies have been performed with alloantisera raised by cross-immunization of strain 2 and strain 13 guinea pigs, and it has been shown that these antisera can specifically inhibit T-cell proliferation by antigens, the responses to which are regulated by histocompatibility-linked immune response (Ir) genes (Shevach et al. 1972). In addition, alloantisera apparently directed against products of the GPLA locus (viz., against antigens B and C) could also block antigen-induced proliferation *in vitro* (Geczy and de Weck 1974). The apparent close relationship between Ir and histocompatibility genes in other species as well as in guinea pigs make further studies of the guinea pig MHS imperative.

The purpose of this chapter is to summarize serologic and genetic studies, including specific absorption experiments, aimed at defining the genetic and serologic composition of the guinea pig MHS.

2. Serology

2.1 Methodology

To detect antibodies specific for histocompatibility antigens present on leukocytes, two methods have been employed: the classical complement-dependent lymphocytotoxicity eosin technique in microplates using peripheral blood lymphocytes as target cells, as described elsewhere (Sato and de Weck 1972), and the ^{51}Cr release technique with lymph node cells as targets (Martin et al. 1970). Other cumbersome procedures such as those described by Walford et al. (1962) have not been used extensively for typing guinea pig lymphocytes.

Whereas the eosin technique is quite suitable for the detection of gene products from the GPLA locus, the ^{51}Cr release technique appears to be more efficient for detecting gene products of the Ia-equivalent region (see below).

Alloantisera were raised by repeated immunization with lymphoid cells or lymphoid cell homogenates in complete Freund's adjuvant. Although some authors (Walford et al. 1962; Brummersted and Franks 1970) have been successful in raising alloantibodies after skin grafting, this procedure was, in our hands, much less effective for the production of suitable typing alloantisera. Further details on the methodology used are given elsewhere (de Weck et al. 1976).

Animals used for investigations of the guinea pig MHC were the inbred strains NIH 2 and 13 and the partially inbred strains R9, BE, and OM3 maintained at the MRC Laboratory Animals Center, Carshalton, England.

Table 5.1. Phenotypes Encountered in Various Strains of Guinea Pigs

		Specificities	
		GPLA B Locus	I Region
Family	Bio. B[a]	B.1	Ia.1,4
	Bio. C	B.2	Ia.1
	Bio. AC	B.2	Ia.1,3
	Bio. AD	B.3	Ia.1,3
Strain	R9	B.3	Ia.1,3
	BE	B.3	Ia.1
	OM3	B.3	Ia.1,3
	2	B.1	Ia.2,4
	13	B.1	Ia.1,3
Colony	RT	B.1,3	Ia.2

[a] *Note on origin of animals:* Animals designated by the prefix Bio (e.g., Bio. B) are taken from a known family line (derived from a closed colony of Himalayan albino spotted guinea pigs, maintained at the Füllinsdorf Institute, Switzerland, for the past 30 years, without any attempt at inbreeding) and are presumed homozygous for their B locus antigens. These families have now been continued by brother-sister matings for over ten generations. The partially inbred strains BE, OM3, R9, were obtained from Dr. M. Festing, MRC Laboratory Animals Center, Carshalton, England. Details of the origins of these strains and the nomenclature used is given in *Guinea Pig Newsletter,* 1971, No. 4, pp. 3–8. Since their arrival from Carshalton in 1971, these animals have been maintained in closed colony without any attempt at inbreeding. Colony RT was obtained from a closed colony maintained at the University of Tübingen and was donated by Dr. G. Riethmüller in 1971. They have since been bred by us in a closed colony.

In addition, outbred guinea pigs from a closed colony (Bio, Fülligsdorf) as well as guinea pig families (designated B, C, AD, and AC) bred to homozygosity for the GPLA antigens B.1 (B), B.2 (C), and B.3 (D),[1] were used. The animal strains used and their detected histocompatibility antigens are given in Table 5.1.

2.2 Serological Characterization of Antigens Governed by Alleles of the First GPLA Locus (Locus B)

Antisera recognizing the GPLA antigens B.1, B.2, and B.3 were prepared by immunization with lymphoid cells among appropriate outbred or inbred animals. For example, an antiserum recognizing the specificity B1 could be prepared by immunization of $B.2^+$ or $B.3^+$ outbreds with $B.1^+$ cells.

[1] In agreement with the NIH Laboratory of Immunology, Bethesda, Maryland, it was decided to adopt a nomenclature based on the recently recommended principles of HLA nomenclature in man. Within the GPLA complex, recognized loci are given symbols, whereas specificities assigned to a locus are given numbers. Therefore, the B, C, and D specificities controlled by a first locus (designated locus B for historical reasons) will hereafter be designated B.1, B.2, and B.3.

Table 5.2. Evidence for the Monospecificity of Anti-B.1 Serum

Antiserum	Absorption with Cells from	Target Lymphocytes			
		Strain 2 (B.1, Ia.2,4)	Strain 13 (B.1, Ia.1,3)	Outbred (B.1,3, Ia.1,3)	Outbred (B.2, Ia.1,3)
Anti-B.1[a]	–	46[b]	33	43	2
Anti-B.1	B.1,3, Ia.1,3	3	2	0	0
Anti-B.1	Strain 2	0	0	0	0
Anti-B.1	Strain 13	0	0	0	0

[a] Raised by immunization of a B.2$^+$ outbred with B.1$^+$ cells.
[b] Percent ^{51}Cr release.

Table 5.3. Evidence for the Monospecificity of Anti-B.2 Serum

Antiserum	Absorption	Target Lymphocytes			
		Outbred (B.2, Ia.1,3)	Inbred 2 (B.1, Ia.2,4)	Inbred 13 (B.1, Ia.1,3)	Outbred (B.1,3, Ia.1,3)
Anti-B.2[a]	0	28[b]	0	0	0
Anti-B.2	Inbred 13	23	0	0	0
Anti-B.2	Inbred 2	25	0	0	0
Anti-B.2	B.1,3, Ia.1,3	27	0	0	0
Anti-B.2	B.1,2, Ia.1,3	1	0	0	0

[a] Raised by immunization of B.1$^+$ cells (B family) with B.2$^+$ cells (C family).
[b] Percent ^{51}Cr release.

The evidence for the monospecificity of this serum is presented in Table 5.2. The absorption of the anti-B.1 serum with B.1$^+$ cells from various sources removes all of the lytic activity for cells from strain 2, strain 13, and outbred B.1$^+$ animals.

Similarly, antisera monospecific for the B.2 antigen were prepared by immunization of individuals from the B family (B.1$^+$) with cells of animals from the C family (B.2$^+$) or by immunization of strain 13 animals (B.1$^+$) with cells from B.2$^+$ outbreds. Both of these alloantisera behaved in similar fashion (Table 5.3); the lymphocytotoxic activity could be removed only by absorption with B.2$^+$ cells. The anti-B.2 serum was not significantly cytotoxic for cells from strain 2, strain 13, and B.3$^+$ animals.

Sera that identified anti-B.3 were raised in similar fashion by immunizing appropriate outbred B.1$^+$ animals with cells from animals of the homozygous AD family (see Table 5.1). These sera reacted only with cells from B.3$^+$ animals and not with inbred strain 2 or strain 13 cells. Absorption studies demonstrated that all cytotoxic activity could be removed by absorption with B.3$^+$ lymphoid cells from various origins but not by inbred strain 13 or outbred B.2$^+$ lymphoid cells. Sera of apparently identical specificity for B.1, B.2, and B.3 may be raised by immunization among various outbred animals of the appropriate phenotype.

The operationally monospecific anti-B.1, B.2, and B.3 sera were used to screen a large number of outbred animals. In our colony, guinea pigs were found to bear one or two of these antigens; a $B.1^+ B.2^+ B.3^+$ animal was never encountered among more than 3000 guinea pigs typed. This finding suggested that antigens B.1, B.2, and B.3 are governed by alleles of a single locus termed the first GPLA or B locus.

During the course of these joint investigations with Dr. E. M. Shevach (NIH), a single outbred animal was identified in the NIH colony that typed as $B.1^- B.2^- B.3^-$. Antisera were raised to the lymphoid cells of this animal by immunization of inbred strain 13 ($B.1^+$) recipients. The resultant antiserum appeared to identify a new and distinct specificity termed B.4. Animals identified as B.4 positive were never found to bear more than one other GPLA antigen. Antigen B.4 is tentatively considered an allelic gene product of the locus coding for antigens B.1, B.2, and B.3.

Because anti-B.1 antiserum coprecipitates membrane antigens of 45,000 and 12,000 daltons (as determined by SDS gel electrophoresis) (Finkelman et al. 1975) and because the B.1 antigen appears to be distributed not only on lymphoid cells but also on sarcoma and hepatoma cells (Forni et al. 1975), it is tempting to consider the GPLA-B locus as an equivalent of the murine H-2D (or K) locus or of the other "serologically defined" loci in other species.

2.3 Serologic Characterization of Antigens Identified by 13 Anti-2 and 2 Anti-13 Sera

The initial studies performed in our laboratory with 2 anti-13 and 13 anti-2 alloantisera using the eosin plate technique revealed that a large number of the outbred animals maintained in our colony were $2^- 13^-$. However, subsequent investigations using the more sensitive ^{51}Cr release assay showed that our animals as well as those maintained in the NIH colony could practically all be classified as $2^+ 13^-$, $2^- 13^+$, or $2^+ 13^+$. It is to be noted that in contrast with alloantisera recognizing GPLA antigens that yield 60 to 90 percent ^{51}Cr release, 2 anti-13 and 13 anti-2 yield only 20 to 40 percent ^{51}Cr release. Another possible reason for the frequent failure in detecting the 2 and 13 antigens using the eosin technique may be the use of peripheral blood lymphocytes instead of lymph node cells as the target tissue. Anti-2 and anti-13 sera have been shown to be preferentially cytotoxic for B lymphocytes. The percentage of B cells in guinea pig peripheral blood is significantly less than the proportion of B lymphocytes in adjuvant-stimulated lymph nodes (Shevach et al. 1973).

Absorption studies with lymphoid cells from animals raised in our colony showed that the 2 anti-13 and 13 anti-2 sera are not monospecific but recognize at least two different specificities. Following absorption of the 2 anti-13

Table 5.4. 2 Anti-13 Serum Identifies Two Distinct Specificities

Antiserum	Absorption with Cells from	Target Lymphocytes		
		Inbred 13	Family B	Inbred 2
2 Anti-13	0	29[a]	12	0
2 Anti-13	Family B	21	0	0
Anti-Ia.3[b]	0	26	0	0

[a] Percent ^{51}Cr release.
[b] Raised by immunization of Family B (B.1, Ia.1,4) animals with cells from strain 13 (B.1, Ia.1,3) guinea pigs.

serum with lymphoid cells from a guinea pig belonging to the B family (Table 5.4) all of the lytic activity was lost for cells from the family B guinea pigs, but significant lytic activity was retained for inbred strain 13 cells (Table 5.4). It is therefore clear that 2 anti-13 serum contains antibodies directed against two distinct specificities, viz., Ia.1 and Ia.3 (previously called 13 and A respectively). An antiserum recognizing Ia.3 (previously A) can also be obtained by immunizing a family B guinea pig with lymphoid cells from an inbred 13 animal.

Further absorption studies with cells from the B family revealed that 13 anti-2 serum also contained antibodies to more than one specificity. Absorption of the 13 anti-2 serum with cells of the B family removed all lytic activity for the B family cells, but significant cytotoxic activity remained for inbred strain 2 cells. This finding demonstrated that the 13 anti-2 serum also recognized two distinct specificities, only one of which was present in the B family. By immunizing a member of the B family with cells from an inbred strain 2, we obtained an antiserum that was lytic for strain 2 but not for strain 13 cells. This serum was also cytotoxic for a large percentage of outbred animals that were also lysed by 13 anti-2 serum (Geczy et al. 1975). The specificity present in family B and strain 2 has been designated Ia.4 and the additional specificity present in inbred strain 2 animals as Ia.2 (previously antigen 2).

Recently, an additional Ia-like specificity was identified by sera prepared in B.1, Ia.1 outbred guinea pigs which had been immunized with strain 13 cells (B.1, Ia.1,3). These sera were cytotoxic for strain 2 (B.1, Ia.2,4) lymph node cells as well as for cells from strain 13 guinea pigs. This specificity, originally designated as 576, has now been termed Ia.5 (Schwartz et al. 1976b).

2.4 The Identification of an Additional Specificity Present in Inbred Strain 2 and Strain 13 Animals

In the course of preparation of antisera that would identify the B.1 antigen (immunization of outbred B.3, Ia.1,3 animals with inbred strain 13 cells), a number of sera were produced that caused appreciable ^{51}Cr release from cells of outbred $B.1^+$ and $B.2^+$ animals as well as from cells of inbred strain 2 and strain 13. The additional specificity identified by this serum has been termed S.1. Absorption studies of antisera that contained both anti-B.1 and S.1 activity with cells from B.2, S.1 animals demonstrated that all of the activity for such cells could be removed, while the cytotoxic activity for B.1 cells remained. Further absorption and immunization studies (Geczy et al. 1975a) have established the existence of the S.1 specificity. To date, it has not been possible to prepare an antiserum that is monospecific for antigen S.1, because all these antisera also possess anti-B.1 activity. Hence, we are unable to determine whether all outbred animals that are $B.1^+$ are also $S.1^+$. Preliminary evidence (E. Shevach, *personal communication*) suggests that antigen S.1 has a molecular weight of 40,000 daltons (see below). Accordingly, it is tempting to speculate that S.1 will ultimately be found to be a gene product of a second GPLA locus (designated locus S) perhaps similar to the H-2D (or K) locus in the mouse.

By cross-immunization among animals of the AD family and various partially inbred strains (R9, OM3, BE) that appear identical with respect to the B.3 and Ia.1,3 specificities, further antisera were raised (de Weck et al. 1976) that are presently under study. It is presumed that such antisera may reveal additional specificities from the I region or from the postulated S or second GPLA locus.

3. Biochemistry

There is a relative dearth of information dealing with the biochemical and chemical nature of the serologically defined antigens in the guinea pig MHS. Water-soluble transplantation antigens have been liberated from lungs, spleens, kidneys, and livers of inbred strains 2 and strain 13 guinea pigs (Kahan 1967; Kahan and Reisfeld 1967). This antigenic material induces a specific state of sensitization such that second-set donor grafts are rejected in accelerated fashion. In addition, the extracted antigenic substance can elicit delayed-type cutaneous hypersensitivity reactions upon intradermal challenge of presensitized allogenic hosts. Later studies by Kahan et al. (1969) showed that water soluble transplantation antigens could be obtained in high yield from tumour cells disrupted by low-intensity sonic energy. However, the antigenic material so obtained was not characterized beyond gel filtration on Sephadex G-200 and electrophoresis in 7.5 percent polyacrylamide gel, in which it was found to have an RF between 0.73 and 0.74.

Finkelman et al. (1975), using lactoperoxidase-catalyzed external labeling of lymphoid cells followed by nonionic detergent extraction and electrophoresis in SDS-polyacrylamide gels, found that lymphoid membrane extracts precipitated by anti-B.1 antiserum produced two peaks: one representing an antigen with a molecular weight of approximately 45,000 daltons and another representing an antigen with a molecular weight of about 12,000 daltons. On the other hand, all anti-2 and anti-13 precipitates produced a single peak when electrophoresed on SDS-polyacrylamide gels. Both the 2 (Ia.2) and 13 (Ia.1) antigens were found by this technique to have molecular weights of about 25,000 to 33,000 daltons. The I region antigens can only be demonstrated on lymphocytes and using indirect immunofluorescence; they could not be detected on two carcinogen-induced hepatomas, one carcinogen-induced sarcoma, and two viral-induced sarcomas (Forni et al. 1975). By molecular weight criteria, as well as by previously investigated tissue distributional criteria, (Shevach et al. 1975) the B.1 antigen is similar to the mouse H-2K or H-2D and the human A and B antigens, whereas the Ia.1 and Ia.2 antigens are similar to the mouse Ia antigens.

Recent detailed structural studies of the alloantigens coded for by the MHC of the guinea pig have been reported by Schwartz et al. (1976a, b). In this procedure tritiated leucine and fucose were internally incorporated into guinea pig lymph node cells. The alloantigens were solubilized by the nonionic detergent Nonidet P-40, purified by affinity chromatography using an immunoadsorbent column of lentil lectin, isolated by immunoprecipitation with alloantisera, and examined by discontinuous polyacrylamide-sodium dodecyl sulfate gel electrophoresis. The B region antigens (B.1, B.2, B.3, and B.4) were shown to be glycoproteins of molecular weight 40,000 daltons and to be non-covalently associated with a protein of 12,000 daltons.

4. Histocompatibility

With the exception of the work of Brummerstedt and Franks (1970), the early studies of Bauer (1960) on the number of histocompatibility antigens responsible for skin transplant rejection between strain 2 and strain 13 guinea pigs have not been followed by similar investigations among outbred animals. In addition to skin grafting, histocompatibility antigens may be detected by serological techniques and mixed lymphocyte reactions (MLR) *in vitro,* and *in vivo* by the intradermal injection of lymphoid cells into normal or presensitized recipients. According to Brent and Medawar (Brent and Medawar 1963, 1966), three types of reactions may be encountered: (1) the *direct reaction* (DR), upon intradermal injection of normal donor leucocytes into a presensitized host; (2) the *immune lymphocyte transfer* (ILT) reaction, developing upon intradermal injection of presensitized donor leucocytes into a normal host; and (3) the *normal lymphocyte transfer* (NLT) reaction developing upon intradermal injection of normal donor leucocytes into a normal host. It has recently been demonstrated (Zakarian and Billingham 1972) that the NLT reaction in guinea pigs is essentially a mixed lymphocyte reaction *in vivo* between donor lymphocytes and leukocytes of the host; the skin transplantation antigens of the host playing little if any part in the reaction.

In our Bio families B and C, disparity in the GPLA antigens does not seem to play a major role in the occurrence and intensity of the NLT reactions.

Table 5.5. Role of GPLA B and I Region Antigens in the NLT Reaction

First GPLA (B Locus)	I Region		Number of Reactions[a]	Average Increase in Skin thickness[b] (in mm)
	Antigens Ia.1,2	Antigens Ia.3,4		
Id.	Id.	Id.	33	0.188±0.117
Id.	Id.	Diff.	12	0.348±0.244
			10	0.575±0.298
Id.	Diff.	Diff.	8	0.738±0.218
Diff. (1 allele)	Id.	Id.	9	0.375±0.151
Diff. (1 allele)	Id.	Diff.	60	0.767±0.289
			5	0.255±0.114
Diff. (1 allele)	Diff.	Diff.	2	0.488
Diff. (2 alleles)	Id.	Id.	8	0.613±0.072
Diff. (2 alleles)	Id.	Diff.	2	0.388

Id. = identical. Diff. = different.

[a] Number of NLT reactions observed among animals differing in B or I antigens as indicated in left-hand columns.

[b] Average of increase in skin thickness measured over the first 4 days after intradermal injection of 5×10^6 peripheral blood lymphocytes. For technical details, see Tötterman et al. (1976).

When all combinations tested up to now are considered in terms of serological disparity and intensity of the NLT reaction (Table 5.5), it is clear that very strong NLT reactions may be elicited among animals with identical GPLA alleles if their I region antigens are different. On the other hand, apparent identity of the I region (judged by two antigens only) may still yield moderate NLT reactions, if the animals differ by one GPLA allele, and strong reactions occur if the animals differ by two GPLA alleles. The impression gained from the overall study is that non-GPLA antigens probably play a major role in NLT reactions, (for further details see Tötterman et al. 1976). These findings are in apparent conflict with our previous report (de Weck et al. 1971) demonstrating that among outbred animals of the Bio-colony a significant prolongation of skin graft survival is observed among animals of identical GPLA phenotypes compared with animals that possess different GPLA phenotypes. As shown elsewhere (de Weck et al. 1976), the polymorphism of the first GPLA locus and I region in our Bio-colony appears very limited. Accordingly, in this colony identical GPLA phenotypes probably indicate identical haplotypes. Even if the GPLA antigens do not play a major role in skin rejection, haplotype identity would be expected to affect survival of skin grafts and to prevent NLT reactions. This interpretation is supported by the observation that no NLT reactions were observed among Bio. B or Bio. C animals, even if these guinea pigs showed a delayed rejection of skin grafts (*unpublished experiments*).

The relationship between MLC reactions *in vitro* and serologically defined antigens controlled by genes in the guinea pig B locus and I region has been investigated in various inbred and partially inbred strains and in guinea pig families homozygous for their GPLA alleles (Geczy and de Weck 1976). No MLC reactions were detected among guinea pig families of a closed colony which had been bred to homozygosity for their GPLA-B locus antigens. However, animals which differed in their I region showed strong MLC reactivity. Animals with identical I regions (based on four serologically-defined specificities) but which differed with respect to B locus determinants yield appreciably lower MLC responses. It appears therefore, that in the guinea pig as in other mammalian species (Shreffler and David 1975) antigenic systems responsible for MLC reactivity are controlled primarily by genes identical with or closely linked to the I region of the MHC.

5. Genetic Control of the Immune Response by Gene Products from the MHS

Following the report by Kantor and corworkers in 1963 (Kantor et al. 1963) that only some Hartley guinea pigs, immunized with 2,4-dinitrophenyl poly-L-lysine copolymer (DNP-PLL), with 2,4-dinitrophenyl glutamic acid lysine copolymer (DNP-GL), or with GL alone, make an immune response to these antigens, subsequent breeding studies quickly established that this ability to respond to DNP-PLL was under the control of a dominant autosomal gene (Levine et al. 1963). It was also demonstrated that all inbred strain 2 guinea pigs are responders, whereas inbred strain 13 guinea pigs are uniformly nonresponders to these antigens. This immune response (Ir) gene has been referred to as the "PLL gene" (McDevitt and Benacerraf 1969). It was later shown that the PLL gene is linked to the serologically defined MHC of strain 2 animals (Ellman et al. 1970). Table 5.6 lists a number of further histocompatibility-linked immune responses in guinea pigs. The linkage of these immune responses to the 2 and 13 MHS antigens was determined in studies in either $F_1 \times 2$ or $F_1 \times 13$ backcross guinea pigs (Green 1974). By contrast, responsiveness to low doses of (T,G)-A–L, penicilloylated bovine IgG (BPO-BGG), aspirin anhydride (ASAN), and phenetidine appears to be under polygenic control. At least one of the Ir genes required for the response to these antigens is linked to either the 13 (Ia.1), B (B.1), or C (B.2) histocompatibility antigen whereas some other genes also required for the response segregate independently in backcross progeny (Geczy and de Weck 1975).

As mentioned earlier (see Introduction), alloantisera directed against products of the GPLA and/or I region loci can specifically block antigen-induced *in vitro* T-cell proliferation. With respect to the *in vitro* proliferative response to the copolymer GA, Shevach et al. (1974) found that 13 anti-2 serum was incapable of blocking the *in vitro* GA response of T cells derived from $2^{-}GA^{+}$ animals (i.e., in outbred animals where the Ir gene controlling the response to GA is no longer associated with the 2-histocompatibility genes), although 13 anti-2 serum could inhibit the *in vitro* T-cell response to GA

Table 5.6. Histocompatibility-Linked Immune Responses in Guinea Pigs

Antigen	Histocompatibility Linkage
Bovine serum albumin (low dose)	2 (Ia.2)
DNP-poly-L-lysine	2 (Ia.2)
DNP-poly-L-arginine	2 (Ia.2)
Copolymer of glutamic acid and alanine	2 (Ia.2)
2,4-Dinitrophenyl guinea pig albumin	13 (Ia.3)
Copolymer of glutamic acid and tyrosine (T,G)-A–L	13 (Ia.1)
	13 (Ia.1) and B (B.1)[a]
Penicilloylated bovine IgG (BPO-BGG)	13 (Ia.1) and B (B.1)[a]
Aspirin anhydride (ASAN)	13 (Ia.1)[a]
Phenetidine	C (B.2)[a]

[a] The responses to these antigens appear to be under polygenic control (Geczy and de Weck 1975). At least one gene required for the response is linked to the histocompatibility complex characterized by the 13 (Ia.1,3), B (B.1), or C (B.2) antigens, whereas the other gene(s) appear to segregate independently.

in 2^+GA^+ outbred animals. In further experiments, it was not possible to dissociate the serologically detected histocompatibility antigens from the blocking of antigen-induced proliferation *in vitro,* suggesting that the Ir gene products are closely associated with the H antigens. Recently we have shown (Geczy et al. 1975b) that antisera, raised against lymphoid cells among various F_2 hybrid guinea pigs in which at least one of the genes involved in the immune response to low doses of ASAN, BPO-BGG, and (T,G)-A–L appeared to be no longer linked to the gene(s) regulating the expression of the serologically-defined 13 MHC, could specifically block the *in vitro* T-cell proliferation of primed (2×13) F_1 cells. In contrast to the inhibition of the GA response, which seems to be mediated by antibodies to strain 2 antigens rather than by antibodies to a product of the GA Ir gene, the *in vitro* suppression of ASAN, BPO-BGG, and (T,G)-A–L is mediated by those Ir gene products not associated with the MHS. Furthermore, the antisera against the "recognition structures" for the three antigens in our system do not appear to contain cytotoxic gene products coded for by the B locus and I region of the guinea pig MHS.

The results obtained in guinea pigs of strain 2 and 13 with antireceptor antisera, led us to speculate that the Ir gene products against which the anti-R sera are directed, are in part similar to immunoglobulin receptors and that our antisera against recognition structures are in fact anti-idiotypic sera. To assess this possibility, immunoadsorbent column-purified anti-BPO-BGG raised in strain 2 and strain 13 guinea pigs, was used to immunize both strain 2 and 13 animals and the resultant antisera tested for their ability to inhibit the BPO-BGG-induced T-cell proliferation of cells from

Table 5.7. Inhibition of T Cell Proliferation by Anti-$R_{BPO\text{-}BGG}$ and Anti-Idiotypic Sera in Primed Low Dose Immunized Strain 13 PEL Capable of Responding to ASP-OVA, BPO-BGG, and (T,G)-A–L

Antigen	Normal Guinea Pig	Serum added to culture:[b]				
		Anti-$R_{BPO\text{-}BGG}$	ā strain 2 BPO-BGG	ā strain 13 BPO-BGG	ā strain 13 BPO-BGG abs with st 13 Cells	ā strain 13 BPO-BGG abs with st 2 Cells
NIL	555[a]	830	1,156	778	356	693
PHA	113,442	89,423	107,980	65,000	94,673	96,527
ASP-OVA	97,673	81,353	89,218	86,124	79,419	77,379
BPO-BGG	93,525	1,129	87,926	1,248	80,687	916
(T,G)-A–L	105,458	68,904	96,712	86,771	86,084	91,979

[a] Results are expressed as counts/minute/tube. Each result represents the mean of three cultures; significantly depressed results are underlined.
[b] Final concentration of serum in culture was 1 percent.

high dose responder strain 2 and low dose responder strain 13 guinea pigs. The following four antisera were tested for their ability to block antigen-induced lymphocyte proliferation: Strain 2 antistrain 2 anti-BPO-BGG (ā strain 2 BPO-BGG), strain 13 antistrain 13 anti-BPO-BGG (ā strain 13 BPO-BGG), strain 2 antistrain 13 anti-BPO-BGG, and strain 13 antistrain 2 anti-BPO-BGG. The first two antisera, presumed to be directed against strain 2 and strain 13 anti-idiotypes, were designated as ā strain 2 BPO-BGG or ā strain 13 BPO-BGG, respectively. To investigate the possibility that the ā strain 2 BPO-BGG and ā strain 13 BPO-BGG sera may be directed against strain-specific idiotypes, the capacity of these sera to inhibit T-cell activation in the syngeneic and allogeneic strains was studied. As shown in Table 5.7, BPO-BGG-pulsed peritoneal exudate lymphocytes (PEL, which are an enriched population of T cells) from primed strain 13 guinea pigs can only be inhibited by an antiserum against ā strain 13 BPO-BGG raised in the isogeneic strain but not by ā strain 2 BPO-BGG raised in the allogeneic strain (Geczy et al. 1976). In addition, the BPO-BGG response of strain 13 cells but not of strain 2 cells is suppressed by anti-$R_{BPO\text{-}BGG}$ raised among (2 × 13) siblings. Furthermore, immune BPO-BGG$^+$ cells from strain 13 are capable of absorbing the inhibitory activity from ā strain 13 BPO-BGG while immune BPO-BGG$^+$ cells from strain 2 animals fail to do so (Geczy et al. 1976). Conversely, BPO-BGG-pulsed PEL from high dose immunised strain 2 guinea pigs can be inhibited by ā strain 2 BPO-BGG but not by ā strain 13 BPO-BGG (Geczy et al. 1976). It is clear therefore, that the antisera (ā strain 2 BPO-BGG and ā strain 13 BPO-BGG) must interact with some gene product(s) characteristic of the syngeneic strain in order to suppress antigen-induced T-cell proliferation *in vitro*. It seems likely that the antisera recognize membrane-associated strain-specific immunoglobulin idiotypes which may function as T cell receptors.

6. Genetic Organization

6.1 Linkage Between the GPLA Locus B and the Ia Region

In order to demonstrate that both the antigens from the GPLA locus B and the I region antigens are products of the same genetic complex the offspring of a number of informative matings were studied (Fig. 5.1). In family 1 the outbred male, which had been typed as B.2,4, Ia.1,2, was mated with both inbred strain 2 and strain 13 females. Analyses of the offspring revealed that antigens B.2 and I.2 on the one hand and antigens B.4 and Ia.1 on the other hand were transmitted as haplotypes. In family 2 a presumed homozygous B.3, Ia.1 animal was mated with an inbred strain 2 (B.1, Ia.2)

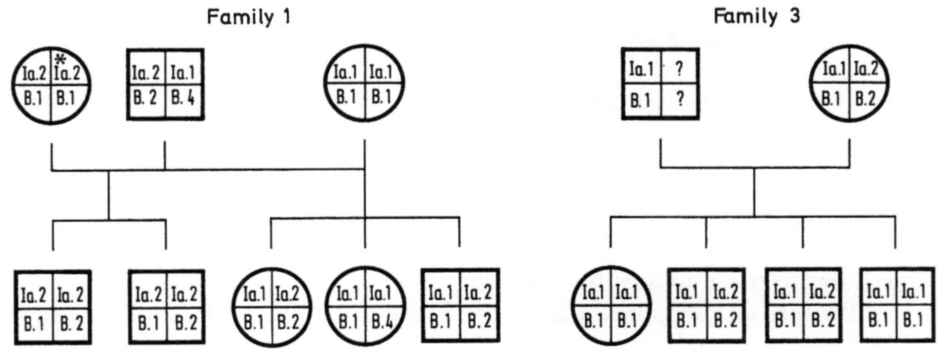

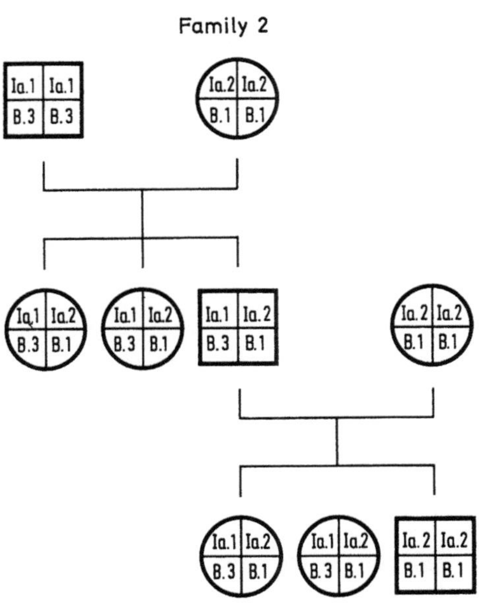

Figure 5.1. Linkage between the GPLA and I region loci (circles denote females and squares denote males.)

female. All of the three male offspring from this mating were B.1,3, Ia.1,2. One of the males was then mated with a strain 2 female. Analysis of the three offspring demonstrated that antigens B.1 and Ia.2 and antigens B.3 and Ia.1 were transmitted together. In family 3, a B.1,2, Ia.1,2 outbred animal was mated to a presumed B.1, Ia.1 homozygote. Analysis of the four offspring revealed that antigens B.1 and Ia.1 and B.2 and Ia.2 were transmitted as haplotypes. These results strongly suggest that the products of the I region and GPLA B locus are linked.

Further linkage studies are in progress. A considerable problem of genetic studies in guinea pigs is the slow rate of reproduction and small litter size so that on the average, genetic studies proceed at the rate of one generation per year.

6.2 Products of the Ia Region and GPLA B Locus Represented on the Lymphoid Cells of Wild Guinea Pigs

To date over 3000 outbred and inbred animals from a variety of sources have been examined for the presence of I region and GPLA specificities. Thus far, practically all animals have been shown to bear some of the antigens identified by 13 anti-2 (Ia.2,4) and 2 anti-13 (Ia.1,3) sera. We have encountered however, a small number of animals (<1 percent) that do not bear the GPLA antigens B.1, 2, 3, and 4, and we are now in the process of raising antisera to these unidentified antigens.

Because all the guinea pigs in Europe and the United States have originated from animals brought back by the Spanish from South America at the end of the sixteenth century, it is possible that the guinea pigs maintained in laboratory colonies have arisen from a relatively small population of animals. It was therefore of interest to examine a number of wild guinea pigs, trapped in villages around Lima, Peru, that had never been maintained in the laboratory. Of the ten animals studied, six had readily identifiable GPLA antigens whereas four of the animals were untypable. The cells of all the animals were lysed by either anti-2, anti-13, or anti-Ia.3 sera; an Ia.1$^-$Ia.2$^-$Ia.3$^-$ animal was not identified.

References

Bauer, J. A. Genetics of skin transplantation and an estimate of the number of histocompatibility genes in inbred guinea pigs. *Ann. N.Y. Acad. Sci. 87*:78–92, 1960.

Brent, L., and Medawar, P. B. Tissue transplantation: a A new approach to the "typing" problem. *Brit. Med. J. II*:269–272, 1963.

Brent, L., and Medawar, P.B. Quantitative studies on tissue transplantation immunity. VII. The normal lymphocyte transfer reaction. *Proc. Roy. Soc. (B) 165*:281–307, 1966.

Brummerstedt, E., and Franks, D. Guinea pig alloantigens studied by a cytotoxic test with lymphocytes. *Transplantation 10*:137–140, 1970.

Dausset, J. Iso-leuco-anticorps. *Acta Haematol. (Basel) 20*:156–166, 1958.

de Weck, A. L., Geczy, A. F., Sato, W., and Mueller, E. Guinea pig histocompatibility antigens.

I. Serologic and genetic characterization of the GPLA antigens. *Transplantation 21*:225–241, 1976.

de Weck, A. L., Polak, L., Sato, W., and Frey, J. R. Determination of histocompatibility antigens by leucocyte typing in outbred guinea pigs and effect of matching on skin graft survival. *Transplantation Proceedings 3*:192–194, 1971.

Ellman, L., Green, I., Martin, J., and Benacerraf, B. Linkage between the poly-L-lysine gene and the locus controlling the major histocompatibility antigens in strain 2 guinea pigs. *Proc. Natl. Acad. Sci.* (USA) *66*:322–328, 1970.

Finkelman, F. D., Shevach, E. M., Vitetta, E. S., Green, I., and Paul, W. E. Guinea pig immune response related histocompatibility antigens. Partial characterization and distribution. *J. Exp. Med. 141*:27–41, 1975.

Forni, G., Rhim, J. S., Pickeral, S., Shevach, E. M., and Green, I. Antigenicity of carcinogen and viral induced sarcomas in inbred and randombred guinea pigs. *J. Immunol. 115*:204–210, 1975.

Geczy, A. F., and de Weck, A. L. Histocompatibility antigens and genetic control of the immune response in guinea pigs. I. Specific inhibition of antigen-induced lymphocyte stimulation by alloantisera. *Eru. J. Immunol. 4*:483–490, 1974.

Geczy, A.F., and de Weck, A. L. Genetic control of sensitization to structurally unrelated antigens and its relationship to histocompatibility antigens in guinea pigs. *Immunology 28*:331–342, 1975.

Geczy, A. F., and de Weck, A. L. The major histocompatibility complex of the guinea-pig. II. Relationship between mixed leucocyte reactivity and serologically-defined phenotypes of the GPLA B locus and I region. *J. Immunogenetics 3*:191–198, 1976.

Geczy, A. F., de Weck, A. L., Schwartz, B.D., and Shevach, E. M. The major histocompatibility complex of the guinea pig. I. Serologic and Genetic studies. *J. Immunol. 115*:1704–1710, 1975a.

Geczy, A. F., Geczy, C. L., and de Weck, A. L. Histocompatibility antigens and genetic control of the immune response in guinea pigs. II. Specific inhibition of antigen-induced lymphocyte proliferation by anti-receptor alloantisera. *Eur. J. Immunol. 5*:711–719, 1975b.

Gorer, P. A. The detection of antigenic differences in mouse erythrocytes by the employment of immune sera. *Brit. J. Exp. Pathol. 17*:42–50, 1936.

Green, I. Genetic control of immune responses. *Immunogenetics 1*:4–21, 1974.

Kahan, B. D. Cutaneous hypersensitivity reactions of guinea pigs to proteinaceous transplantation antigen. *J. Immunol 99*:1121–1127, 1967.

Kahan, B. D., Holmes, E. C., Reisfeld, R. A., and Morton, D. L. Water soluble guinea pig transplantation antigen from carcinogen-induced sarcomas. *J. Immunol. 102*:28–36, 1969.

Kahan, B. D., and Reisfeld, R. A. Electrophoretic purification of a water-soluble guinea pig transplantation antigen. *Proc. Natl. Acad. Sci.* (USA) *53*:1430–1437, 1967.

Kantor, F. S., Ojeda, A., and Benacerraf, B. Studies on artificial antigens. I. Antigenicity of DNP-poly-lysine and DNP-copolymers of lysine and glutamic acid in guinea pigs. *J. Exp. Med. 117*:55–69, 1963.

Levine, B. B., Ojeda, A., and Benacerraf, B. Studies on artificial antigens. III. The genetic control of the immune response to hapten-poly-L-lysine conjugates in guinea pigs. *J. Exp. Med. 118*:953–957, 1963.

Martin, W. J., Ellman, L., Green, I., and Benacerraf, B. Association between poly-L-lysine immune response gene and histocompatibility type of Hartley guinea pigs. *J. Exp. Med. 132*:1259–1266, 1970.

McDevitt, H. O., and Benacerraf, B. Genetic control of specific immune responses. *Adv. in Immuno. 11*:31–74, 1969.

Sato, W., and de Weck, A. L. Leucocyte typing in guinea pigs. *Z. Immunitätsforsch. 144*:49–62, 1972.

Schwartz, B. D., Kask, A. M., Paul, W. E., and Shevach, E. M. Structural characteristics of the alloantigens determined by the major histocompatibility complex of the guinea pig. *J. Exp. Med. 143*:541–558, 1976a.

Schwartz, B. D., Paul, W. E., and Shevach, E. M. Guinea pig Ia antigens: Functional significance and chemical characterization. *Transplant. Rev. 30*:174–196, 1976b.

Shevach, E. M., Ben-Sasson, S. Z., Finkelman, F. D., Paul, W. E., and Green, I. Mechanisms of action of genes controlling the immune response. *Transplant. Proc.* *7*:141–147, 1975.

Shevach, E. M., Green, I., and Paul, W. E. Alloantiserum-induced inhibition of immune response gene product function. II. Genetic analysis of target antigens. *J. Exp. Med.* *39*:679–695, 1974.

Shevach, E. M., Paul, W. E., and Green, I. Histocompatibility linked immune response gene function in guinea pigs. Specific inhibition of antigen-induced lymphocyte proliferation by alloantisera. *J. Exp. Med.* *136*:1207–1221, 1972.

Shevach, E. M., Rosenstreich, D. L., and Green, I. The distribution of histocompatibility antigens on T and B cells in the guinea pig. *Transplantation* *16*:126–133, 1973.

Shreffler, D. C., and David, C. S. The H-2 major histocompatibility complex and the I immune response region: Genetic variation, function and organization. *Adv. Immunol.* *20*:125–198, 1975.

Tötterman, K. J., Mueller, E., and de Weck, A. L. Guinea pig histocompatibility antigens. III. Analysis of normal lymphocyte transfer (NLT) reactions among guinea pigs with serologically defined phenotypes (GPLA locus and I region). *Z. Immunitaetsforsch.* *115*:42–74, 1976.

Walford, R. L., Anderson, E. R., Carter, P. K., and Mihajlovic, F. Leucocyte antibodies in inbred strains of guinea pigs following first- and second-set skin homografts. *J. Immunol.* *89*:427–433, 1962.

Zakarian, S., and Billingham, R. E. Studies on normal and immune lymphocyte transfer reactions in guinea pigs, with special reference to the cellular contribution of the host. *J. Exp. Med.* *136*:1545–1563, 1973.

Chapter 6

The Major Histocompatibility System of the Rat (Ag-B or H-1 System)

E. GÜNTHER and O. ŠTARK

1. Introduction

The experimental use of the laboratory rat, *Rattus norvegicus* (Robinson 1965), resembles in general that of the laboratory mouse, *Mus musculus*. Both species belong to different genera in the family of Muridae.

According to paleontologic evidence, both lines diverged from a common ancestor about 10×10^6 years ago (Simpson 1959). However, hybridization studies on mouse and rat DNA (Laird et al. 1969; Kohne 1970) and comparisons of albumins (Sarich 1972) or C_k region sequences (Gutman et al. 1975) of rat and mouse point to a much greater divergence at the molecular level than could be expected from paleontologic data.

Knowledge of the genetics of the laboratory rat is less advanced than that of the mouse, although more than 100 inbred rat strains are available (Festing and Staats 1973; Festing and Butler 1975). The origin of these strains is as restricted as that of inbred mouse strains, because most rat strains are derived from Wistar rats (Palm and Black 1971).

The karyotype of *Rattus norvegicus* shows $2n = 42$ chromosomes (Committee for a Standardized Karyotype of *Rattus norvegicus* 1973), and several linkage groups have been established (Robinson 1972; Gasser et al. 1973b).

In immunogenetic research, the rats seems to offer some advantages over the mouse for studies of transplantation (Silvers and Billingham 1970), especially that of vascularized organs, disease susceptibility, and lymphocyte function *in vitro*.

There are several studies on the number of histocompatibility systems in the rat using the F_2 test (Billingham et al. 1962b; Ramseier and Palm 1967; Zeiss 1967; Štark and Křen 1967a; Heslop 1968). The greatest number of autosomal histocompatibility genes found segregating between two inbred

---

Abbreviations used

CML	cell-mediated lympholysis
H-antigen	histocompatibility antigen
H-linked	histocompatibility linked
Ir gene	immune response gene
GvH	graft-versus-host
MHS	major histocompatibility system
MLR	mixed lymphocyte reaction (reactivity)

strains was 14 to 16 in the LEW/BN combination (Billingham et al. 1962b). A survey of the non-H-1 alloantigenic systems that have been described so far is given in Table 6.1. The early history of rat blood group systems has been summarized by Owen (1962).

The major histocompatibility system (MHS) of the rat is called the Ag-B system (Elkins and Palm 1966), the RtH-1 system (Štark and Křen, 1967e), or simply the H-1 system (Štark and Křen 1967e). All are different designations for the same system, and the R system (Aizawa et al. 1965) is presumably identical to them. First evidence of a strong histocompatibility system in the rat was given by Bogden and Aptekman (1960), who called it the R-1 system, and by Křen et al. (1960). Allelic antigens of this system were identified serologically by Palm (1962) and were then shown to have histoincompatibility effects (Palm 1964). The first series of four alleles at the H-1 locus was reported by Štark 1966 (Štark et al. 1967a), and the serological analysis of the complex structure of the system was published one year later (Štark et al. 1967b). The scientific history of the MHS of the rat and the problem of nomenclature are discussed by Palm (1970b).

The MHS of the rat has been defined in the same way as that of the mouse and later that of other species:[1] as a histocompatibility system that exhibits a predominant role on allograft survival, incompatibility leading to skin graft rejection in less than 14 days or to tumor graft rejection and to antibody production by means of which an analysis of the system is possible. MHS were later shown to be additionally characterized in that genes determining MLR antigens, genes controlling immune responsiveness (Ir genes), and genes controlling disease susceptibility are linked to the "histocompatibility genes." This is also verified for the MHS of the rat.

Immunogenetic analysis of the H-1/Ag-B system is based almost exclusively on the use of inbred and congenic rat strains and not on data obtained in genetically heterogeneous, more or less random mating populations. At least ten different H-1/Ag-B haplotypes have so far been identified, and in most cases these haplotypes have been genetically isolated by the production of congenic strains. These strains have been bred by repeated backcrossing of the respective haplotypes onto the genetic background of the LEW or BN strains (Iványi 1967; Štark and Křen 1969; Palm 1971; Křen et al. 1973). Our present knowledge of the MHS of the rat is obtained by analysis of these haplotypes, and the congenic strains are taken as the respective reference or typing strains. Because only congenic strains allow a proper analysis of the H-1 system and a differentiation between H-1 and genetic background-determined effects, in the following reference will preferably be made to data obtained with congenic strains.

The different MHS haplotypes are designated by numbers (Ag-B nomenclature) or by letters (H-1 nomenclature). Although a reference testing by direct comparison of anti-Ag-B and anti-H-1 antisera and by exchange of animals has not been performed systematically, the validity of the correspon-

[1] For details on the MHS of various species, the reader is referred to the other chapters of this volume or to Frelinger and Shreffler 1975.

Table 6.1. Non-H-1 Alloantigenic Systems

System or Strain Combination	Tissue	Congenic Strains	Linkage	Remarks	References
Ag-A	RBC[a]			Naturally occurring hemagglutinin, respective rats no longer available	Burhoe 1947; Palm and Black 1971
Ag-C	RBC, liver, spleen not lymphocytes, not platelets		ES-1 ES-2 loci	C/D system of Owen, rabbit antirat typing serum, also detectable by alloantiserum	Owen, 1962; Palm and Black 1971; Poloskey et al. 1975a; Gasser et al. 1973b
Ag-D	RBC			Antigen B2 of Bogden and Aptekman	Bogden and Aptekman 1960; Palm and Black 1971; Palm 1962
Ag-E	Skin			Rats no longer available	Michie and Anderson 1966; Palm and Black 1971
Ag-F	Lymphoid cells		C locus	Probably identical to H-4	DeWitt and McCullough 1975
H-2	RBC, skin	LEW.1W.2W, BP.2W			Křen et al. 1973
H-3	RBC, skin	BP.3W			Křen et al. 1973
H-4	Skin	LEW.C-4A	C locus		Křen et al. 1973
H-5	Skin	LEW.1× -5P	lx locus		Křen et al. 1973
H-X	Skin		X chromosome		Mullen and Hildemann 1972
H-Y	Skin		Y chromosome		Billingham et al. 1962b; Zeiss et al. 1962
BH anti-Lewis	Thymus cells, peripheral T-cells				Lubaroff 1973
Ly-1 (AS anti-Lewis)	Thymus cells, lymphoid cells				Fabre and Morris 1974c
AS anti-Lewis, BH anti-Lewis	(a) Thymus, 20% of lymph node cells (b) 40% of lymph node cells			Two independent antigen systems detected by AS anti-Lewis antiserum, so far AS anti-Lewis identical to BH anti-Lewis	Wonigeit and Stumpenhorst 1975
HO anti-August August anti-HO	Peripheral thymus-derived lymphoid cells				Howard and Scott 1974

[a] Red blood cells.

Table 6.2. Relationships Among H-1 and Ag-B Haplotypes

Original Typing Strains	Congenic Strains[a]	Ag-B Haplotypes[a]	H-1 Haplotypes[a]	Congenic Strains[c, d]	Original Typing Strains	Correspondence Based on Hemagglutination Test with:
LEW		1	l		LEW	LEW
WF	BN.B2	2	w	LEW.1W (L.WP)	WP	WF
BN	AUG.B3	3	n	LEW.1N (L.BN)	BN	BN
DA	BN.B4	4	a	LEW.1A (L.AVN)	AVN	DA
August 28807		5	c	LEW.1C (L.AUG)	CAP	August 28807
BUF		6	b	LEW.1B (L.BP)	BP	BUF
				(L.BUF)	BUF	
KGH		7[b]				
WKA		8[b]				
			d	LEW.1D (L.BD V)	BD V	
			e		BD VII	
			f	LEW.1F (L.AS2)	AS2	
			h	LEW.1H (L.HW)	HW	

[a] Palm 1971.
[b] Kunz and Gill 1974a.
[c] Křen et al. 1973
[d] Two synonymous designations of the congenic strains are used. Either the symbol for the background strain, LEW (=Lewis), is followed by the designation of the H-1 haplotype (Křen et al. 1973), or the abbreviated name of the background strain L (=LEW=Lewis) is followed by the symbol of the H-1 donor strain.

dence of Ag-B and H-1 nomenclature as given in Table 6.2 is beyond doubt.[2] Thus, the six Ag-B haplotypes described by Palm (1971), find counterparts in corresponding H-1 haplotypes. The Ag-B^7 and Ag-B^8 haplotypes (Kunz and Gill 1974a) have not yet been matched with H-1 haplotypes.

Identification of and distinction among the various H-1 and Ag-B haplotypes were originally performed serologically by hemagglutination tests and are therefore based on typing for H-1 antigens that are expressed on red blood cells. Characterization of the H-1 and Ag-B haplotypes has been complemented by MLR and Ir typing (see below). The H-1 haplotypes a, b, c, d, e, f, l, n, and w, and the Ag-B haplotypes 1, 2, 3, 4, 5, 6, and 8, turned out to be associated with individual MLR antigens (Palm and Wilson 1973; Günther et al. 1975; Cramer et al. 1974), and individual immune response patterns (see Table 6.10). The H-1^h haplotype has not yet been studied in this way. The Ag-B^7 haplotype appears to be exceptional in that MLR and Ir-GLT typing data are like that of Ag-B^1 rats, whereas serologically Ag-B^7 represents a new Ag-B haplotype (Cramer et al. 1974). The reference strains for each H-1/Ag-B haplotype are given in Tables 6.2 and 6.3.

In Table 6.4 all inbred strains are listed that reportedly have been typed for their H-1/Ag-B antigens. It must be stressed that H-1/Ag-B identity

[2] Therefore, in the following review only one nomenclature (H-1) will be used except for Ag-B^7 and Ag-B^8.

Table 6.3. Characterization of the Various H-1 (Ag-B) Haplotypes

H-1	Ag-B	Serotype	MLR Type	Ir Pattern	Reference Typing Strain
a	4[a]	a	a	a	L.AVN = LEW.1A
b	6	b	b	b	L.BUF = LEW.1B
c	5	c	c	c	L.AUG = LEW.1C
d		d	d	d	L.BD V = LEW.1D
e		e	e	e	BD VII
f		f	f	f	L.AS2 = LEW.1F
h		h			L.HW = LEW.1H
l	1	l	l	l	LEW
n	3	n	n	n	L.BN = LEW.1N
w	2	w	w	w	L.WP = LEW.1W
	7[b]	7	l	l	KGH
	8[b]	8	8	8	WKA

[a] Ag-B^4 of DA rats differs from H-1^a of L.AVN rats according to F_1 test, but not so far by MLR and Ir typing.
[b] Data taken from Kunz and Gill (1974a) and Cramer et al. (1974). Relation of these haplotypes to the H-1 haplotypes is not yet clarified.

Table 6.4. Ag-B/H-1 Haplotypes of Inbred Rat Strains

Strain	Ag-B	H-1	Reference		H-1-Controlled Immune Responsiveness
			Ag-B	H-1	
A2	2		5		
ACI	4	a	5	2	TGAL h, HGAL l, GLT h, GA l, GT h, LDH l, $(TGAGly)_n$ h
ACP	4		5		HGAL l, GLT h, LDH l, TGProL l
AGA		l		15	
AGUS		l	18		
ALB	6		5		GLT l
AO	2	w	5	2	
AS		l		15	TGAL l, HGAL m, TGProL l
AS2		f		8	TGAL lm, LDH h, TGProL h
AUG 28807	5	c	5	17	TGAL mh, HGAL h, PheGAL h, GLT h, GA h, GT h, LDH h, $(TGAGly)_n$ h
AVN		a		9	TGAL mh, TGProL l
BD I		d		13	LDH h
BD II		w		15	
BD III		l		13	LDH h
BD IV		d		13	
BD V		d		14	TGProL l
BD VI		d		13	
BD VII		e		14	TGAL l, HGAL h, PheGAL h, LDH h, TGProL l
BD VIII		d		13	
BD IX		d		13	
BD X		d		14	
BDE		w		13	LDH h
BH	1		19		
BIRM 4B		w		2	
BIRM 5A		w		2	

Table 6.4 (continued)

Strain	Ag-B	H-1	Reference		H-1-Controlled Immune Responsiveness
			Ag-B	H-1	
BN	3	n	5	14	TGAL l, GLT l, GA l, GT l, LDH h, $(TGAGly)_n$ l, TGProL m
BN.1B		b		3	
BN.B2	2		5		
BN.B4	4		5		
BP		b		10	
BP.1N		n		3	
BROFO		c		18	
BS		l		15	TGAL l, HGAL m, TGProL l
BUF	6	b	5	18	LDH h, GLT l, GA h, GT l, $(TGAGly)_n$ l
CAM		w		2	
CAP		c		14	
CAR	1		5		GLT l
CAS	1		5		GLT l
CB		c		2	
CDF		l		15	
COP	4		5		GLT h, GT h, LDH l
DA	4	a	5	15	TGAL h, HGAL l, GLT h, LDH l, TGProL l
E3		w		17	
F344	1	l	5, 6	17	GA h, GT l, GLT l, LDH h, $(TGAGly)_n$ m
HCS		l		2	
HO (PVG)	5	c	5	2	GLT h
HS		l		15	
HW		h		17	
IW		w?		2	
KGH	7		4		GLT l
LA/N	6		7		
LEP		w		14	TGAL l, HGAL h, PheGAL l, TGProL l
LEW	1	l	15	12	TGAL l, HGAL m, PheGAL h, GLT l, GA h, GT l, Insulin l, LDH h, $(TGAGly)_n$ l, TGProL m
LEW.1A		a		3	TGAL h, HGAL l, PheGAL h, LDH l, TGProL l, PheGProL h, ProL l
LEW.1B		b		3	HGAL l, TGAL l, TGProL h
LEW.1C		c		3	
LEW.1D		d		3	TGAL l, HGAL l, PheGAL h, LDH h, TGProL m, PheGProL mh
LEW.1F		f		3	TGAL lm, HGAL l, PheGAL h, TGProL h, PheGProL h, ProL h
LEW.1H		h		3	
LEW.1N		n		3	TGAL l, HGAL l, PheGAL l, Insulin h, TGProL m, PheGProL m
LEW.1W		w		3	TGAL l, HGAL h, TGProL m, PheGProL m
LIS		c		2	
Long Evans	2		7		GLT m
LOU/C/Wsl	2	w	7	1	HGAL mh, PheGAL l

Table 6.4 (continued)

Strain	Ag-B	H-1	Reference		H-1-Controlled Immune Responsiveness
			Ag-B	H-1	
M520	6	b	4	2	GLT l, GA h, GT l
MAXX	3		7		GLT l, $(TGAGly)_n$ l
MNR/N	4		7		
MNR/Br h		c		2	
MNR/Psy		c?		2	
MR/Psy		d		2	
NBR/1	1		5		GLT l
NBR/2	2		7		GLT m
NH		w		2	
OM	2		5		GLT m
Paralysed/N	1		7		
PD		c		17	
PETH/N	2		7		
PVG	5	c	(5)	2	GLT h
R		w		2	
RHA	2	w	7	2	
RLA	2	w	7	2	
S5B	1		5		
SAL		w		2	
SD	6		5		GLT l
Slonaker	2		5		
VM		w		8	
WA		w		2	
WAG		w		16	TGAL l, HGAL h, TGProL l
WF	2	w	5	18	GLT m, GA h, GT l, LDH h, $(TGAGly)_n$ h
WKA	8		4		GLT l
WP		w		11	
WR		w		15	
Y59		c		8	
YO 38366	2		7		GLT m

Further data (origin, characteristics, holders) of most of the rat strains listed here have been compiled by Festing and Staats (1973) and Festing and Butler (1975).
l = low, m = medium, h = high.

References:

1. Günther et al. 1975
2. Křen 1974
3. Křen et al. 1973
4. Kunz and Gill 1974a
5. Palm 1971
6. Elkins and Palm 1966
7. Poloskey et al. 1975a
8. Štark and Hauptfeld 1969
9. Štark and Křen 1967a
10. Štark and Křen 1967b
11. Štark and Křen 1967c
12. Štark and Křen 1967d
13. Štark and Zeiss 1970
14. Štark et al. 1968a
15. Štark et al. 1968b
16. Štark et al. 1969a
17. Štark et al. 1971
18. Štark, *unpublished data*
19. Wilson and Nowell 1971

For references of Ir gene typing, see Table 6.9. Data for immune responsiveness to (T,G-A–L, (H,G)-A–L, (Phe,G)-A–L of noncongenic strains are taken from Günther et al. 1975.

refers only to serological typing by hemagglutination tests (in some cases by lymphocytotoxic tests) and identity by this criterium does not preclude differences with respect to MLR reactivity or skin graft rejection (F_1-tests). The nomenclature for inbred rat strains as proposed by Festing and Staats (1973) will be followed in this review.

2. Serogenetics of the H-1 System

Serologically detectable antibodies can be elicited against H-1-determined antigens and against non-H-1-determined antigens as well. Thus the prerequisite of a proper serological analysis of the H-1 system is H-1 congenic rat strains.

Analysis is based on alloantisera, although xenoantisera, such as rabbit antirat antisera (Poloskey et al. 1975b), are able to distinguish among different H-1 haplotypes. Alloantisera can be produced by single or repeated skin grafting or by repeated injections of lymphoid cells or by a combination of both (skin grafting followed by several lymphoid cell injections). In most strain combinations anti-H-1 antibodies appear during the second and third week after the first skin graft (see Table 6.8).

Three methods used to obtain potent anti-H-1 alloantisera for typing purposes are the following:

Method I: Skin graft (ear, tail, or abdominal skin grafted to the chest) as first stimulus. After 4 weeks, 3 to 4 doses of 10^8 lymphoid cells (either spleen or lymph node or buffy coat cells) i.p. without adjuvant 2 to 3 days apart. Bleeding between the 4th and 9th day after last dose. Eventually a further stimulation 4 weeks later with lymphoid cells, bleeding after 1 week.

Method II: Intraperitoneal injection of 1 to 5×10^7 lymph node plus spleen cells in saline 2 to 3 weeks apart 3 to 4 times, bleeding 10 days after the last injection.

Method III: Single or repeated inoculations of allogeneic tumor tissues or cell suspensions when the tumor has been proven to carry H-1 antigens. The interval between repeated inoculations depends on the time of regression of the previous inoculum. Bleeding is done in the second to fourth week after the inoculation.

Antisera are stored frozen at -20 or $-80°$C. Some antisera lose activity upon storage, and antisera to be tested in hemagglutination assays should be used only once after having been thawed. During the course of immunization, IgM (19S)-class antibody production is followed by that of IgG (7S) antibodies (Křen et al. 1968; Miller and DeWitt 1974).

Two test systems are used for serological H-1 typing: hemagglutination and complement dependent cytotoxicity assays with lymphoid cells as target cells.

Anti-H-1 alloantibodies are only faintly and irreproducibly detectable when hemagglutination is performed in saline. Therefore "developing" agents must be present, such as 2 percent dextran (Gorer and Mikulska 1954), 1 percent PVP (Palm 1962), or 1 percent Ficoll (Kunz and Gill 1974a). Treatment of red blood cells with enzymes (e.g., papain) and addition of serum albumin have also been proposed (Mitchell et al. 1969; Lucas et al. 1970; Taylor and Morris 1970). (According to the authors' experience it is difficult to determine clearcut negative endpoints under an inverted microscope when using enzyme-treated red blood cells.)

The method used by the authors is the following: Red blood cells: A few drops of blood are obtained in Hepes buffered medium (e.g., Eagle's MEM or RPMI-1640 without $NaHCO_3$) or in saline containing about 10 units/ml of Heparin (e.g., Liquemin, Roche) by cutting the rat tail. Red cells are washed three times in medium, and then a 1 percent suspension in Hepes buffered medium (or saline) containing 50 percent normal rat serum [preferably (Lewis × DA)F1 hybrid serum] is made. Antisera are diluted in 2 percent Dextran (Pharmacia, molecular weight 150,000 to 250,000) solution in Hepes buffered medium (or saline). The test is performed in glass tubes (70 × 6 mm). Fifty microliters of red blood cell suspension are added to 50 µl of antiserum dilution. Tubes are incubated for 120 min at 37° C and then examined under an inverted microscope after suspending the pellet by shaking the tube once. Titers can be as high as or higher than 10^{-6}.

In cytotoxicity tests lymphoid cell death can be scored by ^{51}Cr release or by dye exclusion. As complement source, normal rabbit or guinea pig sera, selected for low antirat antibody titer and high complement titer, as well as rat serum (Thoenes et al. 1970) have been recommended. The test can be done as a semimicromethod using 50- or 30 µl aliquots of reagents or as a microcytotoxicity test, e.g., as has been worked out for H-2 typing in the mouse (Frelinger et al. 1974) or as described by Křen (1974) for the rat. Titers usually are not higher than 10^{-3}.

The preparation of ^{125}I-labeled anti-H-1 antibodies has been described by Shumak et al. (1973).

Anti-H-1 alloantisera produced between H-1 congenic strains are highly cross-reactive serologically. Thus an A anti-B strain antiserum reacts not only with strain B cells but also with those of strains such as C and F. By use of a panel of H-1 congenic strains and of a battery of antisera produced between them, the patterns of cross-reactivity can be elaborated by direct testing and absorption tests. Instances of cross-reactivity define a public specificity, designated by a number, whereas haplotype-specific reactions, i.e., those remaining after absorption of all cross-reactions, represent private specificities, also designated by a number. Thus, an H-1 antigen map can be constructed that reflects the serological interrelationship of the different H-1 haplotypes. This map is based on the assumption of a one-to-one relationship between antibody and antigen and relies on similar principles as the H-2 map of the mouse.

The currently used H-1 antigen maps (Štark et al. 1971; Palm 1971) are based on serological analysis by hemagglutination tests. Table 6.5 presents a revised form of a 1971 map (Štark et al. 1971) describing the H-1 hemagglutinogen interrelationship of eight H-1 congenic strains. It is still incomplete because only 37 of 56 interstrain combinations have been tested so far against a panel of eight congenic strains. (The H-1^{e} and H-1^{h} haplotypes are omitted from the analysis because the respective congenic strains are not yet finished.) It should be stressed that such a table is incomplete principally because it is nothing more than the reflection of one kind of interpretation of a complex serologic system.

Each H-1 haplotype is characterized by one private specificity and a certain number of public specificities. The total number of the latter has increased since 1971 as several public specificities have been split into "shorter" ones. It can also be seen that some haplotypes resemble each other with respect to their cross-reactivity patterns, such as H-1^{a}, H-1^{b}, H-1^{f}, and H-1^{d}. Several public specificities appear together in clusters or even in inclusion groups, such as 4–14, 4–35, 4–20, and 8–18. Some public specificities are detectable only unilaterally. This means that they are found on red blood cells of a given H-1 haplotype only by an antiserum produced in a certain strain combination and not by that produced in another strain combination even though theoretically it should detect it. Some inclusion groups reflect this situation. It is noteworthy that several specificities are detectable only irregularly, which means only by some individuals of a group of immunized rats or only when fresh and not stored antisera are used. On the other hand, red blood cells of some H-1 haplotypes (H-1^{c}, H-1^{b}, H-1^{h}) on Lewis genetic background often exhibit weak agglutinability. "Weakness" or "strongness" of a specificity might not only reflect differences in biochemical structure or expression of the specificities but could also be caused by Ir gene-regulated differences in the antibody response of the antisera producers.

It is so far unknown whether all H-1 specificities that have been detected on red blood cells and that are registered in Table 6.5 are expressed on lymphoid cells was well, although several data indicate that this is true at least for the majority of specificities. H-1 antigens have been detected on heart, kidney, liver, brain, and skin cells by mixed hemagglutination tests using antisera produced between congenic strains (Hausman and Palm 1973). Liver showed less reactivity than heart cells. Among kidney cell cultures, patches of nonreactive cells were detected. H-1 antigens have also been detected on tumors. Immunization with allogeneic tumor cells led to the production of antibodies that reacted against public and private specificities (Křenova et al. 1967, 1969, 1970a, 1970b). These results have been confirmed by indirect immunofluorescence tests (Křenova et al. 1972).

If anti-H-1 alloantisera are absorbed by red blood cells or platelets of the immunizing strain so that the antisera are rendered hemagglutinin-negative, a residual cytotoxic activity nevertheless remains against subpopulations of lymphoid cells (Davies and Alkins 1974; Günther and Bhakdi-Lehnen 1976). A detailed analysis of such antisera for cross-reactivity has not yet been reported. The lack of data on the genetic fine structure of the H-1 system does not permit one to call the H-1 antigens that are detected on

Table 6.5. H-1 Antigen Chart (Based on Dextran Hemagglutinin Testing)

H-1 (Ag-B)	Private Specificities									Public specificities																										
haplo-types	1	3	5	6	10	11	12	19	22	2	4	7	8	9	13	14	15	16	17	18	20	23	24	25	26	27	28	29	30	31	32	33	34	35	36	37
a (4)	1									2	4	7			13	14			17		20											33		35		
b (6)		3								2			8	9						18		23	24													
c (5)					10										13		15					23		25	26	27	28									
d							12				4		8			14		16		18	20			25				29							36	37
f								19			4		8							18	20				26				30	31						37
l (1)			5									7	8					16	17							27				31	32					
n (3)						11											15						24					29	30		32	33	34			
w (2)				6							4			9					17								28						34	35	36	37
h									22	The congenic strain LEW.1H is not yet established																										

Appendix to Table 6.5. Characterization of the Specificity of Alloantisera Produced Between H-1 Congenic Strains, Based on Hemagglutination Tests

Antiserum[a]	Haplotypes Reacting[b]	Specificities Detected[b]
n-a	a, b, d, f, w	1, 2, 4, 14, 20
l-a	a, b, d, f, (w)	1, 2, 14, 20, (4)
w-a	a, b, d, f, l	1, 2, 7, 14, 20
f-a	a, d	1, 14
d-a	a	1
bd-a	a	1
bn-a	a, d	1, 14
dw-a	a, b	1, 2
n-b	a, b, d, f, l, w, (c)	3, 2, 8, 9, 18, (23)
a-b	b, d, f, (c, l, n)	3, 18, (8, 23, 24)
l-b	a, b, d, f	3, 2, 18
d-b	a, b	3, 2
ad-b	b	3,
cl-b	a, b, d, f	3, 2, 18
cl-b/d	a, b	3, 2
n-b/d	a, b	3, 2
n-b/a	b, d, f, l	3, 8, 18
n-b/a+d	b	3
n-b/a+f	b	3
w-c	a, b, c, d, f, l, n	10, 13, 15, 25, 26, 27, 23
b-c	a, c, d, f, n, w	10, 13, 15, 25, 26, 28
l-c	a, c, d, f, n, w	10, 13, 15, 25, 26, 28
n-c	a, c, d, f, l, w	10, 13, 25, 26, 27, 28
al-c	c, n, (f, w)	10, 15, (26, 28)
bn-c	c, (a, d, w)	10, (13, 25, 28)
bw-c	c, n, (a, f)	10, 15, (13, 26)
dn-c	a, c, w	10, 13, 28
ln-c	a, c, d, f, w	10, 13, 25, 26, 28
nw-c	a, c, d, f	10, 13, 25, 26
n-d	a, b, d, f, l, w, (c)	12, 4, 8, 14, 20, (25)
l-d	a, b, d, f, (w)	12, 14, 18, 20, (4)
c-d	a, b, d, f, (l)	12, 14, 18, 20, (16)
a-d	b, d, f	12,18
f-d	a, d, (n)	12, 14, (29)
ab-d	d, (n)	12, (29)
aw-d	d, f, l, (b, c, n)	12, 8, (25, 29)
bn-d	a, d, f	12, 14, 20
fw-d	a, d	12, 14
f-d/a	d	12
l-d/w	a, b, d, f	12, 14, 18, 20
l-d/a	d	12
l-f	a, b, d, f, n	19, 18, 20, 30
a-f	b, d, f, l, (c, n)	19, 8, (26, 30)
d-f	f	19
ad-f	f	19
bn-f	a, d, f	19, 20
bw-f	a, d, f, (c, n)	19, 20 (26, 30)
bn-f/a	f	19
l-f/a+d	f	19

Appendix to Table 6.5 (continued)

Antiserum[a]	Haplotypes Reacting[b]	Specificities Detected[b]
n-l	a, b, d, f, l, w	5, 7, 8, 17
w-l	b, d, f, l,	5, 8, 16
a-l	b, d, f, l	5, 8, 16
b-l	d, l	5, 16
d-l	l, (a, f)	5, (7, 31)
f-l	l, (n)	5, (32)
ad-l	l	5
dw-l	l, (a)	5, (7)
d-l/a	f, l	5, 31
d-l/a+f	l	5
d-l/f	l	5
l-n	a, b, c, d, f, n	11, 15, 24, 29, 30, 33
w-n	c, d, f, n, (a)	11, 15, 29, 30 (33)
b-n	c, n, (a)	11, 15, (33)
d-n	c, n, (a)	11, 15, (33)
al-n	c, n, (d, f)	11, 15, (29, 30)
bd-n	c, n, w	11, 15, 34
cl-n	n, (a, b, d)	11, (24, 29, 33)
cd-n	n	11
cw-n	n	11
al-n/d	c, n	11, 15
b-n/c	a, n	11, 33
b-n/c+a	n	11
l-w	a, d, f, w, (b, c, n)	6, 4/35, 36, 37, (9, 28, 34)
n-w	a, d, f, l, w, (b, c)	6, 4/35, 36, 37, 17, (9, 28)
c-w	a, d, f, l, w	6, 4/35, 36, 37, 17
a-w	d, f, w	6, 36, 37
d-w	w, (a)	6, (35)
f-w	w, (a, d)	6, (35, 36)
bl-w	a, c, d, f, w	6, 4/35, 36, 37, 28
bn-w	a, d, f, w	6, 4/35, 36, 37
cf-w	w, (d)	6, (36)
dl-w	w	6
fl-w/d	c, w	6,28
fl-w	d, w, (a, c)	6, 36, (28, 35)

[a] Designation by the symbols of the H-1 haplotypes involved: n-a = LEW.1N anti-LEW.1A antiserum, bd-a = (LEW.1B × LEW.1D)F_1 anti-LEW.1A antiserum, n-b/a = LEW.1N anti-LEW.1B antiserum absorbed *in vivo* by LEW.1A.

[b] Occasional reactivity given in brackets.

lymphoid cells after platelet absorption Ia antigens. However, it has been shown in the mouse that absorption of anti-H-2 antisera by platelets or red blood cells might be a proper approach to detect Ia antigens (Davies and Hess 1974). Anti-H-1 (plus non-H-1) alloantisera that had been absorbed with platelets or red blood cells have also been reported to inhibit rosetting of IgG-coated red blood cells by Fc receptor-bearing rat spleen cells (Soulillou et al. 1976).

This heterogeneity of MHS antigens that are detectable serologically is well known from the H-2 system of the mouse, including: the H-2D- and H-2K-determined antigens that are detectable on red blood cells and on all lymphocytes and on most other tissues; the Ia antigens that are found only on subpopulations of lymphoid cells, and few other cell types, thereby easily detectable on B lymphocytes; and the H-2G antigen, which is expressed only on red blood cells.

In contrast to the H-2 system, only one private specificity has so far been found for each H-1 haplotype in the rat. Whether this means that the H-1 system possesses only one end "K" or "D" or whether we have so far been unable to split the apparent single private specificity into two is still unanswered. So far no data on intra-H-1 recombinats are available that could help to clarify this point. If among the present panel of H-1 haplotypes there is no recombinant haplotype then it is not surprising that only one private specificity is found for each haplotype. Recently it has been possible to split the private specificity H-1.6 of the H-1^{w} haplotype by absorption with H-1.6 positive cells from a noninbred Wistar rat (Günther et al. 1975). This means either that the anti-H-1.6 antiserum still contains activity against so far unknown public specificities or that there are indeed two private specificities.

Serological typing of 37 wild rats by direct hemagglutination and absorption tests is reported to detect H-1 antigenic specificities and H-1 haplotypes similar if not identical to those present in inbred rat strains (Shonnard et al. 1976). The authors conclude from these results that the polymorphism of H-1 haplotypes in wild rat populations is restricted.

3. Role of the H-1 System in Graft Rejection

3.1 Skin Grafts

The definition of the H-1 system as the MHS of the rat was originally based on the finding that H-1-incompatible skin grafted between parental strains and segregating hybrids was rejected acutely in less than 14 days (Štark et al. 1967a; Palm 1964). This was confirmed in several other studies on the survival of parental skin grafts in backcross or F_2 hybrids (Silvers et al. 1967; Elves 1969; Bildsøe 1972). Only Elves observed exceptionally long-surviving skin grafts—3 out of 24—in spite of H-1 disparity, which was determined by MLR and serological typing. In the case of H-1 compatibility between parent and segregating hybrids, grafts were often rejected in a chronic fashion, and the large scattering of their survival times presumably reflected the more or less cumulative effect of minor histocompatibility antigens. When skin grafts were exchanged between H-1-different congenic strains, acute graft rejection always occurred (Štark et al. 1970, and own unpublished results). It should be noted that in cases of H-1 identity the effect of multiple minor H-loci is usually so strong that acute rejection takes place (Štark et al. 1970). Chronic rejection, however, can be observed between strains that are congenic for minor H systems (Křen et al. 1973).

Some different inbred rat strains that have been reported (according to hemagglutination tests) to be H-1 identical serologically (Table 6.4) have been compared histogenetically by F_1 tests. No rejections have been observed in the following combinations: LEW.1B to (LEW × BUF)F_1, LEW.1C to (LEW × CAP)F_1, LEW.1C to (LEW × PVG)F_1, LEW.1C to (LEW × PD)F_1, LEW.1C to (LEW × BROFO)F_1, LEW.1D to (LEW × BD X)F_1, LEW.1W to (LEW × WAG)F_1, LEW.1W to (LEW × WA)F_1, LEW.1W to (LEW × IW)F_1 (Křen and Štark, *unpublished results*), LEW.1W to (LEW × LEP)F_1, and LEW to (AS × LEW.1A)F_1 (Günther et al. 1975). However, LEW.1A grafts were rejected by (LEW × DA)F_1, and LEW grafts were rejected by (LEW.1A × BS)F_1 (Günther et al. 1975), indicating that $H\text{-}1^l$ of LEW and BS rats are different from each other and that DA and LEW.1A rats carry different $H\text{-}1^a$ genotypes. This leads one to the question of the genetic and functional relationship between the H-1 antigens that induce antibody formation, skin and organ graft rejection, and MLR stimulation. In the case of L.AVN and DA, identity is found for the H-1 antigens that are detectable in the hemagglutination assay, there is no MLR stimulation, but skin grafts are rejected in the F_1 test (Günther et al. 1975) whereas kidney grafts survive permanently (Table 6.6; Wagner, *personal communication*).

Table 6.6. Kidney Allograft Survival in Inbred Rat strains

Donor	Recipient	Graft Survival (days)		References
		Range	MST[a]	
A. *H-1 plus non-H-1 incompatibility*				
AS	AS2		125 (38–412)	Salaman 1971
AS	AS2	7–186		Paris et al. 1976
AS	BD V	8–9	8.0	Thoenes et al. 1974
AS	LEW.1D	6–9	7.2 (6.6–7.9)	Thoenes et al. 1974
AS	LEW.1F	8–171		Paris et al. 1976
(AS × AS2)F_1	AS		11 ±0.6	Sakai 1969
(AS × AS2)F_1	AS2		21.4±0.7	Sakai 1969
(AS × BD V)F_1	AS	46–158		Thoenes et al. 1974
(AS × LEW.1D)F_1	AS	187–336		Thoenes 1975
AS2	AS		8.0 (7–9.2)	Salaman 1971
AS2	AS	10–12		Bildsøe et al. 1970
AS2	DA	7–36		Fabre and Morris 1974a
AUG	AS		8.5	French and Batchelor 1969
(AUG × AS)F_1	AS	8–12	9	French and Batchelor 1972
(AUG × AS)F_1	AS		8.8+1.0	Tilney and Bell 1974
BD V	AS	9–10	9.4	Thoenes et al. 1974
BD V	LEW	10–16	11.0 (8.9–13.5)	Thoenes et al. 1974
BN	LEW		6.8±1.2	Lucas et al. 1970

Table 6.6 (continued)

Donor	Recipient	Graft Survival (days)		References
		Range	MST[a]	
BN	LEW	8–11		Thoenes 1975
BN	WAG	9–55	14	Tinbergen 1968
BUF	LEW		18.9 and 294[b]	Ippolito et al. 1972
BUF	LEW	8–59	18.5 (15.2–22.5)	Mullen and Hildemann 197
DA	LEW	8–10		Fabre and Morris 1974a
(DA × LEW)F_1	DA	13–>300		Fabre and Morris 1975
(DA × LEW)F_1	LEW	9–10		Fabre and Morris 1975
LEW	BD V	8	8.0	Thoenes et al. 1974
LEW	BUF	5–9	7.7 (7.4–8.0)	Mullen and Hildemann 197
LEW	BUF		7.7	Ippolito et al. 1972
LEW	DA	7–21		Fabre and Morris 1974a
LEW.1D	AS	8–10	8.5	Thoenes et al. 1974
LEW	AS2	8–205		Paris et al. 1976
LEW	BN	8–9		Thoenes 1975
(LEW × AS2)F_1	DA	>200		Fabre and Morris 1974b
(LEW × BD V)F_1	LEW	15–146		Thoenes 1975
(LEW × BN)F_1	LEW		17.3 ± 2.7	Stuart et al. 1968
(LEW × BN)F_1	LEW		9.6 + 1.2 and 16 ± 1.0[b]	Lucas et al. 1970
(LEW × BUF)F_1	LEW	7–201	12.5 (9.3–16.8)	Mullen and Hildemann 197
(LEW.1D × AS)F_1	LEW.1D	7–254		Thoenes 1975
(LEW.1D × BD V)F_1	AS	8–10		Thoenes et al. 1974
(LEW.1D × BD V)F_1	LEW	7–10	7.4	Thoenes et al. 1974
B. *H-1 incompatibility (congenic strains)*				
LEW	LEW.1D	6–13	7.4 (6.5–9.1)	Thoenes et al. 1974
LEW	LEW.1F	22–184		Paris et al. 1976
LEW	LEW.1N	9–87		Thoenes 1975
(LEW × LEW. 1D)F_1	LEW	75–293		Thoenes 1975
(LEW × LEW.1D)F_1	LEW.1D	9–> 244		Thones 1975
LEW.1D	LEW	8–13	9.8 (9.1–10.6)	Thoenes et al. 1974
LEW.1D	LEW.1N	7–11		Thoenes 1975
LEW.1F	LEW	5–105		Paris et al. 1976
LEW.1W	LEW	8–172		Thoenes 1975
LEW.1N	LEW.1F	6–>158		Paris et al. 1976
C. *Non-H-1 incompatibility*				
AS	LEW	>300		Thoenes and White 1973
BDV	LEW1D	>480		Thoenes 1975
F344	LEW	76–197	121 (92–158)	Mullen and Hildemann 197
BN	LEW.1N	31–409		Thoenes 1975
LEW	AS	>300		Thoenes and White 1973
LEW	F344	>500	(455–>664)	Mullen and Hildemann 197
LEW.1A	DA	>100		Wagner, *pers. commun.*
LEW.1D	BDSV	>300		Thoenes 1975
LEW.1N	BN	>79–>310		Thoenes 1975

[a] MST = median survival time ± S.D.; in brackets, 95 percent confidence limits.
[b] Two modes of survival times.

3.2 Organ Grafts

As a result of progress in microsurgery (Lee 1967), grafting of primarily vascularized kidney and heart grafts can be performed routinely in the rat. Therefore, a great number of data are available on the influence of the H-1 system on organ graft survival. It is obvious that such data are of great relevance for clinical transplantation in man.

Table 6.6 gives a survey of kidney allograft survival data. It can be seen that, with two exceptions [AS into AS2 and (LEW × AS2)F_1 into DA], kidneys are acutely rejected when grafted across a H-1 plus non-H-1 barrier (group A). H-1 compatibility, on the other hand, leads to long or permanent survival (group C). The major role of the H-1 system for organ graft survival has been proven by transplanting kidneys from AS × (AS × AS2) backcross rats into AS parental rats and (BN × AS)F_2 kidneys into AS recipients (Bildsøe et al. 1970; Bildsøe 1972). There was no graft rejection in cases of non-H-1 incompatibility alone, although in some cases of H-1 difference survival was prolonged.

When kidneys were exchanged reciprocally, in some H-1 different strains rejection times were asymmetric, e.g., BUF-LEW, AS-AS2. It may also be noted that semiallogeneic kidneys often survived longer than homozygous grafts (compare, e.g., LEW and (LEW × DA)F_1 into DA).

The fate of primarily vascularized accessory abdominal heart grafts has also been shown to be strongly influenced by the H-1 system. Hearts from backcross or F_2 hybrids were rejected only in case of H-1 incompatibility (Bildsøe et al. 1970). In the F344-LEW strain combination, which is assumed to be H-1 serologically identical, F344 hearts were as acutely rejected as skin grafts in contrast to prolonged survival of kidney grafts (Freeman and Steinmuller 1969; Barker and Billingham 1970), whereas LEW hearts showed prolonged or permanent survival in F344 rats (Barker and Billingham 1970).

Grafts of different tissue or organ origin but of the same genotype show disparate survival in the same recipient or in recipients belonging to the same inbred strain. Thus H-1-identical kidneys survive permanently, whereas skin is acutely rejected (F344-LEW); AS2 rats take AS kidney for a long time but reject skin acutely, even when having received both grafts at the same time (Salaman 1971). Kidney and heart grafts from F_2 or backcross hybrids survive in the parental strain when they are H-1 compatible, whereas their skin is rejected (Bildsøe et al. 1970; Bildsøe 1972). The greater sensitivity of skin grafts to the rejection reaction is also observed in animals made tolerant to H-antigens by neonatal bone marrow cell injection. In spite of stable chimerism, skin grafts can be rejected normally (Silvers and Billingham 1970), and kidney grafts are accepted while skin is rejected (Feldman et al. 1968).

It has been suggested that organ grafts are less susceptible to the rejection reaction (or more susceptible to enhancement) because of differences in the H-antigen expression or of pathophysiological reasons, such as vascularization, or that there are organ-specific transplantation antigens. However, so far there is no convincing evidence for kidney- or heart-specific antigens playing a dominant role in these transplantation models.

Based on the results obtained with kidney and heart grafts from segregating hybrids (see above), showing organ graft rejection only in H-1-incompatible situations, the "one-locus hypothesis" for organ graft rejection has been put forward (Bildsøe et al. 1970; Bildsøe 1972). However, results obtained with heart grafts in the F344-LEW combination were not in accord with this hypothesis (Freeman and Steinmuller 1969). This concept of an exclusive role of the H-1 system for organ graft rejection becomes still more doubtful in view of data on kidney grafting between H-1-congenic strains (Table 6.6, group B). The LEW ($H\text{-}1^l$) into LEW.1F ($H\text{-}1^f$) combination represents the H-1 haplotype combination, this time on identical background, in which prolonged or permanent kidney graft survival inspite of H-1 difference (AS= $H\text{-}1^l$ into AS2= $H\text{-}1^f$) has been described (Salaman 1971). Because the same effect occurs in the congenic combination, it can be attributed to the H-1 system and not to genetic background genes. However, in the reverse congenic combination, LEW into LEW.1F, prolonged survival is also observed as opposed to the prompt rejection of AS2 kidneys by AS rats in the noncongenic combination. Therefore, non-H-1 genes interfere with the action of H-1 genes. This conclusion is strengthened by the results obtained with LEW into LEW.1N as compared with LEW into BN graftings. In the latter, acute rejection is found regularly; in the former, long survivals occur frequently. In Table 6.6B it can be seen that only some H-1 congenic combinations regularly show acute kidney graft rejection. Also with congenic strains the superior performance of semiallogeneic kidneys is observed.

In all these congenic combinations skin grafts are acutely rejected. It is interesting that, contrary to kidney grafts, LEW hearts are acutely rejected in LEW.1F recipients (Paris et al. 1976).

Among the factors determining kidney graft rejection, the following have to be considered: the structure of the H-1 antigens influencing antigenic strength, H-linked Ir genes, non-H-1 antigens, genetic background genes as modifiers of H-1 antigens or H-1 linked Ir genes, and also environmental factors (health status, surgical technique). The processes of rejection reaction and of (auto)enhancement (see below) compete with each other, and the result may lead to take or rejection. Different tissues or organs can vary for susceptibility to these reactions.

3.3 Immunological Enhancement

Kidney grafting in the rat has become one of the most favored models for investigating immunological enhancement (Stuart et al. 1968; French and Batchelor 1969; White et al. 1969). This is a state of specific sensitization that is serologically transferable and that leads to prolonged or permanent survival of organ (or tissue or tumor) grafts that are otherwise rejected. It can be induced by active or by passive immunization or by a combination of both and can be strengthened by immunosuppression of the host. Whereas H-1-incompatible skin grafts are only slightly enhanceable, enhancement can be achieved readily with kidney grafts. This difference is most obvious when a recipient that has received enhancing serum rejects skin grafts but accepts kidney grafts from the same donor. Enhancement is most readily induced in semiallogeneic combinations (Strom et al. 1973).

Rats carrying enhanced kidneys and tested for their immune competence are found to react normally, or delayed and impaired in MLR, CML, and local GVH assays. However, they are mostly not unresponsive to donor antigens. Skin grafts of kidney donor origin usually are rejected by recipients that carry successfully enhanced kidney grafts. In rare cases they are, however, accepted, especially in long-time enhanced recipients (Mahabir et al. 1969; Salaman et al. 1971; Thoenes and White 1973). Enhanced rats produce anti-H-1 antibodies that are detectable in lymphocytotoxic assays. The mechanism of immunological enhancement is not yet clear (French and Batchelor 1972). It is hypothesized that passively transferred anti-H-1 antibodies block or compete with the cytotoxic response otherwise developing in the normal host and leading to rejection. After some time the host starts to produce its own enhancing (blocking) antibodies, and ultimately even immunological tolerance may be induced. It is reasonable to assume that in cases of spontaneous prolonged or permanent survival of kidneys, i.e., in untreated hosts (AS/AS2 combination, some H-1 congenic strain combinations, non-H-1 different combinations), autoenhancement occurs. That such an enhancement might reflect a delicate balance between different types of competing immune responses is demonstrated by the following experiment (Tilney and Bell 1974): AS rats were hyperimmunized against AUG lymphoid cells. If they were grafted with $(AS \times AUG)F_1$ kidneys, hyperacute rejection was observed. However, if the serum of the ungrafted hyperimmunized rats was transferred to normal AS rats, these took $(AS \times AUG)F_1$ kidneys for more than 100 days (normal MST 9 days).

The role of the H-1 system in induction and maintenance of enhancement is not clear. The following target antigens of immunological enhancement have been cited: (1) classical H-1 transplantation antigens; (2) I region-determined antigens, and (3) idiotypes of H-antigen specific receptor combining sites.

This second possibility has been suggested by Davies and Alkins (1974). Antidonor alloantiserum produced in AGUS rats against $(WAG \times AGUS)F_1$ rats had been exhaustively absorbed with donor red blood cells and was then shown to have the same capacity as the native antiserum to enhance auxiliary vascularized hearts grafts. Similar findings have been reported by Soulillou et al. (1976). In the mouse it was possible to relate enhancement of skin grafts to anti-Ia antibodies (Staines et al. 1974). The involvement of antiidiotypic antibodies in kidney graft enhancement has been suggested by McKearn et al. (1974a) and Stuart et al. (1974). Presence of antiidiotypic antibodies could indeed be shown in rats bearing enhanced kidneys (Stuart et al. 1974). That active immunization against the own idiotypes can lead to prolonged skin graft survival has recently been demonstrated (Binz and Wigzell 1976). LEW rats which were immune to DA-alloantigen-binding receptors of LEW origin showed prolonged survival of DA skin grafts (rejection after 14 to 39 days instead of 9 to 12 days), whereas BN grafts were rejected normally. No side effects of this autoimmunization have been observed so far. (See also section 6.6.)

A role of histocompatibility-linked Ir genes can be supposed in elicitation and maintenance of enhancement but cannot be shown experimentally at present. The observation that enhancement of kidney grafts was more successful in H-1-incompatible congenic combinations than in those that differed for H-1 plus non-H-1 antigens (Thoenes et al. 1974) points to interference of the genetic background with induction and maintenance of immunological enhancement.

3.4 Other Types of Grafts

There are few reports on the influence of the H-1 system on the fate of other types of grafts, such as liver (Lee and Edgington 1968), islets of Langerhans (Reckard and Barker 1973), teeth germ (Iványi 1968), cornea (Gronemeyer and Müller-Ruchholtz 1974), and cartilage (Heyner 1969). For spleen grafts prolonged survival in spite of H-1 incompatibility has been reported in some rat strain combinations without special treatment of donors or recipients (Bitter-Suermann 1974a, 1974b) and was explained by balancing interaction of graft-versus-host and host-versus-graft reactions.

4. Genetic Control of Mixed Lymphocyte Reactivity by the H-1 System

When allogeneic lymphoid cells are cocultured *in vitro* (mixed lymphocyte reaction, MLR), blast transformation and proliferation (determined by ^{3}H-thymidine uptake) of responding cells may be induced by the stimulating cells (blocked by irradiation or mitomycin C). Genetic control of mixed lymphocyte reactivity by the H-1 system has been demonstrated by strain distribution patterns and by testing segregating hybrids and H-1-congenic strains.

Only strains that are serologically H-1 different show a positive MLR, whereas H-1-identical strains are nonstimulatory (Elves 1967; Wilson 1967; Cramer et al. 1974). This means that all H-1-different strains so far tested are MLR positive and all H-1-serologically identical strains are MLR negative. There are three exceptions to this rule: (1) F344 and LEW cells, both Ag-B^1 according to hemagglutinin typing (Palm 1964) and local GvH reaction assay (Elkins and Palm 1966), are reported as weakly MLR positive unidirectionally when F344 lymphoid cells are stimulated by LEW cells (Colley and DeWitt 1969). (2) KGH rats that are Ag-B^7 serologically are MLR nonstimulatory with Ag-B^1 rats (Cramer et al. 1974). (3) Rats of the B strain are reported to be Ag-B^3 serologically and MLR nonstimulatory with Ag-B^4 rats (Gill et al. 1976).

The finding of H-1 dependency of MLR is confirmed by the behavior of H-1-congenic strains. All combinations so far tested are positive (Štark et al. 1971; Palm and Wilson 1973; Günther et al. 1975). Proof of genetic control of MLR by the H-1 system comes from MLR typing of segregating hybrids with parental cells (Silvers et al. 1967; Elves 1969; Bildsøe et al. 1970; Sørensen et al. 1971; Shonnard et al. 1975).

Among 428 F_2 and backcross hybrids of five different parental strain combinations, no phenotype was recorded as being recombinant between the serologically determined H-1 type and the expected type of MLR response. Therefore, gene(s) controlling MLR are closely linked with the H-1 genes. Meanwhile, recombinant H-1 haplotypes have been detected. Among 114 segregant hybrids of the BN/LEW strain combination two recombinants of the above type have been described (Williams and Moore 1976). Furthermore, among (LEW.1A × LEW.1W)F_2 hybrids a rat was found which carried H-1 hemagglutinogens of both parental strains but its MLR and Ir phenotypes were that of the LEW.1W strain (Štark et al. 1977). That this rat carried indeed an H-1 recombinant haplotype was confirmed by progeny testing. Evidence that the MLR gene is separable from other H-1 genes came also from the KGH and B strains which are serologically H-1 different but MLR non stimulatory with respect to certain H-1 haplotypes (Cramer et al. 1974; Gill et al. 1976). Because of lack of data, genetic control of MLR-stimulating antigens and genetic control of MLR responsiveness by H-1 genes are not distinguishable.

Unilateral MLR among some H-1 different strain combinations is reproducibly found to be asymmetric (Sørensen et al. 1971). Homozygous (parental) cells usually have a higher stimulatory effect than semiallogeneic F_1 hybrid cells. This may be due to gene dose effect (Sørensen 1971) or back stimulation in the former case. The F344/LEW strain combination is so far the only reported case of MLR stimulation between serologically H-1 identical strains (Colley and DeWitt 1969). This result might either indicate that both strains differ for their H-1 linked MLR genes or present the first example of the existence of the M locus (Festenstein 1973) in rats. Unilaterality of stimulation would fit this latter interpretation.

MLR phenotypes of wild rat origin appear to be similar or identical to those of inbred strains and the polymorphism of the MLR genes in wild populations, therefore, seems to be rather restricted in the rat (Cramer et al. 1977).

In mouse and man, many data are available on the immunogenetics of the cell mediated lympholysis (CML) reaction that is induced *in vitro* concomitantly with MLR. For the rat, however, similar data have not been reported. Only recently successful generation of cytotoxic lymphocytes in vitro during MLR has been reported (Bruce et al. 1975; Bernstein and Wright 1976).

The stimulator cells in rat MLR can be blocked by anti-H-1 alloantibodies

(Gordon et al. 1971; Larner and Fitch 1973), although the specificity of inhibition remains unclear. Blocking of stimulator and responder cells by alloantiserum (LEW anti-BN) was reported by Soulillou et al. (1976). These authors showed further that exhaustive absorption of the antiserum with BN platelets or red blood cells did not remove the inhibitory activity. Inhibition was H-1 specific only at low antiserum concentrations.

5. Graft-Versus-Host Reactivity and the H-1 System

A graft-versus-host reaction (GvH reaction) occurs when immunocompetent cells are injected into recipients which are unable to reject them. This assay is able to measure antihistocompatibility antigen activity of lymphoid cell populations quantitatively *in vivo*. The initial phase of the GVH response is thought to be an *in vivo* equivalent to the MLR. GvH reaction can be systemic (and is then determined by a spleen weight or mortality assay) or local. The latter is determined by the normal lymphocyte transfer test (Ford 1967), kidney test (Elkins 1964), or popliteal lymph node weight assay (Levine 1968, Ford et al. 1970).

The predominant importance of H-1 incompatibility for elicitation of GvH reaction in rats was demonstrated by the kidney test in backcross and F_2 hybrids (Elkins and Palm 1966). No GvH reaction could be observed in H-1 identical combinations. In the more sensitive popliteal lymph node assay GvH reaction could also be induced across minor histocompatibility barriers in cases of H-1 identity; however, about 100 times more lymphoid cells had to be injected in order to elicit the same lymph node enlargement as was found in H-1 incompatible combinations (Ford et al. 1970). There appeared to be slight quantitative differences between different H-1 strain combinations (Ford et al. 1970; Ford 1973).

Systemic GvH reaction can be elicited by i.v. or i.p. injection of adult spleen cells into neonatal rats, resulting in wasting, exfoliative dermatitis, and even death. In experiments with H-1 congenic strains and respective parental strains, the role of the H-1 system was studied (Křen et al. 1970). Table 6.7 shows some of the results. One can see in combinations with H-1 plus non-H-1 differences, runt syndrome incidence (assayed by death of the recipients) is considerably lower than in pure H-1-different combinations, although the same H-1 haplotypes are involved.

Among the H-1-identical combinations, only one (BP cells into LEW.1B rats) was positive. Thus runt syndrome is always elicited in H-1-incompatible combinations, although to a varying degree that is very much influenced by the genetic background. In H-1-identical combinations, runt syndrome is only rarely induced under the same conditions. It should be noted that in an earlier study (Křen et al. 1969), runt disease was induced by i.p. injection of spleen cell in only some out of 11 H-1 plus non-H-1-incompatible combinations and in all 4 tested H-1 identical combinations, although to a low frequency in the latter group.

Table 6.7. Influence of the H-1 System on Runt Syndrome Incidence (Deaths) After i.v. Administration of Spleen Cells into Neonatal Rats

Donor Strain	Recipient Strain	Incompatibility	Spleen Cell Dose ($\times 10^6$), i.v.	Dead/Total	Mortality (%)
AVN	LEW	H-1 + non-H-1	10	10/25	40
LEW.1A	LEW	H-1	10	10/11	91
LEW	LEW.1A	H-1	10	12/16	75
AVN	LEW.1A	non-H-1	20	0/5	0
BN	LEW	H-1 + non-H-1	30	2/12	17
LEW.1N	LEW	H-1	30	10/10	100
			10	5/5	100
LEW	LEW.1N	H-1	30	7/7	100
			10	2/6	33
BN	LEW.1N	non-H-1	30	0/5	0
			10	0/7	0
WP	LEW	H-1 + non-H-1	20	0/9	0
LEW.1W	LEW	H-1	10	10/10	100
LEW	LEW.1W	H-1	30	5/5	100
			15	5/9	55
WP	LEW.1W	non-H-1	30	0/6	0
BP	LEW	H-1 + non-H-1	20	8/8	100
			5	9/10	90
LEW.1B	LEW	H-1	20	10/10	100
			5	10/12	83
LEW	LEW.1B	H-1	20	7/8	87
			5	21/21	100
BP	LEW.1B	non-H-1	30	6/15	40
			10	1/17	6

From Křen et al. 1970.

Thus H-1 genes and genetic background influence induction of a systemic GvH reaction and several factors may be involved: differences in spleen cell survival, possibly due to variability in immunologic maturation among the recipient strains (Billingham et al. 1962a), differences in the capacity of the spleen cells to mount a GvH reaction, antibody production against host antigens by the inoculated cells. As to the latter point, it is interesting to note that runt syndrom incidence is high in strain combinations in which antibody production is low and vice versa (Štark et al. 1970; see Table 6.8).

When systemic GvH response is studied in adult F_1 hybrids injected with parental cells, antireceptor antibodies against the injected lymphoid cells can be produced and are able to inhibit GvH reaction (McKearn et al. 1974b).

6. Features of the Immune Response to H-1 Antigens

A great variety of different types of immune responses can be elicited against H-1-determined antigens *in vivo* (graft rejection, antibody response, im-

Table 6.8. Antibody Production Against H-1 Antigens Among Congenic Strains After Primary and Secondary Skin Grafting

Strain Combination		H-1 Haplotypes	Mean titer[a]			
			After first Graft		After second Graft	
			h[b]	c[c]	h	c
LEW.1N	anti-LEW	n–l	8.3	2.9	12.2	10.0
LEW.1B	anti-LEW	b–l	6.9	2.9	11.8	6.8
LEW.1A	anti-LEW	a–l	6.6	2.8	5.7	8.6
LEW.1W	anti-LEW	w–l	6.1	3.0	7.3	3.7
LEW.1D	anti-LEW	d–l	< 2.3	0	4.0	2.1
LEW	anti-LEW.1A	l–a	10.8	9.8	12.7	10.0
LEW	anti-LEW.1D	l–d	10.3	4.7	13.2	10.0
LEW	anti-LEW.1N	l–n	10.3	3.6	13.4	9.3
LEW	anti-LEW.1W	l–w	6.3	3.7	11.4	10.0
LEW	anti-LEW.1B	l–b	5.1	< 1.0	11.2	7.2
LEW.1N	anti-LEW.1A	n–a	10.2	8.7	14.4	10.0
LEW.1N	anti-LEW.1D	n–d	12.2	5.9	14.8	10.0
LEW.1N	anti-LEW.1W	n–w	8.6	1.7	12.6	7.2
LEW.1N	anti-LEW.1B	n–b	7.7	< 1.0	7.2	2.2

[a] Groups of 4 to 5 rats, bleeding 11 days after grafting, second graft 4 weeks after first.
[b] Haemagglutinin titer.
[c] Cytotoxic titer.
From Štark et al. (1970).

munological enhancement, tolerance, graft-versus-host reaction) or *in vitro* (MLR, cell-mediated cytotoxicity). This variety presumably reflects several genetically different antigen systems that are determined by the H-1 system and that we cannot differentiate so far.

6.1 Thymus Dependence

Most of the immune reactions against H-1 antigens are thymus dependent. Neonatally thymectomized rats produced only IgM-class anti-H-1 antibodies instead of the IgG-class antibodies that are usually followed by the initial IgM production (Miller and DeWitt 1974). After adult thymectomy followed by irradiation and bone marrow reconstitution, no anti-H-1 antibodies could be elicited (Rolstad et al. 1974).

Skin graft rejection is severely impaired after thymectomy (Arnason et al. 1962; Rolstad and Ford 1974). The responding cells in MLR and GvH reaction are thymus-dependent lymphocytes (Wilson et al. 1967; Johnston and Wilson 1970; Rolstad and Ford 1974).

6.2 Quantity of Anti-H-1 Antibodies

When anti-H-1 antibodies are elicited among congenic strains and are tested by hemagglutination or cytotoxic tests, strong and weak combinations can be distinguished. These differences cannot be overcome by repeated immunizations with lymphoid cells or skin grafts. F_1 hybrids usually produce higher amounts of antibodies than homozygotes. Table 6.8 shows the quantitative differences in anti-H-1 antibody production between some H-1 congenic strain combinations. Whereas the absolute amount of antibodies found may vary according to the sensitivity of the method, the rank order presumably will remain valid. It is difficult so far to identify clearly Ir gene effects and to separate them from effects of different antigen expression on targets cells of different genetic origin.

6.3 Immunological Tolerance to H-1 Antigens

Induction of immunological tolerance against H-1 antigens can be achieved by injecting newborn rats with high doses of bone marrow cells (preferentially of F_1 hybrid origin in order to circumvent GvH response), whereas spleen, lymph node, or even thymus cells are less successful (Silvers and Billingham 1969). In H-1-identical combinations (F344-LEW), low numbers of cells of either source are effective in inducing tolerance even some days after birth (Silvers and Billingham 1969). Tolerance is usually defined operationally by significantly prolonged survival of skin grafts of cell donor strain origin. Although chimerism appears to be a prerequisite for acceptance of these grafts, it does not guarantee it (Silvers and Billingham 1970). In the studies of Křen et al. (1969, 1970), no recipient of H-1-incompatible spleen cells that had survived GvH reaction had become tolerant, but rejected test skin grafts in less than 15 days. However, recipients of H-1-compatible spleen cells—a situation where no GvH reaction can usually be induced—accepted test grafts for more than 15 or even 30 days.

Rats made tolerant neonatally against H-1 antigens will also accept kidney grafts of the cell donor strain origin (Feldman et al. 1968). By neonatal injection of bone marrow cells, rats can also be made specifically areactive in MLR tests (Wilson et al. 1967). This areactivity is also found when tolerance induction does not lead to prolonged acceptance of test skin grafts (Silvers and Billingham 1970). It should be mentioned that after successful induction of "classic" tolerance by neonatal injection of bone marrow cells, serum factors have been observed in the tolerant animals that block their graft-destroying immune response (Bansal et al. 1973a, 1973b).

Thus, the distinction between classical immunological tolerance (Billingham et al. 1956), which is commonly referred to clonal deletion, and the phenomenon of active blockade of an immune response, such as immunological enhancement, may be imprecise. It could be that enhancement leads to tolerance or that both coexist being directed against different antigens (MLR antigens, classical transplantation antigens), different types of lymphocytes being involved. The concepts of immunological tolerance and enhancement are discussed by Elkins et al. (1974). See sections 3.3 and 6.6 for induction of transplantation tolerance by immunization against own idiotypes.

6.4 Effect of Preimmunization

Preimmunization leads to second-set skin graft rejection. In the case of kidney grafts nearly always enhancement is achieved (which was discussed above) and not hyperacute rejection. The MLR changes its profile to an early peak response after preimmunization (Wilson and Nowell 1971); however, source of lymphoid cells and time after immunization appear to be important for the effect of immunization on MLR (Virolainen et al. 1969). After preimmunization, positive, although weak, MLR stimulation can be observed between some H-1-identical strains (Sørensen et al. 1971). Graft-versus-host reactivity against non-H-1 antigens is greatly enhanced (up to 50 times) after preimmunization (Ford and Simonsen 1971). This is not the case in H-1-different combinations. Therefore, the "factor of immunization" is one or less in H-1-different combinations and high in H-1-identical, non-H-1-different combinations.

6.5 "Clone" Size

The number of responding cells has been determined in MLR and GvH reaction and has been found to be rather high. About 1 to 3 percent of parental peripheral blood leukocytes transform and proliferate when stimulated by F_1 hybrid lymphoid cells in MLR (Wilson et al. 1968; Wilson and Nowell 1971). In GvH reaction, 4 to 12 percent of thoracic duct lymphocytes recognize and react against H-1 antigens (Ford et al. 1975).

T-cells that react against different H-1 haplotypes seem to be different and largely nonoverlapping and nonrecruiting (Ford and Atkins 1971; Dorsch and Roser 1974; Wilson and Nowell 1971), although some degree of overlap may exist (Wilson et al. 1972). Thus, the proportion of H-1-reactive cells is rather high when compared to usual clone size. It is not clear to what degree this peculiarity reflects the (complex) nature of the stimulating antigens or the nature of the respective recognition process by T-cells. A detailed discussion of the immune response to MHS antigens is found, e.g., in Simonsen (1970), Wilson et al. (1972), Wilson (1974), Ford et al. (1975), and Nowell et al. (1975).

6.6 Antiidiotypic Antibodies

When $(A \times B)F_1$ hybrids are injected with an alloantiserum (A anti-B) that was produced between the two parental rat strains (A, B), then an antialloantiserum will be produced that is directed against the receptor (idiotype, recognition structure) of A lymphocytes for antigens of B origin (Ramseier and Lindenmann 1972a; Ramseier 1973). Similar or identical antiidiotypic antisera can be obtained in the rat by injection of T-cells of A origin into $(A \times B)F_1$ hybrids (Binz and Wigzell 1975a). Antialloantisera inhibit recognition of antigens on B-cells by A-lymphoid cells in a short-term MLR that is quantitated by the so-called PAR assay (Ramseier 1973). Such antisera also specifically block recognition of fibroblasts by lymphoid cells (Binz et al. 1974), and treatment of MLR-responder cells with antialloantisera plus complement specifically removes reactivity against the respective stimulator antigens (Binz and Askonas 1975). Antiidiotype antisera also specifically abolish GvH reaction activity (Binz et al. 1973; McKearn 1974; McKearn et al. 1974b). Injection of antialloantisera into rats that carry the respective target idiotypes inhibited specifically antibody production (McKearn 1974). During the production of an alloantiserum by repeated injections of lymphoid cells, the recipient started to produce antibodies against the idiotype of his own alloantiserum (autoantiidiotypic antibodies). This process led to the disappearance of that idiotype from the antiserum (McKearn et al. 1974c). Thus, conventional alloantisera may contain antiidiotypic activity. By immunization of rats with alloantigen-binding idiotypic receptors prepared from rats of the same strain a state of specific unresponsiveness could be induced to the set of alloantigens with which the receptors reacted. This kind of autoimmunity against the rat's own idiotypes could be induced during few weeks and was long-lasting. Unresponsiveness was demonstrable for MLR, GvH reaction, and graft rejection (Binz and Wigzell 1976), and could be elicited by material isolated from normal serum or urine (Binz and Wigzell 1976) or by immunization against specifically educated syngeneic T lymphoblasts (Andersson et al. 1976).

By the use of antiidiotypic antibodies it has been possible to visualize and enumerate B- and T-cells that carry the respective idiotype(s) (Binz and Wigzell 1975b). Antisera produced in (LEW × DA)F_1 hybrids against LEW T-cell receptors with anti-DA specificity reacted with about 4 to 6 percent peripheral T-lymphocytes from normal LEW rats and with about 1 percent normal B-cells. This figure agreed well with that obtained for the proportion of MLR- and GvH reaction-responding cells.

By affinity chromatography using antiidiotype antisera, lymphocytes reactive against a given H-1 haplotype can be selectively enriched or removed and then used in functional tests (Binz and Wigzell 1975c).

It is assumed that the antiidiotypic antibodies produced in H-1-different rat strains by immunization with alloantisera or parental T-cells are directed against receptor sites for H-1 antigens: Both types of antiidiotype antisera, produced either against parental T-cells or against parental alloantisera, have a similar specificity. It is therefore concluded that receptors for H-1 antigens on B- and T-cells exhibit the same or similar idiotypes and that, therefore, the same v genes are expressed in B- and T-cells (Binz and Wigzell 1975a; Ramseier and Lindenmann 1972b). Indeed, idiotypes of alloantigen-binding T cells segregate together with allotypes of immunoglobulin heavy chains (Binz et al. 1976). It remains to be established how heterogeneous the specificity of the antiidiotypic antisera produced in F_1 hybrids is and against which antigenic determinants the respective receptors are directed.

7. H-1-Linked Immune Response Genes

The MHS of the rat specifically controls immune responsiveness to a variety of natural and synthetic antigens. In the mouse (Shreffler and David 1975; Klein 1975) and rhesus monkey (Dorf et al. 1975), such genetic control has been proven to be exerted by separate genes of the MHS (H-linked Ir genes).[3] The same applies to the rat, because an H-1 recombinant haplotype has been detected in which Ir genes have been separated from genes determining H-1 antigens and skin grat rejection (Štark et al. 1977).

Table 6.9 lists all antigens for which the immune response by segregation studies and/or by use of H-1-congenic strains has been shown to be H-1 controlled in inbred rat strains.

There is some evidence that antibody responsiveness to LDH_B (Würzburg et al. 1973), GAT (Armerding et al. 1974a), and low doses (1 to 10 μg)

Table 6.9. Antigens for Which Immune Responsiveness Has Been Established to be H-1 Controlled

Antigens	Immune Reaction Reflecting Genetic Control			References
Linear synthetic polypeptides				
$G_{52}L_{33}T_{15}$	ab,[a]	PFC,[b]	DHR[c]	Kunz et al. 1974; Shonnard et al. 1976
$G_{50}A_{50}$	ab,	DHR,	Ly[d]	Armerding et al. 1974b
$G_{50}T_{50}$	ab,	DHR,	Ly	Armerding et al. 1974b
$(T_{25}G_{25}A_{25}Gly_{25})_n$	ab			Luderer et al. 1976
Branched synthetic polypeptides				
(T,G)-A–L	ab		Ly	Günther et al. 1972; Günther and Rüde 1976
(H,G)-A–L	ab		Ly	Günther et al. 1973; Günther and Rüde 1976
(Phe,G)-A–L	ab		Ly	Günther et al. 1973; Günther and Rüde 1976
T_6-A–L	ab			Rüde and Günther 1974
T_4-A–L	ab			Rüde and Günther 1974
(T,G)-Pro–L	ab			Günther et al. 1976
(Phe,G)-Pro–L	ab			Günther et al. 1976
Pro–L	ab			Günther et al. 1976
Natural antigens				
$LDH-A_4$	ab		Ly	Würzburg 1971; Würzburg et al. 1973
Bovine insulin	ab			Günther and Keck, *unpubl. data*
Pig insulin	ab			Günther and Keck, *unpubl. data*

[a] Amount of antibodies.
[b] Number of plaque-forming cells.
[c] Delayed-type hypersensitivity reactivity.
[d] Anamnestic response *in vitro* of *in vivo* primed lymphoid cells.

[3] For general reviews of Ir genes, the reader is referred to Gasser and Silvers (1974) or Benacerraf and Katz (1975).

of BSA (Armerding et al. 1974a) are H-1 controlled. H-1-linked genetic factors also appear to influence the primary IgM plaque-forming cell response to sheep red blood cells *in vivo* (Bhakdi-Lehnen and Günther, *unpublished data*).

Low, high, and in some cases intermediate responder phenotypes can be distinguished operationally. Genetic control is mostly reflected (and determined) quantitatively by the amount of antibodies produced. In some cases high/low responder differentiation is also shown at the cellular level by assaying the anamnestic response *in vitro* or delayed-type hypersensitivity *in vivo*.

Only high and intermediate responders, as defined by antibody production, will show an anamnestic response *in vitro* (assayed by ^{3}H-thymidine uptake of proliferating lymphocytes). Similarly, delayed-type hypersensitivity reactions can be elicited only in the skin of high-responder strains. However, the variability in the intensity of this reaction does not correlate with the quantitative differences in the amounts of antibodies produced by the various high responder strains (Armerding et al. 1974a). Exceptional are the ACI and COP strains (Armerding et al. 1974a). Both are Ag-B^4 and low responding as to the humoral response to GA, but COP rats show an unexpected and pronounced delayed-type hypersensitivity reaction to this antigen. It remains to be established whether two different H-1-linked Ir-GA alleles or genetic background genes are involved.

High (or intermediate) responsiveness is inherited as a dominant, codominant or overdominant trait.

Table 6.10 shows the associations between the immune response phenotypes scored as high, intermediate, and low for the various antigens listed in Table 6.9 and 11 H-1 (Ag-B) haplotypes. Distribution of responsiveness to a given antigen among the different haplotypes can likewise be seen. The patterns can be considered to be consistent in most cases, because the same strains, or even the same H-1 congenic strains have been used.

So far, all serologically H-1 identical strains except one have been found to give the same response pattern (Kunz et al. 1974; Armerding et al. 1974a; Günther et al. 1975). Rats of the B stock, however, are reported to type as Ag-B1 or Ag-B3 serologically but show a high immune response to GLT instead of being low responders (Kunz et al. 1975).

Each H-1 haplotype shows an individual response pattern and, with the exception of Pro—L/(T,G)-Pro—L, each antigen shows a distinct distribution pattern of high, intermediate, or low responsiveness. These data point to a high degree of specificity of Ir gene control and presumably to a great number of different Ir genes. Specificity of Ir gene control is also demonstrated by the findings that the D-isomer of GLT is not immunogenic (Kunz and Gill 1974b) or that the anti-LDH_B response pattern is different from that of LDH_A (Würzburg et al. 1973). However, in spite of the high discriminating power of Ir gene control cross-reactivity can occur. (T,G)-A—L primed lymphocytes could be stimulated *in vivo* (helper function) and *in vitro* (anamnestic response) by (Phe,G)-A—L, but not by (H,G)-A—L, whereas (Phe,G)-A—L primed cells could not be stimulated by (T,G)-A—L (Günther and

Table 6.10. Immune Response Patterns of 11 H-1 Haplotypes[a] to Antigens of Table 6.9

H-1	Ag-B	(T,G)-A – L	(H,G)-A – L	(Phe,G)-A – L	T_6-A – L	T_4-A – L	(T,G)-Pro – L	(Phe,G)-Pro – L	Pro – L	$G_{52}L_{33}T_{15}$[b]	$G_{50}A_{50}$[b]	$G_{50}T_{50}$[b]	$(T_{25}G_{25}A_{25}Gly_{25})_n$[b]	LDH-A_4[b]	Bovine Insulin	Pig Insulin
a	4	H	L	H	H	H	L	H	L	H	L	H	H	L		
b	6	L	L				H			L	H	L	L	H		
c	5	MH	H	H			M			H	H	H	H	H		
d		L	L	H	L	L	M	MH	LM			H		H		
e		L	H	H			L							H		
f		LM	L	H	L		H	H	H			H		H	L	L
h							n.t.[c]									
l	1	L	M	H	L		M			L	H	L	M/L	H	L	L
n	3	L	L	L	L		M	M	M	L	L	L	L	H	H	H
w	2	L	H	L	L		M	M	M	M	H	L	H	H		H
	7									L						
	8									L						

[a] Congenic strains on Lewis genetic background used with exception of H-1[c], H-1[e].
[b] Not the same strains used as for the other antigens. GLT data have been confirmed by use of H-1[w], H-1[n] congenic strains. LDH-A_4 data for H-1[a], H-1[d] have been confirmed by use of congenic strains.
[c] Not tested.

References: (T,G)-A – L: Günther et al. 1972; (H,G)-A – L, (Phe,G)-A – L: Günther et al. 1973; T_6-A – L, T_4-A – L: Rüde and Günther 1974 and unpublished, (T,G)-Pro – L, (Phe,G)-Pro – L, Pro – L: Günther et al. 1976; GLT: Kunz et al. 1974; GA, GT: Armerding et al. 1974a, data for H-1[d], H-1[f] own unpublished results; $(TGAGly)_n$: Luderer et al. 1976; LDH-A_4: Würzburg 1971; bovine, pig insulins: Günther and Keck, *unpublished data.*

Rüde 1976). Thus unilateral cross-reactivity was observed between the two synthetic branched polypeptides under separate control, (T,G)-A – L and (Phe,G)-A – L, at the cellular level of Ir gene control. (It must be noted that cross-reactivity at the antibody level is a very common phenomenon of antigens under different Ir gene control.)

Intermediate anti-(H,G)-A – L responsiveness of the H-1[l] haplotype has been found to be complemented genetically to high responsiveness by the low responder H-1[n] and H-1[d] haplotypes, but not by the low responder H-1[a] and H-1[f] haplotypes (Günther and Rüde 1975). This demonstrates that overdominant responsiveness can occur and that H-1-controlled low responsiveness to (H,G)-A – L is genetically heterogeneous. Most probably, complementation is due to separate genes and is not interallelic. Thus, high responsiveness to antigens as listed in Table 6.9 might not reflect the action of one gene but that of several interacting, not simply additive, H-1-linked Ir genes.

No proven recombination between the genes that determine the serologically detectable H-1 antigens on red blood cells and Ir genes has been reported among more than 400 segregating hybrids tested (Würzburg 1971; Günther et al. 1972, 1975; Kunz et al. 1974; Armerding et al. 1974b; Shonnard et al. 1976). Recently, however, a $(LEW.1A \times LEW.1W)F_2$ hybrid has been analyzed which typed like a heterozygote in hemagglutination tests, but which was a low responder to (T,G)-A–L and (Phe,G)-A–L like the LEW.1W parent and unlike the LEW.1A parent. In addition the MLR phenotype was that of LEW.1W rats (Štark et al. 1977)

H-1-linked Ir genes have been studied in two nonisohistogenic rat populations, NBR/Cr (Kunz et al. 1974) and Wistar/Han (Günther et al. 1975). In both, only two different H-1 haplotypes have been identified serologically by hemagglutination tests. These were indistinguishable from previously known H-1 haplotypes of inbred reference strains. Interestingly, the association of high responsiveness to GLT of NBR rats and to (H,G)-A–L of Wistar rats was the same for each of 81 rats as that expected from responsiveness of the inbred reference strains.

When wild rats, (wild rat × LEW) hybrids, and progeny from backcrossing these hybrids to LEW rats were tested for anti-(T,G)-A–L responsiveness (Günther, *unpublished data*), high and low responders could be detected. Responsiveness was found to be H-1 controlled, some wild rat H-1 haplotypes being associated with the high-responder Ir-(T,G)-A–L allele, others with the low-responder allele.

Immune responsiveness to (T,G)-A–L, (H,G)-A–L, (Phe,G)-A–L, GA, GT, bovine, and pig insulins is controlled by MHS-linked Ir genes in other species also, notably in mouse and guinea pig. Although this is the reason that most antigens have been tested in the rat, the results nevertheless underscore the close homology among H-2-, GPL-A (2/13)-, and H-1-linked Ir genes in the respective rodent species.

It must be noted in this context that anti-Pro–L responsiveness is controlled by MHS-linked Ir genes in the rat (Günther et al. 1976, Table 6.10), whereas in mice anti-Pro–L responsiveness is reported to be controlled by the Ir-3 locus which is neither MHS nor heavy chain allotype-linked (Mozes et al. 1969).

In order to study the actual antigenic determinants in the synthetic branched polypeptide (T,G)-A–L that are under H-1 linked Ir gene control, chemical analogues have been synthesized. These antigens carry oligopeptides of defined numbers of tyrosine residues or of defined sequences of tyrosine and glutamic acid residues at the ends of the DL-alanine side chains. They are abbreviated as T_6-A–L, T_5-A–L, T_4-A–L, T_3-A–L, T_2-A–L, T-A–L, GT-A–L, and T_2G_2-A–L (Rüde and Günther 1974, *unpublished results*). The (T,G)-A–L high responder H-1 congenic rat strain, carrying the $H\text{-}1^a$ haplotype, responded only to the first three of the above mentioned (T,G)-A–L analogous antigens, whereas (T,G)-A–L low responders did not respond to any of them. This indicated that oligopeptides consisting of 4 to 6 tyrosines might be involved in molding the antigenic determinant of (T,G)-A–L that confers genetic control of immune responsiveness. The same antigens were tested in H-2 congenic mice (Rüde and Günther 1974, *unpublished results*). In this case, however the (T,G)-A – L high responder H-2^b haplotype was associated with high responsiveness to the whole series of the above antigens. Therefore, either the specificity of the anti-(T,G)-A – L high responder gene is different in mice and rats, or a set of separate Ir gene loci, having different allelic compositions in the H-2^b and H-1^a haplotypes, control responsiveness to the series of (T,G)-A – L analogues. The latter explanation might imply that there is not merely *one* determinant in the (T,G)-A – L molecule that is responsible for the Ir gene control of immune responsiveness to this polypeptide.

All data available on the function of H-1-linked Ir genes agree that low responsiveness is not caused by unavailability of antigen-specific B cells and lead to similar conclusions as in mice and guinea pigs, i.e. that Ir gene control affects T cell function or T-B-macrophage cooperation (Würzburg et al. 1973; Rüde and Günther 1974).

For many antigens that are under H-1 linked Ir gene control evidence is available that genes of the genetic background are involved in quantitatively controlling the response. Thus, different H-1 (serologically) identical strains that were high responders for a given antigen did not produce equal amounts of antibodies. For the anti-GLT response a second, non-H-1-linked gene has been postulated in order to explain the quantitative differences in the antibody response of segregating (high × low responder) hybrids (Gill and Kunz 1971). A similar result has been reported for anti-$(TGAGly)_n$ responsiveness (Luderer et al., 1976). Involvement of genes that are not linked to the H-1 system has also been postulated for the control of anti-(T,G)-A – L responsiveness (Koch 1974).

A type of genetic control of immune responsiveness that presumably differs from that described is represented by the antibody response to streptococcal group A carbohydrate (Stankus and Leslie 1974, 1975, 1976). Strain differences have been described with respect to the fraction of responding rats and with respect to the frequency of a certain idiotype among the antibodies produced. The idiotypic cross-reactivity between the antistreptococcal carbohydrate antibodies of different individuals, even when belonging to different strains, was remarkably high. Among outbred rats individuals could be found that produced extremely high amounts of antibodies with a restricted degree of heterogeneity. From the data and by analogy to results obtained in rabbits and mice, it can be concluded that this type of genetic control of immune responsiveness may not be associated with the H-1 system but with immunoglobulin allotypes.

Tada et al. (1974, 1976) have described a gene controlling the antibody response against sheep red blood cells which is not H-1 linked and which is expressed in macrophages.

It should be mentioned that the differences that have been observed for MLR and mitogen responsiveness between BN and LEW rats are not controlled by H-1 linked genes (Newlin and Gasser 1973; Williams et al. 1973).

8. The H-1 System and Disease Susceptibility

Susceptibility to a great number of diseases has been shown in man to be associated with the HLA system (Svejgaard et al. 1975). This correlation is assumed to be due to hypothetical disease susceptibility genes that are linked to the HLA genes and found in linkage disequilibrium with certain HLA-A, B, C, D genes at the population level. Experimental animals such as the rat can provide models in order to test the relationship between MHS and disease susceptibility.

Elicitation of two experimental diseases of the rat has so far been shown to be H-1 controlled: experimental allergic encephalomyelitis (EAE) and autoimmune complex nephritis (AIC).

EAE has been elicited with basic protein (Williams and Moore 1973) or spinal cord (Gasser et al. 1973a) from guinea pigs emulsified in Mycobacterium-enriched, complete Freund's adjuvant. Rats of the inbred strain BN (H-1^n) were resistent, whereas LEW (H-1^l) inbred rats and the corresponding F_1 hyprids were susceptible. One gene was found to determine susceptibility in BN × (LEW × BN) backcross hybrids segregating together with the H-1^l haplotype. Among the 68 backcross rats, seven H-1 heterozygotes were exceptional in being resistant. This could either be caused by incomplete penetrance of the EAE gene or could indicate a 10 percent recombination frequency between H-1 and EAE genes (Gasser et al. 1973a; Williams and Moore 1973). Rats that carried the H-1^n gene region on LEW-strain genetic background (congenic strain LEW.1N) were found to be susceptible to EAE induction, although usually less so than Lewis rats (Günther et al. 1975). It is noteworthy that in the DA and BN rat strain combination, segregation tests failed to show a clear association between the H-1 system and EAE susceptibility (Gasser et al. 1975). By use of special immunization procedures (rat spinal cord, carbonyl iron as adjuvant), EAE could also be induced in BN rats (Levine and Sowinski 1975). Strain differences in EAE susceptibility were also described by Hughes and Stedronska (1973).

Autoimmune complex nephritis (AIC) has been elicited by tubular epithelial antigen emulsified in complete Freund's adjuvant (Stenglein et al. 1975). In this case, BN rats were again resistent and LEW rats and F_1 hybrids susceptible. Association with the H-1 system was shown by segregation studies and the differential behavior of H-1-congenic strains. LEW.1N rats were poorly susceptible. The behavior of backcross hybrids, however, also revealed that genetic background genes were involved in controlling susceptibility to AIC (Stenglein, Thoenes, Günther, *unpublished data*).

Both diseases are interpretated as autoimmune. Ir genes controlling immune responsiveness to the basic protein or the tubular antigens could be invoked to play a major role in determining resistance or susceptibility. As such a complex phenomenon as a disease is studied, however, genetic control might also turn out to be complex.

The occurence of anti-glomerular basement antibodies in $HgCl_2$ treated rats has been shown to be H-1 dependent (Druet, *personal communication*),

BN rats developing such antibodies and LEW rats failing to do so. Segregation studies indicated that only few genes were involved one being H-1 linked.

There are reports on strain differences for inducibility of thyroiditis by rat thyroid extracts (Rose 1975; Penhale et al. 1975); in contrast to the mouse (Vladutiu and Rose 1971), association between disease susceptibility and MHS has not yet been established in the rat.

9. Effect of the H-1 System on Fetal-Maternal Interactions

If the H-1 system is involved in maternal-fetal interactions, this might have consequences for the structure of its polymorphism and might suggest the action of natural selection on this polymorphism. Michie and Anderson (1966) reported that in a rat strain tested for isohistogeneity after brother-sister mating for 72 generations, segregation for a strong histocompatibility system still occurred. There was a strong selection against both types of homozygotes, one class still being eliminated before implantation. Thus, selective advantage was observed of rats that were heterozygous at the histocompatibility locus under test. It should be noted that skin graft survival was 14.6 days when rejection occurred among rats of this strain. This acute type of rejection need not necessarily mean that the segregating histocompatibility alleles belong to the H-1 system. As these rats were not available later on, this question could not be answered. Palm favored the interpretation that a non-H-1 system was involved (Palm 1970a) and termed it Ag-E (Palm and Black 1971; see Table 6.1).

Commitment of the H-1 system in fetal-maternal interactions was described by Palm (1970a). Among the progeny from BN♀ × (BN × DA)F_1 and DA♀ × (BN × DA)F_1 matings—and not from the reciprocal matings—a disproportionately high number of H-1 heterozygotes occurred, whereas an excessive number of (male) homozygotes died postnatally from wasting disease. This effect was especially pronounced under adverse environmental conditions. It was suggested that in the strain combinations used, a GvH reaction against non-H-1 antigens was induced in the fetuses by maternal cells and that H-1 incompatibility of the fetus to the mother protected the fetus from the GvH reaction. Support for this interpretation comes from data reported by Beer et al. (1972). Thus, H-1 polymorphism may be under control of natural selection that favors H-1 heterozygotes.

A further argument in favor of selective advantage of H-1 heterozygotes has been presented by the following results (Beer et al. 1975): Litter size, weight of fetuses, and weight of placentas were increased in progeny derived from H-1-incompatible matings (rat strains LEW, DA, BN) as compared to isogeneic matings. These effects had an immunological basis and reflected the (beneficial) maternal immune response in paraaortic lymph nodes against foreign fetal alloantigens. The effect was not due to hybrid vigor of the heterozygous embryos. Whether it is predominantly exerted in H-1-incompatible situations or is also found in non-H-1-incompatible matings remains to be established.

10. Genetic Structure of the H-1 Chromosome

The H-1 genes have not yet been assigned to one of the five established linkage groups (Robinson 1972; Gasser et al. 1973b) and form the provisional linkage group VI. Thus, there is no linkage to the coat color genes A-a (agouti), B-b (brown), C-c (albinism), H-h (hooded), and P-p (pink eyed, yellow) (Palm 1963; Štark et al. 1969b). Also, the H-1 genes have not yet been assigned to an individual chromosome. Because of homologies between the Giemsa banding patterns of mouse and rat chromosomes, it was proposed that chromosome 14 might carry the MHS genes in the rat (Nesbitt 1974).

The genetic fine structure of the H-1 system is still poorly understood. Recombinant H-1 haplotypes that are derived from known parental H-1 haplotypes have been described (Williams and Moore 1976; Štark et al. 1977). These recombinants show that MLR and Ir genes are separable from genes determining H-1 hemagglutinogens and skin graft rejection. Thus the MHS of the rat is determined by a gene complex as is true for other species. So far, however, we do not know whether there is more than one locus determining the serologically detectable H-1 antigens and—if there are two—whether MLR and Ir genes map inside as in the mouse or outside as in the rhesus monkey.

One argument against a complex structure of the H-1 system (Palm and Wilson 1973) was that the rat appears to show no T/t system polymorphism at least as far as being expressed in tail abnormalities. Thousands of wild and laboratory rats have been screened for genes determining taillessness (Dunn et al. 1942, summary of the results by Robinson 1965, pp. 223–227).

Since the T/t system and its polymorphism could have a decisive influence on the genetic structure of the H-2 system in the mouse (Snell 1968; Artzt and Bennett 1975; Hammerberg and Klein 1975), differences in the T/t systems in different species or absence (loss) of the T/t system could have important consequences for the genetic fine structure of the MHS.

The genetic mapping of the Ss-Slp traits inside the H-2 system in the mouse has played a decisive role in establishing the genetic fine structure of the H-2 system. Unfortunately no polymorphism similar to that of the Ss system has been found in the rat. Antimouse Ss antisera cross-react with rat serum (Borovská et al. 1971).

Because the Ss protein is identified as the fourth complement component in the mouse (Meo et al. 1975; Curman et al. 1975; Lachmann et al. 1975) and because linkage between MHS genes and genes controlling the structure or the amount of other complement components of the classical or alternative pathway has been established in several species, it would be interesting to look for a similar genetic relationship in the H-1 system.

There is also no report about a Tla analogous system in the rat. Outside isoenzyme markers such as PGM_3 and glyoxalase (GLO) have not yet been described for the H-1 system both being shown to be on the HLA chromosome in man (Lamm et al. 1971; Mayr et al. 1976). Typing of 17 inbred rat strains and 6 wild rat-derived families have failed to detect GLO polymorphism in rats (Bender and Günther, *unpublished results*).

11. Biochemistry of H-1 Antigens

H-1 antigens have been extracted from lymphoid cells by 3 M KCl and further purified (Stroehmann and DeWitt 1972a, 1972b; Callahan and DeWitt 1975). A molecular weight of 30,000 to 35,000 daltons was determined by SDS-gel electrophoresis (Callahan and DeWitt 1975). In another study H-1 antigens were partially purified from papain digests of liver cell membranes (Katagiri et al. 1975a, 1975b). H-1 specificity was found in 25,000-, 35,000-, and 59,000-dalton molecules. The latter consisted of two noncovalently bound fragments: one (37,000 daltons) carried H-1 activity, the other (11,000 daltons) lacked it and was identified as β_2-microglobulin (cross-reactive with that of man and mouse).

A similar two-component structure is also found for HLA and H-2 antigens and points to a close homology of MHS antigens of different species at the biochemical level.

12. Concluding Remarks

The H-1 system is beyond doubt functionally homologous to the MHS of other vertebrate species, notably to that of the mouse. The data on H-1 recombinants show that there is genetic homology too and that the H-1 system is determined by a gene complex. Several of the MHS-controlled functions and structures have already been assigned to distinct MHS genes in other species and are therefore expected to be determined by separate genes of the H-1 system in the rat. It is an interesting question whether the sequence of MHS constituting genes is functionally important or whether gene rearrangements are of minor significance. If the latter is true, the genetic fine structure of the H-1 system may differ from that worked out for the H-2 system of the mouse, the RhL-A system of the rhesus monkey, or the HLA system of man. Striking examples of the homology between the H-1 and H-2 systems (and also the MHS of other species) are found for the Ir genes and for the biochemical structure of MHS antigens. Serological cross-reactions of rat congenic anti-H-1 antisera with human lymphocytes of different HLA phenotypes and a clear anti-H-1 activity of rat antisera obtained after immunization of LEW rats with human lymphocytes of different HLA phenotypes (Křen et al. 1976; Sachs and Křen 1976) may point to a common ancestral gene product of vertebrate MHS masked by following evolutionary changes.

Further knowledge of the existence and structure of a T/t system in the rat could throw new light on the homology between the H-1 and H-2 systems. Although the homology between the H-1 system and the MHS of other species, especially that of the mouse, has been stressed, it must nevertheless be kept in mind that the divergence of mouse and rat at the molecular level is apparently rather great, as pointed out in the Introduction.

The biological significance of MHS and the mechanism(s) of how such polymorphisms are generated and maintained during evolution are not yet well understood. Some findings in the rat may be used as arguments in favor of natural selection acting on MHS and modeling its polymorphism. Thus, there is complementation of H-1-linked Ir genes and occurrence of overdominance in Ir gene-controlled immune responsiveness. Furthermore, maternal/fetal interactions have been described that would favor H-1 heterozygous progeny.

Further studies on the H-1 system are urgently needed in order to elucidate its genetic fine structure. Such data will help to understand better both evolution and immunogenetic structure of MHS in general.

References

Aizawa, M., Itakura, K., and Katagiri, H. Serologic studies on the histocompatibility hemagglutinogen R-factor of the rat. *Jap. J. Transplants.* *1*:82, 1965.

Andersson, L.C., Binz, H., and Wigzell, H. Specific unresponsiveness to transplantation antigens induced by auto-immunization with syngeneic, antigen-specific T lymphoblasts. *Nature* *264*:778–780, 1976.

Armerding, D., Katz, D. H., and Benacerraf, B. Immune response genes in inbred rats. I. Analysis of responder status to synthetic polypeptides and low doses of bovine serum albumin. *Immunogenetics* *1*:329–339, 1974a.

Armerding, D., Katz, D. H., and Benacerraf, B. Immune response genes in inbred rats. II. Segregation studies of the GT and GA genes and their linkage to the major histocompatibility locus. *Immunogenetics* *1*:340–351, 1974b.

Arnason, B. G., Janković, B. D., Waksman, B. H., and Wennersten, C. Role of the thymus in immune reactions in rats. II. Suppressive effect of thymectomy at birth on reactions of delayed (cellular) hypersensitivity and the circulating small lymphocyte. *J. Exp. Med.* *116*:177–186, 1962.

Artzt, K., and Bennett, D. Analogies between embryonic (T/t) antigens and adult major histocompatibility (H-2) antigens. *Nature* *256*:545–547, 1975.

Bansal, S. C., Hellström, I., Hellström, K. E., and Wright, P. W. Cell-mediated immunity and blocking serum activity before and after breakage of allograft tolerance in rats. *Transplantation* *16*:610–620, 1973a.

Bansal, S. C., Hellström, K. E., Hellström, I., and Sjögren, H. O. Cell-mediated immunity and blocking serum activity to tolerated allografts in rats. *J. Exp. Med.* *137*:590–602, 1973b.

Barker, C. F., and Billingham, R. E. Comparison of fates of Ag-B locus compatible homografts of skin and hearts in inbred rats. *Nature* *225*:851–852, 1970.

Beer, A. E., Billingham, R. E., and Yang, S. L. Maternally induced transplantation immunity, tolerance, and runt disease in rats. *J. Exp. Med.* *135*:808–826, 1972.

Beer, A. E., Scott, J. R., and Billingham, R. E. Histocompatibility and maternal immunological status as determinants of fetoplacental weight and litter size in rodents. *J. Exp. Med. 142*:180–196, 1975.

Benacerraf, B., and Katz, D. H. The nature and function of histocompatibility-linked immune response genes. In B. Benacerraf (ed.), Immunogenetics and Immunodeficiency, pp. 117–177, Medical and Technical Publishing Co., St. Leonard's House, Lancaster, 1975.

Bernstein, I. D., and Wright, P. W. Generation of cytotoxic lymphocytes in mixed leukocyte culture by rat lymphoid cells. *Transplantation 21*:173–178, 1976.

Bildsøe, P., Sørensen, S. F., Petirossi, O., and Simonsen, M. Heart and kidney transplantation from segregating hybrid to parental rats. *Transplant. Rev. 3*:36–45, 1970.

Bildsøe, P. Organ transplantation in the rat. The importance of the Ag-B (or H-1) locus. *Acta Pathol. Microbiol. Scand.* (Section B) *80*:221–230, 1972.

Billingham, R. E., Brent, L., and Medawar, P. B. Quantitative studies on tissue transplantation immunity. III. Actively acquired tolerance. *Phil. Trans. Soc. London* (B) *239*:357–414, 1956.

Billingham, R. E., Defendi, V., Silvers, W. R., and Steinmuller, D. Quantitative studies on the induction of tolerance of skin homografts and on runt disease in neonatal rats. *J. Nat. Cancer Inst. 28*:365–435, 1962a.

Billingham, R. E., Hodge, B. A., and Silvers, W. K. An estimate of the number of histocompatibility loci in the rat. *Proc. Natl. Acad. Sci.* (USA) *48*:138–147, 1962b.

Binz, H., and Askonas, B. A. Inhibition of mixed leukocyte culture by anti-idiotypic antibodies. *Eur. J. Immunol. 5*:618–623, 1975.

Binz, H., Lindenmann, J., and Wigzell, H. Inhibition of local graft-versus-host reaction by anti-alloantibodies. *Nature 246*:146–148, 1973.

Binz, H., Lindenmann, J., and Wigzell, H. Cell-bound receptors for alloantigens on normal lymphocytes. II. Anti-alloantibody serum contains specific factors reacting with relevant immunocompetent T lymphocytes. *J. Exp. Med. 140*:731–741, 1974.

Binz, H., and Wigzell, H. Shared idiotypic determinants on B and T lymphocytes reactive against the same antigenic determinants. I. Demonstration of similar or identical idiotypes on IgG molecules and T cell receptors with specificity for the same alloantigens. *J. Exp. Med. 142*:197–211, 1975a.

Binz, H., and Wigzell, H. Shared idiotypic determinants on B and T lymphocytes reactive against the same antigenic determinants. II. Determination of frequency and characteristics of idiotypic T and B lymphocytes in normal rats using direct visualization. *J. Exp. Med. 142*:1218–1230, 1975b.

Binz, H., and Wigzell, H. Shared idiotypic determinants on B and T lymphocytes reactive against the same antigenic determinants. III. Physical fractionation of specific immunocompetent T lymphocytes by affinity chromatography using anti-idiotypic antibodies. *J. Exp. Med. 142*:1231–1240, 1975c.

Binz, H., and Wigzell, H. Shared idiotypic determinants on B and T lymphocytes reactive against the same antigenic determinants. IV. Isolation of two groups of naturally occuring, idiotypic molecules with specific antigen-binding activity in the serum and urine of normal rats. *Scand. J. Immunol. 4*:591–600, 1975d.

Binz, H., and Wigzell, H. Specific transplantation tolerance induced by autoimmunization against the individual's own naturally occuring idiotypic, antigen-binding receptors. *J. Exp. Med. 144*:1438–1457, 1976.

Binz, H., Wigzell, H., and Bazin, H. T-cell idiotypes are linked to immunoglobulin heavy chain genes. *Nature 264*:639–642, 1976.

Bitter-Suermann, H. Survival of unmodified spleen allografts in rats. *Nature 147*:465–466, 1974a.

Bitter-Suermann, H. Different ways of using graft-versus-host reactivities to achieve acceptance of rat spleen allografts in the same donor-recipient pairing. *Transplantation 18*:515–519, 1974b.

Bogden, A. E., and Aptekman, P. M. The "R-1" factor a histocompatibility antigen in the rat. *Cancer Res. 20*:1272–1282, 1960.

Borovská, M., Kořínek, J., Václavíková, I., and Démant, P. Ss protein: Search for cross-reacting substances in different species. *Folia biol. (Praha) 17*:283–285, 1971.

Bruce, J., Golstein, P., and Mitchison, N. A. Allogenic cytotoxic response by rat cells in vitro. *Transplantation 20*:88–92, 1975.

Burhoe, S. O. Blood groups of the rat *(Rattus norvegicus)* and their inheritance. *Proc. Natl. Acad. Sci. (USA) 33*:102–109, 1947.

Callahan, G. N., and DeWitt, C. W. Rat cell surface antigens. I. Isolation and partial characterization of an Ag-B antigen. *J. Immunol. 114*:776–778, 1975.

Colley, D. G., and DeWitt, C. W. Mixed lymphocyte blastogenesis in response to multiple histocompatibility antigens. *J. Immunol. 102*:107–116, 1969.

Committee for a Standardized Karyotype of *Rattus norvegicus*. Standard karyotype of the Norway rat, *Rattus norvegicus. Cytogenet. Cell. Genet. 12*:199–205, 1973.

Cramer, D. V., Shonnard, J. W., and Gill, T. J., III. Genetic studies in inbred rats. II. Relationship between the major histocompatibility complex and mixed lymphocyte reactivity. *J. Immunogenet. 1*:421–428, 1974.

Cramer, D. V., Shonnard, J. W., Davis, B. K., and Gill, T. J., III. Polymorphism of the mixed lymphocyte response of wild norway rats. *Transplant. Proc. 9*:559–562, 1977.

Curman, B., Östberg, L., Sandberg, L., Malmheden-Eriksson, I., Stalenheim, G., Rask, L., and Peterson, P. H-2 linked Ss protein is C4 component of complement. *Nature 258*:243–245, 1975.

Davies, D. A. L., and Alkins, B. J. What abrogates heart transplant rejection in immunological enhancement? *Nature 247*:294–297 (1974).

Davies, D. A. L., and Hess, M. Isolation and partial characterization of a new alloantigen genetically linked to the major histocompatibility locus of the mouse. *Nature 250*:228–230, 1974.

DeWitt, C. W., and McCullough, M. Ag-F: Serological and genetic identification of a new locus in the rat governing lymphocyte membrane antigens. *Transplantation 19*:310–317, 1975.

Dorf, M. E., Balner, H., and Benacerraf, B. Mapping of the immune response genes in the major histocompatibility complex of the rhesus monkey. *J. Exp. Med. 142*:673–693, 1975.

Dorsch, S., and Roser, B. The clonal nature of allo-antigen-sensitive small lymphocytes in the recirculating pool of normal rats. *Aust. J. Exp. Biol. Med. Sci. 52*:45–66, 1974.

Dunn, L. C., Gluecksohn-Schoenheimer, S., Curtis, M. R., and Dunning, W. F. Heredity and accident as factors in the production of taillessness in the rat. *J. Hered. 33*:65–67, 1942.

Elkins, W. L. Invasion and destruction of homologous kidney by locally inoculated lymphoid cells. *J. Exp. Med. 120*:329–347, 1964.

Elkins, W. L., Hellström, I., and Hellström, K. E. Transplantation tolerance and enhancement. Concepts and questions. *Transplantation 18*:38–45, 1974.

Elkins, W. L., and Palm, J. Identification of a single strong histocompatibility locus in the rat by normal spleen-cell transfer. *Ann. N.Y. Acad. Sci. 129*:573–580, 1966.

Elves, M. W. The mixed lymphocyte reaction in inbred strains of rats. *Vox Sang. 13*:7–11, 1967.

Elves, M. W. The mixed leucocyte reaction. II. A comparison of the MLR with skin graft survival and serological methods of detecting H-antigens using F_2 generation rats. *Transplantation 8*:757–762, 1969.

Fabre, J. W., and Morris, P. J. Passive enhancement of homozygous renal allografts in the rat. *Transplantation 18*:429–435, 1974a.

Fabre, J. W., and Morris, P. J. Passive enhancement of rat renal allografts with only partial cover of the incompatible Ag-B specificities. *Transplantation 18*:436–442, 1974b.

Fabre, J. W., and Morris, P. J. The definition of a lymphocyte-specific alloantigen system in the rat (Ly-1). *Tissue Antigens 4*:238–246, 1974c.

Fabre, J. W., and Morris, P. J. Studies on the specific suppression of renal allograft rejection in presensitized rats. Theoretical and clinical implications. *Transplantation 19*:121–133, 1975.

Feldman, J. D., Pick, E., Lee, S., Silvers, W. K., and Wilson, D. C. Renal homotransplantation in rats. II. Tolerant recipients. *Am. J. Pathol. 52*:687–700, 1968.

Festenstein, H. Immunogenetic and biological aspects of in vitro lymphocyte allotransformation (MLR) in the mouse. *Transplant. Proc. 15*:62–88, 1973.

Festing, M. W. F., and Butler, W. *International Index of Laboratory Animals.* Medical Research Council, Laboratory Animals Center, Carshalton, UK, 1975.

Festing, M. F. W., and Staats, J. Standardized nomenclature of inbred strains of rats. Fourth listing. *Transplantation 16*:221–245, 1973.

Ford, W. L. A local graft-versus-host reaction following intradermal injection of lymphocytes in the rat. *Br. J. Exp. Pathol. 48*:335–345, 1967.

Ford, W. L. Lymphoid cell kinetics in graft-versus-host reactions and allograft rejection. In R. Calne (ed.), *Immunological Aspects of Transplantation surgery*, pp. 39–66, Medical and Technical Publishing Co. St. Leonard's House, Lancaster, 1973.

Ford, W. L., and Atkins, R. C. Specific unresponsiveness of recirculating lymphocytes after exposure to histocompatibility antigen in F1 hybrid rats. *Nature New Biol. 234*:178–180, 1971.

Ford, W. L., Burr, W., and Simonsen, M. A lymph node weight assay for the graft-versus-host activity of rat lymphoid cells. *Transplantation 10*:258–266, 1970.

Ford, W. L., Simmonds, S. J., and Atkins, R. C. Early cellular events in a systemic graft-versus-host reaction. II. Autoradiographic estimates of the frequency of donor lymphocytes which respond to each Ag-B-determined antigenic complex. *J. Exp. Med. 141*:681–696, 1975.

Ford, W. L., and Simonsen, M. The factor of immunization in the rat. The effect of allogeneic immunization on graft-versus-host activity. *J. Exp. Med. 133*:938–949, 1971.

Freeman, J. S., and Steinmuller, D. Acute rejection of skin and heart allografts in rats matched at the major histocompatibility locus. *Transplantation 8*:530–533, 1969.

Frelinger, J. A., Niederhuber, J. E., David, C. S., and Shreffler, D. C. Evidence for the expression of Ia (H-2-associated) antigens on thymus-derived lymphocytes. *J. Exp. Med. 140*:1273–1284, 1974.

Frelinger, J. A., and Shreffler, D. C. The major histocompatibility complexes. In B. Benacerraf (ed.), *Immunogenetics and Immunodeficiency*, pp. 81–116, Medical and Technical Publishing Co., St. Leonhard's House, Lancaster, 1975.

French, M. E., and Batchelor, J. R. Immunological enhancement of rat kidney grafts. *Lancet ii*:1103–1106, 1969.

French, M. E., and Batchelor, J. R. Enhancement of renal allografts in rats and man. *Transplant. Rev. 13*:115–141, 1972.

Gasser, D. L., Newlin, C. M., Palm, J., and Gonatas, N. K. Genetic control of susceptibility to experimental allergic encephalomyelitis in rats. *Science 181*:872–873, 1973a.

Gasser, D. L., Palm, J., and Gonatas, N. K. Genetic control of susceptibility to experimental allergic encephalomyelitis and the Ag-B locus of rats. *J. Immunol. 115*:431–433, 1975.

Gasser, D. L., and Silvers, W. K. Genetic determinants of immunological responsiveness. *Adv. Immunol. 18*:1–66, 1974.

Gasser, D. L., Silvers, W. K., Reynolds, H. M., Jr., Black, G., and Palm, J. Serum esterase genetics in rats: Two new alleles at Es-2, a new esterase regulated by hormonal factors, and linkage of these loci to the Ag-C blood group locus. *Biochem. Genet. 10*:207–217, 1973b.

Gill, T. J., III, and Kunz, H. W. Genetic and cellular factors in the immune response. II. Evidence for the polygenic control of the antibody response from further breeding studies and from pedigree analyses. *J. Immunol. 106*:980–992, 1971.

Gill, T. J., III, and Kunz, H. W. Genetic studies in inbred rats. VII. Tentative model for the major histocompatibility complex. *J. Immunogenetics 3*:139–143, 1976.

Gill, T. J., III, Kunz, H. W., Cramer, D. V., and Shonnard, J. Studies on the major histocompatibility complex of genetically inbred rats. In V. P. Eijsvoogel, D. Roos, W. P. Zeijlemaker (eds.), *Leukocyte Membrane Determinants Regulating Immune Reactivity*, p. 511, Academic Press, New York, 1976.

Gordon, R. O., Stinson, E. B., Souther, S. G., and Oppenheim, J. J. Inhibition of the mixed leukocyte reaction as an assay for enhancing alloantiserum. *Transplantation 12*:484–489, 1971.

Gorer, P. A., and Mikulska, Z. B. The antibody response to tumor inoculation: Improved methods of antibody detection. *Cancer Res. 14*: 651–655, 1954.

Gronemeyer, U., and Müller-Ruchholtz, W. Allogene Hornhauttransplantation bei Inzuchtratten, IV. Bedeutung des Histoinkompatibilitätsgrades zwischen Spender und Empfänger. *Albrecht von Graefes Arch. Klin. Ophthalmol. 190*:309–317, 1974.

Günther, E., and Bhakdi-Lehnen, B. Inhibition of rat lymphocyte function in vitro by alloantisera. In V. P. Eijsvoogel, D. Roos, W. P. Zeijlemaker (eds.), *Leukocyte Membrane Determinants Regulating Immune Reactivity*, pp. 405–414, Academic Press, New York, 1976.

Günther, E., Mozes, E., Rüde, E., and Sela, M. Genetic control of immune responsiveness to poly(LPro) – poly(LLys) derived polypeptides by histocompatibility-linked immune response genes in the rat. *J. Immunol. 117*:2047–2052, 1976.

Günther, E., Odenthal, H., and Wechsler, W. Immunogenetics of EAE in rats. International Workshop: *"Myelin Biology"*, Abstracts, pp. 101–105, 1975.

Günther, E., and Rüde, E. Genetic complementation of histocompatibility-linked Ir genes in the rat. *J. Immunol. 115*:1387–1393, 1975.

Günther, E., and Rüde, E. Cross-stimulation of antigens under separate histocompatibility-linked Ir gene control. *Immunogenetics 3*:261–269, 1976.

Günther, E., Rüde, E., and Hedrich, H.J. Complex structure of the major histocompatibility system of the rat. *Transplant. Proc. 7* (Suppl. 1):147–150, 1975.

Günther, E., Rüde, E., Meyer-Delius, M., and Štark, O. Immune response genes linked to the major histocompatibility system in the rat. *Transplant. Proc. 5*:1467–1469, 1973.

Günther, E., Rüde, E., and Štark, O. Antibody response in rats to the synthetic polypeptide (T,G)-A – L genetically linked to the major histocompatibility system. *Eur. J. Immunol. 2*:151–155, 1972.

Gutman, G. A., Loh, E., and Hood, L. Structure and regulation of immunoglobulins: Kappa allotypes in the rat have multiple amino acid differences in the constant region. *Proc. Natl. Acad. Sci. (USA) 72*:5046–5050, 1975.

Hammerberg, C., and Klein, J. Linkage disequilibrium between H-2 and t complexes in chromosome 17 of the mouse. *Nature 258*:296–299, 1975.

Hausman, S. J., and Palm, J. Variable expression of Ag-B and non-Ag-B histocompatibility antigens on cultured rat cells of different histological origin. *Transplantation 16*:313–324, 1973.

Heslop, B. F. Histocompatibility antigens in the rat: The AS2 strain in relation to the AS, BS and HS strains. *Aust. J. Exp. Biol. Med. Sci. 46*:479–491, 1968.

Heyner, S. The significance of the intercellular matrix in the survival of cartilage allografts. *Transplantation 8*:666–677, 1969.

Howard, J. C., and Scott, D.C. The identification of sera distinguishing marrow-derived and thymus-derived lymphocytes in the rat. *Immunology 27*:903–922, 1974.

Hughes, R. A. C., and Stedronska, J. The susceptibility of rat strains to experimental allergic encephalomyelitis. *Immunology 24*:879–884, 1973.

Ippolito, R. J., Mahoney, R. J., and Murray, I. M. Renal transplantation between histoincompatible rats. I. Acute rejection and prolonged survival of reciprocal renal allografts in immunocompetent rats. *Transplantation 14*:183–190, 1972.

Iványi, D. The role of the major histocompatibility system in tooth germ transplantation of the rat. *Transplantation 6*:594–597, 1968.

Iványi, P. Serological production of congenic lines in rats. *In Polymorphismes biochemiques des Animaux*, pp. 507–510, Ed. Inst. National de la Recherche Agronomique, Paris, 1967.

Jay, G. E., Jr. Genetic strains and stocks II. Rats. In W. J. Burdette (ed.), *Methodology in Mammalian Genetics*, pp. 104–111, Holden-Day, San Francisco, 1973.

Johnston, J. M., and Wilson, D. B. Origin of immunoreactive lymphocytes in rats. *Cell. Immunol. 1*:430–444, 1970.

Katagiri, M., Natori, T., Tanagaki, N., Kreiter, V. P., and Pressman, D. Papain-solubilized Ag-B antigens. I. Isolation and characterization of two components composing Ag-B antigens. *Transplantation 19*:230–239, 1975a.

Katagiri, M., Tanigaki, N., and Pressman, D. Papain-solubilized Ag-B-antigens. II. Characterization of small sized Ag-B molecules. *Transplantation 20*:135–141, 1975b.

Klein, J. *Biology of the mouse histocompatibility-2 complex*. Springer-Verlag, New York, 1975.

Koch, C. Inheritance in the rat of antibody response to two different determinants of (T,G)-A – L. *Immunogenetics 1*:118–125, 1974.

Kohne, D. E. Evolution of higher-organism DNA. *Quart. Rev. Biophys. 3*:327–375, 1970.

Křen, V. The major histocompatibility system (H-1) alleles of some british rat strains. *Transplantation 17*:148–152, 1974.

Křen, V., Brdička, R., and Štark, O. Erythrocyte and transplantation antigens in inbred strains of rats. VIII. The dynamics of 19S and 7S LEW anti-H-1 haemagglutinin production. *Folia biol. (Praha) 14*:274–285, 1968.

Křen, V., Křenová, D., and Štark, O. Runt syndrome incidence and skin graft tolerance in various interstrain combinations of rats differing at a single or multiple histocompatibility loci. *Folia Biol. (Praha) 16*:305–313, 1970.

Křen, V., Sachs, J. A., and Bishop, C. E. Studies on the homology between human and rat MHS. I. Allogeneic effect of xenogeneic rat antihuman immunization. *Folia Biol. (Praha) 22*:60–61, 1976.

Křen, V., Štark, O., Bíla, V., Frenzl, B., Křenová, D., and Kršiaková, M. Rat alloantigenic systems defined through congenic strain production. *Transplant. Proc. 5*:1463–1466, 1973.

Křen, V., Štark, O., and Křenová, D. Tolerance manifestation among inbred rat strains defined in the Rt H-1 antigens. I. Runt syndrome and skin graft tolerance. *Folia Biol. (Praha) 15*:188–196, 1969.

Křen, V., Veselý, P., Frenzl, B., and Štark, O. Inhibition of the runting syndrome in rats. *Folia biol. (Praha) 6*:333–341, 1960.

Křenová, D., Křen, V., and Štark, O. Properties of the rat tumour Fedex-WP during long-term cultivation in vitro. *Neoplasma 15*:379–392, 1967.

Křenová, D., Křen, V., and Štark, O. Properties of spontaneous rat mammary carcinoma CaM-LEW. II. Karyological characteristics and antigenic properties of CaM-LEW tumour, long-term passaged in vivo and in vitro. *Neoplasma 16*:523–530, 1969.

Křenová, D., Křen, V., and Štark, O. Properties of the sarcomas induced by Ferridextran Spofa in inbred rat strain AVN. II. The observation of $H\text{-}1^a$ and B 1 antigenicity of FEDEX-AVN/3 tumour following long term in vitro cultivation. *Neoplasma 17*:505–512, 1970a.

Křenová, D., Křen, V., and Štark, O. H-1 antigenicity of rat tumours after in vivo passage and in vitro cultivation. *In Proceedings of the XIth European Conference on Animal Blood Groups, Biochemistry and Polymorphism*, pp. 557–560. Ed. E.S.A.B.R., PWN-Polish Scient. Publ., Warsaw, 1970b.

Křenová, D., Křen, V., and Štark, O. The detection of alloantigens on rat tumour cells in vitro by membrane immunofluorescence. *Ann. Blood Groups Biochem. Genet.*, Suppl. 1; p. 85, 1972.

Kunz, H. W., and Gill, T. J., III. Genetic studies in inbred rats. I. Two new histocompatibility alleles. *J. Immunogenet. 1*:413–420, 1974a.

Kunz, H. W., and Gill, T. J., III. The effects of antigenic isomerism and antigenic aggregation on the antibody response in inbred rats. *J. Immunogenet. 1*:289–294, 1974b.

Kunz, H. W., Gill, T. J., III, and Borland, B. The genetic linkage of the immune response to poly ($Glu^{52}Lys^{33}Tyr^{15}$) to the major histocompatibility locus in inbred rats. *J. Immunogenet. 1*:277–287, 1974.

Kunz, H. W., Gill, T. J., III, Hansen, C. T., and Poloskey, P. E. Genetic studies in inbred rats. III. Histocompatibility type and immune response of some mutant stocks. *J. Immunogenet. 2*:51–54, 1975.

Lachmann, P. J., Grennan, D., Martin, A., and Démant, P. Identification of Ss protein as murine C4. *Nature 258*:242–243, 1975.

Laird, C. D., MacConaughty, B. L., and McCarthy, B. J. Rate of fixation of nucleotide substitutions in evolution. *Nature 224*:149–154, 1969.

Lamm, L. U., Svejgaard, A., and Kissmeyer-Nielsen, F. PGM_3-HL-A is another linkage in man. *Nature New Biol. 231*:109–110, 1971.

Larner, B. J., and Fitch, F. W. Inhibition of rat mixed lymphocyte culture by hyperimmune alloantiserum. Lack of correlation with allograft-enhancing activity. *Transplantation 16*:54–57, 1973.

Lee, S. An improved technique of renal transplantation in the rat. *Surgery 61*:771–773, 1967.

Lee, S., and Edgington, T. S. Heterotopic liver transplantation utilizing inbred rat strains. I. Characterization of allogeneic graft rejection and the effects of biliary obstruction and portal vein circulation on liver regeneration. *Am. J. Pathol. 52*:649–669, 1968.

Levine, S. Local and regional forms of a graft-versus-host disease in lymph nodes. *Transplantation 6*:799–802, 1968.

Levine, S., and Sowinski, R. Allergic encephalomyelitis in the reputedly resistant Brown Norway strain of rats. *J. Immunol. 114*:597–601, 1975.

Lubaroff, D. M. An alloantigenic marker on rat thymus and thymus-derived cells. *Transplant. Proc. 1*:115–118, 1973.

Lucas, Z. J., Markley, J., and Travis, M. Immunologic enhancement of renal allografts in the rat. I. Dissociation of graft survival and antibody response. *Fed. Proc. 29*:2041–2047, 1970.

Luderer, A. A., Maurer, P. H., and Woodland, R. T. Genetic control of the immune response in rats to the known sequential polypeptide (Tyr-Glu-Ala-Gly)$_n$. *J. Immunol. 117*:1079–1084, 1976

Mahabir, R. N., Guttman, R. D., and Lindquist, R. R. Renal transplantation in the inbred rat. X. A model of "weak histoincompatibility" by major locus matching. *Transplantation 8*:369–378, 1969.

Mayr, W. R., Mayr, D., Kömpf, J., Bissbort, S., and Ritter, H. Possible linkage of HL-A and GLO. *Human. Genet. 31*:241–242, 1976.

McKearn, T. J. Anti-receptor antiserum causes specific inhibition of reactivity to rat histocompatibility antigens. *Science 183*:94–96, 1974.

McKearn, T. J., Finnegan, A., Neu, M., Fitch, F. W., and Stuart, F. P. Suppression of rat renal allograft rejection by antibody against lymphocyte antigen receptors. *Surg. Forum 25*:263–265, 1974a.

McKearn, T. J., Hamada, Y., Stuart, F. P., and Fitch, F. W. Anti-receptor antibody and resistance to graft-versus-host disease. *Nature 251*:648–650, 1974b.

McKearn, T. J., Stuart, F. P., and Fitch, F. W. Anti-idiotypic antibody in rat transplantation immunity. I. Production of anti-idiotypic antibody in animals repeatedly immunized with alloantigens. *J. Immunol. 113*:1876–1882, 1974c.

Meo, T., Krasteff, T., and Shreffler, D. C. Immunochemical characterization of murine H-2 controlled Ss (serum substance) protein through identification of its homologue as the fourth component of complement. *Proc. Natl. Acad. Sci. (USA) 72*:4536–4540, 1975.

Michie, D., and Anderson, N. F. A strong selective effect associated with a histocompatibility gene in the rat. *Ann. N.Y. Acad. Sci. 129*:88–93, 1966.

Miller, C., and DeWitt, C. W. The effect of neonatal thymectomy on antibody responses to histocompatibility antigens in the rat. *Cell. Immunol. 13*:278–287, 1974.

Mitchell, M. S., Bove, J. R., and Calabresi, P. Simplified estimation of mouse isohemagglutinins by microassay. *Transplantation 7*:294–296, 1969.

Mozes, E., McDevitt, H. O., Jaton, J.-C., and Sela, M. The genetic control of antibody specificity. *J. Exp. Med. 130*:1263–1278, 1969.

Mullen, Y., and Hildemann, W. H. Kidney transplantation genetics and enhancement in rats. *Transplant. Proc. 3*:669–672, 1971.

Mullen, Y., and Hildemann, W. H. X- and Y-linked transplantation antigens in rats. *Transplantation 13*:521–529, 1972.

Nesbitt, M. N. Evolutionary relationships between rat and mouse chromosomes. *Chromosoma 46*:217–224, 1974.

Newlin, C. M., and Gasser, D. L. Genetic control of the in vitro responses of peripheral blood lymphocytes to phytohemagglutinin and concanavalin A. *J. Immunol. 110*:622–628, 1973.

Nowell, P. C., Finan, J. B., and Wilson, D. B. Proliferation in vitro of T lymphocytes reactive to histocompatibility alloantigens: a correction. *J. Exp. Med. 142*:230–235, 1975.

Owen, R. D. Earlier studies of blood groups in rats. *Ann. N.Y. Acad. Sci. 97*:37–42, 1962.

Palm, J. Current status of blood groups in rats. *Ann. N.Y. Acad. Sci. 97*:57–68, 1962.

Palm, J. Histocompatibility and linkage relationship of loci determining isoantigens of the rat. *Proceedings of the XIth International Congress on Genetics 1*:198, 1963.

Palm, J. Serological detection of histocompatibility antigens in two strains of rats. *Transplantation 2*:603–612, 1964.

Palm, J. Maternal-fetal interactions and histocompatibility antigen polymorphisms. *Transplant. Proc. 2*:162–173, 1970a.

Palm, J. "Ontogeny" of the major histocompatibility locus in rats. A problem in nomenclature. *Transplantation 9*:161–163, 1970b.

Palm, J. Immunogenetic analysis of Ag-B histocompatibility antigens in rats, *Transplantation 11*:175–183, 1971.

Palm, J., and Black, G. Interrelationships of inbred rat strains with respect to Ag-B and non-Ag-B antigens. *Transplantation 11*:184–189, 1971.

Palm, J., and Wilson, D. B. The Ag-B locus of rats: A major histocompatibility complex? *Transplant. Proc. 5*:1573–1577, 1973.

Paris, A., Bishop, C., Festenstein, E., and Günther, E. Evidence for epistatic gene interaction in rat renal allograft rejection. Submitted for publication, 1976.

Penhale, W. J., Farmer, A., Urbaniak, S. J., and Irvine, W. J. Susceptibility of inbred rat strains to experimental thyroiditis: Quantitation of thyroglobulin-binding cells and assessment of T-cell function in susceptible and non-susceptible strains. *J. Clin. Exp. Immunol. 19*:179–191, 1975.

Poloskey, P. E., Kunz, H. W., and Gill, T. J., III. Genetic studies in inbred rats. V. Xenoantisera against two major histocompatibility antigens raised by immunization with red cells. *J. Immunogenet. 2*:189–193, 1975b.

Poloskey, P. E., Kunz, H. W., Gill, T. J., III, Shonnard, J. W., Hansen, C. T., and Dixon, B. D. Genetic studies in inbred rats. IV. Xenoantisera against rat erythrocyte (Ag-C) antigens. *J. Immunogenet. 2*:179–187, 1975a.

Ramseier, H. Antibodies to receptors recognizing histocompatibility antigens. *Current Topics in Microbiology and Immunology 60*:31–78, 1973.

Ramseier, H., and Lindenmann, J. Aliotypic antibodies, *Transplant. Rev. 10*:57–96, 1972a.

Ramseier, H., and Lindenmann, J. Similarity of cellular recognition structures for histocompatibility antigens and of combining sites of corresponding alloantibodies. *Eur. J. Immunol. 2*:109–114, 1972b.

Ramseier, H., and Palm, J. Further studies of histocompatibility loci in rats. *Transplantation 5*:721–729, 1967.

Reckard, C. R., and Barker, C. F. Transplantation of isolated pancreatic islets across strong and weak histocompatibility barriers. *Transplant. Proc. 5*:761–763, 1973.

Robinson, R. *Genetics of the Norway Rat.* Pergamon Press, London, 1965.

Robinson, R. *Gene Mapping in Laboratory Mammals,* Part B, pp. 365–396, Plenum Press, London, 1972.

Rolstad, B., and Ford, W. L. Immune response of rats deficient in thymus-derived lymphocytes to strong transplantation antigens (Ag-B). Graft-versus-host activity, allograft rejection, and the factor of immunization. *Transplantation 17*:405–415, 1974.

Rolstad, B., Williams, A. F., and Ford, W. L. The alloantibody response to a strong transplantation antigen (Ag-B). Quantitative aspects and thymus dependence of the response. *Transplantation 17*:416–423, 1974.

Rose, N. R. Differing responses of inbred rat strains in experimental autoimmune thyroiditis. *Cell. Immunol. 18*:360–364, 1975.

Rüde, E., and Günther, E. Genetic control of the immune response to synthetic polypeptides in rats and mice. *Prog. Immunol. II, 2*:223–233, 1974.

Sachs, J. A., and Křen, V. Studies on the homology between human and rat MHS. II. Cytotoxic action of congenic rat alloimmune H-1 sera with human lymphocytes. *Folia Biol. (Praha) 22*:62–64, 1976.

Sakai, A. Antigenicity of skin and kidney in the rat, as studied in a transplantation model. *Transplantation 8*:882–889, 1969.

Salaman, J.R. Prolonged survival of renal allografts in rats mismatched at the major histocompatibility locus. *Transplantation 11*:63–70, 1971.

Sarich, V. M. Generation time and albumin evolution. *Biochem. Genet. 7*:205–212, 1972.

Shonnard, J. W., Cramer, D. V., Poloskey, P. E., Davis, B. K., and Gill, T. J., III. Genetic studies in inbred rats. VI. Linkage relationships of mixed lymphocyte reactivity, serologically defined antigens (Ag-B, Ag-C) and the immune response to poly ($Glu^{52}Lys^{33}Tyr^{15}$). *J. Immunogenetics 3*:61–70, 1976.

Shonnard, J. W., Cramer, D. V., Poloskey, P. E., Kunz, H. W., and Gill, T. J., III. Polymorphism of the major histocompatibility locus in the wild Norway rat. *Immunogenetics 3*:193–200, 1976.

Shreffler, D. C., and David, C. S. The H-2 major histocompatibility complex and the I immune response region: Genetic variation, function and organization. *Adv. Immunol. 20*:125–195, 1975.

Shumak, K. H., Batchelor, J. R., and Watts, H. G. ^{125}I-labelled rat transplantation alloantibodies. *Transplantation 15*:70–79, 1973.

Silvers, W. K., and Billingham, R. E. Influence of the Ag-B locus on reactivity to skin homografts and tolerance responsiveness in rats. *Transplantation 8*:167–178, 1969.

Silvers, W. K., and Billingham, R. E. Contributions of the rat to the immunobiology of tissue transplantation. *Transplant. Proc. 2*:152–161, 1970.

Silvers, W. K., Wilson, D. B., and Palm, J. Mixed leukocyte reactions and histocompatibility in rats. *Science 155*:703–704, 1967.

Simonsen, M. On the measurement of antigenic strength. *Transplant. Rev. 3*:22–35, 1970.

Simpson, G. G. The nature and origin of supraspecific taxa. *Cold Spring Harbor Symp. Quant. Biol. 24*:255–271, 1959.

Snell, G. D. The H-2 locus of the mouse: Observations and speculations concerning its comparative genetics and its polymorphism. *Folia Biol. (Praha) 14*:335–358, 1968.

Sørensen, S. F. Evidence for gene dose effect of H-1 (Ag-B) determined antigens in rat mixed lymphocyte culture. *Acta Pathol. Microbiol. Scand. (Section B) 79*:483–488, 1971.

Sørensen, S. F., Bildsøe, P., and Simonsen, M. Effect of strong and weak histocompatibility antigens on the mixed lymphocyte culture reaction in rats. *Acta Pathol. Microbiol. Scand. (Section B) 79*:475–482, 1971.

Soulillou, J.-P., Carpenter, C. B., D'Apice, A. J. F., and Strom, T. B. The role of nonclassical, Fc receptor-associated, Ag-B antigens (Ia) in the allograft enhancement. *J. Exp. Med. 143*:405–421, 1976.

Staines, N. A., Guy, K., and Davies, D. A. L. Passive enhancement of mouse skin allografts: Specificity of the antiserum for major histocompatibility complex antigens. *Transplantation 18*:192–195, 1974.

Stankus, R. P., and Leslie, G. A. Cross-idiotypic specificity of rat antibodies to group A streptococcal carbohydrate. *J. Immunol. 113*:1859–1863, 1974.

Stankus, R. P., and Leslie, G. A. Genetic influences on the immune response of rats to streptococcal A carbohydrate. *Immunogenetics 2*:29–38, 1975.

Stankus, R. P., and Leslie, G. A. Rat interstrain antibody response and cross-idiotypic specificity. *Immunogenetics 3*:65–73, 1976.

Štark, O., Frenzl, B., and Křen, V. Erythrocyte and transplantation antigens in inbred strains of rats. VII. H-1 alleles of the LEP, CAP, BN, BD V, BD VII and BD X strains. *Folia Biol. (Praha) 14*:169–175, 1968a.

Štark, O., Günther, E., Kohoutová, M., and Vojčík, V. Genetic recombination in the major histocompatibility complex (H-1, Ag-B) of the rat. *Immunogenetics*, in press, 1977.

Štark, O., and Hauptfeld, M. Serologically detected Rt H-1 antigens of the AS2, VM and Y59 rats. *Folia Biol. (Praha) 15*:35–40, 1969.

Štark, O., and Křen, V. Erythrocyte and transplantation antigensin inbred strains of rats. II. Antigens of the AVN strain. *Folia Biol. (Praha) 13*:93–99, 1967a.

Štark, O., and Křen, V. Erythrocyte and transplantation antigens in inbred strains of rats. III. Antigens of the BP strain. *Folia Biol. (Praha) 13*:299–305, 1967b.

Štark, O., and Křen, V. Erythrocyte and transplantation antigens in inbred strains of rats. IV. Antigens of the WP strain. *Folia Biol. (Praha) 13*:306–311, 1967c.

Štark, O., and Křen, V. Erythrocyte and transplantation antigens in inbred strains of rats. V. Antigens of the Lewis strain. *Folia Biol. (Praha) 13*:312–316, 1967d.

Štark, O., and Křen, V. Erythrocyte and transplantation antigens in inbred strains of rats. VI. The histocompatibility-1 system and its alleles. *Folia Biol. (Praha) 13*:356–360, 1967e.

Štark, O., and Křen, V. Five congenic resistant lines of rats differing at the rat H-1 locus. *Transplantation 8*:200–203, 1969.

Štark, O., Křen, V., and Frenzl, B. Histocompatibility locus of the rat. Tenth International Conference on Animal Blood Groups and Biochemical Polymorphismes, Paris 1966, *In Polymorphismes Biochemiques des Animaux*, pp. 501–506, ed. Institut Nationale de la Recherche Agronomique, Paris, 1967a.

Štark, O., Křen, V., and Frenzl, B. Erythrocyte and transplantation antigens in inbred strains of rats: I. Serological analysis of strain-specific antigens. *Folia Biol. (Praha) 13*:85–92, 1967b.

Štark, O., Křen, V., Frenzl, B., and Křenová, D. Histocompatibility-1 alleles in inbred rats of the BD II, WR, AGA, CDF, AS, BS, HS and DA strains. *Folia Biol. (Praha) 14*:425–432, 1968b.

Štark, O., Křen, V., Frenzl, B., and Kršiaková, M. Independent segregation of the Rt H-1 alleles and coat color genes in the rat. *Folia Biol. (Praha) 15*:410–473, 1969b.

Štark, O., Křen, V., Křenová, D., and Frenzl, B. Serologically detected antigens in two sublines of the WAG rats. *Folia Biol. (Praha) 15*:259–262, 1969a.
Štark, O., Křen, V., and Günther, E. Rt H-1 antigens in 39 rat strains and six congenic lines. *Transplant. Proc. 3*:165–168, 1971.
Štark, O., Křenová, D., Křen, V., and Frenzl, B. Immunological relationship between five congenic lines of rats and their parental strains. *Folia Biol. (Praha) 16*:1–11, 1970.
Štark, O., and Zeiss, I. Antigene des ersten Histokompatibilitätssystems (H-1) bei den BD-(Berlin-Druckrey) und BDE-Ratteninzuchtstämmen. *Z. Versuchstierkd. 12*:27–40, 1970.
Stenglein, B., Thoenes, G. H., and Günther, E. Genetically controlled autologous immune complex glomerulonephritis in rats. *J. Immunol. 115*:895–897, 1975.
Stroehmann, I., and DeWitt, C. W. Rat transplantation antigens. I. Extraction and partial purification of soluble antigen. *Immunology 23*:921–928, 1972a.
Stroehmann, I., and DeWitt, C. W. Rat transplantation antigens. II. Solubilization of multiple antigenic specificities. *Immunology 23*:929–935, 1972b.
Strom, T. B., Carpenter, C. B., Phillips, S. M., Garovoy, M. R., and Merril, J. P. Rejection and enhancement in an in vitro model of alloimmunity. Comparison of F1 and parental strains. *Transplantation 16*:103–109, 1973.
Stuart, F. P., McKearn, T. J., and Fitch, F. W. Immunological enhancement of renal allografts. *Transplant. Proc.* (Suppl. 1) *6*:53–57, 1974.
Stuart, F. P., Saitoh, T., and Fitch, F. W. Rejection of renal allografts: Specific immunologic suppression. *Science 160*:1463–1465, 1968.
Svejgaard, A., Platz, P., Ryder, L. P., Staub-Nielsen, L., and Thomsen, M. HL-A and disease associations—a Survey. *Transplant. Rev. 22*:3–43, 1975.
Tada, N., Itakura, K., and Aizawa, M. Genetic control of the antibody response in inbred rats. *J. Immunogenetics 1*:265–275, 1974.
Tada, N., Itakura, K., and Aizawa, M. Immune response gene (Ir-SRBC) exerts its effect via macrophages in inbred rats. *J. Immunogenetics 3*:49–60, 1976.
Taylor, H. R., and Morris, P. J. A simple micromethod for detecting isohaemagglutinins in rats using papainized red blood cells. *Aust. J. Exp. Biol. Med. Sci. 48*:245–247, 1970.
Thoenes, G. H. Induction of unresponsiveness to organ transplants in congenic strains of rats and other mammals. In W. H. Hildemann, and A. A. Benedict (eds.), *Immunologic Phylogeny*, pp. 457–466, Plenum Publishing Corp., New York, 1975.
Thoenes, G. H., Urban, G., and Doering, I. Kidney transplantation between congenic versus standard inbred strains of rats. I. The significance of H-1 and non-H-1 gene differences. *Immunogenetics 3*:239–253, 1974.
Thoenes, G. H., and White, E. Enhancement-induced specific nonreactivity in experimental kidney transplantation. *Transplantation 15*:308–311, 1973.
Thoenes, G. H., White, E., and Hildemann, W. H. Alloantibodies induced by weaker histocompatibility antigens in rats. *J. Immunol. 104*:1447–1452, 1970.
Tilney, N. L., and Bell, P. R. F. Studies on enhancement of cardiac and renal allografts in the rat. *Transplantation 18*:31–37, 1974.
Tinbergen, W. J. The effects of some immunosuppressive agents on kidney graft survival in rats. *Transplantation 6*:203–207, 1968.
Virolainen, M., Häyry, P., and Defendi, V. Effect of presensitization on the mixed lymphocyte reaction of rat spleen cell cultures. *Transplantation 8*:179–188, 1969.
Vladutiu, A. O., and Rose, N. R. Autoimmune murine thyroiditis. Relation to histocompatibility (H-2) type. *Science 174*:1137–1139, 1971.
White, E., Hildemann, W. H., and Mullen, Y. Chronic kidney allograft reactions in rats. *Transplantation 8*:602–617, 1969.
Williams, R. M., and Moore, M. J. Linkage of susceptibility to experimental allergic encephalomyelitis to the major histocompatibility locus in rats. *J. Exp. Med. 138*:775–783, 1973.
Williams, M., and Moore, M. J. Genetic recombination between serologically defined antigens and mixed lymphocyte reactivity in the rat major histocompatibility complex. In M. Stephenson and A. Brzytwa (eds.), *Transplantation Abstracts*, Sixth International Congress of the Transplantation Society 1976, pp. 66–67, Grune and Stratton, New York, 1976.
Williams, R. M., Moore, M. J., and Benacerraf, B. Genetic control of thymus-derived cell

function. IV. Mitogen responsiveness and mixed lymphocyte reactivity of thymus cells and lymph node cells from Lewis and Brown Norway rats. *J. Immunol.* *111*:1571–1578, 1973.

Wilson, D. B. Quantitative studies on the mixed lymphocyte interaction in rats. I. Conditions and parameters of response. *J. Exp. Med.* *126*:625–654, 1967.

Wilson, D. B. Immunologic reactivity to major histocompatibility alloantigens: HARC, effector cells and the problem of memory. *Prog. Immunol. II, 2*:145–156, 1974.

Wilson, D. B., Blyth, J. L., and Nowell, P. C. Quantitative studies on the mixed lymphocyte interaction in rats. III. Kinetics of the response. *J. Exp. Med.* *128*:1157–1181, 1968.

Wilson, D. B., Howard, J. C., and Nowell, P. C. Some biological aspects of lymphocytes reactive to strong histocompatibility alloantigens. *Transplant. Rev.* *12*:3–29, 1972.

Wilson, D. B., and Nowell, P. C. Quantitative studies on the mixed lymphocyte interaction in rats. V. Tempo and specificity of the proliferative response and the number of reactive cells from immunized donors. *J. Exp. Med.* *133*:442–453, 1971.

Wilson, D. B., Silvers, W. K., and Nowell, P. C. Quantitative studies on the mixed lymphocyte interaction in rats. II. Relationship of the proliferative response to the immunologic status of the donors. *J. Exp. Med.* *126*:655–665, 1967.

Wonigeit, K., and Stumpenhorst, R. Serologische Charakterisierung von zwei Alloantigensystemen auf Thymus und thymusabhängigen Lymphozyten der Ratte (Abstract). *Z. Immunitaetsforsch.* *150*:257–258, 1975.

Würzburg, U. Correlation between the immune response to an enzyme and histocompatibility type in rats. *Eur. J. Immunol.* *1*:496–497, 1971.

Würzburg, U., Schütt-Gerowitt, H., and Rajewsky, K. Characterization of an immune response gene in rats. *Eur. J. Immunol.* *3*:762–766, 1973.

Zeiss, I. Antigenic interrelationship and number of independently segregating histocompatibility loci in three isohistogenic strains of rats. *Transplantation* *5*:1393–1399, 1967.

Zeiss, I. M., Nisbet, N. W., and Heslop, B. F. A male antigen in rats. *Transplant. Bull.* *30*:161, 1962.

Chapter 7

The Major Histocompatibility System of the Mouse

C.S. DAVID

1. Brief History

The history of the H-2 complex stems from the studies of tumor immunology and represents the foundations of a distinct modern discipline—the immunogenetics of histocompatibility.

In 1936, Gorer identified four blood group antigens in the mouse using heterologous antisera and designated them as I, II, III, and IV. Antigen II was identified by a rabbit antimouse (strain A) serum absorbed in C57BL (B10) strain mice to remove the species-specific antibodies (Gorer 1936). The correlation between antigen II and tumor growth was established using crosses and backcrosses between strains A and B10 (Gorer 1937). The presence of alloantibody against antigen II in B10 mice, which rejected the tumor, suggested that antigen II was an alloantigen (Gorer 1938). These results prompted Gorer to postulate that graft rejection is elicited by alloantigenic differences between the host and the donor.

In the next decade rapid progress was made in the area of transplantation immunology. The terms "histocompatibility genes" and "histocompatibility antigens" were proposed by George Snell in 1948 to denote the genes and antigens involved in tissue compatibility. The identification of individual H loci was greatly accelerated by the production of congenic strains of mice by Snell (1948). Originally congenic lines were developed by the breeding of tumor-resistant animals selected from segregating liters and hence given the term congenic resistant lines. Snell confirmed the previous observation by Gorer that genes controlling resistance to tumor grafts were either the same as or closely linked to genes coding for antigen II. This gene was designated as H-2 and was assigned to the IX linkage group on the basis of its association with the fused tail gene.

In the process of developing congenic resistant lines, Snell discovered several H loci. The products of these loci did not induce cytotoxic alloantibodies, and in terms of graft or tumor rejection were distinctly weaker than the H-2 gene, which eventually emerged as the most potent histocompatibility barrier in the mouse. Gorer (1950) realized that H-2 gene(s) coded for more than the antigen II, and in the next ten years the serological complexity of the H-2 system began to unravel. Use of several congenic lines led to the discovery of several H-2 alleles controlled by the H-2 locus (Snell et al. 1953). Use of better serological techniques revealed that each H-2 allele (designated $H\text{-}2^a$, $H\text{-}2^b$,...) controlled several antigens (designated A, B, C,...) (Amos et al. 1955; Gorer and Mikulska 1959; Hoecker et al. 1959). The designation for antigens were later changed to arabic numerals 1, 2, 3, 4,....

The first evidence for the compound genetic structure of the H-2 locus was shown by Snell et al.'s (1953) observation that H-2^d/H-2^k heterozygotes accepted H-2^a tumor grafts. This led to the hypothesis that H-2^a arose as a recombination between H-2^d and H-2^k, which was later strengthened by the findings of Allen (1955). Screening for recombinants by serological methods yielded one recombinant between H-2^d and H-2^b (Amos et al. 1955) and two recombinants between H-2^a and H-2^b (Gorer and Mikulska 1959), which established that genes controlling H-2 antigens can be separated by crossing over. Further recombinants were identified by Pizarro et al. (1961) and Stimpfling and Richardson (1965). On the basis of these recombinational events, genetic maps were constructed for the H-2 genes by standard multipoint genetic mapping procedures, consisting of five H-2 regions: D, C, V, E, and K. The mapping was done under the following assumptions: (1) Recombinants arose from single crossing over; (2) the H-2 genetic regions of different strains have the same subdivisions, the same length, and are in the same order; (3) an individual specificity is controlled by a gene mapping in the same subdivision of every chromosome on which it occurs.

As new recombinants were being analyzed, the multiregional control of H-2 antigens became difficult to interpret. For example, the expression of specificity H-2.3 in several recombinants was inconsistent with genetic expectation (Stimpfling and Richardson 1965; Shreffler et al. 1966). These inconsistencies became even more evident after the discovery of a genetically controlled quantitative variant in the serum of normal mice (Ss), the genes for which mapped between H-2 regions determining H-2 antigens (Shreffler and Owen 1963; Shreffler 1965). The classification of several recombinants for the Ss locus was further strengthened by the identification of a new variant of the Ss system, a sex-limited allotype antigen designated as Slp (Passmore and Shreffler 1970). Detailed analysis for these regions indicated mapping inconsistencies for several H-2 antigens (Shreffler 1970; Demant et al. 1971). These inconsistencies prompted Shreffler et al. (1971) to propose a bypartite model where genetic determinant for some of these specificities could have duplicated during evolution, thereby locating them on two different positions on the same chromosome. This suggests at least two H-2 subregions on either side of the Ss-Slp locus, where some of the same specificities could be expressed in each of these regions.

As the understanding of the complexity of the H-2 genes increased, some new H-2 terminology was introduced. The segment of the chromosome comprising the H-2 genes and associated traits was called the H-2 gene complex. The H-2 phenogroups previously recognized as alleles were designated as H-2 haplotypes. H-2 specificities limited to a putatively independent haplotype or its crossover derivative were termed "private," and those that exhibited cross-reactivity with several haplotypes were termed "public." Snell et al. (1971 a) found that private H-2 specificities can be arranged into two segregant series, H-2K and H-2D, separated by the Ss-Slp determinant. H-2K and H-2D loci could have evolved by duplication of an ancestral locus, with the S gene by chance included within the duplication. This could account for some of the specificities being expressed on both the K and D regions. To test for the existence of the central regions C, V, E, and A, an extensive set of grafts was performed. No skin graft rejections were seen that could be attributed to the central region differences (Demant et al. 1971; Stimpfling 1971; Klein and Shreffler 1972; Demant and Graff 1973). These results strongly suggested the existence of only the H-2K and the H-2D regions controlling histocompatibility.

Under the duplication model it was proposed that serological cross-reaction occurred between the H-2K and H-2D antigens. This assumption gained further support when preliminary data by David et al. (1973b) showed serological cross-reactivity of antisera directed against either of these regions with the antigens of the other regions. In an extention of these studies, Murphy and Shreffler (1975a, 1975b) demonstrated extensive cross-reactivity between K and D regions from several haplotypes. These results eliminated the necessity of postulating additional regions to code for H-2 specificities and substantiated the structural similarity between H-2K and H-2D regions. Further evidence for the two-region model was obtained from studies on the biochemical properties of the serologically detected H-2K and H-2D antigens (Davies 1969; Nathenson and Cullen 1974). Two distinct polypeptides with molecular weights of approximately 45,000 (detergent solubilization) can be identified in cell membrane preparations. These polypeptides are glycoproteins and carry one or more H-2 specificities assigned to the K or D regions. In an H-2 heterozygote, two different H-2K and H-2D polypeptides have been demonstrated (Cullen et al. 1972). "Capping" studies also gave similar results (Neauport-Sautes et al. 1973). Peptide mapping shows a remarkable homology between the K and D products (Nathenson and Cullen 1974). These findings strongly support the view that H-2 antigens are controlled by two loci, H-2K and H-2D, which arose by duplication from an ancestral H-2 locus.

During this period of the genetic definition of the H-2 antigens, a series of discoveries were being made linking the H-2 system to several biologically important functions. Susceptibility of different strains of mice to Gross virus was found to be controlled by a gene located within the H-2 complex (Lilly 1970). McDevitt and Sela (1965) first discovered that immune responses to certain synthetic polypeptides in mice were under genetic control and linked to the H-2 system. The gene, designated Ir-1, was later found to be located within the H-2 gene complex between the K and S regions (McDevitt et al. 1972). Since then responses to several antigens have been found to be linked to the H-2 system. The work of Lyon et al. (1968) and Klein (1970) showed that the H-2K region is closer to the centromere of the 17th chromosome. According to accepted genetic practice, the genetic markers are ordered from left to right starting from the centromere, as H-2K, Ir-1, Ss-Slp, and H-2D. The regions were designated as K, I, S, and D (Klein et al. 1974). A new region between S and D, designated G, has recently been identified (David et al. 1975; Klein et al. 1975). A new set of serologically identified antigens

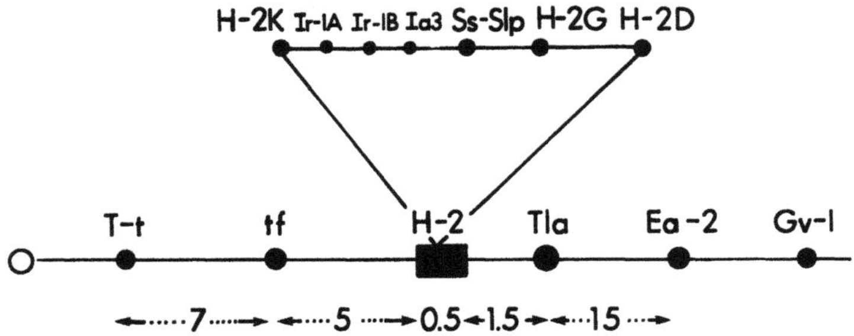

Fig. 7.1. IX Linkage group. T-t, brachyury complex; tf, tufted; H-2, histocompatibility-2; Tla, thymus leukemia antigens; Ea-2, erythrocyte antigen-2; Gv-1, Gross virus-1. Map distance is shown below

controlled by the I region was identified and designated as the Ia antigens (Shreffler et al. 1974). Figure 7.1 shows the map of the IX linkage group with the composition of the H-2 gene complex.

This brief historical section is intended to bring the reader up to date on nearly 40 years of research leading to the current status of the understanding of the H-2 gene complex. It is not intended as an exhaustive survey of the literature. Detailed information on the H-2 system can be found in a recent book by Jan Klein, titled *Biology of the Mouse Histocompatibility-2 Complex* (Klein 1975b). The rest of this chapter will focus on the current state of knowledge of the H-2 gene complex.

2. Serology

The serological aspects of antigens coded by genes in the five major regions of the H-2 gene complex will be discussed in this section.

2.1 K and D Regions

The K and D regions determine the classical histocompatibility-2 antigens. Approximately 56 H-2 antigens in inbred strains and six antigens in the wild population of mice have been identified (Klein 1975b). Those specificities that serve as markers for the widely used inbred strains will be discussed here (Table 7.1).

H-2.2: Specificity 2 was originally identified by Amos et al. (1955). This specificity is a marker for the D region of H-2^b strains and its derivatives. Haplotype H-2^j seems to express H-2.2, suggesting that the D region of H-2^j and H-2^b could have had a common origin. The specificity can be detected by hemagglutination as well as cytotoxic texts. However, when antisera are produced in certain combinations, only cytotoxic antibodies are elicited. This raises the question of whether the H-2.2 specificity identified by hemagglutination is controlled by a locus closely linked to the D region rather than within

Table 7.1. H-2 Antigen Markers for Independent Strains

H-2 Haplotype	K End				D End	
	Private	Public			Private	Public
b	33	39			2	
d	31			8	4	13
f	9(a)	37	39	8	9b	7
j	15	38			2	7
k	23	11	25	8	32	7
p	16(a)	37	38	8	16(b)	7
q	17	11			30	13
r	18(a)	11	25	8	18(b)	
s	19				12	7
u	20				4	13
v	21				30	13

the region. Antiserum $(B10.D2 \times A)F_1$ anti-B10.A(4R) yields cytotoxic as well as hemagglutinating anti-2, whereas $(B.10.D2 \times A)F_1$ anti-B10.A(2R) yields only cytotoxic antibodies.

H-2.4: Specificity 4 was identified by Gorer et al. (1948) with the absorbed antiserum C3H anti-Balb/C. It is a marker for the D region of $H\text{-}2^d$ haplotypes. Antigen 4 induces very strong hemagglutinating and cytotoxic antibodies. Antiserum $(B10 \times AKR.M)F_1$ anti-B10.A produces a good anti-4 but could also contain anti-Ia antibodies. Antiserum $(C3H.OL \times B10)F_1$ anti-B10.A(5R) contain anti-H2.4 and also antibodies against public specificity H-2.3, but lacks anti-Ia antibodies.

H-2.9: Specificity 9 was identified by Hoecker et al. (1959) with an antiserum A.SW anti-A.CA absorbed in strain A and is a private specificity of the $H\text{-}2^f$ haplotype. Recent studies suggest that antigen 9 can be subdivided into two specificities, one controlled by a K-region gene and the other by a D-region gene (David, *unpublished data*). Antiserum $(A \times B10.S)F_1$ anti-A.CA contains hemagglutinating as well as cytotoxic anti-9 antibodies.

H-2.11: Specificity 11 was identified by Amos et al. (1955). It is not a private specificity but has a narrow distribution, present in haplotypes k, q, and r, and is mapped in the K region. These three haplotypes could have had a common ancestor. Antigen 11 is a strong antigen and can be detected both by hemagglutination and cytotoxic methods. Anti-H-2.11 can be produced by immunization with cells from any one of three haplotypes: (1) $(C3H.OH \times A.SW)F_1$ anti-C3H; (2) $(Balb/c \times B10.P)F_1$ anti-B10.RIII; (3) $(Balb/c \times B10.P)$ anti-B10.T(6R). All three antisera contain cytotoxic anti-Ia antibodies along with antibodies against the private H-2 antigen of the donor strain. Combination A.TL anti-A.AL produces a good anti-11 without anti-Ia but also contains anti-23.

H-2.12: Specificity 12 was identified by Snell and Cherry (1974) and is a marker for the D region of the $H\text{-}2^s$ allele. The anti-12 serum-$(DBA/1 \times SWR)F_1$ anti-DA also contains non-H-2 antibodies. Congenic combina-

Table 7.2. H-2 Specificities in Independent Haplotypes

H-2 Haplo-type	Type Strain(s)	H-2 Antigens															
		1	2	3	4	5	6	7	8	9	11	12	13	15	16	17	18
b	B10 (A.BY)		2			5	6										
d	B10.D2 (Balb/C) (DBA/2)			3	4		6		8				13				
f	B10.M (A.CA)						6	7	8	9							
j	B10.WB (JK)		2				6	7						15			
k	B10.K (C3H) (AKR)	1		3		5		7	8		11						
p	B10.P (P/J) (C3H.NB)	1		3		5	6	7	8						16		
q	B10.G (C3H.Q) (DBA/1)	1		3		5	6				11		13			17	
r	B10.RIII (LP.RIII)	1		3		5	6		8		11						18
s	B10.S (A.SW) (SJL)	1		3		5	6	7				12					
u	B10.PL (PL)			3	4	5			8				13				
v	B10.SM (SM)	1		3													

tions (A.TH anti-A.SW) used to produce anti-H-2.12 yield very low-titer cytotoxic antibodies.

H-2.13: Specificity 13 was identified by Amos (1959) and is defined by the cross-reaction of anti-H-2^q against H-2^d strains. Antigen 13 maps in the D end, and is expressed in haplotypes q and d. Antiserum (C3H × B10)F_1 anti C3H.Q has a good hemagglutinating and cytotoxic anti-H-2.13 along with antibodies against H-2.17 and H-2.30.

H-2.15: Specificity 15 was identified by Snell et al. (1971b) and Klein (1971). It is a private specificity of haplotype H-2^j and is presumed to map in the K end. Antiserum [B10.A(2R) × A.CA] anti-B10.WB contains hemagglutinating and cytotoxic anti-15 antibody.

H-2.16: Specificity 16 was identified by Hoecker et al. (1954) and is a private specificity of the haplotype H-2^p presumed to map in the K region. A good hemagglutinating and cytotoxic anti-16 can be produced in the com-

H-2 Antigens																		
19	20	21	23	24	25	27	28	29	30	31	32	33	35	36	37	38	39	40
						27	28	29				33	35	36			39	
						27	28	29		31			35	36				40
						27									37		39	
							28	29								38		
			23	24	25						32							
				24									35		37	38		
						27	28	29	30									
					25													
19							28							36				
	20					27	28	29					35	36				40
		21							30									

bination (B6 × A)F_1 anti-B10.P. This antiserum also contains a hemagglutinating anti-7, antibodies against I region antigens, and possibly antibodies against D region antigens.

H-2.17: Specificity 17 was identified by Hoecker et al. (1954). It is a private specificity of H-2^q and is a marker for the K region. Antiserum (AKR.M × C3H.B10) anti-C3H.Q contains a strong cytotoxic but weak hemagglutinating anti-17 along with antibodies against I region antigens. A specific but weak anti-17 can be produced in the combination B10.A anti-B10.AQR.

H-2.18: Specificity 18 was identified by Shreffler and Snell (1969) and is a private specificity of haplotype H-2^r. Antigen 18 is presumed to map in the K region, but anti-18 sera [C3H.NB × B10.A(2R)]F_1 anti-B10.RIII probably contains antibodies against I region antigens and D region antigens.

H-2.19: Specificity 19 was identified by Hoecker et al. (1954). It is a private

Table 7.3. Donor-Recipient Combinations for Production of Selected Anti-H-2 Sera

Specificity		Recipient	Donor	Target Strain	Other Antibodies Present
2	(a)	(B10.D2 × A)F_1	B10.A(4R)	B10	
	(b)	[B10.A(5R) × LP.RIII]F_1	B10	B10	
4	(a)	(B10 × AKR.M)F_1	B10.A	B10.D2	
	(b)	(B10.AKR × 129)F_1	B10.A	B10.D2	
7	(a)	(B6 × A)F_1	B10.P	B10.M	
					H-2.16, Ia.13
	(b)	(A × B10.A)F_1	A.SW	B10.M	H-2.19, Ia.4
	(c)	(A × B10)F_1	B10.M	B10.S	H-2.9, Ia.14
8	(a)	(B10 × A.SW)F_1	A.CA	B10.RIII	H-2.9, Ia.14
	(b)	(B10 × A.SW)F_1	B10.M	B10.RIII	H-2.9, Ia.14
9	(a)	(B10.A × A.SW)F_1	A.CA	B10.M	Ia.14
	(b)	(B10.D2 × SJL)F_1	B10.M	B10.M	Ia.14
11	(a)	(C3H.OH × A.SW)F_1	C3H	C3H.Q	H-2.1, 23, Ia.1,2
	(b)	(Balb/C × B10.P)F_1	B10.RIII	C3H.Q	H-2.18, 25, Ia.12
	(c)	(SJL × DBA/2)F_1	DBA/1	B10.BR	H-2.17, 30, Ia.10
12	(a)	(B10 × DBA/1)F_1	DA	B10.S	Non-H-2
13	(a)	(C3H × B10)F_1	C3H.Q	B10.D2	H-2.17, 30, Ia.10
	(b)	(B10 × LP.RIII)F_1	B10.A(5R)	C3H.Q	H-2.4
15	(a)	[A.CA × B10.A(2R)]F_1	B10.WB	B10.WB	Ia?
16	(a)	(A × B10.S)F_1	B10.P	B10.P	Ia.13, W21
	(b)	(A.CA × B10.A)F_1	B10.Y	B10.P	H-2.7, Ia.13, W21
17	(a)	(AKR.M × C3H.B10)F_1	C3H.Q	C3H.Q	Ia.10
	(b)	(DBA/2 × B10.AKM)F_1	B10.Q	B10.Q	Ia.10
18	(a)	[C3H.NB × B10.A(2R)]F_1	B10.RIII	B10.RIII	Ia.12
	(b)	(B10 × C3H)F_1	B10.RIII	B10.RIII	Ia.12
19	(a)	(A.CA × DA)F_1	A.SW	A.SW	Ia.4
	(b)	(A × B10)F_1	A.TL	A.SW	–
20	(a)	(B10.D2 × C3H.NB)F_1	B10.PL	B10.PL	Ia?
	(b)	(DBA/2 × B10.BR)F_1	B10.PL	B10.PL	Ia?
23	(a)	(C3H.Q × B10.D2)F_1	C3H	C3H	Ia.1, 2, ...
	(b)	(B10.AQR × 129)F_1	B10.A	B10.A	–
25	(a)	(B10.D2 × C3H.NB)F_1	B10.RIII	B10.BR	H-2.18, Ia.12
	(b)	(DBA/2 × B10.Q)F_1	B10.RIII	B10.BR	H-2.18, Ia.12
30	(a)	(B10.A × AKR)F_1	AKR.M	AKR.M	–
	(b)	(C3H.B10 × B10.A)F_1	B10.AKM	B10.AKM	–
31	(a)	(B10 × A)F_1	B10.D2	B10.D2	Ia.11, 16
	(b)	(B10.A × A)F_1	B10.D2	B10.D2	Ia.11, 16
32	(a)	(B10.A × A)F_1	B10.K	B10.K	–
	(b)	[C3H.SW × B10.A(2R)]F_1	C3H	C3H	–
33	(a)	(B10.D2 × A)F_1	B10.A(5R)	B10	H-2.39, Ia.9, W20
	(b)	(C3H.Q × HTH)F_1	C3H.B10	B10	H-2.39, Ia.8, W20

specificity of haplotype H-2^{s} and is a marker for the K region. Antiserum (A × B10)F_1 anti-B10.S contains good hemagglutinating and cytotoxic anti-19 along with antibodies against I region antigens. Specific anti-H-2.19 can be made in the combination (B10 × A.AL)F_1 anti-A.TL.

H-2.20: Specificity 20 was identified by Demant et al. (1971). It is a private specificity of H-2^{u} and is presumed to map in the K region. Antiserum

(B10.D2 × C3H.NB)F_1 anti-B10.PL contains hemagglutinating and cytotoxic anti-20 antibodies.

H-2.21: Specificity 21 was identified by Snell et al. (1971 b). It is a private specificity of haplotype H-2^v and is presumed to map in the K region. A good anti-21 is found in the antiserum (B10.A × C3H)F_1 anti-B10.SM.

H-2.23: Specificity 23 was identified by Hoecker et al. (1959). It is a private specificity of haplotype H-2^k and is a marker for the K region. Anti-23 serum (C3H.Q × B10.D2) anti-C3H usually contains additional cytotoxic antibodies against I region antigens. A specific but weak anti-H-2.23 can be produced in the combination B10.AQR anti-B10.A.

H-2.25: Specificity 25 was identified by Hoecker et al. (1959). It is shared between haplotypes H-2^k and H-2^r and maps in the K region. Immunization of (B10.D2 × C3H.NB)F_1 with B10.RIII yields an anti-25 antibody.

H-2.30: Specificity 30 was identified by Stimpfling and Pizarro (1961). It is a D region marker for the H-2^q haplotype, but is also present in haplotype H-2^v. The antiserum (B10.A × AKR)F_1 anti-AKR.M contains a good anti-30 along with a weak anti-17.

H-2.31: Specificity 31 was identified by Amos et al. (1955). It is a private specificity of haplotype H-2^d and is a marker for the K region. Anti-31 antisera usually contains antibodies against I region antigens. Antigen 31 induces strong cytotoxic and weak hemagglutinating antibodies. Good anti-31 antibodies are elicited in (B10 × A)F_1 by immunization with B10.D2.

H-2.32: Specificity 32 was first identified by Gorer and Mikulska (1959) and is most often detected by cytotoxic test. It is a private specificity of haplotype H-2^k and is a marker for the D region. Specificity 32 is a weak antigen and anti-32 can be made in the combination (B10.A × A)F_1 anti-B10.K.

H-2.33: Specificity 33 was identified by Gorer and Mikulska (1959) and is again predominantly a cytotoxic specificity. It is a private specificity of haplotype H-2^b and is a marker for the K region. Antigen 33 induces strong cytotoxic antibodies, but the antiserum usually contains antibodies against I region antigens. A good combination for the preparation of anti-33 is (B10.D2 × A)F_1 anti-B10.A(5R).

The H-2 specificities discussed so far provide markers for the K and D regions of most of the commonly used H-2 haplotypes (Table 7.1). Most of the other specificities are public specificities and will not be discussed individually, but are included as part of the H-2 chart in Table 7.2. Specificities beyond H-2.40 are not included because several of them are I region antigens. Table 7.3 gives the recipient-donor combinations for production of antisera against the specificities discussed in this section.

2.2 H-2G Region

Specificity H-2.7 was first defined by Hoecker et al. (1959), with an A anti-A.CA antiserum tested by hemagglutination against A.SW (H-2^s) cells. H-2.7 was found to be expressed on haplotypes H-2^p, H-2^j, H-2^f, and H-2^s. Recombinants involving H-2^f suggested localization of H-2.7 to the left of the D region (Stimpfling and Richardson 1965). Analyses of other recombinants by cytotoxic test suggested localization of the antigen to the right of S region (David and Shreffler 1972). Extensive analyses of several anti-7 sera have shown that H-2.7 is predominantly an erythrocyte antigen and is controlled by an independent locus, designated H-2G, which maps between regions S and D (David et al. 1975; Klein et al. 1975). The antigen detected in the cytotoxic test is not H-2.7 but an antigen coded by the I region genes and designated as Ia.13 (David et al. 1976). Haplotype H-2^k tissues were shown to be positive for 7 by virtue of their ability to absorb anti-7 sera. Immunization combinations (B6 × A)F_1 anti-B10.P and (C3H.SW × B10.A) anti-C3H.NB make good anti-7 antibodies along with anti-H-2.16, and these antisera also contain antibodies against I region antigens.

2.3 I Region

The I region was first described when the genes controlling immune response to synthetic polypeptides—(T,G)-A—L, (H,G)-A—L—designated Ir-1 was mapped in the chromosomal segment between the K and S regions (McDevitt et al. 1972). The Ir-1 locus was subdivided into Ir-1 and Ir-IgG by the demonstration by Lieberman et al. (1972) that the response to a specific IgG allotype was controlled by a locus other than Ir-1. Reciprocal immunization of strains differing in the I region led to production of antibodies detecting a set of lymphocyte antigens (David et al. 1973a; Hauptfeld et al. 1973) which were designated I region associated or Ia antigens (Shreffler et al. 1974). Ia antigens were also identified in several other laboratories about the same time (Sachs and Cone 1973; Götze et al. 1973; Hämmerling et al. 1974). Ia antigens differed from H-2K and H-2D antigens in the limitation of their expression to a subpopulation of lymphocytes. Anti-Ia sera kill only 50 to 60 percent of cells, whereas anti-H-2 kill 100 percent of cells. In this section the identification, map localization, and strain distribution of the Ia specificities will be discussed.

Ia.1,2,3,7: Strains A.TL and A.TH have identical K and D regions. The I region of A.TL is derived from the H-2^k haplotype, whereas A.TH is derived from the H-2^s haplotype. A.TH anti-A.TL contained antibodies not only against I^k strains but also against I^f, I^b, I^q, I^p, I^d, I^r strains (David et al. 1973a). Ia.1 is defined by the cross-reaction of anti-I^k with I^f strains, Ia.3 by the cross-reaction of anti-I^k with I^b and I^q strains, Ia.7 by the cross-reaction of anti-I^k with I^d and I^p strains, and Ia.2 is a private specificity of I^k (David and Shreffler 1974).

The strain distribution of Ia.7 suggested a new I subregion to the right of Ir-IgG, because strain B10.A(5R) was positive for Ia.7. The Ir-1 and Ir-IgG regions of 5R were derived from H-2^b, and suggested an I^d subregion to the right of Ir-IgG. Further evidence was obtained when antiserum B10 anti-B10.A(5R) contained anti-7 antibodies, and the subregion was designated

I-C (David et al. 1975). The designation for Ir-1 and Ir-IgG was changed to I-A and I-B (Klein et al. 1974).

By analyzing several H-2 recombinants, specificities Ia.1 and 2 were mapped in the I-A region while Ia.3 was tentatively mapped in the I-B region and Ia.7 in the I-C region. The distribution of these Ia specificities has been confirmed by several other anti-K(I)^k sera. Further confirmation of the distribution of Ia.1, 3, and 7 was provided by *in vitro* absorptions and reactions of restricted antisera made in F_1 combinations.

Ia.4,5: Antiserum A.TL anti-A.TH identifies two specificities in I^s bearing strains. Ia.4 is a private I^s specificity and Ia.5 is defined by the cross reaction of anti-I^s with I^f- and I^q-bearing strains. Both these specificities seem to map either in the I-A or I-B region. A.TL anti-A.TH antiserum also contained antibodies against Tla antigens. Ia.4, 5 were again confirmed with other antisera, by absorption, and by reactions of restricted antisera in F_1 combinations.

Ia.6: Antiserum B10.A(4R) anti-B10.A(2R) is directed against the I-B^k and I-C^d regions but reacts only with I-C^d-bearing haplotypes (David et al. 1974). This specificity was designated Ia.6.

Ia.8,9, W20: Antiserum B10.A anti-B10 contains anti-H-2.33 antibodies but gave Ia-like reactivity against H-2^d and H-2^q haplotypes that were designated Ia.8 and Ia.9 respectively (Sachs et al. 1975). Ia.9 is also expressed in the H-2^s haplotype. Both these specificities were mapped in the I-A region by analyzing relevant recombinants. Absorption of the antisera for Ia.8, Ia.9, and H-2.33 still left reactivity with H-2^b targets, suggesting the presence of a private Ia specificity of H-2^b that has been designated Ia.W20 because recombinants at present are not available to map the specificity to the right of K region (Sachs and Cone 1975).

Ia.10: Specificity 10 was identified by Hauptfeld et al. (1973) with the antisera B10.AQR anti-B10.T(6R), which identifies a private specificity in I^q strains. This antibody is very weak.

Ia.11,16: Specificity 11 was identified by Davies and Hess (1974) by exhaustive absorption of anti-H-2K^d (anti-H-2.31) serum with erythrocytes and is a private specificity of H-2^d haplotype. The same specificity was also identified by other methods, absorption with Ia negative tumor, and cells from a recombinant strain, LG/Ckc (David, *unpublished data*). Several of the anti-H-2.31 sera cross-react with H-2^q strains and were previously defined as H-2.34 (Davies 1969). Recent studies by Staines et al. (1974) and David (*unpublished data*) have shown that this reaction is due to an Ia specificity designated Ia.16. Ia.11 and 16 map in the I-A subregion.

Ia.12: Specificity 12 was defined by David et al. (1976) by the cross-reaction of antiserum B10.A(2R) × C3H.NB anti-B10.RIII (anti-H-2.18) with H-2^s strains and is mapped in the I-A or I-B subregion.

Ia.13, W21: Specificity 13 was defined by David et al. (1976) by the cross-reaction of antiserum (B6 × A)F_1 anti-B10.P (anti-H-2.16) with H-2^q strains. Ia.13 was found to coprecipitate with Ia.5, suggesting a localization in the I-A/I-B regions (Cullen et al. *in preparation*). The antisera also identifies another specificity that coprecipitates with Ia.7, suggesting a localization in the I-C subregion. This specificity has been tentatively designated Ia.W21, a private specificity of H-2^p.

Ia.14: Specificity 14 was defined by David et al. (1976) with the antiserum A.TFR1 anti-A.CA (anti-H-2.9) after absorption of anti H-2 antibodies with platelets. This is a private specificity of H-2^f strains. The same specificity was also identified by Archer et al. (1974).

Ia.15: Specificity 15 was defined by David (*unpublished data*) by the reaction of antiserum (A.TH × B10.HTT)F_1 anti-A.TL with H-2^d strains. This specificity seems to map to he left of the I-C subregion.

Ia.17,18,19: Specificity 17 was defined by the reaction of antiserum (C3H.Q × B10.D2) anti-A.QR with H-2^s strains (Colombani et al. 1975) or (DBA/1 × B10.D2)F_1 anti-AQR with H-2^s (Götze 1976). Ia.17 is also present in H-2^r, H-2^t, and H-2^j and maps in the I-A/I-B regions. Absorption of this antiserum with H-2^r leaves residual activity for k, s, and f that is designated Ia.18. Absorption with H-2^s leaves residual activity for k and r that is designated Ia.19.

Ia.22: Antiserum (C3H.Q × B10.D2) anti-AQR was shown to contain antibodies against Ia 2, 17, 18 and 19 (Colombani et al. 1975). These specificities were all later mapped to the I-A subregion. This antiserum reacted with cells from recombinants B10.A(3R) and B10.A(5R) (both K^b A^b B^b C^d S^d D^d), even though these two antisera were unreactive with cells from strains B10 (H-2^b) and B10.D2 (H-2^d). This suggested that these strains may be carrying a segment of H-2^k origin that had been contributed by one of their parents, H-2^a haplotype. This required that recombination in 3R and 5R must have occurred between I-B and I-C regions, and Ia.22 was coded by this new region which was designated as I-E (Shreffler et al. 1977). Later results showed that recombinant strains B10.HTT and B10.S(9R) also carried the I-E^k region expressing Ia.22 which is a private specificity.

2.4 I-J Region

An antigen specific suppressive T cell factor produced by Tada and his associates was found to be an I region gene product (Tada et al. 1976). Anti-Ia sera directed against different I subregions were utilized in absorption experiments to map the gene(s) coding for the suppressor molecule. Initial attempts were ambiguous since certain antisera localized the gene to the I-A subregion, while others indicated the I-C subregion. At the same time, Murphy et al. (1976) showed that Ia antigens on the allotype suppressor T cells are controlled by genes which map between I-B and I-C subregions. Strain B10.HTT and B10.S(9R), until then thought to be identical, had different Ia determinants on the allotype suppressor T cells, B10.HTT having the H-2^s type and B10.S(9R) having the H-2^k type. Tada's results also suggested a region between I-B and I-C controlling suppressor factor. This region controlling specific T cell suppression was designated as "I-J". Recombinants B10.A(3R) and B10.A(5R) were found to code for different suppressor genes, 3R having

Table 7.4. Distribution of Ia Specificities in Haplotypes of Independent Origin

H-2 Haplo-type	Type Strain	Ia Specificities																				
		1	2	3	4	5	6	7	8	9	10	11	12	13	14	15	16	17	18	19	W20	W21
b	C57BL/10			3					8	9						15					W20	
d	B10.D2						6	7	8			11				15	16					
f	B10.M	1				5									14			17	18			
k	B10.K	1	2	3				7								15		17	18	19		
p	B10.P					5	6	7						13								W21
q	B10.G			3		5				9	10			13			16					
r	B10.RIII	1		3		5		7					12					17		19		
s	B10.S				4	5				9			12					17	18			

Table 7.5. Ia Specificities in Recombinant Haplotypes

Strain	Haplo-type	1	2	3	4	5	6	7	8	9	10	11	12	13	14	15	16	17	18	19	W20	W21
A	a	1	2	3			6	7								15		17	18	19		
A.AL	a1	1	2	3				7								15		17	18	19		
HTG	g						6	7	8			11				15	16					
D2.GD	g2								8			11				15	16					
B10.A(2R)	h2	1	2	3			6	7								15		17	18	19		
B10.A(4R)	h4	1	2	3												15		17	18	19		
HTI	i			3					8	9						15					W20	
B10.A(5R)	i5			3			6	7	8	9						15					W20	
A.KRM	m	1	2	3				7								15		17	18	19		
C3H.OL	01, 02						6	7	8			11				15	16					
C3H.OH																						
A.TL	t1	1	2	3				7								15		17	18	19		
A.TH	t2, t5				4	5				9			12					17	18			
BSVS																						
B10.HTT	t3				4	5		7		9			12					17	18			
B10.S(9R)	t4				4	5	6	7		9			12					17	18			
AQR	y1	1	2	3			6	7								15		17	18	19		
B10.T(6R)	y2			3		5				9	10			13			16					
A.TFR1	an1	1	2	3				7								15		17	18	19		
A.TFR2	ap2)	1				5									14			17	18			
A.TFR5	ap5)																					
LG/Ckc	ar1)																					
A.QSR1	sq1				4	5				9			12					17	18			
B10.A(8R)	as1	1	2	3												15		17	18	19		

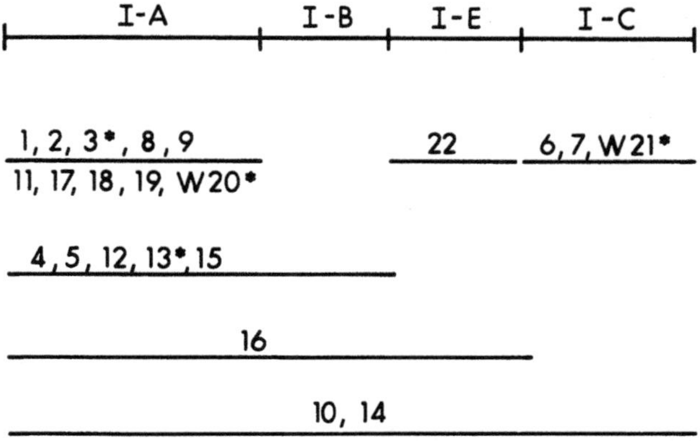

Fig. 7.2. Map positions for Ia specificities. Ia.3 and W21 are mapped by molecular association

the I-J^b locus and 5R having the I-J^k locus. A B10.A(3R) antisera absorbed the suppressor molecules from H-2^k strains.

Since strains B10.S(9R), B10.A(3R) and B10.A(5R) are identical at the I-E subregion expressing specificity Ia.22, I-J regions had to map to the left of I-E. Recombination in B10.HTT and B10.A(3R) occurred between I-J and I-E, while in B10.S(9R) and B10.A(5R) it occurred between I-B and I-J.

Tables 7.4 and 7.5 shows the distribution of Ia specificities in independent and recombinant haplotypes. Figure 7.2 shows the localization of Ia specificities within the different I subregions.

2.5 S Region

The serological markers for the S region are the Ss and Slp serum proteins. Ss (serum substance) protein was identified in the immunodiffusion test by an antiserum made in rabbits against the mouse serum betaglobulin (Shreffler and Owen 1963). This antiserum detected a quantitative difference in the Ss antigen of up to 20-fold in sera of different H-2 haplotypes. The high level is controlled by the Ss^h gene whereas the low level is controlled by the Ss^l gene. Recently, additional quantitative variations associated with the Ss^h alleles of different H-2 haplotypes have been shown by a radial immunodiffusion assay (Hansen et al. 1974).

The slp (sex-limited protein) was first demonstrated with an alloantiserum produced by the immunization of RF/J male mice with betaglobulin of DBA/2 male mice (Passmore and Shreffler 1970). The antiserum gave a precipitation line in the immunodiffusion test with serum of selected strains that were classified as Slp positive. The Slp antigen is generally androgen dependent and is expressed only in males of the positive strains, but could be induced in females or castrated males carrying the dominant gene by administration of testosterone (Passmore and Shreffler 1970). Subsequently a feral female

Table 7.6. Ss and Slp Levels in Sera from Different Strains and Sexes

Strain	Ss Allele	Ss Units ± SE (No.)	Slp Units ± SE (No.)
A male	Ss^d	0.97 ± 0.04 (11)	1.01 ± 0.03 (18)
A female	Ss^d	0.43 ± 0.02 (10)	0
A.BY male	Ss^b	0.56 ± 0.04 (5)	0
A.SW male	Ss^s	0.95 ± 0.05 (5)	0.35 ± 0.06 (12)
A.SW female	Ss^s	0.60 ± 0.08 (5)	0
B10 male	Ss^b	0.65 ± 0.04 (10)	0
B10 female	Ss^b	0.47 ± 0.04 (10)	0
B10.A male	Ss^d	0.90 ± 0.05 (18)	0.68 ± 0.04 (25)
B10.A female	Ss^d	0.46 ± 0.04 (12)	0
B10.D2 male	Ss^d	0.87 ± 0.07 (8)	0.67 ± 0.04 (8)
B10.M male	Ss^f	0.91 ± 0.03 (10)	0
B10.M female	Ss^f	0.48 ± 0.03 (10)	0
B10.P male	Ss^p	0.73 ± 0.03 (8)	0.03 ± 0.03 (8)
B10.S male	Ss^s	0.84 ± 0.06 (6)	0.18 ± 0.03 (25)
(B10 × B10.D2) male	Ss^b/ss^d	0.62 ± 0.07 (7)	0.33 ± 0.05 (7)
B10.K male	Ss^k	0.06 ± 0.01 (5)	0
C3H male	Ss^k	0.05 ± 0.01 (5)	0

Reproduced with permission from T. H. Hansen, Ph.D. dissertation, University of Michigan, 1975.

mouse was found that normally expressed the Slp antigen and transmitted it in a simple dominant fashion without sex limitation (Klein 1975a). Recent quantitative analyses suggest that Slp-positive strains may differ in levels of Slp antigens (Hansen et al. 1974). Table 7.6 shows the Ss and Slp types of several independent haplotypes.

The mapping of the Ss and Slp traits within the H-2 gene complex was first regarded as a chance occurrence, and the functions of the protein were thought to be independent of those of the other H-2 regions. But a finding by Demant et al. (1973) that differences in serum levels of hemolytic complement were associated with the S region of H-2 gene complex suggests a functional relationship with the other regions. Recent studies by Hansen et al. (1975) strongly support the involvement of Ss protein in the hemolytic complement activity. Goldman and Goldman (1975) showed that the levels of C′1, C′2, and C′4 activities are correspondingly lower in Ss-low than in Ss-high strains. Recently Meo et al. (1975b) identified a component of human plasma that cross-reacts with anti-mouse Ss and that also displays electrophoretic and size similarities to the mouse Ss protein. This component was isolated and characterized immunochemically as the fourth component of human complement (C′4 or beta IE globulin). Monospecific antisera made against human C′4 cross-react and differentiate the quantitative variation in mouse Ss protein. Recent results also suggest that the S region may be associated with the C3 receptor on B cells (Arnaiz-Villena et al. 1975).

Several studies suggest that genes of the HLA complex in humans plays a role in the genetic control of the human complement (Fu et al. 1974), and there is also evidence that a C′4-deficient gene in the guinea pig is closely linked to the major histocompatibility system (MHS) of that species (Shevach, *personal communication*). The interspecies homology in the association of genes controlling early complement components with the MHS of man, mouse, and guinea pig suggest a functional relationship between the S region genes and the genes controlling other immune mechanisms and thereby a rather intriguing functional homogeneity in the genetic organization of the MHS.

3. Tissue Distribution

H-2 antigens have a very wide tissue distribution. Highest concentrations of H-2 antigens are found in lymphoid organs—spleen, lymph nodes, bone marrow, and thymus (Edidin 1972). A relatively high concentration of H-2 antigens is also present in the liver, where their activity is primarily associated with Kupffer cells. Lower amounts of H-2 antigens are found in epidermis, lung, kidney, heart, muscle, and red cells. Considering that most of the H-2 antigens were defined by the hemagglutination test, the amount of H-2 antigens on erythrocytes in relation to spleen (less than 10 percent) is surprising. Probably a small amount of H-2 is present on mouse sperm (Johnson and Edidin 1972). There is no evidence for the expression of H-2 on nervous tissue, ova, and trophoblasts.

Immunofluorescence assays with anti-Ss sera on frozen liver tissue sections showed specific staining in the parenchymal cells of the liver (Saunders and Edidin 1974). The cytoplasm of peritoneal macrophages, bone marrow, and peripheral blood stain specifically for Ss. Cultured fibroblasts seem to stain on the cell membrane. Studies by Saunders and Edidin (1974) suggest that peritoneal macrophages and liver parenchymal cells may be the site of Ss synthesis. It is worth noting that the macrophage has been shown to be the major site of synthesis of C′4 in the guinea pig and in man (Muller-Eberhard 1975).

H-2.7 antigen, controlled by genes in the G region, seems to be expressed predominantly on erythrocytes (David et al. 1975; Klein et al. 1975). *In vitro* absorptions using a large number of lymphocytes removes antibodies to H-2.7, suggesting a low density of expression of H-2.7 on those cells.

Ia antigens are easily detectable on splenic and lymph node lymphocytes but are very weakly expressed on normal thymocytes (David et al. 1973a). The antigens were found to be absent from erythrocytes, brain tissue, kidney cells, and liver cells (Frelinger et al. 1974). Tissue distribution studies indicate that Ia antigens are present on macrophages, fetal liver cells, epidermal cells, bone marrow cells, and spermatozoa (Delovitch and McDevitt 1975; Hämmerling et al. 1975). Some tumor cells also express Ia antigens (David, *unpublished data*).

In contrast to anti-H-2 sera, which kill 100 percent of lymphocytes, anti-Ia sera kill only 50 to 70 percent of lymphocytes, suggesting the expression of Ia only on a subpopulation of lymphocytes. The weak reactivity of Ia on

Table 7.7. Tissue Distribution of MHS Antigens

Tissues	H-2K,D	Ia	Ss	G.7
Spleen	+++	++	−	±[a]
Lymph node	++	++	−	−
Thymus	+	+[a]	−	−
Liver	+	−	±	−
Kidney	+	−	−	−
Erythrocytes	+	−	−	++
Sperm	±	±	−	−
Serum	−	−	++	−

[a]Detected by absorption only.

thymocytes suggests their absence on T cells. Experiments with purified T- and B-cell populations showed that the reactivity is due mainly to B-cells (Sachs and Cone 1973; Hämmerling et al. 1974), but Götze (1975) identified an Ia specificity expressed both on T- and B-cells. Studies by indirect ferritin labeling in the electron microscope have shown up to 70 to 80 percent labeling of lymph node lymphocytes by anti-Ia, much too high a frequency for B-cells only (Schultz et al. 1975). Detailed studies by Frelinger et al. (1974) showed that Ia antigens are expressed on both T- and B-cells. Wagner et al. (1975a) showed that Ia antigens are expressed on 100 percent of LPS-induced blast cells and 30 to 40 percent of Con A-induced blast cells and absent on PHA-induced blast cells. Recent studies with mitogen-induced blasts have shown that (1) most of the Ia specificities are expressed on T- and B-cells, (2) the specificities on the two cell populations are either similar or identical, and (3) Ia antigens are detected on a subpopulation of Con A-stimulated cells (David et al. 1976). Table 7.7 gives a summary of the tissue distribution of different components of the MHS.

4. Biochemistry

4.1 K and D Products

Current knowledge about the biochemical properties of the serologically detected H-2K and H-2D antigens and their genetic control has been thoroughly covered in a recent review by Nathenson and Cullen (1974). It is now generally accepted that H-2 antigens are glycoprotein molecules with the antigenicity residing in the protein portion of the molecule. Evidence has mounted that contradicts the earlier theories of the involvement of lipid and carbohydrates in the H-2 antigenic site.

Two distinct polypeptides, carrying specificities assigned to the K or D regions, can be isolated and separated from each other. Cullen et al. (1972) have shown that pretreatment of a preparation of NP-40 detergent solubilized

H-2 antigen with anti-H-2K sera did not affect its reactivity with anti-H-2D sera in an indirect immunoprecipitation assay. They demonstrated four separable polypeptides in an heterozygote, two H-2K peptides and two H-2D peptides. Some of these products have been shown to carry one private specificity along with one or more public specificity. Serological evidence that only two loci control serologically detected H-2 alloantigens has been reinforced by the inability to find a third polypeptide expressing H-2 specificity. Pancake and Nathenson (1973), working with the H-2^b antigens, have shown that specificities 33 and 5, which reside in the same molecule, occupy two separate sites. Further confirmation on the association of public and private specificities at the molecular level has been shown by Hauptfeld et al. (1975).

The H-2 antigen molecule isolated from cell membranes by detergent solubilization has an approximate molecular weight of 45,000 daltons and consists of a single polypeptide chain with two carbohydrate chains attached to it (Schwartz et al. 1973). Nathenson and Muramatsu (1971) have shown that carbohydrates are covalently linked to the protein portion of the H-2 glycoprotein and has a molecular weight of approximately 3300 daltons. The polysaccharide is composed of galactose, mannose, glucosamine, fucose, and sialic acid, and appears to be invariant in products from different H-2 haplotypes. Isolated glycopeptides fail to inhibit anti-H-2 sera, and enzymatic removal of the sugar groups fails to destroy H-2 activity, indicating no major role for the carbohydrate in the antigenic site. Nathenson and Muramatsu (1971) have suggested that the carbohydrate chain could be involved in either biosynthesis and turnover of the H-2 glycoprotein or positioning of the antigens in the membrane.

The evidence showing that H-2 antigenic variations are due to differences in the primary structure of the protein are (1) destruction of H-2 activity to protein-denaturing agents or agents that specifically modify certain amino residues and (2) differences in peptide maps of products from different haplotypes. Peptide mapping studies have shown considerable homology between the H-2K and H-2D products, further supporting the duplication model (Nathenson and Cullen 1974).

4.2 I Region Antigens

The NP-40 solubilization and immunoprecipitation assay used so successfully in the chemical characterization of H-2 antigens (Schwartz and Nathenson 1971) was applied in the identification of I region antigens or Ia antigens (Cullen et al. 1974). When specific anti-Ia sera was used in this assay, a 30,000-molecular-weight peak was detected. When antisera containing both anti-H-2 and anti-Ia were used, both the 45,000-mol.-wt. and 30,000-mol.-wt. peaks were observed. Specific anti-H-2K or H-2D sera gave only the H-2 peak (45,000 mol.-wt.). When anti-Ia sera were tested in the precipitation assay with a panel of H-2 congenic strains, complete concordance was found between anti-Ia cytotoxic activity and presence of the 30,000-mol.-wt. peak. These results strongly suggest that the 30,000-mol.-wt. peak contains Ia specificity. Preprecipitation with anti-H-2K did not remove the 30,000-mol.-wt. peak, indicating that H-2 and Ia specificities are located on different molecules. This has also been confirmed by Vitetta et al. (1974) and Goding et al. (1975). Ia antigens have been shown by "co-capping" analysis to be independent of the immunoglobulins and the H-2K and H-2D antigens (Unanue et al. 1974).

It was shown that Ia antigens incorporated not only ^{3}H-leucine, but also ^{3}H-fucose, ^{3}H-galactose, ^{3}H-glucosamine, and ^{3}H-mannose (Cullen et al. 1974). Because of this pattern of labeling, it was tentatively concluded that the Ia antigens are glycoproteins. Further analysis by Cullen et al. (1975) showed that specificity Ia.7 can be destroyed by protein denaturation and protease digestion but not by removal of some or most of the nonsaccharide residues of the glycoprotein. This suggests that the antigenic determinant for Ia antigens is in the protein portion of the molecule.

When antiserum against the whole I region was used for immunoprecipitation, rather broad peaks were observed, suggesting that multiple, somewhat heterogeneous antigen molecules might be precipitated within each peak. Sequential precipitation experiments with antisera directed against different subregions demonstrated the existence of two separable Ia molecules. Specificities Ia.4 and Ia.9, determined by the I-A subregion, were shown to be located on the same molecule distinct from the location of Ia.7, determined by the I-C subregion (Cullen et al. 1974; Sachs et al. 1975). Recent studies by Cullen et al. (1976) have shown that specificities mapping in the same subregion are found on the same molecule. These results suggest that at least two molecules are determined by I region genes ranging in molecular weight from 25,000 to 33,000.

4.3 S Region Antigens

Very little data are available on the physical-chemical properties of Ss and Slp antigens. On sephadex G-200 column, mouse Ss protein segregates into two peaks, the first eluting with the excluded volume (molecular weight greater than 200,000), the second at a molecular weight of approximately 180,000 (Hansen et al. 1974). Capra et al. (1975) have reported that Ss protein has a molecular weight of 120,000 composed of two basic subunits of 23,000 and 14,000. Recent results suggest that the Ss has a molecular weight of 180,000 in plasma but in serum form aggregates with molecular weight of up to 900,000 (Krasteff et al., *in preparation*).

5. Histocompatibility

This section will be concerned mainly with the histocompatibility factors associated with the MHS. The H-2 complex poses the most potent histocompatibility barrier in the mouse. Incompatibility for H-2 genes causes rapid skin graft rejection within 10 to 15 days (Billingham et al. 1954; Graff and Bailey 1973). Primary grafts are normally rejected within 6 to 8 days after a second graft. There is some variation in the potency of histocompatibility antigens mapping in the different subregions.

K Region: There are only two recombinants between the K and I regions (A.TL, AQR), so most grafts across K region barriers also include the I and S region incompatibility. The results of these grafts (Klein 1972; McKenzie and Snell 1973) suggested that K region differences are more potent than D region differences. But when combinations involving K incompatibilities only are tested, the average rejection time was 15 days (Klein 1975b).

D Region: Even though there are several strains that differ only in the D region, most test combinations include the G region and/or the Tla region incompatibility. Grafting across a D end barrier results in rejection at 15 to 18 days (Klein 1972; McKenzie and Snell 1973).

I Region: The central portion of the H-2 complex between the K and D regions were originally considered to be free of histocompatibility genes (Klein and Shreffler 1972). However, when recombinants that differ only in the I (and S) regions A.TH-A.TL, B10.AQR-B10.T(6R) were tested, rejection was rapid (Shreffler, *unpublished data;* Klein et al. 1974). Using intra-I region recombinants, the histocompatibility gene was localized to the I-A or I-B subregion and designated H-2I (Klein et al. 1974). H-2I-A incompatibility causes a graft rejection in 15 to 17 days. Recently, a weak histocompatibility locus was also demonstrated for recipient-donor differences in the I-C subregion [B10.HTT-B10.S(7R)]. The skin rejection occurred between days 20 and 55 after grafting (Götze et al. 1976).

G Region: G region differences do not cause first-set skin graft rejection (Shreffler, *unpublished data*). However, when the mice are presensitized, G region barrier causes graft rejection in approximately 60 days (Stimpfling, *personal communication*). These results suggest that the G region possibly contains a minor histocompatibility locus.

S Region: So far no known histocompatibility gene has been found mapping in the S region (Shreffler, *unpublished data*).

An important question to be answered was whether the histocompatibility genes are the same genes that control the serologically defined antigens. The evidence available at present indicates the involvement of K and D region antigens in skin graft rejection. However, genes in the K and D regions other than those determining serologically identifiable products could also be involved. Similarly, whether Ia antigens are involved in skin graft rejection across H-2I loci has not been resolved. The production of anti-Ia antibodies following skin graft rejection across the H-2I barrier could be due to passenger lymphocytes (Klein et al. 1974). Preliminary evidence suggests that Ia antigens might have an enhancing role (Staines et al. 1974). Klein and Murphy (1973) have shown cross-reactivity for histocompatibility antigens similar to the cross-reactivity that has been demonstrated between serologically determined products of the K and D region.

6. Immune Response

The first clearcut demonstration of an immune response gene in mice came from studies on the response of inbred strains to the branched, synthetic polypeptide antigen (H,G)-A—L (McDevitt and Sela 1965). The autosomal dominant gene controlling this response was designated Ir-1 and was mapped within the H-2 gene complex between the K and S regions (McDevitt et al. 1972). The region in which the Ir-1 gene maps is now designated the I-A subregion (Klein et al. 1974), and is known to control immune response to several antigens (Benacerraf and Katz 1975) (Table 7.8). The responses controlled by these genes are dependent on thymus-derived lymphocytes or T-cells and are thought to code for the antigen recognition system of the T-cell (Benacerraf and McDevitt 1972). However, some recent experiments have placed the site of the action of the Ir genes on the B-cells also (Mozes et al. 1975).

Taussig (1974) produced an antigen-specific molecule termed a T-cell "factor" that is capable of replacing T-cells in thymus-dependent antibody responses. Taussig et al. (1974) found that strains that were low responders to the (T,G)-A—L antigen produced the cooperative T-cell factor as efficiently as high responders. On the other hand, the factor, whether of high- or low-responder origin, would only cooperate effectively with bone marrow cells of high-responder origin. These data suggest that the defect in low-responder strains is in the B-cells and not in the T-cells. Further experiments by Taussig and Munro (1975) show that among the low responders, $H\text{-}2^f$ strains were unable to produce the T-cell factor, but their B-cells were capable of cooperation with high-responder T-cells. The nonresponder state in this case appears to be caused by a T-cell defect. Another low-responder strain, $H\text{-}2^s$, is not able to produce the factor nor to respond in the presence of the factor—a T-cell plus B-cell defect. These findings made it very likely that immune res-

Table 7.8. Immune Responses of Independent Haplotypes

H-2 Haplotype	Collagen	GLØ^5	(T,G)-A—L	(H,G)-A—L	GAT^{10}	GLØ	IgA	IgG	LDH^B	OA	OM	BGG	RE	NASE	GLT^5
b	h	l	h	l	h	l	l	h	h	h	l	l	l	l	l
d	l	l	m	m	h	h	l	l	h	h	l	l	h	h	h
f	h	l	l	l	h	l	—	h	h	h	l	—	l	—	l
j	l	h	m	l	h	h	l	—	l	h	—	—	l	—	h
k	l	l	l	h	h	l	h	l	l	l	h	h	h	h	l
p	l	h	l	l	l	l	h	h	h	h	—	—	h	—	h
q	—	h	l	l	l	h	l	l	h	h	l	l	—	l	h
r	l	h	l	—	h	h	h	h	l	h	—	—	—	—	h
s	h	l	l	l	l	l	h	h	h	l	l	l	—	l	l

From Shreffler and David (1975); Klein (1975b).

Table 7.9. Two-Gene Control of (T,G)-A—L Response

H-2 Haplotype	Strains	Response	T-cell Defect	B-cell Defect
b	B10, C3H.SW	High	No	No
d	B10.D2, Balb/c	High	No	No
k	B10.BR, C3H	Low	No	Yes
q	DBA/1	Low	—	Yes
j	I/st	Low	No	Yes
f	B10.M	Low	Yes	No
s	SJL	Low	Yes	Yes
j/f	$(I \times B10.M)F_1$	High	No	No
k/f	$(B10.BR \times B10.M)F_1$	High	No	No

From Munro and Taussig (1975).

ponse to (T,G)-A—L is controlled by two genes, one expressed on T-cells and one on B-cells. Munro and Taussig (1975) added further evidence for this two-gene model by an elegant complementation experiment where a cross between a T-cell-defective strain B10.M ($H\text{-}2^f$) and a B-cell-defective strain B10.BR ($H\text{-}2^k$) produced high-responder offspring. Both the genes seem to map in the I-A region. The molecule carrying the T-cell receptor as well as the molecule carrying the B-cell acceptor seem to express Ia antigenic specificity (Taussig and Munro 1975) (Table 7.9).

Is the immune response to other antigens also controlled by two genes? Response to synthetic polypeptide GLPhe was mapped in the I-C region (Maurer and Merryman 1974). Recently, Dorf et al. (1975) have shown that two genes control response to GLPhe, one mapping in the I-C region and the other one in the I-A region. Studies of the genetic control of immune response to other thymus-dependent antigens may indeed demonstrate that this is a general phenomenon. Figure 7.3 gives the current state of knowledge regarding map positions of Ir genes within different I subregions.

Kapp et al. (1974) have shown that in the GAT system, suppressor T-cells may be generated in situations where low response results from an acceptor defect. A soluble expression of the suppressor T-cells that is antigen specific and functionally suppressive in the KLH antigen system has been described by Takemori and Tada (1975). This T-cell factor also expresses Ia antigens (Tada, *personal communication*). Armerding et al. (1974) have described an Ia-positive T-cell factor (allogeneic effector) that lacks antigen specificity.

6.1 T-Cell, B-Cell Cooperation

Katz et al. (1975) have shown that for optimal cooperative interactions to occur between carrier-specific helper T-lymphocytes and hapten-specific B-lymphocytes in the development of antibody response, identity for the I region of the major histocompatibility system is required. The genes controlling T,B-

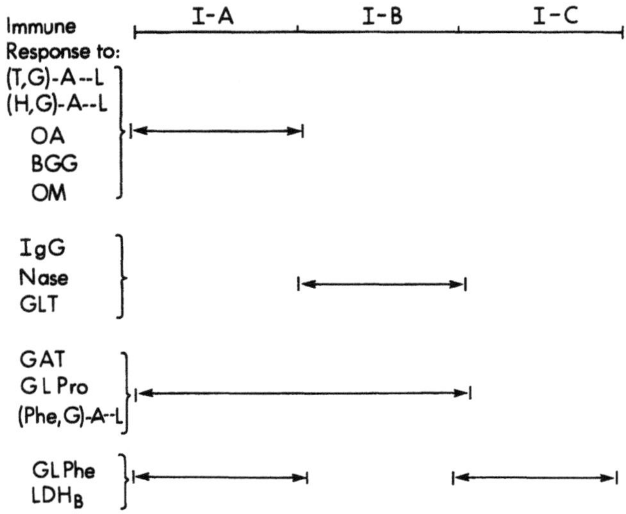

Fig. 7.3. Map positions for Ir genes

cell cooperative interactions (designated CI genes) map in the I-A and/or I-B subregions. Are the CI genes and the genes controlling the T-cell factor and B-cell acceptor identical? Although T,B-cell cooperation requires identity for the I region, T-cell factor is able to interact with allogeneic bone marrow cells as effectively as with syngeneic bone marrow cells (Taussig et al. 1975). This suggests that the histocompatibility restriction on cooperation between cells may not be related to the triggering event itself. Possibly, identity of I region is required for the production of T-cell factor. But once the factor is produced, it can interact in allogeneic conditions. Frelinger et al. (1975) have shown that antisera directed at products coded by the I region could inhibit the secondary IgG plaque-forming response of primed mouse spleen cell cultures responding to xenogeneic erythrocytes. More specific inhibition of response to (T,G)-A – L and GAT can also be obtained by using appropriate anti-Ia sera (R. Schwartz et al., *in preparation*).

What is the role of Ia antigens in immune response? With the available data we can only speculate. The anti-Ia antibodies are probably not directed at the antigen receptor. Ia most likely serves as a recognition structure that mediates cooperation between subclasses of lymphoid cells or between lymphoid cells and macrophages.

6.2 Viral Oncogenesis

Lilly (1970) showed by analyses of H-2 recombinant congenic strains that susceptibility to viral oncogenesis is associated with the K end of the H-2 complex, and has postulated (Lilly 1972; Lilly and Pincus 1973) that an Ir gene influences the level of immune response to virus-induced cell surface antigens. There is therefore ample although as yet inconclusive evidence that resistance to tumor virus is another expression, biologically probably a very significant expression, of the action of the Ir genes.

6.3 Mixed Leukocyte Reaction

In the mixed leukocyte reaction (MLR),lymphocyte proliferation is stimulated by exposure to allogeneic lymphocytes *in vitro*. Dutton (1966) first showed the association between MLR response and H-2 gene complex, using congenic strains of mice. Rychlikova et al. (1970, 1971) further localized the association to the K end of the H-2 complex, and finally Bach et al. (1972) and Meo et al. (1973) established that the major gene controlling MLR stimulation by antigens of the H-2 complex is controlled by the I region. Current data suggest that the strongest MLR determinants are found in the I-A and/or I-B subregion, moderately strong determinants in the I-C subregion, and weak determinants in the K and D regions. S and G region stimulation are almost negligible.

Serologically detectable I region antigens are most probably responsible for stimulation in the MLR. In support of the view that Ia gene products are involved in MLR stimulation are data of Meo et al. (1975a) and Götze et al. (1975). Anti-Ia sera specifically inhibits MLR stimulation, whereas anti-H-2K and anti-H-2D do not. Anti-Ia sera do not inhibit the responding cells in MLR. In several cases of one-way stimulation (2R-4R; 5R-18R; 7R-9R), MLR occurs only when the stimulating cells are Ia incompatible with the responding cells. In the reverse direction, the stimulating cells have no known Ia incompatibility with the responding cells and also no MLR (Dorf et al. 1975a). These MLR-stimulating structures are designated lymphocyte-activating determinants (Lad). The ability of a cell population to respond to the allogeneic stimulation of a Lad gene product is probably under the control of an Ir gene, as first suggested by Yunis and Amos (1971).

6.4 Graft-Versus-Host Reaction

Demant (1970) first reported an effect of differences in the K end of the H-2 complex on the graft-versus-host (GvH) reaction measured by a splenomegaly assay. Later, Livnat et al. (1973) and Klein and Park (1973) found that GvH reaction behaved in a manner similar to the MLR. They found strong GvH reaction for I region differences, moderate GvH reaction for K and D region differences, and a negligible effect of S region differences. These results suggest that the stimulating determinants in GvH reaction and MLR may be the Lad gene products and that MLR is an *in vitro* equivalent of GvH reaction.

6.5 Cell-Mediated Lympholysis

6.5.1 Allogeneic Response

Although the mixed leukocyte reaction represents the recognition phase of *in vitro* allograft reaction, cell-mediated lympholysis represents the destructive phase of the reaction. Specific cytotoxic T-cells are generated in the course of a mixed leukocyte reaction (MLR). If these cells are placed in culture with phytohemagglutinin (PHA)-stimulated target cells, the target antigens for the killer cells are specificities identical with (or genetically and physically closely linked to) the molecules carrying the H-2K and H-2D specificities (Alter et al. 1973; Abbasi and Festenstein 1973; Nabholz et al. 1974). Either killer cells are not generated against I region-associated antigens or these antigens are not expressed on PHA-stimulated cells. Nabholz et al. (1975) and Wagner et al. (1975a) showed that T-cell-mediated lysis against I region determinants can be detected on LPS-stimulated target cells, suggesting that I region antigens present on LPS-stimulated cells are absent or weakly expressed on PHA-stimulated cells. Wagner et al. (1975b) also demonstrated that cytotoxic T-lymphocytes can be generated across I region differences that kill Con A-stimulated target cells.

6.5.2 Specificity of Virus-Immune Effector T Cells

A great amount of experimental evidence has accumulated during recent years that in mice, specific thymus derived lymphocytes (T cells) and the cells with which they interact must share part of the major histocompatibility (H-2) gene complex to be functional (Zinkernagel and Doherty 1976). Specific cytolytic interactions occur in vitro between immune T cells and virus infected or chemically modified targets (Zinkernagel and Doherty 1975; Shearer et al. 1975). Such immune T cells can also be generated against targets expressing minor histocompatibility antigens and the male Y antigen (Bevan 1977; Gorden et al. 1975). Such interactions are efficient only when T cells and targets share either K or D regions of H-2. I region compatibility is neither sufficient nor required for cytolysis. By using H-2K mutants, it was possible to map the locus coding for the relevant cell surface markers for cytolytic interactions of LCMV or pox-virus immune T cells and infected target cells in the K region (Zinkernagel 1976).

The original H-2 restriction results from the LCMV model have been confirmed for ectromelia virus (mouse pox), vaccinia virus, paramyxovirus, Friend leukemia virus and probably also murine sarcoma virus (reviewed in Zinkernagel and Doherty 1976). Two hypotheses were proposed to explain this apparent K and D region associated restriction of virus-specific cytotoxic T cells.

1. Physiological interaction model: According to this model, T cells are specific for viral antigens expressed on the cell surface and for lysis to occur, a second physiological (self-self-like) interaction is necessary. Such interaction structures would have to be coded within H-2K or H-2D. The fact that F_1

or H-2 recombinant T cells can lyse both parental type targets could thus be explained with a minimal one set of specificities of T cells directed against viral surface antigens. Although this model was originally proposed to explain the need for H-2I compatibility between T helper cells and B cells for cooperation, it differs from it because interaction structures would have to be coded in K or D.

2. "Altered self": Altered self could be envisaged as a complex of virus (or other antigens) with K or D coded structures as a modification of self structures, as a biochemical alteration, or as derepression of a genetic mechanism regulating expression of multigenic H antigens (Zinkernagel and Doherty 1976). A minimum of two sets in homozygotes and four sets in heterozygotes, of T cell specificities directed against altered H-2K or D would have to exist to explain the fact that infected F_1 and H-2 recombinants can generate T cells cytotoxic for either parental type infected target (Doherty and Zinkernagel 1975).

Experimental proof for either of the above hypotheses is not available now. But overall most of the phenomenon can be explained by the "altered self" hypothesis better than the physiological interaction model. Biochemical analysis should yield further insight into the story. The TNP model leans more toward the "altered self" hypothesis. Cytotoxicity to alloantigens can also be explained by this model. On the other hand, the H-2K and D restriction of cytotoxic T cell activity against minor histocompatibility antigens or the male Y antigen are difficult to reconcile with the idea of altered self. Perhaps the major transplantation antigens (modified) are the targets in most T cell effector systems, and this may be their most relevant biological function.

7. Genetic Organization

The H-2 gene complex is comprised of five regions, K, I, S, G, D, and the I region is further separated into three subregions, I-A, I-B, I-C. Each of these regions is separated by known recombinants. In this section, recombinants defining these regions and the recombination frequencies will be discussed. Table 7.10 lists the recombinants and their H-2 composition.

H-2K-I-A: Three recombinants have been identified that arose from crossover events between K and I-A regions. Two of them A.TL (t1) and AQR (y1) are well-established recombinants, whereas the third one LG/Ckc (ar1) is postulated on the basis of H-2 and Ia typing, but has not been typed for Ir genes. The recombination frequency between K and I-A has been calculated to be approximately 0.023 percent (Klein 1975b).

I-A—I-B—I-J: Crossing over in four recombinants (B10.A(4R), D2.GD, B10.S(9R), B10.A(5R)) have been established to have occurred between I-A and I-J. Results based on Ir-IgG typing suggest that recombination in 4R and D2.GD occurred between A and B while in 5R it was between B and J.

I-J and I-E. Recombination in strains B10.A(3R) and B10.HTT occurred at this interval.

Table 7.10. Recombinant H-2 Haplotypes

Strain(s)	H-2 Haplo-type	Parental Haplo-type	H-2 Regions						
			K	I-A	I-B	I-C	S	G	D
A, B10.A	a	k/d	k	k	k	d	d	d	d
A.AL	al	k/d	k	k	k	k	k	k	d
C3H.OL	o1	d/k	d	d	d	d	k	k	k
C3H.OH	o2	d/k	d	d	d	d	d	d	k
HTG, B10.HTG	g	d/b	d	d	d	d	d	?	b
B10.D2(R101)	g1	d/b	d	d	d	d	d	?	b
B10.D2(R103)	g3	d/b	d	d	d	d	d	?	b
B10.BDR1	g4	d/b	d	d	d	d	d	?	b
B10.BDR2	g5	d/b	d	d	d	d	d	?	b
D2.GD	g2	d/b	d	d	?	b	b	b	b
HTH	h	a/b	k	k	k	d	d	?	b
B10.A(1R)	h1	a/b	k	k	k	d	d	?	b
B10.A(2R)	h2	a/b	k	k	k	d	d	?	b
B10.A(15R)	h15	a/b	k	k	k	d	d	?	b
B10.A(4R)	h4	a/b	k	k	b	b	b	b	b
B10.AM	h3	k/b	k	k	k	k	k	k	b
HT1	i1	b/a	b	b	b	b	b	?	d
B10.A(18R)	i18	b/a	b	b	b	b	b	?	d
B10.A(3R)	i3	b/a	b	b	b	d	d	d	d
B10.A(5R)	i5	b/a	b	b	b	d	d	d	d
B10.D2(R106)	i6	b/d	b	b	b	b	b	?	d
B10.D2(R107)	i7	b/d	b	b	b	b	b	?	d
A.TL	t1	s/a1	s	k	k	k	k	k	d
A.TH, B10.S(7R)	t2	s/a	s	s	s	s	s	s	d
B10.HTT	t3	s/t1	s	s	?	k	k	k	d
B10.S(9R)	t4	s/a	s	s	?	d	d	d	d
BSVS	t5	s/a?	s	s	s	s	d	d	d
B10.M(17R)	aq1	a/f	k	k	k	d	d	d	f
B10.M(11R)	ap1	a/f	f	f	f	f	f	f	d
A.TFR2	ap2	f/t2	f	f	?	?	s	s	d
A.TFR3	ap3	f/t2	f	f	?	?	s	s	d
A.TFR4	ap4	f/t2	f	f	?	?	s	s	d
A.TFR5	ap5	f/t1	f	f	f	f	k	k	d
A.TFR1	an1	t1/f	s	k	k	k	k	f	f
DA	qp1	q/s	q	q	q	q	q	q	s
A.QSR1	sq1	s/q	s	s	s	s	q	q	q
B10.QSR-2	sq2	s/2	s	s	?	?	q	q	q
AQR, B10.AQR	y1	q/k	q	k	k	d	d	d	d
B10.T(6R)	y2	q/k	q	q	q	q	q	?	d
AKR.M, B10.AKM	m	k/q	k	k	k	k	k	k	q
LG/Ckc	ar	d/f?	d	f	f	f	f	f	?
B10.S(8R)	as	a/s	k	k	?	s	s	s	s
B10.F(13R)		p/b	p			?			b
B10.R(20R)		t2/r	s	s	s	s	r	r	r
B10.S(21R)	i21	b/t2	b	b	b	b	b	?	d

From Shreffler and David (1975), Klein (1975b), and Stimpfling *(personal communication)*.

I-E and I-C. Two recombinants are identified in this interval, B10.S(8R) obtained during recombinant screening and a presumed recombinant at this interval, B10.A.

I-C—S: Well-established crossovers in this segment are C3H.OL (o1) and A.TFR5 (ap5). Haplotypes ap2, ap3, ap4, sq1, sq2, and t5 also probably contain crossovers at this point. Recombination in the interval IB—S is 0.102 percent (Klein 1975b).

S—G: Only one recombinant, A.TFR1 (an1), separates regions S and G. As more antigens mapping within the G region are identified, other recombinants between S and D will most likely be identified.

G—D: Established recombinants within this segment are A.AL(a1), C3H.OH(o2), B10.AM(h3), A.TH(t2), and B10.AKM(m). Other recombinants cannot be classified for this interval because of lack of markers.

Numerous recombinants have been identified in the interval S-D to yield recombination frequency of 0.193 percent (Klein 1975b). This suggests that there are probably unidentified loci in the S-D segment. I postulate that this interval contain 1–5 closely linked loci controlling erythrocyte antigens now assigned to the D region. Production of monospecific antisera against D region public specificities should elucidate some of these loci. The average recombination frequency between K and D is 0.329 percent (Klein 1975b). Higher recombination frequencies are found in some combination of H-2 haplotypes, such as a/b heterozygotes. Conversely almost negligible recombination is detected in b/k heterozygotes. In certain heterozygotes, recombination frequencies is much higher in females than males. The presently estimated recombination frequency between the K and D regions is a minimal estimate. Numerous recombinants have doubtlessly been overlooked due to limitation in screening procedures.

Mutations: Several mutations have been reported in the H-2 gene complex, some spontaneous, some induced. Most of the mutations reported so far have been localized to the K end. Extensive studies are underway to determine the serological, immunological, and biochemical properties of these mutants. In general, they behave as new haplotypes and have not greatly increased the understanding of the major histocompatibility system, primarily because both the localization of the mutational event as well as its extent (point mutation or more complex mutation) are difficult to ascertain.

8. Concluding Remarks

The evolution of the H-2 gene complex went through several phases. The years 1935–1945 represented the identification of the H-2 locus and the recognition that it is correlated with tumor rejection. The production of the congenic resistant strains in the years 1945–1955 enabled identification of several antigenic specificities and the understanding of the allelic system of the H-2 locus. The occurrence of recombination within the H-2 loci indicated the complexity of the system resulting in the postulation of multiple loci within the system

(1955–1965). The past decade has seen the identification of several traits linked to the mouse MHS, which offset the simplification derived from the two-locus model for the control of histocompatibility antigens.

The "H-2 gene complex" in 1975 consists of six regions, K and D region genes controlling the major histocompatibility antigens, I region genes controlling traits associated with immune response, S region genes controlling complement components, G region controlling genetic markers on erythrocytes, and TL region containing genes for antigens on normal and leukemic thymocytes. This segment of chromosome contains the most characterized genes and gene products on a mammalian genome. The mouse MHS not only represents an ideal system for the study of fundamental gene action in higher animals but controls traits of major biological significance. If the progress in the past decade is an indication, the next decade will result in better understanding of the immune response genes and their products and their association with the other genes in the complex.

Acknowledgments. The author is greatly indebted to Dr. Jane Schultz for her critical reading of the manuscript. I also thank Drs. T. Meo and D. C. Shreffler for valuable suggestions and Ms. Janey Jackson for secretarial assistance. The support of American Cancer Society grants IM-80 and IM-74 is greatly appreciated.

References

Abbasi, K., and Festenstein, H. Antigenic strength investigated by cell-mediated lympholysis in mice. *Eur. J. Immunol. 3*:430–435, 1973.

Allen, S. L. *H-2*^{f}, a tenth allele at the histocompatibility-2 locus in the mouse as determined by tumor transplantation. *Cancer Res. 15*:315–319, 1955.

Alter, B. J., Schendel, D. J., Bach, M. L., Bach, F. H., Klein, J., and Stimpfling, J. H. Cell-mediated lympholysis: Importance of serologically defined H-2 antigens. *J. Exp. Med. 137*:1303–1313, 1973.

Amos, D. B. Some iso-antigenic systems of the mouse. *Proc. 3rd Can. Cancer Res. Conf. 3*:241–248, 1959.

Amos, D. B., Gorer, P. A., and Mikulska, Z. B. An analysis of an antigenic system in the mouse (the H-2 system). *Proc. R. Soc. B 144*:369–380, 1955.

Archer, J. R., Smith, D. A., Davies, D. A. L., and Staines, N. A. A skin graft enhancing antiserum which recognizes two new B-cell alloantigens determined by the major histocompatibility locus of the mouse. *J. Immunogenet. 1*:337–344, 1974.

Armerding, D., Sachs, D. H., and Katz, D. H. Activation of T and B lymphocytes in vitro. III. Presence of Ia determinants on allogenic effect factor. *J. Exp. Med. 140*:1717–1727, 1974.

Arnaiz-Villena, A., Halloran, P., and David, C.S. Specific inhibition of lymphoid complement receptors by anti-H-2 sera: Evidence for a new H-2 tinked polymorphism. *J. Immunogen. 2*:415–425, 1975

Bach, F. H., Widmer, M. B., Bach, M. L., and Klein, J. Serologically defined and lymphocyte defined components of the major histocompatibility complex in the mouse. *J. Exp. Med. 136*:1430–1444, 1972.

Benacerraf, B., and Katz, D. H. The histocompatibility-linked immune response genes. *Adv. Cancer Res. (in press)*, 1975.

Benacerraf, B., and McDevitt, H. O. Histocompatibility-linked immune response genes. *Science* *175*:273–279, 1972.

Bevan, M. J. Recognition of minor histocompatibility antigens by cytotoxic T lymphocytes. *In* J. Watson (ed.), *Origins of Lymphocyte Diversity (in press)*, 1977.

Billingham, R. E., Brent, L., Medawar, P. B., and Sparrow, E. M. Quantitative studies on tissue transplantation immunity. The survival times of skin homografts exchanged between members of different inbred strains of mice. *Proc. R. Soc. (Lond.) B 143*:43–58, 1954.

Capra, J. D., Vitetta, E. S., and Klein, J. Studies on the murine Ss protein. 1. Purification, molecular weight and sub-unit structure. *J. Exp. Med. 142*:664–672, 1975.

Colombani, J., Colombani, M., Shreffler, D. C., and David, C. S. Separation of anti-Ia (I-region associated antigens) from anti-H-2 antibodies in complex sera, by absorption on blood platelets. Description of three new specificities. *Tissue Antigens 7*:74–85, 1975.

Cullen, S. E., David, C. S., Cone, J. L., and Sachs, D. H. Evidence for more than one Ia antigenic specificity on molecules determined by the I-A sub region of the mouse major histocompatibility complex. *J. Immunol. 116*:549–553, 1976.

Cullen, S. E., David, C. S., Shreffler, D. C., and Nathenson S. G. Membrane molecules determined by the H-2 associated immune response region: Isolation and some properties. *Proc. Natl. Acad. Sci. (USA) 71*:648–652, 1974.

Cullen, S. E., Freed, J. H., Atkinson, P. H., and Nathenson, S. G. Evidence that protein determines Ia antigenic specificity. *Transplant. Proc. 7*:237–242, 1975.

Cullen, S. E., Schwartz, B. D., Nathenson, S. G., and Cherry, M. The molecular basis of codominant expression of the histocompatibility-2 genetic region. *Proc. Natl. Acad. Sci. (USA)* *69*:1394–1397, 1972.

David, C. S., Colombani, J., Colombani, M., and Cullen, S. E. Murine I region associated antigen system: Identification and chemical characterization of specificities Ia. 12, 13 and 14. *Transplantation 21*:520–30, 1976.

David, C. S., Frelinger, J. A., and Shreffler, D. C. New lymphocyte antigens controlled by the Ir-IgG region of the H-2 gene complex. *Transplantation 17*:122–125, 1974.

David, C. S., and Shreffler, D. C. Studies on recombination within the H-2 complex. II. Serological analyses of four recombinants, H-2^{a1}, H-2^{o1}, H-2^{t1}, and H-2th. *Tissue Antigens 2*:241–249, 1972.

David, C. S., and Shreffler, D. C. The *Ir* region associated antigen system Ia (formerly Lna) of the mouse H-2 gene complex. Further definition with restricted antisera. *Transplantation* *18*:313–323, 1974.

David, C. S., Shreffler, D. C., and Frelinger, J. A. New lymphocyte antigen system (Lna) controlled by the Ir region of the mouse H-2 complex. *Proc. Natl. Acad. Sci. (USA)* *70*:2509–2514, 1973a.

David, C. S., Shreffler, D. C., Murphy, D. B., and Klein, J. Serological cross-reaction between H-2D and H-2K region antigens. *Transplant. Proc. 5*:287–293, 1973b.

David, C. S., Stimpfling, J. H., and Shreffler, D. C. Identification of specificity H-2.7 as an erythrocyte antigen: Control by an independent locus, H-2G, between the S and D region. *Immunogenetics 2*:131–139, 1975.

Davies, D. A. L. The molecular individuality of different mouse H-2 histocompatibility specificities determined by single genotypes. *Transplantation 8*:51–70, 1969.

Davies, D. A. L., and Hess, M. New Alloantigen genetically linked to the major histocompatibility locus of the mouse. *Nature 250*:228–230, 1974.

Delovitch, T. L., and McDevitt, H. O. Isolation and characterization of murine Ia antigens. *Immunogenetics 2*:39–52, 1975.

Demant, P. Genetic requirements for graft-versus-host reaction in the mouse. Different efficacy of incompatibility at D- and K-ends of the H-2 locus. *Folia Biol. (Praha) 16*:273–275, 1970.

Demant, P., Capkova, J., Hinzova, E., and Vovacova, B. The role of the histocompatibility-2 finked Ss-Slp region in the control of mouse complement. *Proc. Natl. Acad. Sci. 70*:863–864, 1973.

Demant, P., and Graff, R. J. Transplantation analysis of the H-2 system. *Transplant. Proc.* *5*:267–270, 1973.

Demant, P., Snell, G.D., and Cherry, M. Hemagglutination and cytotoxic studies of H-2. II. A family of 3-like specificities not in the C crossover region. *Transplantation 11*:242–249, 1971.

Doherty, P., and Zinkernagel, R. H-2 compatibility requirement for T cell mediated lysis of target cells infected with lymphocytic choriomeningitis virus. Different cytotoxic-T-cell specificities are associated with structures coded for in H-2K or H-2D. *J. Exp. Med. 141*:1427–1436, 1975.

Dorf, M. E., Plate, J. M. D., Stimpfling, J. H., and Benacerraf, B. Characterization of immune response and mixed lymphocyte reactions in selected intra-H-2 recombinant strains. *J. Immunol. 114*:602–620, 1975a.

Dorf, M. E., Stimpfling, J. H., and Benacerraf, B. Requirement for two H-2 complex Ir genes for the immune response to the L-Glu, L-lys, L-phe terpolymer. *J. Exp. Med. 141*:1469–1473, 1975b.

Dutton, R. W. Spleen cell proliferation in response to homologous antigens studied in congenic resistant strains of mice. *J. Exp. Med. 123*:665–671, 1966.

Edidin, M. The tissue distribution and cellular location of transplantation antigens. *In* B. D. Kahan and R. A. Reisfeld (eds.), *Transplantation Antigens*, pp. 125–140, Academic Press, New York, 1972.

Frelinger, J. A., Niederhuber, J. E., David, C. S., and Shreffler, D. C. Evidence for the expression of Ia (H-2I associated) antigens on thymus derived lymphocytes. *J. Exp. Med. 140*:1273–1284, 1974.

Frelinger, J. A., Niederhuber, J. E., and Shreffler, D. C. Inhibition of immune responses in vitro by specific antiserums to Ia antigens. *Science 188*:268–270, 1975.

Fu, S. M., Kunkel, H. G., Brusman, H. G., Allen, F. H., and Fotino, M. Evidence for linkage between HL-A histocompatibility genes and those involved in the synthesis of the second component of complement. *J. Exp. Med. 140*:1108–1112, 1974.

Goding, J. W., Nossal, G. J. V., Shreffler, D. C., and Marchalonis, J. J. Cellular localisation of an I-associated (Ia) antigen. *J. Immunogenet. 2*:41–48, 1975.

Goldman, M. B., and Goldman, J. N. Relationship of levels of early components of complement to the H-2 complex of mice. *Fed. Proc. 34*:979, 1975 (Abstract).

Gorden, R. D., Simpson, E., and Samelson, L. E. In vitro cell mediated immune responses to the male specific (H-Y) antigen in mice. *J. Exp. Med. 142*:1108–1121, 1975.

Gorer, P. A. The detection of antigenic differences in mouse erythrocytes by the employment of immune sera. *Br. J. Exp. Pathol. 17*:42–50, 1936.

Gorer, P. A. The genetic and antigenic basis of tumor transplantation. *J. Pathol. Bacteriol. 44*:691–697, 1937.

Gorer, P. A. The antigenic basis of tumor transplantation. *J. Pathol. Bacteriol. 47*:231–252, 1938.

Gorer, P. A. Studies in antibody response of mice to tumor inoculation. *Br. J. Cancer 4*:372–379, 1950.

Gorer, P. A., Lyman, S., and Snell, G. D. Studies on the genetic and antigenic basis of tumor transplantation: Linkage between a histocompatibility gene and "fused" in mice. *Proc. R. Soc. B135*:499–505, 1948.

Gorer, P. A., and Mikulska, Z. B. Some further data on the H-2 system of antigens. *Proc. R. Soc. B151*:57–69, 1959.

Götze, D. T(Iat) and B (Iab)-Cell alloantigens determined by the H-2 linked I region in mice. *Immunogenetics 1*:495–507, 1975.

Götze, D. Serological characterization of Ia antigens of the H-2^u, H-2^s, and H-2^q haplotypes by antisera produced against skin lymphocytes and lymphoblasts. Strain distribution pattern of Ia antigens and their relationship to Ir genes. *Immunogenetics 3*:139–156, 1976.

Götze, D., Grosse-Wilde, H., and Netzel, B. The effect of anti-Ia sera on mixed lymphocyte reaction in mice. *Folia Biol. (Praha) 21*:424–426, 1975.

Götze, D., Reisfeld, A., and Klein, J. Serological evidence for antigens controlled by the Ir-region in mice. *J. Exp. Med. 138*:1003–1008, 1973.

Götze, D., Rössler, R., and Thierfelder, S. A minor H locus within the H-2 complex in mice. *Transplant. Proc.* 1976.

Graff, R. J., and Bailey, D. W. The non-H-2 histocompatibility loci and their antigens. *Transplant. Rev. 115*:26–49, 1973.
Hämmerling, G. J., Deak, B.D., Mauve, G., Hämmerling, U., and McDevitt, H. O. B lymphocyte alloantigens controlled by the I region of the major histocompatibility complex in mice. *Immunogenetics 1*:68–81, 1974.
Hämmerling, G. J., Mauve, G., Goldberg, E., and McDevitt, H. O. Tissue distribution of Ia antigens: Ia on spermatozoa, macrophages and epidermal cells. *Immunogenetics 1*:428–438, 1975.
Hansen, T. H., Krasteff, T. N., and Shreffler, D. C. Quantitative variations in the expression of the mouse serum antigens Ss and its sex limited allotype Slp. *Biochem. Genet. 12*:281–293, 1974.
Hansen, T. H., Shin, H. S., and Shreffler, D. C. Evidence for the involvement of the Ss protein of the mouse in the hemolytic complement system. *J. Exp. Med. 141*:1216–1220, 1975.
Hauptfeld, M., Hauptfeld, V., and Klein, J. A method for detection of Ia antigens in the absence of appropriate H-2 recombinants. *J. Immunol. 115*:351–355, 1975.
Hauptfeld, V., Klein, D., and Klein, J. Serological identification of an Ir-region product. *Science 181*:167–169, 1973.
Hoecker, G., Counce, S., and Smith, P. The antigens determined by the H-2 locus: A rhesus-like system in the mouse. *Proc. Natl. Acad. Sci. (USA) 40*:1040–1051, 1954.
Hoecker, G., Pizarro, O., and Ramos, A. Some new antigens and histocompatibility factors in the mouse. *Transplant. Bull. 6*:407–411, 1959.
Johnson, M. H., and Edidin, M. H-2 antigens on mouse spermatozoa. *Transplantation 14*:781–786, 1972.
Kapp, J., Pierce, C. W., and Benacerraf, B. Genetic control of immune responses in vitro. III. Tolerogenic properties of the terpolymer L-glutamic acid^{60}-L-alanine^{30}-L-tyrosine^{10} (GAT) for spleen cells from non-responder ($H\text{-}2^s$ and $H\text{-}2^q$) mice. *J. Exp. Med. 140*:172–184, 1974.
Katz, D. H., Graves, M., Dorf, M. E., Dimuzio, H., and Benacerraf, B. Cell interactions between histoincompatible T and B lymphocytes. VII. Cooperative responses between lymphocytes are controlled by genes in the I-region of the H-2 complex. *J. Exp. Med. 141*:263–268, 1975.
Klein, J. Order of loci in the 2nd linkage of the mouse with respect to the centromere. *Genetics* 64:s35, 1970 (Abstract).
Klein, J. Private and public antigens of the mouse H-2 system. *Nature 229*:635–637, 1971.
Klein, J. Histocompatibility-2 system in wild mice. I. Identification of five new H-2 chromosomes. *Transplantation 13*:291–299, 1972.
Klein, J. A case of no sex limitation of Slp in the murine H-2 complex. *Immunogenetics 2*:297–299, 1975a.
Klein, J. *Biology of the Mouse Histocompatibility-2 Complex*. Springer-Verlag, New York, 1975b.
Klein, J., Festenstein, H., McDevitt, H., Shreffler, D., Snell, G., and Stimpfling, J. Genetic nomenclature for the *H-2* complex of the mouse. *Immunogenetics 1*:184–188, 1974.
Klein, J., Hauptfeld, V., and Hauptfeld, M. Evidence for a fifth region (G) in the H-2 complex of the mouse. *Immunogenetics 2*:141–150, 1975.
Klein, J., and Murphy, D. B. The role of "private" and "public" H-2 antigens in skin graft rejection. *Transplant. Proc. 5*:261–266, 1973.
Klein, J., and Park, J. M. Graft-versus host reaction across different regions of the H-2 complex of the mouse. *J. Exp. Med. 137*:1213–1255, 1973.
Klein, J., and Shreffler, D. C. The H-2 model for the major histocompatibility systems. *Transplant. Rev. 6*:3–29, 1971.
Klein, J., and Shreffler, D. C. Evidence supporting a two-gene model for the H-2 histocompatibility system of the mouse. *J. Exp. Med. 135*:924–937, 1972.
Lieberman, R., Paul, W. E., Humphrey, W., Jr., and Stimpfling, J. H. H-2-linked immune response *(Ir)* genes. Independent loci for *Ir-IgG* and *Ir-IgA* genes. *J. Exp. Med. 136*:1231–1240, 1972.
Lilly, F. The role of genetics in Gross virus leukemogenesis. *Bibl. Haematol. 36*:213–220, 1970.
Lilly, F. Mouse leukemia: A model of a multiple-gene disease. *J. Natl. Cancer Inst. 49*:927–934, 1972.

Lilly, F., and Pincus, T. Genetic control of murine viral leukemogenesis. *Adv. Cancer Res. 17*:231–277, 1973.

Livnat, S., Klein, J., and Bach, F. H. Graft versus host reaction in strains of mice identical for H-2K and H-2D antigens. *Nature New Biol. 243*:42–49, 1973.

Lyon, M. F., Butler, J. M., and Kemp, R. The positions of the centromeres in linkage groups II and IX of the mouse. *Genet. Res. (Camb.) 11*:193–199, 1968.

Maurer, P. H., and Merryman, C. F. Genetic control of immune responses of inbred mice: Responses against terpolymers Poly (Glu^{57} Lys^{36} Ala^{10}) and Poly (Glu^{54} Lys^{36} Ala^{10}). *Immunogenetics 1*:174–183, 1974.

McDevitt, H. O., Deak, B. D., Shreffler, D. C., Klein, J., Stimpfling, J. H., and Snell, G. D. Genetic control of the immune response: Mapping of the Ir-1 locus. *J. Exp. Med. 135*:1259–1278, 1972.

McDevitt, H. O., and Sela, M. Genetic control of the antibody response. 1. Demonstration of determinant-specific differences in response to synthetic polypeptide antigens in two strains of inbred mice. *J. Exp. Med. 122*:517–531, 1965.

McKenzie, I. F. C., and Snell, G. D. Comparative immunogenicity and enhanceability of individual H-2K and H-2D specificities of the murine histocompatibility-2 complex. *J. Exp. Med. 138*:259–277, 1973.

Meo, T., David, C. S., Rijnbeck, A. M., Nabholtz, M., Miggiano, V., and Shreffler, D. C. Inhibition of mouse MLR by anti-Ia sera. *Transplant. Proc. 7*:127–129, 1975a.

Meo, T., Krasteff, T., and Shreffler, D. C. Immunochemical characterization of murine H-2 controlled *Ss* protein through the identification of its human homologue as the fourth component of complement. *Proc. Natl. Acad. Sci. (USA) 72*:4536–4540, 1975b.

Meo, T., Vives, J., Miggiano, V., and Shreffler, D.C. A major role for the Ir-l region of rhe mouse H-2 complex in the mixed leucocyte reaction. *Transplant Proc. 5*:1507–1517, 1973.

Mozes, E., Isac, R., and Taussig, M. J. Antigen-specific T cell factors in the genetic control of the immune response to poly (Tyr, Glu)-poly DL Ala-poly lys. Evidence for T and B cell defects in SJL mice. *J. Exp. Med. 141*:703, 1975.

Muller-Eberhard, H.J. Complement. *Ann. Rev. Biochem. 44*:697–724, 1975.

Munro, A.J., and Taussig, M.J. Two genes in the major histocompatibility complex control immune response. *Nature 256*:103–106, 1975.

Murphy, D. B., and Shreffler, D. C. Cross reactivity between H-2K and H-2D products. I. Evidence for extensive and reciprocal serological cross reactivity. *J. Exp. Med. 141*:374–391, 1975a.

Murphy, D. B., and Shreffler, D. C. Cross reactivity between H-2K and H-2D products. III. Effect of H-2K – H-2D cross sensitization on skin graft survival. *Transplantation 20*:38–48, 1975b.

Nabholz, M., Vives, J., Young, H. M., Meo, T., Miggiano, V., Rijnbeck, A., and Shreffler, D. C. Cell mediated cell lysis in vitro: Genetic control of killer cell production and target specificities in the mouse. *Eur. J. Immunol. 4*:378–387, 1974.

Nabholz, M., Young, H., Rijnbeck, A., Boccardo, R., David, C. S., Meo, T., Miggiano, V., and Shreffler, D. C. I-region associated determinants: Expression on mitogen stimulated lymphocytes and detection by cytotoxic T cells. *Eur. J. Immunol. 5*:594–603, 1975.

Nathenson, S. G., and Cullen, S. E. Biochemical properties and immunochemical-genetic relationships of mouse H-2 alloantigens. *Biochem. Biophys. Acta 344*:1–25, 1974.

Nathenson, S. G., and Muramatsu, T. Properties of the carbohydrate portion of mouse H-2 alloantigen glycoproteins. *In* G. A. Jamieson and T.J. Greenwalt (eds.), *Glycoproteins of Blood Cells and Plasma*, pp. 245–262, Lippincott, Philadelphia, 1971.

Neauport-Sautes, C., Lilly, F., Silvestre, D., and Kourilsky, F.M. Independence of H-2K and H-2D antigenic determinants on the surface of mouse lymphocytes. *J. Exp. Med. 137*:511–526, 1973.

Pancake, S. J., and Nathenson, S. G. Selective loss of H-2 antigenic reactivity after chemical modification. *J. Immunol. 111*:1086–1092, 1973.

Passmore, H. C., and Shreffler, D. C. A sex-limited serum protein variant in the mouse: Inheritance and association with the H-2 region. *Biochem. Genet. 4*:351–365, 1970.

Pizarro, O., Hoecker, G., Rubinstein, P., and Ramos, A. The distribution in the tissues and development of H-2 antigens of the mouse. *Proc. Natl. Acad. Sci. (USA) 47*:1900–1906, 1961.

Rychlikova, M., Demant, P., and Ivanyi, P. The predominant role of the K-end of the H-2 locus in lymphocyte transformation in mixed cultures. *Folia Biol. (Praha) 16*:218–221, 1970.

Rychlikova, M., Demant, P., and Ivanyi, P. Histocompatibility gene organization and mixed lymphocyte reaction. *Nature New Biol. 230*:271–272, 1971.

Sachs, D. H., and Cone, J. L. A mouse B-cell alloantigen determined by gene(s) linked to the major histocompatibility complex. *J. Exp. Med. 138*:1289–1304, 1973.

Sachs, D. H., and Cone, J. L. Ir-Associated murine alloantigens: Demonstration of multiple Ia specificities in H-2 alloantisera after selective absorptions. *J. Immunol. 114*:165–169, 1975.

Sachs, D. H., Cullen, S. E., and David, C. S. Immune response associated lymphocyte antigen system (Ia). Definition of specificities Ia.8 and Ia.9 controlled by the I^b region. *Transplantation 19*:388, 1975.

Saunders, D., and Edidin, M. Sites of localization and synthesis of Ss protein in mice. *J. Immunol. 112*:2210–2218, 1974.

Schultz, J. S., Frelinger, J. A., Kim, S. K., and Shreffler, D. C. The distribution of Ia antigens of the H-2 complex on lymph node cells by immuno ferritin labelling. *Cell. Immunol. 16*:125–134, 1975.

Schwartz, B. D., Kato, K., Cullen, S. E., and Nathenson, S. G. H-2 histocompatibility alloantigens. Some biochemical properties of the molecules solubilized by NP-40 detergent. *Biochemistry 12*:2157–2164, 1973.

Schwartz, B. D., and Nathenson, S. G. Isolation of H-2 alloantigens solubilized by the detergent NP-40. *J. Immunol. 107*:1363–1367, 1971.

Shearer, G. M., Rehn, T. G., and Garbarino, C. A. Cell-mediated lympholysis of trinitrophenyl-modified autologous lymphocytes. Effector cell specificity to modified cell surface components controlled by the H-2K and H-2D serological regions of the murine major histocompatibility complex. *J. Exp. Med. 141*:1348–1364, 1975.

Shreffler, D. C. The Ss system of the mouse—A quantitative serum protein difference genetically controlled by the H-2 region. *In* J. Palm (ed.), *Isoantigens and Cell Interactions*, pp. 11–19, Wistar Institute Press, Philadelphia, 1965.

Shreffler, D. C. Immunogenetics of the mouse H-2 system. *In* D. Aminoff (ed.), *Blood and Tissue Antigens*, pp. 85–99, Academic Press, New York, 1970.

Schreffler, D.C., and David, C.S. The H-2 major histocompatibility Complex and the I immune response region. Genetic Variation, function and Organization. *Adv. Immunol. 20*:125–179, 1975.

Shreffler, D. C., Amos, D. B., and Mark, R. Serological analysis of a recombination in the H-2 region of the mouse. *Transplantation 8*:435–450, 1966.

Shreffler, D. C., David, C. S., Passmore, H. C., and Klein, J. Genetic organization and evolution of the mouse H-2 region: A duplication model. *Transplant. Proc. 3*:176–179, 1971.

Schreffler, D.C., David, C.S., Gotze, D., Klein, J., McDevitt, H., and Sachs, D.H. Genetic nomenclature for new tymphocyte antigens Controlled by the Ir region of the H-2 Complex. *Immunogenetics 1*:189–191, 1974.

Shreffler, D. C., and Owen, R. D. A serologically detected variant in mouse serum: Inheritance and association with the histocompatibility-2 locus. *Genetics 48*:9–25, 1963.

Shreffler, D. C., and Snell, G. D. The distribution of thirteen H-2 alloantigenic specificities among the products of eighteen H-2 alleles. *Transplantation 8*:435–450, 1969.

Snell, G. D. Methods for the study of histocompatibility genes. *J. Genet. 49*:87–108, 1948.

Snell, G. D., and Cherry, M. Hemagglutination and cytotoxic studies of H-2. IV. Evidence that there are 3-like antigenic sites determined by both the K and the D crossover regions. *Folia Biol. (Praha) 20*:81–100, 1974.

Snell, G. D., Cherry, M., and Demant, P. Evidence that the H-2 private specificities can be arranged in two mutually exclusive systems possibly homologous with the two subsystems of HL-A. *Transplant Proc. 3*:183–186, 1971a.

Snell, G. D., Demant, P., and Cherry, M. Hemagglutination and cytotoxic studies of H-2. I. H-1 and related specificities in the EK crossover regions. *Transplantation 11*:210–237, 1971 b.

Snell, G. D., Russell, E., Fekete, E., and Smith, P. Resistance of various inbred strains of mice to tumor homoiotransplants, and its relation to the H-2 allele which each carries. *J. Natl. Cancer Inst. 14*:485–491, 1953.

Staines, N. A., Guy, K., and Davies, D. A. L. Passive enhancement of mouse skin allografts. Specificity of the antiserum for major histocompatibility complex antigens. *Transplantation 18*:192–195, 1974.

Stimpfling, J. H. Recombination within a histocompatibility locus. *Ann. Rev. Genet. 5*:121–142, 1971.

Stimpfling, J. H., and Pizarro, O. On the antigenic products of the $H\text{-}2^m$ allele in the laboratory mouse. *Transplant. Bull. 28*:102–106, 1961.

Stimpfling, J. H., and Richardson, A. Recombination within the histocompatibility-2 locus of the mouse. *Genetics 51*:831–846, 1965.

Takemori, T., and Tada, T. Properties of antigen-specific suppressive T cell factor in the regulation of antibody response of the mouse. 1. In vivo activity and immunochemical characterizations. *J. Exp. Med. 142*:1241–1250, 1975.

Taussig, M. J. T cell factor which can replace T cells in vivo. *Nature (Lond.) 248*:234–236, 1974.

Taussig, M. J., Mozes, E., and Isac, R. Antigen-specific thymus cell factors in the genetic control of the immune response to poly-(tyrosyl, glutamyl)-poly-DL-alanyl—poly-tysyl. *J. Exp. Med. 140*:30–40, 1974.

Taussig, M. J., and Munro, A. J. In immune recognition. *In* A. Rosenthal (ed.), *Proc. 9th Leucocyte Culture Conference,* Academic Press, New York, 1975.

Taussig, M. J., Munro, A. J., Campbell, R., David, C. S., and Staines, N. A. Antigen specific T-cell factor in cell cooperation. Mapping within the I region of the H-2 complex and ability to cooperate across allogeneic barriers. *J. Exp. Med. 142*:694–700, 1975.

Unanue, E., Dorf, M. E., David, C. S., and Benacerraf, B. The presence of Ia antigens on the B cells in molecules distinct from Ig and H-2K and H-2D. *Proc. Natl. Acad. Sci. (USA) 71*:5014–5016, 1974.

Vitetta, E.S., Klein, J., and Uhr, J.W. Partial Characterization of Ia antigens from murine lymphoid Cells. *Immunogenetics 1*:82–90, 1974.

Wagner, H., Götze, D., Ptschelinzew, L., and Rollinghoff, M. Induction of cytotoxic T lymphocytes against I-region coded determinants: In vitro evidence for a third histocompatibility locus in the mouse. *J. Exp. Med. 142*:1477–1487, 1975a.

Wagner, H., Hämmerling, G., and Rollinghoff, M. Enhanced in vitro cytotoxic anti-H-2 responses in the presence of Ia antigens. *Immunogenetics 2*:257–268, 1975b.

Yunis, E. J., and Amos, D. B. Three closely linked genetic systems relevant to transplantation. *Proc. Natl. Acad. Sci. (USA) 12*:3031–3035, 1971.

Zinkernagel, R. M., and Doherty, P. C. H-2 compatibility requirement for T cell mediated lysis of targets infected with lymphocytic choriomeningitis virus. Different cytotoxic T cell specificities are associated with structures coded in H-2K or H-2D. *J. Exp. Med. 141*:1427–1436, 1975.

Zinkernagel, R. M., and Doherty, P. C. Major transplantation antigens, virus and specificity of surveillance T cells: The "altered self" hypothesis. *In Contemporary Topics in Immunology,* Plenum Press, New York 1976 *(in press).*

Zinkernagel, R., and Doherty, P. H-2 antigens and specificity of virus-immune T cells: Altered self or physiological interaction? *In* J. Watson (ed.), *Origins of Lymphocyte Diversity,* 1977 *(in press).*

Chapter 8

The Major Histocompatibility System of the Chicken

K. HÁLA

1. Introduction

Gallus gallus domesticus, one of the species of the class Aves, occupies an important position in experimental biology. Throughout their ontogeny, chickens provide suitable experimental material for various scientific disciplines, for example, virology, genetics, immunology, and immunogenetics. Experiments carried out in chickens have contributed much to the discovery and analysis of immunological tolerance (Hašek 1953), graft-versus-host (GvH) reaction (Simonsen 1957), and to the discovery of the T- and B-cell systems in animals (Warner 1967). They provided one of the first indications of an effect of the genotype at the major histocompatibility system (MHS) on a variety of physiological traits (Gilmour 1960; Briles 1960, 1964).

The advantages of using chickens for experimental work include having large numbers of offspring from the same parents, and having readily accessible embryos which, unlike mammalian embryos, can be incubated under sterile conditions. The fact that two primary lymphoid organs—the bursa of Fabricius, responsible for the humoral immune response, and the thymus, responsible for the cellular immune response—are anatomically separated is a great asset in many immunological studies. Finally, the nucleated erythrocytes are more similar to "red" cells than are the mammalian red blood cells.

Studies on chickens, which are so different from mammals in phylogeny (Ohno 1967), are important for comparative biology. A chicken model sometimes reveals certain aspects more clearly than does a corresponding mammalian model. Thus, studies of the MHS in chickens may also be useful for a better understanding of the structure and function of the MHS of mammals.

2. The B System of the Chicken

Thirteen blood group systems have been described in the chicken: A, E, B, C, D, L, N, H, I, J, K, P, and R (Gilmour 1960; Briles 1962; Briles and Crittenden 1971). Among these, the B system, which is associated with the major histocompatibility system of chickens, occupies a special position. Originally this system was given the designation D (Briles et al. 1948), but since 1950 it has been named B (Briles et al. 1950). From the very beginning

Table 8.1. Chart of B Specificities

Antigens	1	2	3	4	5	6	7	8	9	10	11	12	13	14	15	16	17	18	19	20	21	22	23	24	25	26	27	28
	Individual Antigenic Factors																											
B1					5	6	7	8	9			12	13	14							21			24	25	26	27	28
B2	1	2	3	4					9				13	14							21				25		27	
B9		2		4			7	8		10	11	12	13	14	15			18		20	21							
B10			3	4				8							15	16	17	18			21			24		26	27	
B13				4		6					11	12	13		15		17		19	20		22						
B17					5	6	7	8	9	?	?	?	?	?	?					?	?	22				26	27	

After Hála et al. (1974) and unpublished results.

it has been clear that antigens determined by the alleles of this genetic system are complex, i.e., that they are composed of a number of antigenic factors. Therefore, numerals were used to designate the antigens, B_{15}, B_{25}, B_3, etc., or alleles, B^{15}, B^{25}, etc., or a combination of letters and numerals, for example, $K_1K_2B_2$ or $B_1B_2YK_2$ (Gilmour 1959). In later work numerals indicated individual alleles and their products (Briles et al. 1957; Gilmour 1959), in contrast to the original designation where each figure represented a hypothetical antigenic factor (Briles et al. 1950).

Recently, attempts have been made to determine the antigenic factors of which a particular antigen is composed (Tab. 8.1) in order to define more precisely the antigens present in the chicken lines (Hála and Knížetová 1970; Oosterlee and Bouw 1970).

Schierman and McBride (1969) and Hála et al. (1975, 1976) have found serological evidence of crossing over within the MHS, thus indicating the presence of at least two loci. Hála et al. screened systematically for crossing-

Production of Hybrids for Detection of Recombination

CB (B^1/B^1) × CC (B^2/B^2)
↓
F_1 (B^1/B^2) × WB (B^{10}/B^{10})
↙ ↘
B^1/B^{10} B^2/B^{10}

Preparation of Specific Antisera Used in the Analysis

Antiserum B2 CB (B^1/B^1) × WB (B^{10}/B^{10})
↓
F_1 (B^1/B^{10}) ← immunized with RBC from CC (B^2/B^2)

Antiserum B1 CC (B^2/B^2) × WB (B^{10}/B^{10})
↓
F_1 (B^2/B^{10}) ← immunized with RBC from CB (B^1/B^1)

Fig. 8.1. Scheme of experiment for detection of crossing over in the B chromosome region

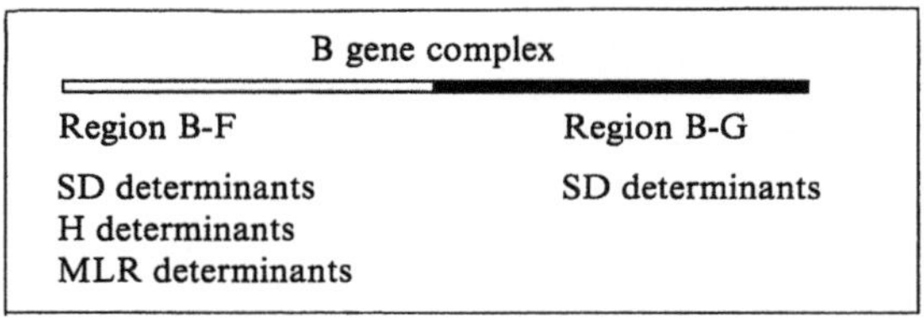

Fig. 8.2. Structure of the MHS (B system) of chickens

over events in experiments in which F_1 hybrids obtained by reciprocal crosses of the congenic lines CB and CC were crossed with the WB line. Anti-B1 and anti-B2 sera were prepared that did not cross-react with WB (Fig. 8.1), and they were applied to a total of 1206 offspring from the cross (CB × CC) × WB. All but two birds showed positive reactions with either the B1 or the B2 antiserum. The two exceptional birds reacted with both. One of these, cock 744, contained a recombinant haplotype, R1, which had arisen as a result of crossing over between the B^1 and B^2 chromosomes. In the other bird the mechanism of the dual reactivity is still unknown.

In the case of R1, the graft-versus-host reaction with lymphocytes from cock 744 or its R1-containing offspring revealed that the locus B-G determined only the serologically detected (SD) specificities of the B antigen, whereas the locus B-F determined, in addition, the GvH reaction. Also, skin graft rejections were determined by B-F (Vilhelmová et al., *to be published*) (Fig. 8.2). It is not yet known whether the latter locus is identical with the locus AA (Simonsen 1973, 1975), or whether two or more loci are involved.

Furthermore, the immune response (Ir) genes, controlling the ability of chickens for immune response against various defined antigens, are linked to the MHS. One of these antigens, the 2,4-dinitrophenol group conjugated to chicken gamma globulin (DNP-CGG), elicits low antibody levels in the WB line and high antibody levels in the CB line after immunization. Birds from the first backcross (CB × WB) × WB, carrying the allele B^1 derived from the CB line, produced significantly more antibody against this antigen than birds B^{10}/B^{10} (Balcarová et al. 1974). Another antigen, a synthetic polypeptide, (T,G)-A — L, also showed that the Ir gene, which controls the immune response against it, was linked to the B allele (Günther et al. 1974). In both cases, it has been demonstrated that a strong immune response is inherited in F_1 hybrids as a dominant trait.

2.1 Biochemical Characterization of B Antigens

The B antigens contain two polypeptide chains with molecular weights of 40,000 to 45,000 and 11,000 to 12,000, which are not covalently linked (Pink et al. 1975; Ziegler and Pink 1975).

The antigens have been isolated from peripheral blood leukocytes labeled with tritiated leucine and lysine. Their purification from the lysate was performed by a two-step indirect immunoprecipitation technique, and the precipitate was separated by electrophoresis on polyacrylamide gels. The authors further found a difference in molecular weight of the B antigen between the WA and WB lines (42,000 and 45,000, respectively).

2.2 Distribution of B Antigens

Antigens of the B system were demonstrated for the first time on erythrocytes (RBC) (Briles et al. 1948). Later, they were detected on lymphocytes (Schierman and Nordskog 1962; David et al. 1966), fibroblasts from 12-day embryos grown in tissue culture (Hložánek and Hála 1969; Benda et al. 1970), spleen cells and bone marrow cells (Benda 1971; Benda and Hála 1972), and liver cells (Waters and Bennett 1971). They were not detectable on cells of the brain and muscles (Waters and Bennett 1971). They were not found in a soluble form in the abdominal fluid (McDermid 1964).

The ability for absorption can be expressed as "absorption units" (one unit is the amount of tissue that inhibits on absorption 50 percent of the haemagglutinating activity of the reagent employed). The relative constants of such units were for RBC 2.4, spleen cells 0.7, bone marrow cells 0.5, and liver cells 0.3. However, when individual cell suspensions were used for immunization, the highest antibody titers (measured by agglutination of RBC) were obtained after immunization with bone marrow cells (Benda 1971). According to both criteria, the lowest antigenicity was exhibited by liver cells.

The results obtained showed that, in contrast to the H-2 system (Basch and Stetson 1962), the B system antigens had the highest concentration on erythrocytes (Benda and Hála 1972). The reason for this difference is not clear.

The B antigens present on cells of the skin and on erythrocytes were also studied by means of immunological tolerance. Like other investigators (Hašek et al. 1955; Billingham et al. 1955), Schierman and Nordskog (1964) found that RBC were not capable of inducing tolerance to skin grafts. On the other hand, Kinsky and Mitchison (1963) demonstrated the ability of RBC to induce tolerance to skin grafts. Because in these works it is not possible to exclude the importance of the difference in additional H antigens, which may cause skin graft rejection, the experiments should be repeated using congenic lines differing only in the B complex.

2.3 Development of B Antigens

In contrast to the blood group antigen A, which has been demonstrated on embryonic erythrocytes as early as 72 hr of incubation (Johnson 1956),

Table 8.2. Detection of Antigens B9 in Four Embryos of the Same Age (14 Days of Incubation) with Different anti-B9 Sera in Reciprocal Titer Values

Serum	Chicken Embryo				Adult Chicken
	First	Second	Third	Fourth	
6928	2	4		8	16
6691					4
6401	2	2		2	64
6725					8
6912					64
334/8410					32
377/2247					64
458/401	2	8	8	16	32
392/2029					8
404/2411	2	2			4
407/2065		4	4	4	4
357/8429		2	2	2	16
375/179/8	4	32	32	32	128
443/2411	2	4	4	4	32
395/179	4	32	32	32	64
481/anti-B9		2	2	4	16

After Pöschl and Hála (1974).

individual B antigens are demonstrated in embryos of different ages. For example, antigen B1 (given the symbol D1 in the paper of Briles et al. 1948) has been detected as early as the third day of incubation, whereas additional three antigens have been identified as late as the sixth day after hatching (Briles et al. 1948). Furthermore, a gradual "maturation" is characteristic for the B antigens, that is, RBC of chickens reach the agglutinability of RBC of adult hens as late as the fifth (Johnson 1956) to the 30th day of life (Briles and Lee 1970). The B antigens can be detected earlier in homozygous embryos than in the heterozygous ones (Drobná 1967; Briles and Lee 1970).

The differences in the ontogenic development of B antigens may be due to the fact that different B antigens have been studied by various investigators. Additional important differences may be caused by the different B alloantisera used. Pöschl and Hála (1974) found that 6 of the 16 anti-B9 test sera used for agglutination of erythrocytes from four embryos of the inbred WA line (genotype B^9/B^9) did not agglutinate these erythrocytes, although the sera reacted with erythrocytes from adult birds of the same genotype in titers of 1:4 to 1:64 (Tab. 8.2). The authors believed that "the detection of B antigens on embryonic erythrocytes depended on the quality of antiserum apparently determined by the content of antibodies against individual antigenic factors and not on serum titers". Further, they found that erythrocytes from embryos of the same genotype, though of the same age, did not react identically with the sera used.

3. Methods for the Detection of B Antigens

3.1 In vitro Demonstration of B Antigens

3.1.1 Demonstration by Means of Antibodies

The B antigens can be determined by means of an alloantiserum or antiserum prepared by immunization of a different animal species with chicken erythrocytes. However, heteroimmune sera prepared mostly in rabbits were not extensively used. Landsteiner and Miller (1924) employed them for the first time, and by their absorption identified eight different types of erythrocytes in ten chickens.

The most widely used method is the agglutination of RBC by alloantisera (Gilmour 1960; Briles 1962; McDermid 1964). The agglutination tests are performed either in the classical form, i.e., in the tubes (Briles, Gilmour), or especially in the recent times, on plastic plates (Oosterlee). The open glass slide is seldom used (Simonsen). The 2 to 5 percent washed erythrocyte suspensions in 0.75 or 0.9 percent saline are mixed with antiserum in appropriate dilutions. Although the reactions are often seen immediately after the contact of RBC with the serum [according to Keily et al. (1966), this is typical mainly for B antigens], the readings are usually made 30 to 60 min later. First the sediment is evaluated, and after resuspension, the agglutination is assessed macroscopically or semimicroscopically. After another 60 min at room temperature, or the following day (the mixtures are stored at $+4°C$ in a refrigerator), a second reading is made. Also, the mixtures can be incubated at 37°C (Matsumoto and Okada 1961).

Because the agglutination tests give standard and reliable results, other methods, such as the antiglobulin technique (Dunsford et al. 1961), Chown capillary method (McDermid 1964), and/or enzyme-treated RBC (Borel 1963) are used only in special cases. Simonsen (1975) described massive agglutination on glass slides after the addition of 20 percent fresh normal chicken serum. Lymphocytes (Schierman and Nordskog 1962), instead of RBC, can be used in agglutination to identify the B antigens. The B antigens on lymphocytes were also detected by immunofluorescence (David et al. 1966), and by allofixation (Wong et al. 1972). On fibroblasts, these antigens were detected by mixed agglutination (Hložánek and Hála 1969).

The cytotoxicity test using chicken complement was not suitable because of the peculiarities of the chicken complement. Neither was guinea pig complement effective, because avian antibodies do not activate its first component, C1 (Benson et al. 1961). Stolfi et al. (1971) used with success a mixture consisting of the C1 component of the chicken complement and guinea pig complement devoid of the C1 component to identify chicken antiviral antibodies. This method was used by Gilmour (1975) for the demonstration of alloantigens on cells of the bursa of Fabricius in the avian system.

3.1.2 Mixed Lymphocyte Reaction

The mixed cultivation of lymphocytes from two genetically different individuals of the same species leads to the transformation of these cells into blast cells (Hirschhorn et al. 1963; Bain et al. 1963), particularly in dependence on the differences in the MHS (Iványi et al. 1967). This reaction is considered to be analogous to the GvH reaction (Klein 1973). The intensity of the reactions is measured by incorporation of radioactively labeled thymidine during the final phase of incubation.

In chickens, spleen cells (Skopińska and Skamene 1968; Alm 1971) and peripheral blood lymphocytes (Skopińska and Skamene 1968; Miggiano et al. 1974a, 1974b) were used for mixed lymphocyte reaction (MLR). The methods of MLR differ (the number of cells used, the time of incubation, etc.) between various investigators. We shall keep here to the method used by Miggiano et al. (1974a). The reactions are performed in macrocultures in the tubes (in a volume of about 1 ml), microcultures (total volume of 10 μl/well), or minicultures. The latter are most appropriate with regard to the amount of medium and the number of cells used and the results obtained. They are performed as a two-way MLR (1.5×10^6 lymphocytes from two birds mixed in 200 μl of medium RPMI 1640), or a one-way MLR (0.75×10^6 untreated lymphocytes mixed with aliquots of X-irradiated or mitomycin-treated cells). In micro- and minicultures the cells are cultivated on hemagglutinating plates and incubated at 37°C in a 5 percent CO_2 in humidified air atmosphere for 5 days. Twenty hours before cell harvesting, radioactively labeled thymidine is added (Miggiano et al. 1974a).

Miggiano and his collaborators (1974a) showed that birds within an inbred line did not stimulate their lymphocytes reciprocally, but they observed that the stimulation always occurred between birds from different inbred lines. In six F_2 hybrids from the cross of the CB and WB lines, this reaction depended only on the genotype in the MHS. They did not demonstrate the influence of additional histocompatibility antigens in which these two lines differ (Hála 1969). With an identical B antigen in F_2 hybrids, the stimulation index was less than 1.7, whereas with a different antigen it was greater than 2.2.

An analysis of the recombinant chromosome Rl in the MLR revealed that this reaction was also determined by the B-F region, whereas the B-G region had no effect on stimulation in MLR (Miggiano and Vilhelmová, *in preparation*).

3.2 In vivo Demonstration of B Antigens

3.2.1 Transplantation

The genetic aspects of transplantation have been studied by many investigators (Craig and Hirsch 1957; Craig et al. 1960; Polley et al. 1960), but their work was directed to demonstrating the genetic similarities or differences without any relation to the blood groups.

The evidence that the B blood group antigen was also a histocompatibility antigen was provided by Schierman and Nordskog (1961). They found in 16-day-old chickens that skin grafts exchanged between B-incompatible birds were rejected within 12 days, whereas grafts between B-identical individuals all survived to the 12th day. This finding was confirmed and developed further by other investigators on different populations of birds (Craig and McDermid 1963; Gleason and Fanguy 1964; Crittenden et al. 1964; Hašek et al. 1966; Hála et al. 1966). Because different congenic lines differing in individual transplantation loci are not available, the data on comparison of graft survival with the difference at the B locus and additional transplantation loci are lacking.

In contrast to the results obtained in mice, where both the H-2K and H-2D ends of the H-2 locus determine the antigens capable of eliciting the graft rejection (Démant 1973), of the two B chromosome regions in chickens, only the B-F determines the transplantation determinants (H).

3.2.2 Graft-Versus-Host Reaction

As described by Simonsen (1957), the donor lymphoid cells react immunologically against foreign antigens expressed in the recipient that are incapable of immune reaction. In embryos, the spleen and in part the liver is enlarged and the body weight is decreased (Elkins 1971). After hatching, the reaction is apparent as a GvH disease (runt disease) (Cock and Simonsen 1958). There is a direct relationship between the spleen enlargement and the log dose of cells injected (Simonsen 1967), although the recipient's cells also participate in the spleen enlargement. Therefore control birds must be derived from the same population of the same age, genotype, etc.

For the induction of splenomegaly, 13- or 14-day embryos are most suitable to be injected with lymphoid cells (Solomon 1971; Solomon and Tucker 1962), and the spleen is weighed from the fourth to the eighth day after the inoculation of donor cells (Elkins 1971). The ability of donor cells to induce a GvH reaction develops, depending on the age of the donor (Seto 1967; Solomon and Tucker 1962) and the cell type (Seto 1968). Full details on this reaction have been reported by Solomon (1971) and Elkins (1971).

The GvH reaction can be studied not only by splenomegaly but also by pock formation on dropped chorioallantoic membranes of 12-day embryos after inoculation of competent cells (Boyer 1960; Burnet and Burnet 1960). The number of pocks is determined on the fourth or fifth day after inoculation. It has been demonstrated that one pock results from the activity of one lymphoid cell (Coppleson and Michie 1965, 1966; Simons and Fowler 1966). This model allows the counting of cells capable of reacting against the recipient's antigens.

Another modification is the local GvH reaction after intradermal injections of the donor's lymphoid cells into the recipient's wattle. The positive reactions are evident as a swelling of the wattle, with a maximum within 4 days of injection. At about 7 days, the reactions begin to recede (Warner 1964; Jaffe 1965).

The genetic analysis of GvH reactions was performed in inbred lines of chickens and their crosses. The major histocompatibility locus and a number of the weaker ones causing slight enlargement were found to be responsible for the reactions (Jaffe and Payne 1962).

In the experiments on embryos from parents with known blood groups the major locus has been identified as the B system of the chicken (Jaffe and McDermid 1962; Schierman and Nordskog 1963; Bacon et al. 1973). One locus (Burnet and Burnet 1961), which has been recognized again as the B system (Schierman and Nordskog 1963), is responsible for pock formation.

As in the case of splenomegaly, in pock formation the reactions can be induced even with a non-B difference, and their size is only one-third that of pocks formed with a B incompatibility (Longenecker et al. 1970; Knížetová et al. 1970). For the induction of splenomegaly in B-incompatible birds, large amounts of lymphoid cells are required (Simonsen 1967; Nisbet and Simonsen 1967). In no case was this additional locus/loci causing the weak GvH reaction identified. It was considered that a smaller number of antigen-reactive cells present in the donor and capable of reacting with the corresponding antigen of the recipient might be responsible for the weak reaction in the non-B difference (Nisbet et al. 1969).

Using appropriately diluted sera, a donor-recipient combination can be selected where no GvH reactions occur (Simonsen 1973, 1975). It is assumed that the alleles of the AA (alloaggression) locus, which is closely linked to or identical with the B chromosome region, are responsible for the GvH reactions. In Simonsen's experiments the anti-B allosera were absorbed with erythrocytes from different outbred hens. In special cases, after the removal of agglutinating activity against some erythrocytes, the positive reactions were seen with erythrocytes of other birds whose lymphocytes were inhibited by these sera and were not capable of eliciting GvH reactions. On the basis of the results obtained, Simonsen postulated that the agglutinating activity remaining after absorption with certain erythrocytes was directed against antigenic products of the AA locus responsible for the GvH reaction.

There is still another involvement of the B complex in the GvH reactions. Independently from the Japanese investigators (Mikami et al. 1969), Longenecker et al. (1970, 1972) found that chickens with the B14 allele had the ability to elicit differently strong reactions determined genetically and that this ability was associated or controlled by the MHS of chickens. The alleles of this system seem to regulate the duration of the intermitotic period and/or the number of mitoses during the differentiation of cells capable of initiating the GvH reactions. Okada and Mikami (1974) showed that genes controlling the GvH competence are additive in nature.

3.2.3 Elimination of ^{51}Cr-Labeled Erythrocytes

In analogy to mice (Möller 1963), this test can be used to study the antigens of the MHS in chickens (Hartmanová, *in preparation*). In chickens, the tolerance induced by RBC (Mitchison 1962) and the ontogeny of immunity against erythrocyte antigens (Solomon and Tucker 1963) was studied by this test.

The erythrocytes are labeled with sodium chromate (^{51}Cr) in the form of hexovalent chromium ions, which become bound to hemoglobin when they penetrate into the erythrocytes where a reduction into the trivalent form takes place. The chromium in the trivalent form can leave the erythrocytes only when the membrane is ruptured. Sixty minutes after injection of labeled erythrocytes, a sample is collected and its value constitutes 100 percent. How many of the originally injected RBC survive in the recipients is assessed from blood samples collected at regular intervals (Solomon and Tucker 1963).

This sensitive method was used to select chickens during the preparation of syngeneic lines (Hašek et al. 1966).

4. Definition of B Antigens

Briles and his collaborators demonstrated that some antigenic substances are common to several antigens. Originally they used numerals to indicate the similarity of the antigens (for example, B_{15} and B_{25}), the numeral 5 indicating the antigenic factor shared in common by the antigens B_{15} and B_{25} and the numerals 1 and 2 indicating the different antigenic factors. They used the term antigen only in referring to the "total antigenic product of an allele" and the term antigenic factor in referring to the "serological components of which the antigen appears to be composed" (Briles et al. 1950).

With increasing numbers of populations studied, the number of the described alleles increased. Because of the cross-reactions between individual sera, the original terminology appeared to be too complicated and it was abandoned. Numerals were used to indicate the alleles (for example, B^{16}, B^{17}, etc.); this did not reflect the degree of similarity between individual antigens but indicated the whole antigenic product of the allele (Briles et al. 1957; Gilmour 1959). The antigen was determined on the basis of its specific pattern on agglutination with a broad spectrum of typing reagents (Briles 1960, 1964; Fanguy et al. 1961).

Various factors played a role in changing the nomenclature:

1. Extensive polymorphism of B antigens (Briles et al. 1957),
2. Sharing of the factors by different antigens, i.e., considerable cross-reactivity,
3. The fact that small amounts of antiserum obtained from one producer do not allow thorough analysis by absorption,
4. The fact that the immune response of individuals of the same genotype against an antigen is generally different, i.e., the sera produced differ in individual antibody populations and give different cross-reaction patterns with the same antigen (Hála and Knížetová 1966; Drobná 1970), and
5. The fact that for various experiments it was sufficient to determine homozygosity and/or heterozygosity in the B system.

When testing a new chicken population the B antigens are defined on the basis of the reactions with various anti-B sera produced in another population. The structure of the new population is estimated according to the cross-reaction pattern (Fanguy 1961; Fanguy et al. 1961). Because the antisera are prepared against the whole product of the allele, which is precisely not defined, it is difficult to determine the degree of similarity between the B antigens prepared by various investigators who, in addition, work with different chicken populations. Also, an international comparison of the specificity of B antisera by individual investigators was not successful (McDermid and Oosterlee 1970; Okada and McDermid 1970; Oosterlee and Hála 1972), and so the investigators use their own nomenclature to designate the B antigens.

Attempts to define more precisely the individual products of the B alleles resulted in the adoption of the original Briles nomenclature and in the analysis of antigenic factors composing these products (Oosterlee and Bouw 1970; Hála and Knížetová 1970). At the present time 41 antigenic specificities are described in the laboratory in Edmonton (Pazderka et al. 1975a) and 27 antigenic factors in Prague (Hála et al. 1974). Some of the described factors (Tab. 8.1) are private antigens (for example, 1, 16, 19). Those that are common to various antigens may be designated as public antigens (13, 21, 27, etc.). The term "shared antigens" is suggested for antigens common to two alleles (Pazderka et al. 1975a).

The B system was found to be extensively polymorphic, with considerable cross-reactivity of its products (Briles et al. 1957; McDermid 1964). However, a number of similar B antigens were detected, using antisera against private antigens (Pazderka et al. 1975a). These investigators analyzed chickens from ten inbred or semiinbred lines in which 15 B alleles were present. Of these, 12 alleles reacted with one of the seven test sera prepared against private antigenic factors. In a number of them, Pazderka et al. (1975a) further confirmed the identity of the new alleles with their own alleles by the GvH reaction on the chorioallantoic membranes. It remains to be elucidated whether this similarity also involves the serologically defined antigens of the B complex.

In conclusion, we can say that:

1. The best definition of the B antigen is provided by designating the inbred or semiinbred line in which it is present. In contrast to these lines, the B antigens in outbred birds are mostly defined only by the cross-reaction pattern of a limited number of typing test sera.
2. While analyzing the product of the B alleles and while stating the cross-reactions, it is necessary to distinguish between conceptual and operational cross-reactions (Hirschfeld 1974). The introduction of new B alleles onto the genetic background of known lines is the most effective way of definition.
3. An analysis of the recombinant birds may contribute to a better understanding of the structure of the B region of the chromosome and to a better definition of its products.

5. Preparation of Antisera

Typing antisera are mostly alloimmune, capable of agglutinating in saline the RBC carrying the corresponding antigen. The selected recipients are immunized with washed RBC suspensions or with whole blood from appropriate donors. Approximately 1 to 4 ml of whole blood are injected, depending on the investigators. One course of immunization consists of four to five intravenous injections (two to three injections per week). The interval between immunizations may be 14 days (Briles 1962) or more than one month (Gilmour 1959; McDermid 1964).

During immunization and on the day after the last immunizing injection, blood samples are collected for the determination of antibody titers. If the titers are high enough (more than 1:32), larger amounts of blood are collected, either without an anticoagulation solution for the preparation of serum, or with citrate (one part citrate and four parts of blood) for the preparation of plasma. Poor coagulation of chicken blood and the resulting low yields of serum are conducive to using plasma for the preparation of the reagents.

Because of the adjuvant capacity of the B antigens (Schierman and McBride 1967), anti-B sera often contain antibodies against other non-B antigens after random immunization. In the case of B compatibility, antibodies against these antigens would not be formed, or would have lower titers. The incidence of non-B antibodies can be reduced by the choice of donor-recipient pairs within one family.

The specificity of the test serum prepared is tested by absorption. With a large number of progeny from one female, the progeny tests can be used. With an appropriate choice of parents, one-half of the offspring lack the respective antigen and the other half inherit the desired antigen and react positively with the operatively monospecific serum analyzed. If several antibodies against different antigens are present in the serum prepared, it is more convenient to select a donor-recipient combination that differs only in the desired antigen and to prepare newly the antiserum of desired specificity.

The genotype of the B system in a new chicken population is determined by various anti-B reference test sera produced in other populations of chickens. The use of the parents and their offspring will facilitate the initial analysis of the cross-reactions of the antisera used and the determination of the B antigens, or the genotype of the birds under study. On the basis of these preliminary results, appropriate donor-recipient pairs are selected and antisera for the determination of the B antigens segregating in this population are prepared by immunization. Thus, the tentatively determined genotype in the B system is confirmed (Fanguy 1961; Fanguy et al. 1961). Also, antisera against private antigens can be used with success (Pazderka et al. 1975b).

The methods employed for the preparation of test sera and in typing of B antigens in birds of semiinbred and outbred populations can be compared with those used, for example, in cattle, pigs, and/or man. A more simple method of preparing anti-B sera is provided by the use of inbred lines. If such lines are not homozygous for the B chromosome region, reciprocal immunizations between birds of the line can be performed (Gilmour 1959; Hašek et al. 1966; Hála et al. 1966). With congenic lines, reciprocal immunizations between birds of different lines are possible. In this case, the procedure is similar to that used in inbred mouse lines.

Individual test sera from birds of the same genotype against one B antigen differ in their ability to react (cross-react) with other B antigens (Hála and Knížetová 1968; Drobná 1970). Of the 12 anti-B2 sera under study, prepared by immunization of birds of the CB line with erythrocytes from a congenic CC line, only two sera reacted identically with outbred birds. These 12 sera were found to contain antibodies against two to eight antigenic factors (Hála and Knížetová 1966). Despite the difference between individual antisera, which must be kept in mind, the congenic lines yield more standard test sera than outbred birds reacting specifically only with the B antigens.

6. Chicken Populations Used for the Study of MHS

In the studies concerned with the relationship between the blood groups and the important production characters, most investigators used the lines of particular economical importance in their countries. As an international comparison of individual B antigens among different investigators has not been done, and in addition, some of the investigators now work on other projects, it is impossible to give the number of hitherto known B alleles and to make attempts to characterize the populations used, mostly the outbred chicken lines. The greatest number of alleles of the B system as determined by one working group is 21 (Briles et al. 1957).

The determination of gene composition of the B locus revealed a similarity between Barred Plymouth Rock and Rhode Island Red; these two breeds are more closely related than Rhode Island Red and New Hampshire (Natsume et al. 1972).

A list of the lines typed, giving only the number of segregating alleles, without attempts to identify the respective B alleles in most cases, was included in the paper of Briles et al. (1957). Furthermore, a registry of genetic stocks in the United States was published by Somes (1971) where some lines used for immunogenetic studies were also reported. In this chapter we shall concentrate mainly on the lines used for the study of MHS. Insofar as a particular line has been included in the list of Briles or Somes, it will be referred to. We are aware of the possible gaps in this table, because some authors describe the lines in general with only some B antigens, but do not give their designation nor the source of the animals. The lines listed in the table (Tab. 8.3) can be roughly divided into three groups:

1. Inbred lines (homozygous for the blood group and transplantation loci, syngeneic),

Table 8.3. Chicken Lines Used for the Study of the MHS (B) of Chickens

Line	Characteristics	B System	Established Place	Citation	Notes
CH	Inbred, WL	B^{R6}, B^{R7}	1932 Reaseheath	Gilmour 1959	
CA	Inbred (from CH)	B^{1}	1964 Prague	Hašek et al. 1966	IP isogenic
CB	Inbred (from CH)	B^{1}	1964 Prague	Hašek et al. 1966	Congenic to CA (non-B antigen)
CC	Inbred (from CH)	B^{2}	1964 Prague	Hašek et al. 1966	Congenic to CB
CD	Inbred (from CH)	B^{2}	1964 Prague	Hašek et al. 1966	Congenic to CC (no longer available)
IA	Inbred, WL	B^{R8}, B^{R9}	1938 Reaseheath	Gilmour 1959	
IA	Inbred (from IA)	B^{13}	1964 Prague	Hála et al. 1966	IP isogenic
IB	Inbred (from IA)	B^{13}	1964 Prague	Hála et al. 1966	Congenic to IA (non-B antigen)
IC	Inbred (from IA)	B^{13}	1966 Prague	Hála et al. 1966	Congenic to IA (non-B antigen)
WA	Inbred, Cuckoo Leghorn	B^{R4}, B^{R5}	1938 Reaseheath	Gilmour 1959	
WA	Inbred (from WA)	B^{9}	1962 Prague	Hála et al. 1966	IP isogenic
WB	Inbred (from WA)	B^{10}	1964 Prague	Hála et al. 1966	Congenic to WA
M	Inbred, Black Minorca	B^{5}	1963 Prague	Hála et al. 1966	Isogenic
F	Inbred, Silky Leghorn	B^{17}	1963 Prague	Hála et al. 1974	Isogenic: closed bred since 1971
RE	Inbred, BL	B^{R1}, B^{R2}, B^{R3}	1940 Reaseheath	Gilmour 1959	
50	Closed flock, WL	B^{1}, B^{2}, B^{3}, B^{7}, B^{9}, B^{10}		Fanguy et al. 1961	Closed for seven generations
X	Closed flock, WL	B^{19}, B^{21}	Thornbers (England)	McDermid 1964	
Y	Closed flock, WL	B^{2}, B^{14}	Thornbers (England)	McDermid 1964	
C	Closed flock	B^{8}, B^{9}, B^{13}	1944	Mikami et al. 1969	
N	Closed flock	B^{8}, B^{11}, B^{13}	1957	Mikami et al. 1969	
G	Partially inbred	B^{1}, B^{2}	Iowa State Univ.	Schierman and Nordskog 1964	Sublines G-B1 and G-B2
H	Partially inbred			Schierman and Nordskog 1964	
9	Partially inbred		Iowa State Univ.	Schierman and Nordskog 1964	

AA	Inbred		1946–1948 Australia	Burnet and Burnet 1961	
M	Inbred, Rhode Island Red		Reaseheath	Cock and Clough 1956	
Texas line 24	Inbred, WL	B^2, B^7, B^8		Briles et al. 1957	
OS	Closed bred			Wick et al. 1974	
P	Closed bred	B^2	Hy-line	Toivanen et al. 1974	Pazderka et al. (1975a) gives the existence of five alleles
N	BL	B^{21}		Craig 1963; Pazderka et al. 1975a	
22	Partially inbred	B^2, B^7, B^9	Texas	Briles et al. 1957, 1963	
23	Partially inbred	B^2, B^6, B^7	Texas	Briles et al. 1957, 1963	
6	Inbred	2 alleles?	East Lansing	Crittenden et al. 1964	Pazderka et al. (1975a) determines only one allele, B^2, which is also present in line 7
7	Inbred	Homozygous	East Lansing	Crittenden et al. 1964	
9	Inbred	Homozygous	East Lansing	Crittenden et al. 1964	
100	Inbred	2 alleles?	East Lansing	Crittenden et al. 1964	
15	Inbred	B^9, B^{10}, B^{11}	East Lansing	Crittenden et al. 1964	Pazderka et al. (1975a) determines only two alleles
15I	Inbred (from 15)	B^9, B^{10}	East Lansing	Crittenden et al. 1964	
—	Inbred	B^2		Longenecker et al. 1970	
—	Inbred	B^{14}		Longenecker et al. 1970	
—	Closed, Single Comb WL	9 alleles	1957	Matsumoto and Okada 1961	

WL = White Leghorn.
BL = Brown Leghorn.

2. Histocompatible in B antigens (inbred or partially inbred, homozygous for the B system; but skin grafts are not accepted permanently, because they often segregate even in erythrocyte antigens),
3. Blood group-typed (often partially inbred, mostly closed populations. The alleles segregating in the B system are known, and sometimes information on the situation in the blood group loci is available).

Because the project of Prof. R. F. Ruth and his collaborators (Pazderka et al. 1975a) has the purpose of assembling all important lines and comparing their B alleles, it can be expected that the similarity between individual B antigens will be determined in the near future. This will help introduce a unified nomenclature for the antigens of this system that will be valid for the most important lines.

7. MHS in Other Species of Birds

The blood groups have been studied in various species of Aves. Pigeons and doves are among the best-studied species thanks to the work of Irwin and his collaborators (Irwin 1939; Shaw 1962). However, all data refer only to antigenic properties of the erythrocytes, and no attempts have been made as yet to identify the major histocompatibility locus.

A similar situation is encountered in turkeys (Law et al. 1965; Briles 1964), ducks (McGibbon 1945; Drobná et al. 1964; Podliachouk 1964), geese (Losonczy 1970), and quail (Perramon 1970). In all these species a number of antigens or blood group systems are known, but the data on transplantation analysis are lacking.

8. Conclusions

The B system of chickens, which has been described as the blood group system, is the major histocompatibility system, with a number of features similar to the MHS of other animals and man (Iványi 1970; Hála and Hašek 1971). Its antigens have been detected on various cells (for example, lymphocytes and fibroblasts), but they are mostly present on nucleated erythrocytes. Alloantibodies are demonstrated by agglutination of erythrocytes or lymphocytes.

The characteristic feature of the alloantisera produced is considerable cross-reactivity, which reflects the overlapping of antigenic mosaicism of the products of individual B alleles. Maximally 50 antigenic factors have been demonstrated in one laboratory so far. The described antigenic factors can be divided into private and shared or public.

More than 30 alleles are known to determine the individual complexes of antigenic factors (McDermid 1964). Maximally 21 alleles have been described in one laboratory (Briles et al. 1957).

In recent years, the genetic structure of the B chromosome region has received increasing attention. Two regions, B-F and B-G, have been described. The B-F region is responsible for the histocompatibility (H) antigens and the serologically defined (SD) antigens, whereas the B-G region determines only the SD antigens and has no effect on the fate of skin grafts, graft-versus-host, and mixed lymphocyte reactions. The difference at the B-F region is responsible for these reactions.

It has been found that Ir genes, determining the immune response against the synthetic polypeptide (T,G)-A–L (Günther et al. 1974) and against the DNP (Balcarová et al. 1974) are localized in the B region of the chromosome. Studies of Ir genes may disclose the effect of the B chromosome region on spontaneous autoimmune thyroiditis in the obese strain of chickens (Bacon et al. 1974; Wick et al. 1974) and on susceptibility to Marek's disease (Hanson et al. 1967; Brewer et al. 1969; Pazderka et al. 1975b).

In addition to the effect of the B complex on the preparation of antibody formation in bursectomized chickens (Toivanen et al. 1974) and on the intensity of the GvH reaction (Longenecker et al. 1972), an association with various quantitative indicators has been described (for a review, see Gilmour 1960; Briles 1964; McDermid 1964). It has also been demonstrated that natural and artificial selection prefers heterozygotes in this complex (Shultz and Briles 1953; Gilmour 1954, 1959; Okada and Matsumoto 1962).

A number of theories (Sheppard 1953; Snell 1968; Jerne 1971; Bodmer 1972; Burnet 1973) try to explain the importance and role of the MHS from different aspects. However, its role is not yet clear. It is generally accepted that this system has an adaptive value and that its polymorphism is maintained by selection. It is noteworthy that systems with a number of similarities exist in both mammals and birds. This may prove their effect throughout the phylogenesis of these two animal classes.

The concentrated efforts of several laboratories will certainly provide many new findings within the next few years that will contribute to a better understanding of the structure of this complex. The prerequisite is international cooperation together with an exchange of experimental animals, semiinbred lines, and test sera, and the introduction of more modern methods.

References

Alm, G. V. In vitro studies of chicken lymphoid cells. 3. The mixed spleen leucocyte reaction with special reference to the effect of bursectomy. *Acta Pathol. Microbiol. Scand. (Section A)* *79*:359–365, 1971.

Bacon, L. D., Kite, J. H., and Rose, N. R. Immunogenetic detection of B locus genotypes in chickens with autoimmune thyroiditis. *Transplantation 16*:591–598, 1973.

Bacon, L. D., Kite, J. H., and Rose, N. R. A relationship between the major histocompatibility [B] locus and autoimmune thyroiditis in obese chickens. *Science 186*:274–275, 1974.

Bain, B., Vas, M. R. and Lowenstein, L. A reaction between leucocytes in mixed peripheral blood cultures. *Fed. Proc. 22*:428, 1963.

Balcarová, J., Derka, J., Hála, K., and Hraba, T. Genetic control of immune response to the dinitrophenol group in inbred lines of chickens. *Folia Biol. (Praha) 20*:346–349, 1974.

Basch, R. S., and Stetson, C. A. The relationship between hemagglutinogens and histocompatibility antigens in the mouse. *Ann. N.Y. Acad. Sci. 97*:83–94, 1962.

Benda, V. Identification of B antigen on chicken somatic cells. *Proceedings of the VIIth International Symposium on Laboratory Animals,* pp. 49–55. Hrubá Skála, 1971.

Benda, V., and Hála, K. Relative distribution of B antigens in erythrocytes and some other chicken tissues. *Folia Biol. (Praha) 18*:301–304, 1972.

Benda, V., Hála, K., and Hlōzánek, I. Detection of antigens on the surface of chick fibroblasts. *In Proceedings of the XIIth European Conference on Animal Blood Groups and Biochemical Polymorphism,* pp. 437–440, Akademiai Kiado, Budapest, 1970.

Benson, H. N., Brumfield, H. P., and Pomeroy, B. S. Requirement of avian C'1 for fixation of guinea pig complement by avian antibody-antigen complexes. *J. Immunol. 87*:616–622, 1961.

Billingham, R. E., Brent, L., and Medawar, P. B. Tolerance of red cell antigens and transplantation immunity in chickens. *Experientia 11*:444, 1955.

Bodmer, W. F. Evolutionary significance of the HL-A system. *Nature 237*:139–145, 1972.

Borel, J. F. Recherches sur la détermination de l'individualité génétique du poulet au moyen de certaines substances spécifiques localisées dans le sang et dans l'oeuf. Thesis, Swiss Federal Institute of Technology, 1963. Cited by McDermid (1964).

Boyer, G. Chorioallantoic membrane lesions produced by inoculation of adult fowl leukocytes. *Nature 185*:327–328, 1960.

Brewer, R. N., Moore, C. H., and Johnson, L. W. Effects of blood group antigens on resistance to Marek's disease. *Poult. Sci. 48*:1970 (abstr.), 1969.

Briles, W. E. Blood groups in chickens, their nature and utilization. *World's Poult. Sci. J. 16*:223–242, 1960.

Briles, W. E. Additional blood group systems in the chicken. *Ann. N.Y. Acad. Sci. 97*:173–183, 1962.

Briles, W. E. Current status of blood groups in domestic birds. *Z. Tierzüchtung Züchtungsbiol. 79*:371–391, 1964.

Briles, W. E., Allen, C. P., and Millen, T. W. The B blood group system of chickens. I. Heterozygosity in closed populations. *Genetics 42*:631–648, 1957.

Briles, W. E., and Crittenden, L. B. The immunogenetic identification of an isoantigen associated with susceptibility to an avian leukosis-sarcoma virus. *Poult. Sci. 50*:1558 (abstr.), 1971.

Briles, W. E., and Lee, K. E. Time of appearance of the B system red cell antigens in the chicken. *In Proceedings of the XIIth European Conference on Animal Blood Groups and Biochemical Polymorphism,* pp. 451–454, Akademiai Kiado, Budapest, 1970.

Briles, W. E., McGibbon, W. H., and Irwin, M. R. Studies of time of development of cellular antigens in the chicken. *Genetics 33*:97 (abstr.), 1948.

Briles, W. E., McGibbon, W.H., and Irwin, M.R. On multiple alleles affecting cellular antigens in the chicken. *Genetics 35*:633–652, 1950.

Burnet, D., and Burnet, F. M. Analysis of major histocompatibility factors in a stock of closely inbred White Leghorn fowls using a graft-versus-host reaction on the chorioallantoic membrane. *Aust. J. Exp. Biol. Med. Sci. 39*:101–110, 1961.

Burnet, F. M. Multiple polymorphism in relation to histocompatibility antigens. *Nature 245*:359–361, 1973.

Burnet, F. M., and Burnet, D. Graft versus host reactions on the chorioallantoic membrane of the chick embryo. *Nature 188*:376–379, 1960.

Cock, A. G., and Clough, M. Successful skin homografts in inbred chickens. *Nature 178*:136–137, 1956.

Cock, A. G., and Simonsen, M. Immunological attack on newborn chickens by injected adult cells. *Immunology 2*:103–110, 1958.

Coppleson, L. W., and Michie, D. Comparison of the chorioallantoic membrane and splenomegaly systems of graft-versus-host assay in the chick embryo. *Nature 208*:53–54, 1965.

Coppleson, L. W., and Michie, D. A quantitative study of the chorioallantoic membrane reaction in the chick embryo. *Proc. R. Soc. B. 163*:555–563, 1966.

Craig, J. V., and Hirsch, L. J. Genetic relationship and reactions to skin grafts. *J. Hered. 48*:235–238, 1957.

Craig, J. W., and McDermid, E. M. Prolonged skin homograft survival and erythrocyte (B locus) antigens in young chicks. *Transplantation 1*:191–200, 1963.

Craig, J. V., Polley, C. R., and Wearden, S. Estimation of genetic diversity by skin-graft reactions in young chicks. *Poult. Sci. 39*:1533–1540, 1960.

Crittenden, L. B., Johnson, L. W., and Okazaki, W. Histocompatibility and erythrocyte antigen variability within highly inbred lines of White Leghorns. *Transplantation 2*:362–374, 1964.

David, L. A., Law, G. R. J., and Ruth, R. F. Specific detection of cellular transplantation antigens by fluorescent antibody. *Ann. N.Y. Acad. Sci. 129*:46–75, 1966.

Démant, P. H-2 gene complex and its role in alloimmune reactions. *Transplant Rev. 15*:162–200, 1973.

Drobná, V. Some data on the development of blood group antigens in chickens. *In Works of the Research Institute for Poultry Breeding*, pp. 187–193, Ivanka pri Dunaji, 1967 (in Slovak).

Drobná, V. The study of the complex blood group systems in chickens. *Sci. Works—Poult. Ser. 9*:163–169, 1970.

Drobná, V., Hort, J., Ivãnyi, P., and Mardiak, J. A contribution to the problem of blood groups in ducks. *In Blood Groups of Animals. Proceedings of the 9th European Animal Blood Group Conference*, pp. 467–468, Prague, 1964.

Dunsford, I., Lodge, T., McDermid, E. M., and Gilmour, D. G. Incomplete antibodies to chicken red cell antigens. *Nature 190*:544, 1961.

Elkins, W. L. Cellular immunology and the pathogenesis of graft versus host reactions. *Prog. Allergy 15*:78–187, 1971.

Fanguy, R. C. Blood typing techniques in poultry. *Texas Agr. Exp. Sta. Bull. MP-551*, 1961.

Fanguy, R. C., Ferguson, T. M., and Quisenberry, J. H. The blood group spectrum of a non-inbred population as determined from cross-reactions with antisera produced in non-related populations. *Poult. Sci. 40*:848–853, 1961.

Gilmour, D. G. Selective advantage of heterozygosis for blood group genes among inbred chickens. *Heredity 8*:291, (abstr.), 1954.

Gilmour, D. G. Segregation of genes determining red cell antigens at high levels of inbreeding in chickens. *Genetics 44*:14–33, 1959.

Gilmour, D. G. Blood groups in chickens. *Br. Poult. Sci. 1*:75–100, 1960.

Gilmour, D. G., Donnelly, N., Brand, A., and Stone, H. A. Two loci determining alloantigens of bursal or thymic cells in the chicken. *In International Symposium on Laboratory Animals*, Hrubá Skála, 1975. *Folia Biol. (Praha) 21*:359 (abstr.), 1975.

Gleason, R. E., and Fanguy, R.C. The relationship of blood groups to skin graft survival in chickens. *Transplantation 2*:509–514, 1964.

Günther, E., Balcarová, J., Hála, K., Rüde, E., and Hraba, T. Evidence for an association between immune responsiveness of chicken to (T,G)-A—L and the major histocompatibility system. *Eur. J. Immunol. 4*:548–553, 1974.

Hála, K. Syngeneic lines of chickens. III. The number of different histocompatibility loci between the lines. *Folia Biol. (Praha) 15*:136–140, 1969.

Hála, K., and Hašek, M. Comparative aspects of the B system in chickens and the H-2 system in mice. *In Proceedings of the Symposium on Immunogenetics of the H-2 System*, Liblice-Prague, 1970, pp. 334–340, Karger, Basel, 1971.

Hála, K., Hašek, M., Hložánek, I., Hort, J., Knížetová, F., and Mervartová, H. Syngeneic lines of chickens. II. Inbreeding and selection within the M, W and I lines and crosses between the C, M and W lines. *Folia Biol. (Praha) 12*:407–421, 1966.

Hála, K., and Knížetová, F. The analysis of complex B phenogroups in inbred lines of chickens. *In 10th European Conference on Animal Blood Groups and Biochemical Polymorphisms*, pp. 217–221, Paris, 1966.

Hála, K., and Knížetová, F. Complex antigens of the B system in inbred lines of chickens. *Proceedings of the 11th European Conference on Animal Blood Groups and Biochemical Polymorphism*, Warsaw, 1968, pp. 385–387, Junk, The Hague–PWN, Polish Scientific Publishers, Warsaw, 1970.

Hála, K., Vilhelmová, M., and Hartmanová, J. Probable crossing-over between 2 alleles of the B system of chickens. *XIIIth International Symposium on Laboratory Animals*, Hrubá Skála, 1975. *Folia Biol. (Praha) 21*:363–365, 1975.

Hála, K., Vilhelmová, M., and Hartmanová, J. Probable crossing-over in B blood group system of chickens. *Immunogenetics 3*:91–103, 1976.

Hála, K., Vilhelmová, M., Hašek, M., Kratochvílová, J., Plachý, J., Benda, V., and Karakoz, I. Syngeneic lines of chickens. V. The inbred F line. *Folia Biol. (Praha) 20*:378–385, 1974.

Hanson, M. P., VanZandt, J. N., and Law, G. R. J. Differences in susceptibility to Marek's disease in chickens carrying two different *B* locus blood group alleles. *Poult. Sci. 46*:1268 (abstr.), 1961.

Hašek, M. Parabiosis of birds during embryogenesis. *Čsl. Biol. 2*:25–26, 1953 (in Czech).

Hašek, M., Knížetová, F., and Mervartová, H. Syngeneic lines of chickens. I. Inbreeding and selection by means of skin grafts and tests for erythrocyte antigens in C line chickens. *Folia Biol. (Praha) 12*:335–353, 1966.

Hašek, M., Lengerová, A., and Maternová, E. Analysis of the role of the blood cells in overcoming experimentally the incompatibility of skin grafts in warm-blooded animals. *Čsl. Biol. 4*:564–565, 1955 (in Czech).

Hirschfeld, J. Some notes on the concept of cross-reactivity. *Vox Sang. 27*:254–264, 1974.

Hirschhorn, K., Bach, F. H., Kolodny, R. L., Firschein, I. L., and Hashem, N. Immune response and mitosis of human peripheral blood lymphocytes in vitro. *Science 142*:1185, 1963.

Hložánek, I., and Hála, K. The detection of B red blood cell allele in chick embryo fibroblasts. *Folia Biol. (Praha), 15*:474–477, 1969.

Irwin, M. R. A genetic analysis of species differences in Columbidae. *Genetics 24*:709–721, 1939.

Iványi, D., Rychlíková, M., Sassportes, M., Iványi, P., and Dausset, J. Leukocyte antigens and the mixed lymphocyte culture reaction. *Vox Sang. 12*:186–198, 1967.

Iványi, P. The major histocompatibility antigens in various species. *Curr. Top. Microbiol. Immunol. 53*:1–90, 1970.

Jaffe, W. P. The relationship between the blood group locus and the intradermal reaction in chickens. *Vet. Rec. 77*:388–389, 1965.

Jaffe, W. P., and McDermid, E. M. Blood groups and splenomegaly in chick embryos. *Science 137*:984, 1962.

Jaffe, W. P., and Payne, L. N. The genetic basis for the graft-against-host reaction between inbred lines of fowls. Differences between the Reaseheath C and I inbred lines. *Immunology 5*:399–413, 1962.

Jerne, N. K. The somatic generation of immune recognition. *Eur. J. Immunol. 1*:1–19, 1971.

Johnson, L. W. Studies on the role of chicken blood groups A and B in the induction of anemia in chicks. Ph.D. Thesis, Texas Agricultural and Mechanical College Library, College Station, Texas, 1956. Cited by Briles (1964).

Keily, S. D., Schierman, L. W., and Nordskog, A. W. Molecular weight differences in chicken isoantibodies. *Proc. Soc. Exp. Biol. Med. 121*:137–139, 1966.

Kinsky, R., and Mitchison, N. A. Tolerance of skin induced by erythrocytes in poultry. *Transplantation 1*:224–231, 1963.

Klein, J. The H-2 system: Past and present. *Transplant. Proc. 5*:11–21, 1973.

Knížetová, F., Longenecker, B. M., Law, G. R.J., and Ruth, R. F. Discrimination between major and minor histoincompatibility in the GVHR: Effects of genotype, X ray dose rate and immunization. *Fed. Proc. 29*:651 (abstr.), 1970.

Landsteiner, K., and Miller, C. P. On individual differences in chicken blood. *Proc. Soc. Exp. Biol. Med. 22*:100–102, 1924.

Law, G. R. J., Miller, W. J., Asmundson, V. S., and Stormont, C. Blood groups of turkeys. *Genetics 51*:253–261, 1965.

Longenecker, B. M., Pazderka, F., Law, G. R. J., and Ruth, R. F. Genetic control of graft-versus-host competence. *Transplantation 14*:424–431, 1972.

Longenecker, B. M., Sheridan, S., Law, G. R. J., and Ruth, R. F. Measurement of graft-versus-host reactions on the chorallantoic membrane of the chicken. *Transplantation 9*:544–547, 1970.

Losonczy, S. On the blood groups and the appearance of natural antibodies in the goose.

In Proceedings of the XIIth European Conference on Animal Blood Groups and Biochemical Polymorphism, pp. 501–507, Akademiai Kiado, Budapest, 1970.
Matsumoto, K., and Okada, I. The blood group systems in the chicken. *Jap. J. Genet. 36*:257–267, 1961.
McDermid, E. M. Immunogenetics of the chicken. *Vox Sang. 9*:249–267, 1964.
McDermid, E. M., and Oosterlee, C. C. Development on comparison of chicken blood typing reagents. *In Proceedings of the XIIth European Conference on Animal Blood Groups and Biochemical Polymorphism*, pp. 419–423, Akademiai Kiado, Budapest, 1970.
McGibbon, W. H. Further division of contrasting antigens in species hybrids in ducks. *Genetics 30*:252–265, 1945.
Miggiano, V. C., Birgen, I., and Pink, J. R. L. The mixed leukocyte reaction in chickens. Evidence for control by the major histocompatibility complex. *Eur. J. Immunol. 4*:397–401, 1974a.
Miggiano, V. C., Meo, T., Birgén, I., and Nabholze, M. Further miniaturization and automatization of in vitro lymphocyte cultures. *Tissue Antigens 5*:173–185, 1974b.
Mikami, H., Okada, I., and Hachinohe, Y. Genetic differences in the homologous splenomegaly reaction in chickens due to the donor. *Jap. J. Genet. 44*:81–87, 1969.
Mitchison, N. A. Tolerance of erythrocytes in poultry: Induction and specificity. *Immunology 5*:341–358, 1962.
Möller, G. Survival of mouse erythrocytes in histocompatible recipients. *Nature 199*:573–575, 1963.
Natsume, N., Fujio, Y., and Kondo, K. The B blood group polymorphism in the chicken. II. The distribution of the alleles in several breeds. *Jap. J. Zootech. Sci. 43*:712–718, 1972.
Nisbet, N. W., and Simonsen, M. Primary immune response in grafted cells-dissociation between proliferation of cells. *J. Exp. Med. 125*:967–981, 1967.
Nisbet, N. W., Simonsen, M., and Zaleski, M. The frequency of antigen-sensitive cells in tissue transplantation. *J. Exp. Med. 129*:459–467, 1969.
Ohno, S. *Sex Chromosomes and Sex-Linked Genes*. Springer-Verlag, Berlin-Heidelberg-New York, 1967.
Okada, I., and Matsumoto, K. Fitness of the genotypes at the B locus determining the blood group of chickens. *Jap. J. Genet. 37*:267–275, 1962.
Okada, I., and McDermid, E. M. Some aspects of international comparison test for blood grouping of chickens. *Jap. J. Zootech. Sci. 41*:319–325, 1970.
Okada, I., and Mikami, H. Three generations of selection for high and low donor competences of splenomegaly in chickens. *Br. Poult. Sci. 15*:1–10, 1974.
Oosterlee, C. C., and Bouw, J. Detection of alleles in chicken strains and hybrids. *In Proceedings of the 11th European Conference on Animal Blood Groups and Biochemical Polymorphism*, pp. 389–395, Junk, The Hague-PWN, Polish Scientific Publishers, Warsaw, 1970.
Oosterlee, C. C., and Hála, K. The 9th comparison test of chicken blood typing reagents (comparison of selected B locus reagents). *Anim. Blood Groups Biochem. Genet. 3* (Suppl. 1):24–25, 1972.
Pazderka, F., Longenecker, B. M., Law, G. R. J., and Ruth, R. F. The major histocompatibility complex of the chicken. *Immunogenetics 2*:101–130, 1975a.
Pazderka, F., Longenecker, B. M., Law, G. R. J., Stone, H. A., and Ruth, R. F. Histocompatibility of chicken populations selected for resistance to Marek's disease. *Immunogenetics 2*:93–100, 1975b.
Perramon, A. Argument in favor of a hypothesis of gametic incompatibility concerning blood groups in domestic quail. *In Proceedings of the XIIth European Conference on Animal Blood Groups and Biochemical Polymorphism*, pp. 517–521, Akademiai Kiado, Budapest, 1970.
Pink, J. R. L., Ziegler, A., and Buder, A. Characterisation of chicken B blood group antigens. *XIIIth International Symposium on Laboratory Animals*, Hrubá Skála, 1975. *Folia Biol. (Praha) 21*:363 (abstr.), 1975.
Podliachouk, L. The blood groups of chicks. In *Blood Groups in Animals. Proceedings of the 9th European Animal Blood Group Conference*, pp. 187–191, Prague, 1964.
Polley, C. R., Grosse, A. E., and Craig, J. V. A skin grafting technique for use in genetic studies with chickens. *Transplant Bull. 7*:425–428, 1960.

Pöschl, M., and Hála, K. Development of chicken erythrocyte alloantigens in ontogenesis. *Folia Biol. (Praha) 20*:168–176, 1974.

Schierman, L. W., and McBride, R. A. Adjuvant activity of erythrocyte isoantigens. *Science 156*:658–659, 1967.

Schierman, L. W., and McBride, R. A. Evidence for a mutational event at the B blood group histocompatibility locus in chickens. *Transplantation 8*:515–516, 1969.

Schierman, L. W., and Nordskog, A. W. Relationship of blood type to histocompatibility in chickens. *Science 134*:1008–1009, 1961.

Schierman, L. W., and Nordskog, A. W. Relationship of erythrocyte to leukocyte antigens in chickens. *Science 137*:620–621, 1962.

Schierman, L. W., and Nordskog, A. W. Influence of the B blood group histocompatibility locus in chickens on a graft-versus-host reaction. *Nature 197*:511–512, 1963.

Schierman, L. W., and Nordskog, A. W. Immunogenetic studies with fowl: Relationship of blood groups to transplantation immunity and tolerance. *Ann. N.Y. Acad. Sci. 120*:348–355, 1964.

Seto, F. Graft-versus-host and host-versus-graft reaction in the chick embryo. *Transplantation 5*:1280–1288, 1967.

Snell, G. D. The H-2 locus of the mouse: Observations and speculations concerning its comparative genetics and its polymorphism. *Folia Biol. (Praha) 14*:335–358, 1968.

Somes, R. G. *Gallus domesticus. Registry of Genetic Stocks in the United States.* Storrs Agr. Exp. Sta., The University of Connecticut, Storrs, 1971.

Stolfi, R. L., Fungmann, R. A., Jensen, J. J., and Siegel, M. M. A Cl-fixation method for the measurement of chicken anti-viral antibody. *Immunology 20*:299–306, 1971.

Toivanen, P., Toivanen, A., and Vainio, O. Complete restoration of bursa-dependent immune system after transplantation of semiallogeneic stem cells into immunodeficient chicks. *J. Exp. Med. 139*:1344–1349, 1974.

Warner, N. L. Immunological reactions produced by the local injection of adult fowl leucocytes in chickens. *Aust. J. Exp. Biol. Med. Sci. 42*:417–428, 1964.

Warner, N. L. The immunological role of avian thymus and bursa of Fabricius. *Folia Biol. (Praha) 13*:1–17, 1967.

Waters, L. D., and Bennett, J. An attempt to demonstrate erythrocyte antigens in brain, liver and muscle tissue in White Leghorns. *Poult. Sci. 50*:975–976, 1971.

Wick, G., Sundick, R. S., and Albini, B. The obese strain (OS) of chickens: An animal model with spontaneous autoimmune thyroiditis. *Clin. Immunol. Immunopathol. 3*:272–300, 1974.

Wong, S. Y., Pazderka, F., Longenecker, B. M., Law, G. R. J., and Ruth, R. F. Immobilization of lymphocytes at surfaces by alloantibodies. *Immunol. Commun. 1*:597–613, 1972.

Ziegler, A., and Pink, J. R. L. Characterisation of major histocompatibility (B) antigens of the chicken. *Transplantation 20*:523–527, 1975.

Chapter 9

Major and Minor Histocompatibility Systems of Ectothermic Vertebrates

N. Cohen and N.H. Collins

1. Introduction

Every mammalian and avian species that has been rigorously examined possesses a homologous system of closely linked genes designated as its major histocompatibility complex or system (MHS). Certain products of some of the genes within this complex are serologically detectable as alloantigens on the surface of cells; others can be visualized by their abilities to elicit lymphocyte transformation and mitosis in the *in vitro* mixed lymphocyte culture reaction (MLR). In several endothermic (warm-blooded) species, component genes of this complex have been associated with acute allograft rejection, intense graft-versus-host (GvH) reactivity, susceptibility and resistance to a variety of pathogens, the quantitative ability to produce antibodies to a spectrum of antigenic determinants, the physiologic cooperation between T- and B-cells, and the regulation of the level of some serum complement components (Klein 1975; this volume).

All ectothermic (cold-blooded) vertebrates are similar to birds and mammals with respect to fundamental expressions of immune competence. Primitive as well as phylogenetically advanced fishes, amphibians, and reptiles reject allogeneic tissue transplants, synthesize specific antibodies in response to confrontations with particulate and soluble antigens, and exhibit at least some manifestations of immunologic memory. In each species examined, lymphoid cells participate in these immunologic happenings. Moreover, *in vitro* studies point out that lymphocytes from teleosts (Etlinger 1975; Lopez et al. 1974; Sigel et al. 1973) and amphibians (Goldshein and Cohen 1972; Du Pasquier et al. 1975; Goldstine et al. 1975) undergo blast transformation and proliferation when they are exposed to specific antigens, selective T- and B-cell mitogens, or allogeneic cells. GvH reactivity in reptiles (Sidky and Auerbach 1968; Borysenko and Tulipan 1973) and amphibians (Clark and Newth 1972; Murakawa 1968) and the carrier hapten effect in amphibians (Ruben 1975) and fishes (Yocum et al. 1975; Stolen and Mäkelä 1975) have also been reported. For comprehensive reviews on the phylogeny of these various facets of immunity, the reader should consult recent papers and books by Cohen (1975), Du Pasquier (1973), Hildemann (1972), Marchalonis and Cone (1973), Marchalonis (1976), and Manning and Turner (1976).

The detection of certain immune phenomena in ectotherms that appear to be predominantly under the genetic control of the MHS in endotherms is provocative. Indeed, it has encouraged the speculation (Bodmer 1972;

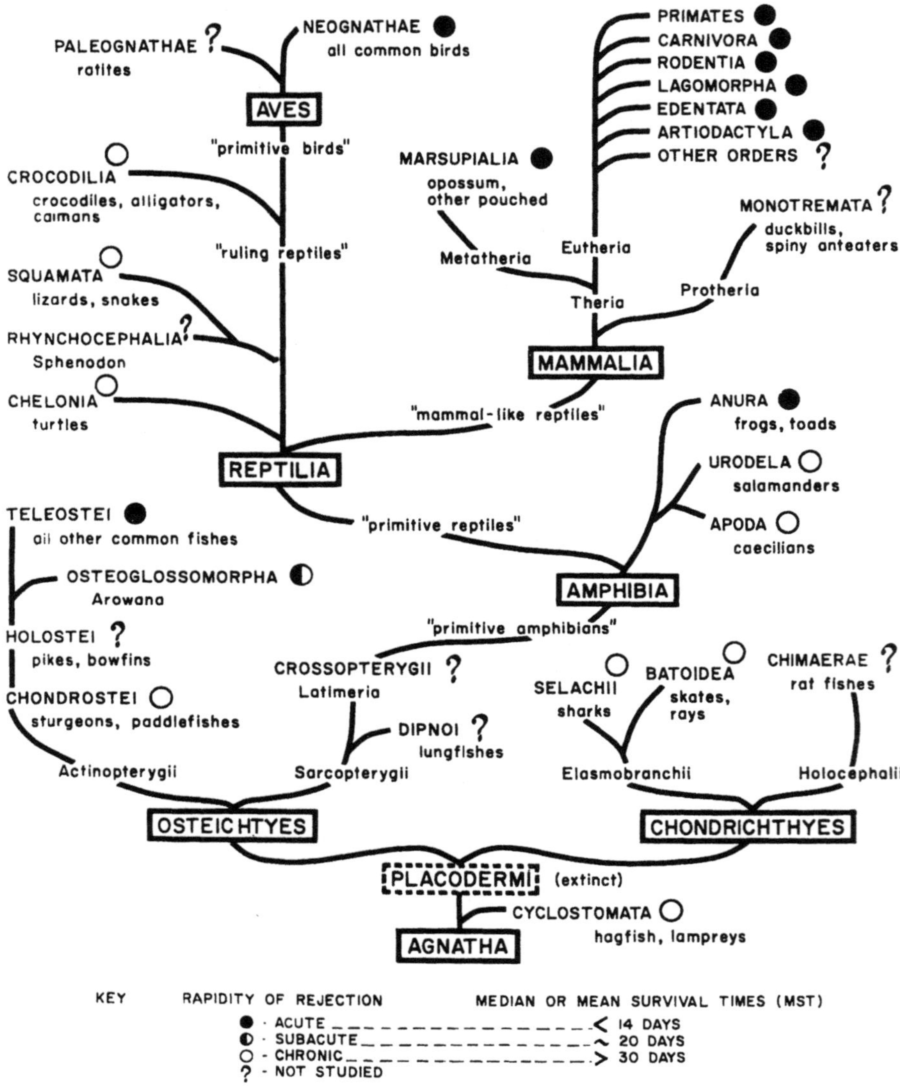

Fig. 9.1. Evolutionary trends in the rapidity of allograft rejection in the Vertebrata. Temperature at which allograft rejection in ectothermic species studied was ~20 to 25°C in most instances. From Cohen and Borysenko (1970); copyright by Henry M. Stratton, New York

Burnet 1973; Miggiano et al. 1974) that this important cluster of linked genes evolved quite early and might be detectable as a true homologue in modern representatives of some, if not all, of the five classes of vertebrates phylogenetically distal to birds (Reptilia, Amphibia, Osteichthyes, Chondricythyes, Cyclostomata; Figure 9.1). In recent years, a few investigators have tried to come to experimental as well as theoretical grips with this hypothesis

(Du Pasquier et al. 1975; DeLanney et al. 1975; Collins et al. 1975). However, the development of a precise flow sheet of the phylogeny of the MHS has been severely hampered by significant obstacles. These include: a paucity of investigators, the diversity of vertebrates that must be studied, the lack of inbred strains of critical species, the long (>1 year) period between each generation of such animals, animal husbandry, and the problems of deciphering evolution with living descendents of long extinct species. These obstacles have made it impossible, at this time, to demonstrate the *unequivocal* presence (or absence) of the *complete* functional and structural homologue of the mammalian MHS in any ectothermic vertebrate. On the other hand, the collation of those data that deal with acute graft rejection, significant stimulation in MLR, and severe GvH reactivity in ectotherms does make it possible to sketch out roughly what may prove to be the real phylogenetic history of the MHS. Each of these phenomena has been associated with one or more of the genes that constitute the MHS of endotherms; each has been sought after in more than a single order of ectotherms. The purpose of this chapter is to review this information in the context of the phylogeny of diverse histocompatibility systems.

2. The MHS and the Phylogeny of Transplantation Immunity

2.1 Rapidity of First-Set Allograft Reactions: Immunogenetic Considerations

Rejection of first-set skin transplants exchanged between two outbred members of the same mammalian or avian species is invariably rapid. Typically, such grafts are destroyed within 2 weeks after they are transplanted (Klein and Bailey 1971). Comparable acute rejection also occurs when grafts are exchanged between two strains of mice that are congenic at all loci save those that constitute their MHS (Démant 1973). This barrier imposed by disparities within the MHS is said to be "strong" (Counce et al. 1956). On the other hand, when grafts are transplanted between individuals from two strains of mice (or other endotherms) that share all MHS specificities but differ at one or more of the so-called minor or weak histocompatibility (H) loci, the tempo of rejection is radically slowed. Depending on the particular minor H barrier(s) transgressed, such grafts may survive for weeks, months, or even indefinitely, despite the fact that they are genetically and antigenically dissimilar from their hosts (Hildemann and Cohen 1967; Graff and Bailey 1973).

Like endotherms, all ectothermic vertebrates reject allografts but not autografts and mount a specific second-set memory response (Hildemann 1972). These observations provided the earliest and simplest (but indirect) demonstration that transplantation immunity in ectotherms is elicited by alloantigenic products of at least one multiallelic H locus.

The macroscopic and the histologically recorded events associated with graft rejection are remarkably similar for all vertebrates. However, the rapidity with which a given vertebrate rejects a transplant correlates with its position on the classic phylogenetic tree. Acute graft rejection—the typical response of outbred endotherms—is the atypical response of outbred ectotherms (Cohen and Borysenko 1970). In fact, allografts exchanged between representatives of all but two orders of lower vertebrates (Figure 9.1) are rejected chronically (median survival times, MST$\geqq$4 weeks) or in some instances, subacutely (MST$\sim$3 weeks). An analysis of the genetic basis of chronic and acute rejection in these creatures, therefore, is quite relevant to the phylogeny of the MHS.

2.1.1 Acute Rejection

Of the many orders of ectothermic vertebrates examined, only advanced teleost fishes (Hildemann 1970a) and anuran amphibians (Cohen, 1971a) routinely exhibit acute reactivity toward histoincompatible allografts. These responses are comparable to the vigorous alloimmune response triggered by and directed against alloantigens of the MHS of endotherms. Based on the uniformly rapid rejection of multiple allografts exchanged between outbred, F_1, or F_2 siblings, Hildemann and Owen (1956) estimated that goldfish have from four to seven unlinked H loci. Kallman and his co-workers' (1964, 1970) classic immunogenetic analyses of the survival times of grafts between inbred parental strains of platyfish and from parental–F_1, parental–F_2, and parental–backcross progeny revealed from 10 to 15 H loci in different species of *Xiphophorus*. These studies also validated application of the genetic laws of transplantation (Snell and Stimpfling 1966) to teleosts. Gene dosage effects, exaggerated by using low temperature and cardiac allografts, further pointed out the codominance of alleles at a given locus (Kallman 1970). Because the genetic principles of segregation, association, mutation, and isolation (Bailey 1970) have not been fully applied to these teleosts (or to any ectotherm), we cannot state with certainty that differences at only one H locus are sufficient to lead to acute rejection whereas differences at any of the other H loci will result in chronic reactions. Nevertheless, circumstantial evidence analogous to that obtained from murine systems makes at least partial homology of major and minor H systems in teleosts and endotherms a plausible argument.

A few years ago, our knowledge of the genetic basis of rapid graft rejection in another ectotherm—the anuran amphibian (frogs, toads)—was restricted to general statements pointing out significant H-antigen polymorphism in outbred and sibling populations of Ranid frogs (Hildemann and Haas 1959, 1961). This important fact was derived from comparisons of the survival times of true second-set grafts with those of unrelated third-party test grafts placed on animals sensitized by a first-set transplant. Subsequent experiments involving grafts between diploid and triploid members of clones obtained by nuclear transplantation provided evidence for multiple H loci and for the codominance of H-alleles (Roux and Volpe 1974). It was not until the publication of a series of critical experiments by Du Pasquier and his associates, however, that we were provided with the first substantive genetic evidence for a causal relationship between a single histocompatibility system and relatively rapid graft rejection in the South African clawed frog, *Xenopus laevis* (Du Pasquier and Miggiano 1973; Du Pasquier et al. 1975). Like fish, all F_1 siblings produced from a mating of outbred *Xenopus* parents reject grafts from their brothers and sisters over the range typical of acute to subacute rejection reactions (15 to 31 days). When such siblings were typed by the mixed lymphocyte culture reaction (MLR), the result of 25 percent MLR identical sibs and 75 percent MLR nonidentical sibs fits with a classic Mendelian 1:4 segregation pattern (see Section 3 for more details). An analysis of survival times of grafts exchanged between such typed siblings makes it apparent that the 1:4 segregation ratio observed in MLR is reflected by significant variations in the rapidity of graft rejection. Thus, Du Pasquier et al. (1975) found that the time rejection began and the time it was completed were each significantly longer when grafts were transplanted between MLR-identical sibs rather than between MLR-nonidentical animals within the same sibship. The very observation that all MLR-identical siblings rejected allografts, but did so chronically (MST ~ 31 days), argues convincingly for the existence of a minimum of three rather than two multiallelic loci concerned with histocompatibility interactions in this amphibian. By applying the original temporal guidelines for calling a particular H barrier "strong" or "weak" (Counce et al. 1956), one H barrier in *Xenopus* is "strong" or major whereas the others are "weak" or minor.

Additional evidence for the involvement of major and minor H systems in the transplantation reactivities of anurans has been gleaned from analyzing the survival times of skin allografts transplanted to *Xenopus* that are either undergoing metamorphosis or that have recently transformed into juveniles (Du Pasquier and Chardonnens 1975; Chardonnens and Du Pasquier 1973). Only during this perimetamorphic period does a genetically and statistically significant number of grafts (approximately 25 percent) exchanged between siblings born from heterozygous parents enjoy indefinite survival. The percent of grafts reflecting this apparent host tolerance in the F_2 as well as the F_1 generation supports the hypothesis that the rejection of grafts during this period primarily reflects incompatibility at a single genetic region (i.e., the MHS). The same phenomenon of prolonged survival of 22 percent (< 30 days) of grafts on frogs in the perimetamorphic period has recently been confirmed by Chardonnens *(personal communication)* for *Rana delmatina*. Subsequent studies with MLR and serologically typed *Xenopus* siblings (Du Pasquier and Chardonnens 1975) dovetail with the supposition that, during the perimetamorphic period, "tolerance" is preferentially induced to weak H antigens (i.e., antigens that are products of genetic regions other than those associated with rapid graft rejection and reproducibly strong

MLR). Thus, by definition, *Xenopus* must now be immunogenetically characterized by a minimum of three multiallelic H systems, one of which is functionally homologous with part of the MHS of man and mouse. It should be noted parenthetically that Wachtel et al. (1975) presented serologic evidence that sperm of two anuran species possess antigenic determinants that are either identical to or cross-reactive with the H-Y antigens of the mouse. Whether these determinants function as transplantation antigens in frogs as they do in mice is unknown.

2.1.2 Chronic Rejection

Recent years have witnessed a resurgence of interest in immune potentials of invertebrates as well as vertebrates (Cooper 1974; Hildemann 1974; Hildemann and Reddy 1973). Allograft rejection, characterized as immunologic by the hallmarks of specificity and memory, has now been documented in annelids (Cooper 1970; Duprat 1967; Valembois 1974) and echinoderms (Hildemann and Dix 1972; Karp and Hildemann 1976). In both invertebrate classes, rejection has proved to be chronic.

Long-term graft survival also describes transplantation immunity of the most primitive living vertebrates known – the hagfish (Hildemann and Thoenes 1969) and the lamprey (Perey et al. 1968). Because chronicity also typifies graft rejection by the chondrichthyean (Borysenko and Hildemann 1970) and chondrostean (Perey et al. 1968) descendants of the now extinct Placodermi (Figure 9.1), the evolution of modern teleosts is marked by a progression from species that reject chronically to those that reject acutely.

The rapidity with which any amphibian rejects a first-set allograft is also predictably related to its taxonomic position (Cohen 1971a). Members of the orders Urodela (salamanders and newts) and Apoda (caecelians) routinely reject allografts chronically between 20 and 100 days (Cohen 1968; Cooper and Garcia-Herrera 1968). With respect to the order Anura, rejection reactions of a primitive frog, the Discoglossid *Bombina,* are temporally similar to reaction rates of diverse urodeles (Charlemagne, *personal communication;* Cohen and Richards, *unpublished data*). More advanced pipid frogs such as *Xenopus* reject subacutely whereas acute rejection characterizes the fate of allografts on members of the families Ranidae and Bufonidae (Cohen 1973). Thus, the mechanisms (genetic and other) that control the rate of allograft rejection in the Anura appear to have evolved within the contemporary members of this vertebrate order themselves rather than in some transitional form (e.g., Crossoptergyrii) that gave rise to both reptiles and amphibians.

All representatives of the three reptilian orders also reject chronically (Cohen 1971b). Thus, we must emphasize (Cohen and Borysenko 1970) that acute rejection not only emerged independently during the evolution of amphibians and fishes but must also have appeared independently a third and fourth time in phylogeny – once in the Aves and then again in the Mammalia (or in the lines leading to them).

Does chronic rejection in outbred ectothermic vertebrates (and invertebrates) signify the activities of alloantigenic products of minor H loci acting in the absence of a MHS, or does it simply reflect the lack of the physiologic and immunologic machinery necessary to effect rapid graft recognition and destruction? At least for vertebrates, this former possibility is supported by experimental observations whereas the latter is not. We now recognize that, like anurans, salamanders are also quite capable of mounting vigorous alloimmune responses *in vivo*. We (Cohen 1968, 1973; Cohen and Hildemann 1968) and others (Tournefier et al. 1969, 1970) have repeatedly (albeit occasionally) observed acute and subacute rejection of first-set allografts on newts that have apparently been confronted with particularly immunogenic combinations of alloantigens. It is most important that shortened survival times are also typical of transplants on salamanders that have been selectively immunosuppressed so as to delay the functional appearance of their normal enhancing humoral immune reactivities to weak H antigens (Manickavel and Cohen 1975a, 1975b; Section 2.2).

The following immunogenetic analyses (plus the data in Sections 2.2 and 3) support the hypothesis that the histocompatibility systems of at least one order of chronically rejecting ectotherms—the Urodela—display marked functional homology with the minor rather than the major systems of endotherms. Much genetic insight has been derived from evaluating the survival times of first-set, second-set, and third-party test grafts transplanted within and between populations of newts *(Notophthalmus v. viridescens)*. These studies have repeatedly revealed a substantial diversity of H antigens distinguishing animals within a population. In one such study (Hildemann and Cohen 1967), newts from population A rejected first-set grafts chronically. Unexpectedly, newts from population B rejected intrapopulation allografts much more quickly. Nearly 40 percent of population B allografts were destroyed by day 20; another 30 percent were completely rejected by day 25. Not only did this observation underline the fact that newts are capable of mounting vigorous alloimmune responses, but it afforded the opportunity to test functionally whether newts have the components of a MHS involved in acute rejection. The following reasoning is based on the "devil's advocate" hypothesis that acute and subacute rejection in newts is, in fact, a manifestation of an "H-2 type" of multiallelic system. If we assume that population B animals rejected rapidly because they differed from each other by many "strong" antigens and that such diversity was lacking in population A, we would then expect rapid rejection of A grafts on B newts. On the other hand, if population A animals rejected chronically because they were homozygous for the same alleles at a major locus but these alleles were present in much lower frequency in population B (i.e., allelic polymorphism at a "strong" locus would be necessary to account for rapid rejection in this population), then grafts from population B on population A newts should reflect this disequilibrium by exhibiting a high incidence of rapid rejection. In point of fact, chronic rejection characterized the fate of *both* sets of interpopulation allografts. Indeed, the number of grafts rejected during the same postoperative interval was strikingly similar in each combination. Thus, these results and those obtained from estimates of antigen sharing in these and several other populations argue that acute and subacute rejection in urodeles does not reflect a multiallelic "strong" H locus. It is probable that these more rapid rejections are partly attributable to the cumulative effects of multiple weak specificities, as they are in murine systems (Graff et al. 1966). However, it is known that the degree of chronicity encountered in any population study is, in part, a statement of the extent to which these weak alloantigens are effectively shared between any donor-host pair of animals. Typical survival times of 35 to 50 days speak to a moderate degree of antigen sharing; more prolonged survivals reflect increased sharing; and more rapid rejections are invariably associated with minimum antigen sharing, as detected by the technique of third-party test grafting (Cohen and Hildemann 1968; Cohen, *unpublished observation*).

As previously discussed, all existing transplantation studies argue that urodeles lack that part of the MHS of any endothermic species whose products serve as an effective trigger for rapid cytotoxic reactions and/or as a target for visualizing such reactivities. They also point out that urodeles possess multiple (number unknown) minor histocompatibility systems. In the mouse, alloantigenic products of such minor loci vary significantly with respect to the rapidity with which they evoke basically chronic reactions (Hildemann 1970b; Graff and Bailey 1973). Thus, DeLanney and Blackler's (1967) proposals that, like the mouse, (1) the minor H systems of salamanders are of unequal "strength" and (2) within the framework of chronic rejection, one of these systems may be relatively strong (i.e., predominant or major *for the species*) seem most reasonable. We could further envisage that incompatibility at this predominant locus would invariably result in rejection, whereas incompatibility only at the other loci might favor prolonged or even indefinite survival due to active enhancement or the induction of tolerance. Of course, incompatibilities at all H loci could result in a wide range of acute to chronic survival times due to the cumulative interactions of multiple weak H antigens. A straightforward way to test this simple hypothesis would be to exchange reciprocally relatively large skin grafts between F_1 progeny of a mating between field-collected heterozygous parents. If 25 percent of the grafts exhibited indefinite or even unusually prolonged survival while the remaining 75 percent were rejected within the typical survival range, we would have to assume that not only did one-quarter of the F_1 siblings share the same alleles at least at one H locus, but, with respect to transplant survival, this locus was the predominant minor H locus of the species. This simple experiment has yet to be carried out with field-collected animals. However, results identical to those described above were obtained by Tournefier et al. (1969) with F_1-sibling *Pleurodeles waltlii* derived from parents that had been raised in the laboratory for several years. To obtain the predicted segregation ratios, the original parents must have been heterozygous at a minimum of one locus and between them carried at least three different alleles of this locus. However, the possibility that the parents themselves might have been derived from a closed breeding colony and therefore might have been homozygous for the same alleles at several loci would provide an explanation of the survival of 22 percent of the intrasibling grafts which is independent of the single "predominant" minor H-locus concept. There are additional experiments with partially inbred strains of axolotls where a 1:2:1 segregation ratio of alleles at one predominant locus is sufficient to explain the genetic basis of the survival patterns of parental strain grafts on F_2 hybrids (DeLanney et al. 1975). It is also important to point out that survival patterns of grafts from F_2 on parental-strain animals provide evidence for at least two minor H systems in these neotenic animals. That the axolotls used to develop several inbred strains may have originated from a closed population collected in Mexico (DeLanney and Blackler 1967) again limits our interpretation of these data. Obviously, it is important not only to continue developing and exploiting inbred strains of axolotls (DeLanney et al. 1975) and *Pleurodeles* (Charlemagne and Tournefier 1974), but to carry out F_1 and F_2 grafting experiments with the progeny of wild caught specimens.

The origins of a predominant minor H-locus system in chronically rejecting ectothermic vertebrates might trace back to the Invertrebrata. Du Pasquier (1974) recently reviewed and reanalyzed some literature dealing with the genetic basis of nonconfluence phenomena in sponges, colony fusion in tunicates, and incompatibility reactions in cnidarians. He pointed out that, in these systems, recognition appears to be under the control of such a predominant minor locus and that the "weaker" the locus, the more obvious the haplotype effect.

2.2 Immunobiology of Major and Minor Histoincompatibility Interactions in Outbred Ectotherms and in Inbred Endotherms: Selected Parallel Observations

In the previous section we reviewed the limited immunogenetic data favoring the hypothesis that (1) acute first-set graft rejection in outbred ectotherms accurately marks the presence of a polymorphic MHS homologue, (2) chronic rejection marks the lack of a MHS, and (3) the MHS has evolved repeatedly during vertebrate phylogeny. If these hypotheses are valid, then we would predict that a range of transplantation phenomena uniquely associated with incompatibilities at "strong" or "weak" H barrier in warm-blooded vertebrates should have their parallel counterparts in the transplantation reactions of acutely and chronically rejecting ectotherms. The following data substantiate this prediction.

2.2.1 First-Set Rejection Phenomena

The postulate—the later the time of onset of graft rejection, the greater the interval between onset and complete rejection—was derived from descriptions of chronic rejection in congenic H-2-compatible strains of mice (Hildemann and Cohen 1967). It describes graft rejection in outbred urodeles as well (Cohen 1968). Equally valid for the murine and urodelean systems of chronic rejection is the clearcut relationship between breadth of the survival time range and the chronicity of the MST. As mentioned earlier, a cumulative effect of multiple weak specificities, first observed under genetically controlled conditions in mice (Graff et al. 1966), also appears to account for acute and subacute rejection in newts. Finally, it is most significant that, regardless of the species studied (e.g., salamander, hagfish, iguana, mouse), the survival times of chronically rejected first-set grafts frequently fail to fall into the normal distribution pattern that describes vigorous rejection across a strong H barrier in fishes, frogs, and H-2-incompatible strains of mice. Rather, the pattern of chronic rejection is marked by multiple alternating episodes of destruction and recovery (Cohen et al. 1975). As will be described shortly, this pattern appears to reflect alternating waves of those immunoprotective and immunocytotoxic responses to weak H-alloantigens that determine the eventual chronicity of skin allograft rejection.

2.2.2 Second-Set Rejection Phenomena

Repeat second-set grafts transplanted across a major histocompatibility barrier are often rejected very rapidly as white grafts or as transplants marked by a severe inflammation (Eichwald et al. 1966). Accelerated and vigorous rejection, often of the white graft type, characterizes the response of *Rana pipiens* (Bovbjerg 1966) and *Rana catesbeiana* (Hildemann and Haas 1959, 1961) to most second-set transplants. In these species, the range of second-set survival times rarely overlaps that of the first set. Such rapid and vigorous second-set reactivity, however, is not observed in those warm- or cold-blooded vertebrates that reject their initial grafts chronically. Indeed, it is not uncommon to observe in hagfish (Hildemann and Thoenes 1969), apodans (Cooper and Garcia-Herrera 1968), salamander (Cohen 1968, 1971), and iguanas (Cooper and Aponte 1968) that second-set transplants may survive as long as or even longer than first-set grafts. Similar data have been collected for mammals where weak histoincompatibility interactions prevail (Hildemann and Cooper 1967; Hildemann and Walford 1960). In both urodeles and mice, this phenomenon appears to result from active enhancement elicited by the "weak" specificities carried on both the initial and repeat grafts (Cohen et al. 1975).

Studies in mammals point out that repeated immunization of MHS-incompatible hosts with skin grafts fails to reduce test graft survival times below those recorded for second-set transplants (Solowey and Rapaport 1966). This observation is equally valid for teleosts (Hildemann 1958, 1970a) and frogs (Hildemann and Haas 1959, 1961). It does *not* apply to MHS-compatible mammals (Hildemann and Walford 1960), chronically rejecting hornsharks (Borysenko and Hildemann 1970), and salamanders (Cohen 1968, 1970), where third- or fourth-set grafts may be rejected significantly more rapidly than the preceding transplant. Thus, for recipients of weakly histoincompatible grafts, the second-set response to weak alloantigens need not mirror the maximum destructive host response capable of being generated against a given set of alloantigens.

2.2.3 Differential Survival of Organ and Skin Grafts

Rejection of a variety of first-set tissue and organ transplants grafted across a MHS barrier to immunosuppressed rodents is usually as rapid as skin graft rejection (Hildemann and Mullen 1973; Guttman 1974). Comparable transplants between rodents matched at the MHS, however, often enjoy extended survival times relative to skin (Hildemann and Mullen 1973; Barker and Billingham 1971). These basically unexplained survival differences, which relate to the "strength" of H antigens, have their counterpart in ectotherms. In several species of salamanders, heterotopic allografts and xenografts of heart, pituitaries, gonads, and several other tissues survive far longer (even indefinitely) than skin transplants (Cohen 1971 a). In the case of heart allografts, differential susceptibility of cardiac tissue to cytotoxic or enhancing components of the immune response and tissue specific transplantation antigens may each explain the fact that such grafts survive much longer than skin transplants on hosts that have been hyperimmunized by repeated grafts of integument from the original donor (Cohen and Rich 1970).

2.2.4 Nonspecific Immunosuppression

It is generally held that the weaker the histocompatibility barrier, the easier it is to obtain nonspecific immunosuppression with drugs or X-rays. We know that 6-mercaptopurine, antibiotics (Cooper 1964), and azathioprine (Stutzman, 1967) delay scale allograft rejection in teleosts by only a few days. Although these drugs have not been screened for suppressive activity in chronically rejecting ectotherms, *certain* doses of cytosine arabinoside (ara-c) effectively prolong survival of salamander skin allografts (Manickavel and Cohen 1975a; see below for opposite effects of low doses of ara-c). Salamanders' destructive alloimmune responses are also much more sensitive to the suppressive effects of X-irradiation and low temperature (Cohen 1966, 1971 a) than are those of fishes and frogs (Hildemann and Cooper 1964).

2.2.5 Specific Immunosuppression: Tolerance and Enhancement

As a general rule, transplant tolerance and/or enhancement is most easily evoked in endotherms by a challenge with the products of minor rather than major histocompatibility systems (Voisin 1971). The following demonstrations that it is also easier to induce specific unresponsiveness in salamanders than frogs support the genetic data favoring the lack of a MHS homologue in urodeles.

1. It is possible to produce viable adult chimeric salamanders that carry tissues or even the intact head and trunk of two species or genera by exchanging the relevant parts during embryonic life (Goujon 1974; Houillon 1964).

In turtles, extra limbs differentiate from allogeneic limb buds heterotopically transplanted to young embryos (Yntema and Borysenko 1971). In the limited number of cases tested, skin grafts from the original donor animals or strain were tolerated by the adult chimeras, whereas third-party grafts were not (Goujon 1974). Creation of chimeric frogs by similar procedures involving allogeneic and xenogeneic transplants in anuran embryos, however, is often unsuccessful. Nonlymphoid tissues that differentiate from such grafts are rejected once the immune response capacity of the host develops during larval life (Volpe 1964).

2. Brephloplastic allotransplants (grafts from embryonic donors to adult hosts) invariably differentiate into huge teratoma-like masses in newts (Fankhauser and Stonesifer 1956; Cohen 1969). Such a procedure is less successful in *Xenopus laevis* (Simnett 1966) and *Rana pipiens* (Harris 1941; Rafferty 1961). Similarly, fetal grafts in adult mice are most successful when the donors and hosts are H-2 compatible (Wachtel and Silvers 1971).

3. In a parallel series of experiments utilizing congenic H-2-compatible mice and field-collected salamanders, specific unresponsiveness to skin allografts was induced by alloantigenic pretreatment with tissue fragments (Baldwin and Cohen 1970, 1971, 1972, 1974; Cohen and Latorre 1975). This appears to be a property of the response to weak H antigens (Kornblum and Silvers 1968; Linder 1962). Moreover, the passive transfer of sera from appropriately treated mice (Baldwin and Cohen 1973, 1974) and newts (Cohen et al. 1975) adoptively enhanced test skin graft survival on the secondary recipients. These results led to the hypothesis (Baldwin and Cohen 1974) that, regardless of species, weak H alloantigens are in fact quite immunogenic because they elicit an early and effective enhancing antibody response. The data also suggested the corollary that chronic rejection elicited by antigenic products of defined minor H genes in mice and putatively minor H genes in salamanders reflects active enhancement. Both the hypothesis and its corollary have been supported by the demonstration in mice and newts that the selective functional elimination or delay of putative B-cell responses (enhancing antibody) by *certain* doses of cytosine arabinoside (Heppner and Calabresi 1972) leads to the dramatic shortening of normally chronic graft survival times (Manickavel and Cohen 1975a, 1975b, *unpublished observations*).

3. The MHS and the Phylogeny of Mixed Lymphocyte Reactivities

In the previous section, we selected one facet of the MHS of endotherms—its association with rapid graft rejection—and suggested that the transition from chronic to acute graft destruction that apparently accompanied the phylogeny of fishes, amphibians, birds, and mammals might reflect the evolutionary history of at least part of the mammalian MHS. This "argument by analogy" would be strengthened considerably if we could describe other functions of the mammalian and avian MHS components that have been looked for in all key primitive species but found only in those that display acute allograft reactivities. The behavior of allogeneic lymphocytes in the MLR provides just such a second marker of MHS evolution. When lymphocytes from two individuals selected at random from outbred mammalian or avian species are cocultured, a strong two-way stimulation/response reaction occurs that is characterized by blast cell transformation and cell proliferation (Bach and Hirschhorn 1964). Invariably, disparities at MLR loci of the MHS of chickens, mice, rats, man, and other warm-blooded vertebrates (this volume) are always equated with intense reactivities. In the face of MHS compatibility, however, stimulation of chicken, rat, and human lymphoid cells in MLR is either undetectable by current techniques (Miggiano et al. 1974; Thorsby 1974; Cramer et al. 1974) or is significantly less than that recorded when MHS disparities prevail (Colley and DeWitt 1969).

In the mouse, where immunogenetic definition of the strains providing the allogeneic cells is more precise, a less black and white picture emerges. In the face of MHS compatibility, stimulation in MLR ranges from that which is comparable to control syngeneic cultures, through weak responses, to stimulation indexes that are similar to those obtained in the presence of MHS incompatibilities (Dutton 1966; Häyry and Defendi 1970; Rychilikova and Ivanyi 1969; Mangi and Mardiney 1971; Peck and Click 1973). The extent of stimulation is very much dependent on the culture conditions and on the particular minor H loci or M locus (Festenstein 1973) disparities that are involved. Regardless of whether weak or even strong stimulation *can* occur as a response to multiple minor loci or gene products of the M locus, it *always* occurs with a MHS difference (e.g., with cells from outbred endotherms). Thus, if acute rejection in fishes and frogs means that these animals have a MHS homologue whereas chronic rejection in primitive fish and salamanders means that they do not, MLR should be intense in the first group of vertebrates and either minimal or undetectable in the second.

3.1 Fishes

In very general terms, the currently available information about the presence or absence of MLR in primitive and advanced fishes fits elegantly with those results predicted by the rejection of integument graft. MLR has either not been observed or is at best marginal with cells from the hagfish (Cooper and Du Pasquier 1974) and the lamprey (Cooper 1971). Cells from an elasmobranch are also MLR negative (Sigel et al. 1973), whereas those from the teleost (trout) are quite reactive (Etlinger 1975). However, much more effort with several species from each of the above classes must be expanded before we shall feel entirely comfortable with the generalization with which this paragraph begins. For example, peripheral blood leukocytes from the MLR-negative nurse shark were responsive to high doses of Con A but not to PHA (over a wide dose range). Ficoll hypaque separation of the peripheral cells revealed a PHA-reactive population whose response could be abrogated when cells from other layers were added (Sigel et al. 1973; Lopez et al. 1974). Thus, we shall not know with certainty whether MLR negativity in the nurse shark reflects the lack of part of the MHS or the activity of suppressor cells until further experiments are carried out. Similarly, the question of whether cells from agnathans display MLR is also open ended. Cooper (1971) reported positive reactivity of cells from larval lampreys to specific antigens and to mitogens but not to alloantigens. However, the culture conditions (15° C, 4-day cultures) and the assay technique (counting blast cells) that detected mitogen reactivity may have been less than optimal for visualizing MLR in this chronically rejecting species. Moreover, for some but not all combinations of allogeneic cells, the addition of PHA to the culture media appeared to potentiate an MLR. Finally, a full report on the behavior of hagfish lymphocytes *in vitro* has not been published. Thus, it is only our interpretation of preliminary studies of Reddy and Hildemann [summarized by Cooper and Du Pasquier (1974)] that leads us to the provisional conclusion of marginal or negative MLR in this agnathan species.

3.2 Amphibians

The first definitive studies revealing that lymphocytes from any ectotherm respond to alloantigens *in vitro* were carried out with lymphoid cells from the toad, *Bufo marinus*. Incubation of allogeneic splenic lymphocytes under conditions of macroculture (with homologous sera) resulted in stimulation indexes (S.I.) of 11 to 19 (Goldshein and Cohen 1972). Stimulation is also obvious in allogeneic microcultures of cells from other anuran species (*Rana pipiens* and *Xenopus laevis*). Indeed, for the latter species there is now decisive evidence provided by Du Pasquier and colleagues that the MLR is under control of a single region that is functionally homologous to the MHS of the mouse (Du Pasquier and Miggiano 1973; Du Pasquier et al. 1975; Du Pasquier and Chardonnens 1975). Their first critical observation compared the low (3 percent) incidence of MLR-negative reactions between cells from unrelated animals with the genetically significant incidence of 22 percent MLR negativity when the cocultured cells were derived from F_1 siblings of outbred parents. This single finding suggested that the MLR in *Xenopus* is under the control of one locus (or closely linked loci) that segregates in a Mendelian fashion within a sibship. Further evidence that the MLR is under the control of a single region in this species was provided by the fact that MLR-identical individuals within each of three families (sibships) distributed themselves into four different classes or haplotypes. Moreover, a gene dose or haplotype effect was obvious and predictable within a sibship (i.e., stimulation was stronger when the cells differed by two haplotypes rather than by one). As mentioned earlier, MLR-identical sibs reject skin allografts more slowly than do MLR-incompatible ones. During the perimetamorphic period—when tolerance to new self-antigens must occur—this haplotype effect is also sharply defined for skin allografts; only large grafts between MLR-identical sibs survive indefinitely. Thus, those antigens involved in eliciting rapid graft rejection and clearcut stimulation in MLR in *Xenopus* are products of either the same or closely linked genes. It is equally important that appropriately absorbed alloantisera, raised by immunizing MLR-incompatible animals with skin and erythrocytes, exclusively detect antigens coded for by a genetic region that segregates with MLR genes (DuPasquier et al. 1975). Because this linkage of serologically defined specificities with rapid graft rejection with MLR describes the MHS of the mouse as well as that of *Xenopus laevis,* it presents a powerful argument for the phylogenetic emergence of an MHS in anuran amphibians. The extent to which the two systems are functionally homologous awaits detection of immune response genes in the MHS of *Xenopus*. Similarly, the extent to which both systems are structurally homologous at the chromosomal level (e.g., duplicate loci) and biochemically homologous at the level of the gene products remains conjectural.

Just as decisive MLR and rapid rejection are genetically linked in Pipid frogs, weak or negative MLR and chronic rejection are at least phenomenologically linked in salamanders. Early studies in our laboratory with the mudpuppy, *Necturus,* and in DuPasquier's (1974) laboratory with *Triturus,* did not reveal a MLR with cells from these outbred salamanders. Because such negative data might mirror technical rather than immunobiological limitations of the system, we recently initiated a comprehensive comparative study of MLR and mitogen reactivity of cells from partially inbred strains of axolotls, random bred newts, and frogs (Collins et al. 1975; DeLanney et al. 1975). Our attention has focused primarily on optimizing our culture procedures. Frogs and mitogens were to provide us with positive control reactivities, axolotls with the opportunity to study the genetics of MLR, and newts with the maximum diversity of allelic combinations found in outbred animals. Frog cells *(Rana pipiens, Xenopus laevis)* respond quite well to the B-cell mitogens LPS and PPD, and to the T-cell mitogens PHA and Con A (Goldstine et al. 1975) as well as to allogeneic cells. The marked response (S.I. = 18) of salamander cells to LPS and PPD, however, is in striking contrast to the consistently low (S.I. = 2 to 3) and delayed responses to T-cell mitogens. To date, we have been unable to reproducibly increase these poor responses of axolotl cells by supplementing our standard L-15 culture medium with 2-mercaptoethanol, various lots of heat-inactivated fetal calf serum, homologous serum, nucleotides, or $NaHCO_3$, or by carrying the cultures for a week or more. Parallel experiments with cells from *Rana* and axolotl reaffirmed the ease with which an earlier and significantly higher stimulation occurs for anuran cells. Although newt and axolotl cells reacted in a poor but similar fashion to Con A, newt cells were, in fact, unresponsive to PHA.

These striking differences between mitogen reactivity of anuran and urodele cells to T-cell mitogens under comparable and variable culture conditions make it clear that there are fundamental quantitative and/or qualitative differences between subpopulations of frog and salamander lymphocytes. For example, salamanders may have many more B- than T-cells in their spleens and blood (reactivities of thymocytes have not been studied). Salamander LPS reactive cells (B-cells?) may survive better than T-cells in our culture conditions and/or these conditions may favor B-cell responses and inhibit reactivities of numerous T-cells. These possibilities, as well as the existence of a suppressor population that checks reactivity to T-cell mitogens, are all currently being investigated. Until the necessary data are generated, however, it is still permissible to speculate that B-cell responses may have evolved earlier than T-cell responses, perhaps because preferential stimulation activated by bacterial polyclonal activators afforded primitive animals an excellent survival value.

Those culture conditions that permit detection of marked stimulation of urodele lymphocytes to LPS and low responses to Con A also permit detection of MLR with axolotl cells provided that the cell donors are not from the same strain (Collins et al. 1975; DeLanney et al. 1975). However, MLRs of axolotl or newt cells are not always positive, and those that are, are consistently characterized by lower S.I. (1.6 to 3) than those often obtained with cocultured frog cells (Du Pasquier and Chardonnens 1975). Thus, it is certainly plausible that the stimulation we do observe in urodeles reflects differences at minor loci rather than at a MHS. However, our current inability to detect high stimulation of urodele cells to T-cell mitogens under conditions that promote excellent reactivity to LPS places an obvious restriction on this interpretation. We may not yet have refined our culture conditions to visualize a T-cell response such as the MLR, or T-cells in these animals may differ from those of the frog or mouse. If future experiments reveal excellent stimulation with T-cell mitogens but not with allogeneic cells, strong evidence for the absence of a MHS homologue in urodele amphibians will be provided. On the other hand, it would be equally exciting and satisfying to try to fathom the relationship between poor T-cell mitogen responsiveness, minimal MLR, presence of only one Ig class (Marchalonis and Cohen 1973; Tournefier 1975; Houdayer and Fougereau 1973), and delayed antibody responses (all of which characterize urodeles, not frogs) to the phylogeny of lymphocyte structure and function.

4. The MHS and the Phylogeny of Graft-Versus-Host Reactivities

Parental strain lymphocytes injected into F_1 hybrid hosts, newborn hosts, or immunosuppressed hosts home to the lymphoid organs of the recipient where, in response to host alloantigens, they proliferate and differentiate into killer cells. These events excite proliferation of host reticuloendothelial and lymphoid cells in the spleen and liver. Characteristic of such intense reactions is the eventual destruction of the host lymphoid system, the runting syndrome, and eventual host death.

Like rapidity of graft rejection and the intensity of MLR stimulation, variations in the intensity and symptomology of the GvH reactivity can measure the strength of a given histocompatibility barrier (Cantrell and Hildemann 1972). GvH reactivity is most demonstrable when allogeneic lymphoid cells are injected into recipients that do not share the same alleles of the MHS. However, Cantrell and Hildemann (1972) recently pointed out that GvH reactivity can be effected across almost any minor H barrier provided that certain variables are properly manipulated (e.g., preimmunization, large number of cells, intravenous route).

We are unaware of any GvH reactivity studies in primitive or advanced fishes. Indeed, the only detailed investigations of GvH reactivity in an ectothermic species were performed with snapping turtles which, like all reptiles, reject allografts chronically (Borysenko 1970; Cohen 1971 a). GvH reactivity was first observed in explants of spleens from newly hatched turtles cultured with allogeneic adult splenocytes (Sidky and Auerbach 1968). In a subsequent *in vivo* experiment (Borysenko and Tulipan 1973), immunoincompetent hatchlings, unfortunately from several sibships (Borysenko, *personal communication*), were injected i.p. with 5×10^6 spleen or kidney (control) cells from adults. The intensity and incidence of the GvH reactivity (percent lethality postinjection time and extent of splenomegaly) were dependent on the age of the recipient, the geographical origins of the donors and hosts, and the temperature at which the hosts were kept. At 30° C, 73 percent of newly hatched New York State recipients of spleen cells from a single Wisconsin donor died. The remaining seven turtles recovered from their initial weight loss. Of 19 deaths, about 50 percent were recorded within the first week after inoculation; the other occurred more chronically during the 4-month observational period. At 20° C, mortality associated with cells from the same donor decreased to 35 percent.

Splenomegaly associated with loss in white pulp lymphocytes and increased activity of macrophages and numbers of eosinophils occurred only with acute GvH reactivity. When donors and hosts were both from New York State, the incidence of lethality at 30° C and 20° C was significantly reduced (48 and 19 percent, respectively). Associated with this apparent decrease in genetic disparity among outbred animals was the lessened incidence (20 percent) of acute lethal GvH reaction. The fact that acute GvH reaction can be visualized in immunoincompetent turtles is, by itself, insufficient for us to argue that it is controlled by a single genetic region. Similarly, the fact that not all the hosts succumbed to this GvH reaction cannot be taken as evidence for the lack of such a locus. Clearly, further studies dealing with the genetic basis of GvH reactivity in this species as well as basic MLR data in reptiles are sorely needed. They may yield an invaluable opportunity to dissect different evolutionary rates of MHS in this chronically rejecting vertebrate class.

Attempts to induce GvH reactivity in newly hatched lizards by injecting them with adult splenocytes or thymocytes have been unsuccessful (Kanakambika and Muthukkaruppan 1972). However, unlike the turtle, the immune response of the garden lizard is already developed within 24 hr of hatching, as judged by the ability of such hatchlings to mount an immune response against sheep erythrocytes.

A recent investigation of GvH reactivity in sibling frogs *(Xenopus laevis)* was made possible by subcutaneously implanting an allogeneic spleen into a recipient that had been rendered tolerant to the donor's H antigens during embryonic life (Clark and Newth 1972). Prior to implantation, but during the perimetamorphic period, the spleen donor had rejected two immunizing skin grafts from the tolerant partner. In 7 of 9 clearly tolerant animals (78 percent), the spleen implant was the focus of a local GvH reaction. Skin over the implant became inflamed, and vasodilation and hemorrhaging were progressive. Two of these animals died (day 15 and 17); the others recovered and the grafted spleens disappeared. These data suggest that: (1) like the MLR, the GvH reaction in *Xenopus* is under the control of a single genetic region and (2) host death or recovery reflects a haplotype effect. Whether this GvH reactivity segregates with the MLR is presently unknown.

Unfortunately, the data describing GvH reactivity in salamanders are also quite minimal. DeLanney (1958) transplanted fragments of adult spleens into the coelem or tail fin of immunoincompetent salamander larvae. That no splenomegaly or lethality was recorded is consistent with, but by no means proves, the general theme that urodeles lack a MHS homologue. As part of a comprehensive description of transplantation immunity in another species, *Cynops pyrrhogaster,* Murakawa (1968) joined pairs of adult animals together by their tails. Approximately 80 percent of these animals died between 50 and 100 days postsurgery from chronic parabiotic disease. Surviving animals were tolerant to skin grafts from each other but not from third parties. Acute rather than chronic parabiotic intoxication is typical of MHS incompatibilities in rodents.

5. Concluding Remarks

A set of multiple genetically linked functions (e.g., acute graft rejection, reproducible and intense MLR and GvH reactivity permits one histocompatibility system of diverse mammalian and avian species to be functionally singled out as its MHS. A functional homologue of the MHS has yet to be discerned in any invertebrate. Yet, for many of these phylogenetically disparate creatures, several investigators have reported the activities of cell-associated recognition signals that appear under the control of a single gene locus and that serve to mark self from nonself by immunologic or nonimmunologic means (DuPasquier 1974). Current data provisionally argue that the functional homologue of the MHS is also lacking in primitive fishes (agnathans, elasmobranchs), primitive amphibians (caecelians, salamanders, perhaps primitive Discoglossid frogs), and all reptiles. We assume that this means that the genetic homologue of the MHS is also lacking in these species. However, we cannot yet rule out the possibility that multiple linked loci are present but that the functional expression of their gene products is somehow blocked or masked. In this regard it is noteworthy that in mice, a single point mutation in the MHS can provide a sufficient phenotypic alteration in the mutant strain so that it can be distinguished from the strain of origin by graft rejection, GvH reactivity, and MLR (Egorov 1974). On the other hand, primitive fishes, salamanders, and reptiles do have more than one genetically controlled polymorphic histocompatibility system that, at the functional level, appears homologous with minor histocompatibility systems of endotherms. There is also the critical suggestion from studies with urodeles that for each of these species, one minor H system serves as a predominant or major system of that species. A MHS homologue is functionally and genetically detectable in advanced anuran amphibians and will most probably be identified genetically in advanced Osteichthyes (teleosts).

Although there is a clear need for more information to confirm the previous statements, those data that do exist suggest that the phylogeny of the MHS is a classic example of convergent evolution. The MHS independently appeared on four different occasions during evolution. The first was during the evolution of the fishes. It appeared again during the evolution of modern anuran amphibians from their labyrinthodontian ancestors; during the emergence of birds from the Thecodonts; and during the phylogeny of mammals from the Therapsids. In his recent book, *Evolution by Gene Duplication,* Ohno (1970) discusses convergent evolution at the levels of allelic mutation and gene duplication. Essential to his concept of convergent evolution is that divergent species maintain homologous gene loci. He states that "at a homologous gene locus natural selection may independently favor similar types of tolerable mutations to cope with particular demands imposed by similar environments." We suggest that for each vertebrate that lacks a MHS (and indeed in every invertebrate species) there exists such a requisite homologous locus. Eventually it may well be recognized as the predominant minor H locus of that species. According to Ohno, convergent evolution, in this case of the MHS, could simply reflect the recurrence of homologous mutations at each of these homologous loci. On the other hand, it is currently held that the MHS evolved by gene duplication (Shreffler et al. 1971; Klein 1975). The current data arguing in favor of convergent evolution of the MHS would also be compatible with this gene duplication theory. According to Ohno, "as long as divergent organisms have the homologous gene locus which can serve as an ancestor, duplication can independently create a new gene locus with the same basic characteristics."

One of our goals in reviewing histocompatibility systems of primitive vertebrates was to provide a broader base of fact from which speculations and testable hypotheses concerning the phylogeny and true functions of the MHS could be developed. A second goal was to chart those areas where a lack of knowledge makes such speculations tenuous. It concerns us that the minimal literature available for review at this time made it quite easy to meet our second objective. We hope that it will not take as long to fathom the phylogeny of the MHS as it did for this unique genetic system to evolve.

Acknowledgments. This review was written during the senior author's sabbatical leave from the University of Rochester at the Basel Institute for Immunology. The hospitality of this institute and the interest and assistance of its members Drs. L. DuPasquier, V. C. Miggiano, M. Nabholz, and J. R. L. Pink in the preparation of this manuscript are gratefully appreciated.

Research cited from the authors' laboratory at the University of Rochester was supported by U.S. Public Health Service Grant HD-07901. N.C. is a recipient of U.S. Public Health Service Research Career Development Award AI-70736. N. H. C. was a predoctoral trainee supported by U.S. Public Health Service Training Grant 5 TO 1-GM-00591.

References

Bach, F. H., and Hirschhorn, K. Lymphocyte interaction: A potential histocompatibility test *in vitro. Science 142*:813–814, 1964.

Bailey, D. W. Four approaches to estimating number of histocompatibility loci. *Transplant. Proc. 2*:32–38, 1970.

Baldwin, W. M., III, and Cohen, N. Liver-induced immunosuppression of allograft immunity in urodele amphibians. *Transplantation 10*:530–537, 1970.

Baldwin, W. M., III, and Cohen, N. Effects of diverse tissue implants on the survival of subsequent skin allografts transplanted across weak histocompatibility barriers in newts and mice. *Transplant. Proc. 3*:217–219, 1971.

Baldwin, W. M., III, and Cohen, N. Immunosuppression of subacute skin allograft rejection in the newt *Diemictylus v. dorsalis* by alloantigenic pretreatment with kidney and liver implants. *Folia Biol. (Praha) 18*:181–188, 1972.

Baldwin, W. M., III, and Cohen, N. Immune serum implements either accelerated rejection or prolonged survival of murine skin grafts. *Transplantation 15*:633–637, 1973.

Baldwin, W. M., III, and Cohen, N. "Weak" histocompatibility antigens generate functionally "strong" humoral immunity. *Immunogenetics 1*:33–44, 1974.

Barker, C. F., and Billingham, R. E. Histocompatibility requirements of heart and skin grafts in rats. *Transplant. Proc. 3*:172–175, 1971.

Bodmer, W. F. Evolutionary significance of the HL-A system. *Nature 237*:139–145, 1972.

Borysenko, M. Transplantation immunity in Reptilia. *Transplant. Proc. 2*:299–306, 1970.

Borysenko, M., and Hildemann, W. H. Reactions to first-set skin allografts in the horn shark, *Heterodontis francisci. Transplantation 10*:545–551, 1970.

Borysenko, M., and Tulipan, P. The graft-versus-host reaction in the snapping turtle, *Chelydra serpentina. Transplantation 16*:496–504, 1973.

Bovbjerg, A. M. Rejection of skin homografts in larvae of *Rana pipiens. J. Exp. Zool. 161*:69–80, 1966.

Burnet, F. M. Multiple polymorphism in relation to histocompatibility antigens. *Nature 245*:359–361, 1973.

Cantrell, J. L., and Hildemann, W. H. Characteristics of disparate histocompatibility barriers in congenic strains of mice. I. Graft-versus-host reactions. *Transplantation 14*:761–770, 1972.

Chardonnens, X., and DuPasquier, L. Induction of skin allograft tolerance during metamorphosis of the toad *Xenopus laevis:* A possible model for studying generation of self tolerance to histocompatibility antigens. *Eur. J. Immunol. 3*:569–573, 1973.

Charlemagne, J., and Tournefier, A. Obtention of histocompatible strains in the urodele amphibian *Pleurodeles waltlii* Michah (Salamandridae). *J. Immunogenet. 1*:125–129, 1974.

Clark, J. C., and Newth, D. R. Immunological activity of transplanted spleens in *Xenopus laevis*. *Experientia 28*:951–953, 1972.

Cohen, N. Tissue transplantation immunity in the adult newt, *Diemictylus viridescens*. III. The effects of X-irradiation and temperature on the allograft reaction. *J. Exp. Zool. 163*:231–240, 1966.

Cohen, N. Chronic skin graft rejection in the Urodela. I. A Comparative study of first- and second-set allograft reactions. *J. Exp. Zool. 167*:37–48, 1968.

Cohen, N. Immunogenetic and developmental aspects of tissue transplantation immunity in urodele amphibians. *In* M. Mizell (ed.), *Biology of Amphibian Tumors, Recent Results in Cancer Research*, pp. 153–168. Springer-Verlag, Berlin, Heidelberg, New York, 1969.

Cohen, N. Immunological memory involving weak histocompatibility barriers in urodele amphibians. *Transplantation 10*:382–388, 1970.

Cohen, N. Amphibian transplantation reactions: A review. *Am. Zool. 11*:193–205, 1971 a.

Cohen, N. Reptiles as models for the study of immunity and its phylogenesis. *J. Am. Vet. Med. Assoc. 159*:1662–1671, 1971 b.

Cohen, N. Predictable variability in the response of two newt subspecies *(D. v. viridescens* and *D. v. dorsalis)* to first-set allografts. *Folia Biol. (Praha) 19*:169–173, 1973.

Cohen, N. Phylogeny of lymphocyte structure and function. *Am. Zool. 15*:119–133, 1975.

Cohen, N., Baldwin, W. M., III, and Manickavel, V. Phylogeny of functional humoral transplantation immunity: Comparative studies in amphibians and rodents. *Adv. Exp. Med. Biol. 64*:411–420, 1975.

Cohen, N., and Borysenko, M. Acute and chronic graft rejection: Possible phylogeny of transplantation antigens. *Transplant. Proc. 2*:333–336, 1970.

Cohen, N., and Hildemann, W. H. Population studies of allograft rejection in the newt, *Diemictylus viridescens*. *Transplantation 6*:208–217, 1968.

Cohen, N., and Latorre, J. A. The influence of histocompatibility and anti-thymocyte serum on the ability of alloantigenic pretreatment to prolong the survival of mouse skin grafts. *Folia Biol. (Praha) 21*:33–42, 1975.

Cohen, N., and Rich, L. C. Exceptionally prolonged survival of allogeneic heart implants in untreated and previously skin grafted salamanders. *Am. Zool. 10*:536, 1970.

Colley, D. G., and Dewitt, C. W. Mixed lymphocyte blastogenesis in response to multiple histocompatibility antigens. *J. Immunol. 102*:107–116, 1969.

Collins, N. H., Manickavel, V., and Cohen, N. *In vitro* responses of lymphoid cells: Mitogenic and mixed lymphocyte culture reactivities. *Adv. Exp. Med. Biol. 64*:305–314, 1975.

Cooper, A. J. Ammocete lymphoid cell population *in vivo*. *In* O. R. McIntyre (ed.), *Proceedings of the 4th Annual Leukocyte Conference*, pp. 137–147, Appleton Century-Crofts, New York, 1971.

Cooper, E. L. The effects of antibiotics and X-irradiation on the survival of scale homografts in *Fundulus heteroclitus*. *Transplantation 2*:2–20, 1964.

Cooper, E. L. Transplantation immunity in helminths and annelids. *Transplant. Proc. 2*:216–221, 1970.

Cooper, E. L. (ed). *Invertebrate Immunology: Contemporary Topics in Immunobiology 4*:299, Plenum Press, New York, 1974.

Cooper, E. L., and Aponte, A. Chronic allograft rejection in the iguana, *Ctenosaura pectinata*. *Proc. Soc. Exp. Biol. Med. 128*:150–154, 1968.

Cooper, E. L., and DuPasquier, L. Primitive vertebrate immunology: *Workshop Rep. in Prog. Immunol. 2*:297–301, 1974.

Cooper, E. L., and Garcia-Herrera, F. Chronic skin allograft rejection in the apodan, *Typhlonectes compressicanda*. *Copeia 2*:224–229, 1968.

Counce, S., Smith, P., Barth, R., and Snell, G. D. Strong and weak histocompatibility gene differences in mice and their role in the rejection of homografts of tumors and skin. *Ann. Surg. 144*:198–204, 1956.

Cramer, C. V., Shonnard, J. W., and Gill, T. J., III. Genetic studies in inbred rats. II. Relationship between the major histocompatibility complex and mixed lymphocyte reactivity. *J. Immunogenet. 1*:421–428, 1974.

DeLanney, L. E. Influence of adult amphibian spleen on the development of embryos and larvae: An immune response? *In* W. D. McElroy and B. Glass (eds.), *Chemical Basis of Development*, pp. 562–568, The Johns Hopkins Press, Baltimore, Md., 1958.

DeLanney, L. E., and Blackler, K. Acceptance and regression of a strain specific lymphosarcoma in Mexican axolotly. *In* M. Mizell (ed.), *Biology of Amphibian Tumors, Recent Results in Cancer Research*, pp. 399–408, Springer-Verlag, New York, 1967.

DeLanney, L. E., Collins, N. H., Cohen, N., and Reid, R. Transplantation immunogenetics and MLC reactivities of partially inbred strains of salamanders *(A. mexicanum)*: Preliminary studies. *Adv. Exp. Biol. Med. 64*:315–324, 1975.

Démant, P. H-2 gene complex and its role in alloimmune reactions. *Transplant. Proc. 15*:162–200, 1973.

DuPasquier, L. Ontogeny of the immune response in cold-blooded vertebrates. *Curr. Top. Microbiol. Immunol. 61*:37–88, 1973.

DuPasquier, L. The genetic control of histocompatibility reactions: Phylogenetic aspects. *Arch. Biol. 85*:91–103, 1974.

DuPasquier, L., and Chardonnens, X. Genetic aspects of tolerance to allografts induced at metamorphosis in the toad *Xenopus laevis. Immunogenetics 2*:431–440, 1975.

DuPasquier, L., Chardonnens, X., and Miggiano, V. C. A major histocompatibility complex in the toad *Xenopus laevis* (Daudin). *Immunogenetics 1*:482–494, 1975.

DuPasquier, L., and Miggiano, V. C. The mixed leukocyte reaction in the toad *Xenopus laevis:* A family study. *Transplant. Proc. 5*:1457–1461, 1973.

Duprat, P. Etude de la prise et du maintien d'un greffon de paroi du corps chez le Lombricien *Eisenia foetida typica. Ann. Inst. Pasteur 113*:867–881, 1967.

Dutton, R. W. Spleen cell proliferation in response to homologous antigens: Studies in congenic resistant strains of mice. *J. Exp. Med. 123*:665–671, 1966.

Egorov, I. K. Genetic control of H-2 alloantigens as inferred from analysis of mutation. *Immunogenetics 1*:97–107, 1974.

Eichwald, E. J., Wetzel, B., and Lustgraff, E. C. Genetic aspects of the second-set skin graft in mice. *Transplantation 4*:260–273, 1966.

Etlinger, H. M. Function and structure of rainbow trout leukocytes. *Doctoral dissertation*, University of Washington, Seattle, 1975.

Fankhauser, G., and Stonesifer, G. L., Jr. The fate of newt embryos implanted with or without jelly under the skin of adults. *J. Exp. Zool. 132*:85–104, 1956.

Festenstein, H. Immunogenetic and biological aspects of *in vitro* lymphocyte allotransformation (MLR) in the mouse. *Transplant. Proc. 15*:62–88, 1973.

Goldshein, S. J., and Cohen, N. Phylogeny of immune competent cells. I. *In vitro* blastogenesis and mitosis of toad *(Bufo marinus)* splenic lymphocytes to phytohemagglutinin and in mixed lymphocyte cultures. *J. Immunol. 108*:1025–1033, 1972.

Goldstine, S. N., Collins, N. H., and Cohen, N. Mitogens as probes of lymphocyte heterogeneity in anuran amphibians. *Adv. Exp. Med. Biol. 64*:343–352, 1975.

Goujon, P. Induction de la tolérance aux allogreffes de peau dans les chimères de l'amphibien urodèle, *Pleurodeles waltlii* Michah. *J. Embryol. Exp. Morphol. 32*:805–815, 1974.

Graff, R. J., and Bailey, D. W. The non-H-2 histocompatibility loci and their antigens. *Transplant. Rev. 15*:26–49, 1973.

Graff, R. J., Silvers, W. K., Billingham, R. E., Hildemann, W. H., and Snell, G. D. The cumulative effects of histocompatibility antigens. *Transplantation 4*:605–617, 1966.

Guttman, R. D. Genetics of acute rejection of rat cardiac allografts and a model of hyperacute rejection. *Transplantation 17*:383–386, 1974.

Harris, M. The establishment of tissue specificity in tadpoles of *Hyla regilla. J. Exp. Zool. 88*:373–397, 1941.

Häyry, P., and Defendi, V. Allograft immunity *in vitro*. II. Induction of DNA-synthesis in mixed cultures of mouse peripheral lymphocytes from inbred strains differing at non-H-2 Loci. *Transplantation 9*:410–416, 1970.

Heppner, G. H., and Calabresi, P. Suppression by cytosine arabinoside of serum blocking factors of cell-mediated immunity to syngeneic transplants of mouse mammary tumors. *J. Natl. Cancer Inst. 48*:1161–1167, 1972.

Hildemann, W. H. Tissue transplantation immunity in goldfish. *Immunology 1*:46–53, 1958.

Hildemann, W. H. Transplantation immunity in fishes: *Agnatha, Chondrichthyes* and *Osteichthyes. Transplant. Proc. 2*:253–259, 1970a.

Hildemann, W. H. Components and concepts of antigenic strength. *Transplant. Rev. 3*:5–19, 1970b.

Hildemann, W. H. Phylogeny of transplantation reactions. *In* B. D. Kahan and R. A. Reisfeld (eds.), *Markers of Biologic Individuality: The Transplantation Antigens*, pp. 3–73, Academic Press, New York, 1972.

Hildemann, W. H. Phylogeny of immune responsiveness in invertebrates. *Life Sci. 14*:605–614, 1974.

Hildemann, W. H., and Cohen, N. Weak histoincompatibilities: Emerging immunogenetic rules and generalizations. *In* E. S. Curtoni, P. L. Mattiuz, and R. M. Tosi (eds.), *Histocompatibility Testing* 1967, pp. 13–20, Munksgaard, Copenhagen, 1967.

Hildemann, W. H., and Cooper, E. L. Immunogenesis of homograft reactions in fishes and amphibians. *Fed. Proc. 22*:1145–1151, 1964.

Hildemann, W. H., and Cooper, E. L. Transplantation genetics: Unexpected histoincompatibility associated with skin grafts from F_2 and F_3 hybrid donors to F_1 hybrid recipients. *Transplantation 5*:707–720, 1967.

Hildemann, W. H., and Dix, T. Transplantation reactions of tropic Australian echinoderms. *Transplantation 15*:624–633, 1972.

Hildemann, W. H., and Haas, R. Homotransplantation immunity and tolerance in the bullfrog. *J. Immunol. 83*:478–485, 1959.

Hildemann, W. H., and Haas, R. Histocompatibility genetics of bullfrog populations. *Evolution 15*:267–271, 1961.

Hildemann, W. H., and Mullen, Y. The weaker the histoincompatibility, the greater the effectiveness of specific immunoblocking antibodies. *Transplant. Proc. 5*:617–620, 1973.

Hildemann, W. H., and Owen, R. D. Histocompatibility genetics of scale transplantation. *Transplant. Bull. 4*:132–134, 1956.

Hildemann, W. H., and Reddy, A. L. Phylogeny of immune responsiveness: Marine invertebrates. *Fed. Proc. 32*:2188–2194, 1973.

Hildemann, W. H., and Thoenes, G. H. Immunological responses of Pacific hagfish. I. Skin transplantation immunity. *Transplantation 7*:506–521, 1969.

Hildemann, W. H., and Walford, R. L. Skin homograft rejection in the Syrian hamster. *Ann. N.Y. Acad. Sci. 85*:56–71, 1960.

Houdayer, M., and Fougereau, M. Phylogénie des immunoglobulines: La réaction immunitaire de l'axolotl *Ambystoma mexicanum* cinétique de la réponse immunitaire et characterisation des anticorps. *Ann. Inst. Pasteur (Paris) 123*:1–28, 1973.

Houillon, M. C. Chimères xénoplastique entre les urodèles, *Pleurodeles waltlii* Michah et *Triturus alpestris* Laur. *C. R. Acad. Sci. (Paris) 258*:3901–3903, 1964.

Kallman, K. D. An estimate of the number of histocompatibility loci in the teleost *Xiphophorus maculatus. Genetics 50*:583–595, 1964.

Kallman, K. D. Genetics of tissue transplantation in Teleostei. *Transplant. Proc. 2*:263–271, 1970.

Kanakambika, P., and Muthukkaruppan, V. R. Immunological competence in the newly hatched lizard, *Calotes versicolor. Proc. Soc. Exp. Biol. Med. 140*:21–23, 1972.

Karp, R. D., and Hildemann, W. H. Specific rejection of integumentary allografts by the sea star, *Dermasterias imbricata. Adv. Exp. Med. Biol. 64*:137–147, 1976.

Klein, J. *Biology of the Mouse Histocompatibility-2 Complex*. Springer-Verlag, New York, 1975.

Klein, J., and Bailey, D. W. Histocompatibility differences in wild mice. *Genetics 68*:287–297, 1971.

Kornblum, J., and Silvers, W. K. Modification of the homograft response following intrasplenic exposure to ovarian or testicule tissue. *Transplantation 6*:783–786, 1968.

Linder, O. E. Modification of the homograft response after pretreatment with ovarian grafts. *Ann. N.Y. Acad. Sci. 99*:680–688, 1962.

Lopez, D. M., Sigel, M. M., and Lee, J. C. Phylogenetic studies on T cells. I. Lymphocytes of the shark with differential responses of phytohemagglutinin and concanavalin A. *Cell. Immunol. 10*:287–293, 1974.

Mangi, R. J., and Mardiney, M. R., Jr. The mixed lymphocyte reaction. Detection of single histocompatibility loci and the correlation to skin graft survival in mice. *Transplantation 11*:369–373, 1971.

Manickavel, V., and Cohen, N. Does chronic rejection elicited by weak histocompatibility antigens in mice and salamanders result from active enhancement? *Transplant. Proc. 7*:451–453, 1975a.

Manickavel, V., and Cohen, N. Chronicity of graft rejection across weak barriers is a function of active enhancement. *Fed. Proc. 34*:4622, 1975b.

Manning, M. J., and Turner, R. J. *Comparative Immunobiology*. Blackie and Son, Glasgow, 1976 184 pp.

Marchalonis, J. J. (ed.). *Comparative Immunology*, Blackwell, England, 1976 470 pp.

Marchalonis, J. J., and Cohen, N. Isolation and partial characterization of immunoglobulin from a urodele amphibian *(Necturus maculosus)*. *Immunology 24*:395–407, 1973.

Marchalonis, J. J., and Cone, R. E. The phylogenetic emergence of vertebrate immunity. *Aust. J. Exp. Biol. Med. Sci. 51*:461–488, 1973.

Miggiano, V. C., Birgen, F., and Pink, J. R. L. The mixed leukocyte reaction in chickens: Evidence for control by the major histocompatibility complex. *Eur. J. Immunol. 4*:397–401, 1974.

Murakawa, S. Studies on the transplantation immunity in the Japanese newt, *Cynops pyrrhogaster. SABCO J. 4*:17–32, 1968.

Ohno, S. *Evolution by Gene Duplication*, p. 160. Springer-Verlag, New York, 1970.

Peck, A. B., and Click, R. E. Immune responses *in vitro* VII. Differentiation of H-2 and non-H-2 alloantigens of the mouse by a dual mixed leukocyte culture. *Transplantation 16*:331–338, 1973.

Perey, D. Y. E., Finstad, J., Pollara, B., and Good, R. A. Evolution of the immune response. VI. First and second-set skin homograft rejection in primitive fishes. *Lab. Invest. 19*:591–597, 1968.

Rafferty, N. S. Fate of implanted embryos in frog eyes. *J. Exp. Zool. 147*:33–42, 1961.

Roux, K. H., and Volpe, E. P. Expression of histocompatibility loci in the leopard frogs. *J. Hered. 65*:341–344, 1974.

Ruben, L. N. Ontogeny, phylogeny, and cellular cooperation. *Am. Zool. 15*:93–106, 1975.

Rychilikova, M., and Ivanyi, P. Mixed lymphocyte cultures and histocompatibility antigens in mice. *Folia Biol. (Praha) 15*:126–135, 1969.

Schreffler, D. C., David, C. S., Passmore, H. C., and Klein, J. Genetic organization and evolution of the mouse H-2 region: A duplication model. *Transplant. Proc. 3*:176–179, 1971.

Sidky, Y. A., and Auerbach, R. Tissue culture analysis of immunological capacities of snapping turtles. *J. Exp. Zool. 167*:187–196, 1968.

Sigel, M. M., Ortiz-Muniz, G., Lee, J. C., and Lopez, D. M. Immunobiological reactivities at the cellular level in the nurse shark. *In Proceedings of the Symposium on Phylogenetic and Ontogenetic Study of the Immune Response and Its Contribution to the Immunological Theory*, pp. 113–119, INSERM, Paris, 1973.

Simnett, J. D. Factors influencing the differentiation of amphibian embryos implanted into homologous immunologically competent hosts *(Xenopus laevis)*. *Dev. Biol. 13*:112–143, 1966.

Snell, G. D., and Stimpfling, J. F. Genetics of tissue transplantation. *In* E. L. Green (ed.), *Biology of the Laboratory Mouse*, 2nd ed., pp. 457–491, McGraw-Hill, New York, 1966.

Solowey, A. C., and Rapaport, F. T. The immunologic response to repeated individual-specific skin allografts. *Transplantation 4*:178–181, 1966.

Stolen, J. S., and Mäkelä, O. Carrier preimmunisation in the anti-hapten response of a marine fish. *Nature 254*:718–719, 1975.

Stutzman, W. J. Combined effects of temperature and immunosuppressive drug therapy on allograft rejection in goldfish. *Transplantation, 5*:1344–1346, 1967.

Thorsby, E. The human major histocompatibility system. *Transplant. Rev. 18*:51–129, 1974.

Tournefier, A. Incomplete antibodies and immunoglobulin characterization in adult urodeles, *Pleurodeles waltlii* Michah and *Triturus alpestris* Laur. *Immunology 29*:209–216, 1975.

Tournefier, A., Charlemagne, J., and Houillon, C. Evolution des homogreffes cutanées chez l'amphibien urodèle *Pleurodeles waltlii* Michah: Réponse immunitaire primaire et secondaire. *C. R. Acad. Sci. (Paris) 268*:1456–1459, 1969.

Tournefier, A., Charlemagne, T., and Houillon, C. Réponse immunitaire aux homogreffes cutanées et absence d'histocompatibilité liée sexe chez *Triturus alpestris* Laur. *C. R. Acad. Sci. (Paris) 270*:1057–1060, 1970.

Valembois, P. Cellular aspects of graft rejection in earthworms and some other metazoa. *Contemp. Top. Immunol. 4*:121–126, 1974.

Voisin, G. A. Immunological facilitation, a broadening of the concept of the enhancement phenomenon. *Prog. Allergy 15*:328–485, 1971.

Volpe, E. P. Fate of neural crest homotransplants in pattern mutants of the leopard frog. *J. Exp. Zool. 157*:179–196, 1964.

Wachtel, S. S., Koo, G. C., and Boyse, E. A. Evolutionary conservation of H-Y ('male') antigen. *Nature 254*:270–272, 1975.

Wachtel, S. S., and Silvers, W. K. Skin homografts: Tolerogenic versus immunogenic influences in mice. *J. Exp. Med. 133*:921–937, 1971.

Yntema, C. L., and Borysenko, M. Survival of embryonic limb bud transplants in snapping turtles. *Experientia 27*:567–569, 1971.

Yocum, D., Cuchens, M., and Clem, L. W. The hapten-carrier effect in teleost fish. *J. Immunol. 114*:925–927, 1975.

Chapter 10

Evolution and Function of the Major Histocompatibility System: Facts and Speculations

J. KLEIN

1. Introduction: The Tower of Babel

Leafing through this extraordinary collection of review articles, I am reminded of the painting hanging in the Kunsthistorisches Museum in Vienna. On that painting is a monumental structure built to reach heaven. Looking from a distance, one does not see more than a dark, towering object, monstrous in a way, yet, at the same time, strangely beautiful. But when one looks more closely, one sees the object to be alive with myriads of tiny workers, busying themselves in an ant-like fashion, adding yet another story to the structure, improving stories already built, or repairing parts damaged by the passing of time. The painting is, of course, the famous Tower of Babel by the unsurpassed Flamish master of fantasy, Pieter Breughel.

The accumulation of knowledge on the major histocompatibility system (MHS) is very much like the building of the Tower of Babel: a daring attempt to reach the immunobiological skies on the one hand, a monstrous labyrinth of confusion on the other hand. Because the individual chapters of this book are close-up views of the MHS tower, I shall step back from the painting and view the tower from a distance, ignoring details and tracing only its outline, its architectonic plan, its general design. And where hard facts fail, I shall help myself with speculations. To comply with the assigned number of pages, I shall have to keep the number of references to a minimum and many times—as much as I hate to do so—shall refer the reader to reviews rather than to original reports.

2. Facts

2.1 Genetic Organization

The major histocompatibility system (MHS) is a cluster of loci occupying a single chromosomal area, the products of which are involved in the following immunological phenomena:

1. *Induction of B-cell differentiation* leading to the production of humoral antibodies detectable by a variety of serological methods.
2. *Induction of T-cell differentiation* leading to blast transformation and production of cytotoxic effector cells. The blast transformation can be detected by mixed lymphocyte reactions *in vitro* or certain types of graft-versus-host

(GvH) reactions *in vivo*. The tests for the effector T-cells are cell-mediated lymphocytotoxicity (CML) *in vitro*, certain other forms of GvH reactions *in vivo*, allograft reactions, and delayed-type hypersensitivity (DTH) reactions *in vivo*.

3. *Regulation of the immune response* to a variety of antigens. Because of this regulation, the response is either high or low. The regulation pertains either to the humoral response, as measured by humoral antibody production, or to the cellular response as measured by DTH reactions, allograft reactions, or T-cell proliferation *in vitro*.
4. *Complement biosynthesis and activation*. Several complement components have been demonstrated to be controlled by the MHS. The nature of this control (structural versus regulating loci) is not known.

There is no unity in designating the MHS of different species. The following designations are most commonly used: H-2 (mouse), HLA (man), RhL-A (rhesus monkey), ChL-A (chimpanzee), RtH-1 or AgB (rat), RbH-1 or RL-A (rabbit), DLA (dog), SL-A (pig), GPL-A (guinea pig), B (chicken), the MHS and Hm-1 (syrian hamster) clawed toad remain undesignated.

Genetically, the MHS can be divided into regions and the regions can be grouped into classes. An MHS *region* is a portion of the complex delimited by genetic crossing over and consisting of at least one marker locus; the existence of additional loci in a given region is often presupposed. Regions are sometimes divided into *subregions*, which are portions of the MHS identified by distinct but functionally related marker loci and separated by crossing over. The need for this peculiar genetic nomenclature is dictated by the ignorance of the fine-structure organization of the MHS. Should the day ever arrive when this structure is known, the term *locus*, defined as a portion of the genetic material coding for a single polypeptide chain, would be adequate to describe it. The term *class*, in reference to the MHS, is introduced here for the first time. It is meant to designate regions related by their genetic origin and/or function. The products of different classes differ in their biochemical properties, phenotypic expression, and function. Three major classes of MHS regions have been recognized so far. I shall designate them simply class I, class II, and class III.

2.1.1 Class I Regions

Class I regions correspond to what has been termed serologically defined or SD regions (Bach et al. 1976). However, the SD designation is misleading because it is now evident that *all* MHS regions can be defined serologically; for this reason the designation should be abandoned. As far as is known, class I regions occur in pairs with the two members of each pair closely linked but separated by other loci. Shreffler and co-workers (1971) suggested that members of a pair originated from an ancestral gene by gene duplication, and this suggestion—as I shall discuss below—has recently been corroborated by biochemical analysis of class I products. The hypothesis that class I regions of different species also have common evolutionary origin has been favored by many investigators for some time, but again it has been only recently that the hypothesis received direct support in the form of amino acid sequence homology between class I products of mouse and man (see below). There is no unity in the designation of class I regions for different species. In the mouse, the regions are designated K and D, in man A and B, in the rhesus monkey SD_1 and SD_2, and so forth. Because of the interspecies homology of class I regions, it would seem proper to designate the regions by the same symbol in all the species, for example, A and B. However, such nomenclatorial change may prove to be too much to put up with, at least for the mouse immunogeneticists.

The products of class I regions are glycoproteins, the monomers of which have a molecular weight of some 45,000 daltons, and are noncovalently associated with a single chain of β_2-microglobulin. The class I antigens are expressed in the plasma membrane of all cells except some cells in terminal stages of differentiation, early embryonic cells, and some neoplasias. The highest concentration of class I products is found on mature lymphocytes (both T and B) and macrophages; other cell types contain much lesser quantities of these molecules.

In an allogeneic situation, class I molecules induce production of humoral antibodies and can, therefore, be detected by serological methods. The serologically detectable antigens are complex, consisting of several antigenic determinants, some unique for a molecule controlled by a particular allele, others shared with molecules controlled by different alleles. The serologically detectable sites are quite variable, and this variability is presumed to reflect variability (genetic polymorphism) of the corresponding genes. Serologically detectable class I molecules have been described in mouse (Gorer 1936), man (Dausset 1958), rat (Frenzl et al. 1960; Bogden and Aptekman 1960), rabbit (Levine and Landsteiner 1929), rhesus monkey (Balner et al. 1971; Rogentine et al. 1971), chimpanzee (Balner et al. 1967), guinea pig (Sato and de Weck 1972), dog (Cleton et al. 1967), pig (Vaiman et al. 1970), possibly cattle (for a discussion, see Chapter 4), chicken (Briles et al. 1948), and clawed toad (Du-Pasquier et al. 1975). Of these species, two class I regions have been identified in man, mouse, rhesus monkey, guinea pig, and dog. In the remaining species, the serologically detectable class I products behave as if controlled by a single region; but this behavior is very likely the result of inadequate analysis of the class I products in these species.

Class I molecules also induce T-cell proliferation and the production of effector T-cells. The T-cell proliferation is often weak and so far has been unequivocally demonstrated only for class I molecules of the mouse. In man, rhesus monkey, dog, and rat, class I molecules are claimed to be incapable of inducing MLR or GvH reactions. This discrepancy, however, is probably caused by differences in methodology used for the different species, for even in the mouse, the stimulation is demonstrable easily only in certain strain combinations. (For the discussion of why this might be so, see Klein 1976a.) Becaus a positive result usually bears more weight than a negative one, it would not come as a surprise if eventually T-cell stimulation by class I molecules were to be demonstrated also in species other than the mouse.

In contrast to their meager MLR- and GvH-reaction-stimulatory capacity, class I molecules are potent stimulators of effector T-cell production, as manifested by their capability of inducing acute allograft reaction *in vivo* and CML *in vitro*. Recent studies of H-2 mutants of the mouse indicate that the sites responsible for effector cell production are composed of multiple determinants, some shared by products of different alleles, others restricted to a product of a single allele (Klein and Forman 1976).

Thus, class I molecules carry three types of determinants: those detected serologically by antibodies, those causing lymphocyte proliferation, and finally those responsible for generation of effector cells. The relationship of the last two types of determinants is unknown, but it would not be surprising if they were to turn out to be identical. The determinants defined serologically by antibodies, on the other hand, are most likely distinct from determinants inducing pure T-cell responses. The distinctiveness of the determinants is supported by the fact that H-2 mutations often change the T-cell-stimulating determinants without qualitatively changing the serologically detectable determinants (Klein 1976a). However, the two types of determinants are nevertheless present on the same molecule and in at least some instances may overlap.

2.1.2 Class II Regions

Class II regions roughly correspond to the lymphocyte-defined or LD regions in the nomenclature of Bach and his colleagues (1976). Again, the term "LD" is misleading and inappropriate, as will be apparent from the discussion which follows. The number of class II regions, their interrelationships, and their genetic organization are at present unresolved issues. The regions appear to be clustered in a single chromosomal area, which can best be designated—following the example of the mouse studies—as the I region. Currently four types of loci, as defined by their phenotypic manifestations, are known to belong to class II regions: Ia, Ir, Lad, and H.

The I region-associated antigen or Ia loci code for molecules the precise size of which has not yet been determined. The molecular weight estimates of the Ia monomers range from 25,000 to 35,000 daltons (fragments of less than 6000 daltons have been reported in normal mouse serum, cf. Parish et al. 1976). Part of the difficulty in estimating the Ia molecular weight may be in the heterogeneity of these molecules. In contrast to class I molecules, membrane-bound Ia molecules do not seem to be associated with β_2-microglobulin chains (Vitetta et al. 1976a). Ia molecules are part of the plasma membrane of lymphocytes (predominantly B-cells, and to a lesser degree also T-cells), macrophages, epidermal cells, and spermatozoa. Other cell types that have been investigated have been claimed to be Ia negative, but the presence on these cells of a low concentration of Ia molecules has not been excluded (Klein and Hauptfeld 1976). The serologically detectable antigens carried by Ia molecules are complex (one molecule may carry several antigenic determinants, cf. Shreffler and David 1975), and the loci coding for Ia molecules are polymorphic (Klein et al. 1976c).

Ia or Ia-like loci have been demonstrated so far in the mouse (David et al. 1973b; Hauptfeld et al. 1973), man (Wernet et al. 1975), guinea pig (Walford et al. 1962; Finkelman et al. 1975), and rhesus monkey (Balner et al. 1976). In the mouse, firm evidence is available for the existence of two Ia loci, Ia-1 in the IA subregion and Ia-2 in the IC subregion (Shreffler and David 1975); in addition, claims are constantly made of the existence of more Ia loci (David et al. 1974, 1975; Dorf and Benacerraf 1975; Lindahl 1975; Götze 1976), but the existence of such loci is poorly documented and, in at least some cases, the claims were later retracted (Shreffler et al. 1976). In all other species, the number of Ia loci remains undetermined.

The immune response or Ir loci control the level of immune response to thymus-dependent antigens. Their mode of expression and the cell types in which they are expressed are still matters of controversy (Mozes 1975). MHS-linked Ir or Ir-like loci have been described in the mouse (McDevitt and Chinitz 1969), guinea pig (Ellman et al. 1970), rhesus monkey (Dorf et al. 1974), rat (Günther et al. 1972), possibly man (Levine et al. 1972; Marsh et al. 1973), and chicken (Günther et al. 1974; Karakoz et al. 1974). In the mouse, the existence of three Ir loci has been claimed, Ir-1A in the IA subregion (McDevitt et al. 1972), Ir-1B in the IB subregion (Lieberman et al. 1972), and Ir-1C in the IC subregion (Merryman and Maurer 1975). In all other species, no information is available about the number of *Ir* loci. In the mouse, complementation is known to occur between genes located in different subregions (Zaleski and Milgrom 1973).

The lymphocyte-activating determinant or Lad loci are defined by the capacity of their products to stimulate MLR or GvH reaction. They must be expressed on B-lymphocytes because most investigators agree that these cells are good stimulators of MLR or GvH reaction; they are probably also expressed on T-lymphocytes (Lonai and McDevitt 1976) and macrophages (Schirrmacher et al. 1975; Greineder and Rosenthal 1975), because these cells also have been implicated in MLR stimulation by at least some investigators; whether or not they are also expressed on other cell types is presently unknown. MHS-associated Lad loci have been demonstrated in the mouse (Humer et al. 1968), man (Bach and Amos 1967), rat (Cramer et al. 1974), rhesus monkey (Appelman and Balner 1972; Neefe et al. 1973), dog (Serre and Clot, 1968; Rudolph et al. 1969), rabbit (Tissot and Cohen 1974; Chai and Lerner 1975), Syrian hamster (W. R. Duncan and J. W. Streilein, *personal communication*), probably guinea pig (Greineder and Rosenthal 1975), chicken (Schierman and Nordskog 1961; Jaffe and McDermid 1962; Miggiano et al. 1974), and clawed toad (DuPasquier et al. 1975). In the mouse, there are at least two Lad loci in the I region, Lad-1 in the IA subregion and Lad-2 in the IC subregion (for references see Klein 1975). Multiple Lad loci are suspected in man and the rhesus monkey, but no firm mapping data confirming this suspicion are available. In the other species tested, the data are too scanty to allow any predictions about the number of Lad regions.

Class II histocompatibility or H loci have so far been demonstrated only in the mouse and guinea pig. In the mouse, two H loci are associated with the I region, H-2A and H-2C. The H-2A locus, residing in the IA subregion, is responsible for acute rejection of skin grafts (Klein et al. 1974), heart fragments (Klein et al. 1976a), and adenocarcinomas (J. Klein, *unpublished data*), and for CML lysis of LPS and Con A blasts (Nabholz et al. 1975; Wagner et al. 1975). The H-2C locus, residing in the IC subregion, causes chronic rejection of first-set skin grafts (Klein et al. 1976b) and CML lysis of LPS and Con A blasts in the CML assay (Klein et al. 1976b; Nabholz et al. 1975). In the guinea pig, only one class II H locus has been identified so far. The products of this locus initiate acute skin graft rejection, delayed hypersensitivity reactions, and CML (see Geczy et al. 1975 for discussion and references).

The interrelationship of the class II loci is not understood. The Ia, Lad, and H loci appear to be very similar, if not identical. These three types of loci map in the same subregions, display the same genetic polymorphism, and their products appear to have similar tissue distribution. Furthermore, the MLR can be inhibited by exposing stimulating cells to Ia antibodies (Meo et al. 1975a), and the graft rejection is accompanied by the production of Ia antibodies (Klein et al. 1974, 1976a, b). The Ir loci, on the other hand, appear to be distinct, but this might be only because we know so little about their products. In fact, one can make a case—as is discussed elsewhere (Klein and Hauptfeld 1976)—for the Ia antigens being the products of the Ir loci. According to this unifying hypothesis, most of the diverse traits currently attributed to distinct class II loci, in fact, would be controlled by the same loci.

2.1.3 Class III Regions

Class III regions are those concerned with the complement pathway, i.e., with the control of complement components or receptors for these components. MHS loci coding for complement components have been demonstrated in man, mouse, rhesus monkey, guinea pig, and chicken. In man, evidence exists for close linkage with HLA of the structural gene for the C2 component (Fu et al. 1975; Day et al. 1975; Wolski et al. 1975; Friend et al. 1975) and for the C3 proactivator (C3Pa or properdin factor B, also called the glycine-rich β-glycoprotein or GBG protein, cf. Allen 1974). In the mouse, the Ss protein, encoded by the S region in the middle of the H-2 complex, has been recently shown to be probably the C4 component (Meo et al. 1975b; Lachman et al. 1975; Curman et al. 1975). In addition, the H-2 complex also has been reported to control the time of appearance of the C3 receptor on B cells (Gelfand et al. 1974), and the gene controlling the level of the C3 component itself has been claimed to be loosely linked to H-2 (Ferreira and Nussenzweig 1975). In the rhesus monkey, as in man, the C3 proactivator gene is also known to be part of the MHS (Ziegler et al. 1975). In the guinea pig, recent data suggest linkage between C4 deficiency and the MHS of this species (Shevach et al. 1976). And finally, in the chicken, Chanh and co-workers (1976) found the total complement levels to be controlled by a dominant gene linked to the MHS. Thus, it appears that in each MHS there are probably several class III loci. Whether these loci belong to a single region or are distributed over a large portion of the MHS chromosome is not yet known.

2.1.4 Arrangement of MHS Regions

Class I regions have been genetically separated from class II regions in the following species: mouse, man, rhesus monkey, rat, guinea pig, dog, and possibly chicken (Figure 10.1). However, in all these species the two classes are closely linked, being separated by crossing over frequency of between 0.5 and 2 percent. In the mouse, class II regions are located between the two class I regions; in all other species tested, class II regions are outside

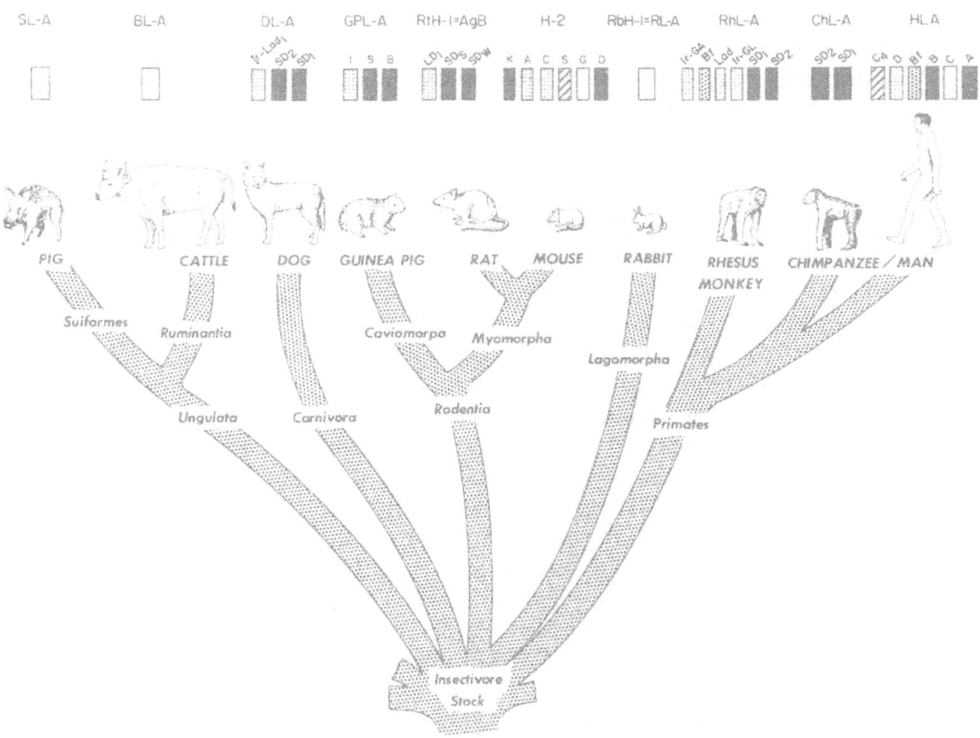

Figure 10.1. Genetic organization of the MHS in various species of mammals. ■ Class I regions; ▭ Class II regions; ▭ and ▨ Class II regions; ▭ MHS has not been genetically divided into regions

of class I regions. Class III regions seem to be more closely linked to class II than to class I regions, but the data in this regard are still preliminary.

2.2 Function

It is simply frustrating! One knows so much about the MHS that one can write a 600-page book about the MHS of a single species—yet, when it comes to the question of the MHS function, there is no answer. All the traits described in preceding paragraphs are surely somehow related to the MHS function, but they probably are not the true physiological function of this complex. They are like the shadows on the wall of Plato's cave—a mere reflection of the function. What, then, is the true MHS function? Because this is a section of facts and not of speculations, there is not much I can report to answer the question. All I can do is to describe two phenomena, the DZSB and the KK phenomenon, which I consider most relevant to the MHS function, and hope that they may provide some clues to help to resolve this problem.

2.2.1 The DZSB Phenomenon

Three variants of the phenomenon have been described by three different laboratories. The first variant was described by Doherty and Zinkernagel and their co-workers (for a review and references, see Doherty et al. 1976), and its principle is this. A mouse injected with lymphocyte choriomeningitis (LCM) virus develops effector T-lymphocytes which kill *in vitro* (but also *in vivo*) target cells infected with LCM virus. However, there is an important restriction to this effect: The killing occurs only if the effector and the target cells share the same allele at least at one of the two class I loci (H-2K or H-2D). Sharing or nonsharing of other H-2 loci appears to be irrelevant for the effect, and so does the sharing or nonsharing of all other histocompatibility loci. Similar observation has since been made with other viruses, in fact, with all viruses that have been tested. Thus, it appears not to be some freak exception, but rather a general phenomenon.

The second variant of the DZSB phenomenon was described by Shearer and his colleagues (Shearer et al. 1975) and Forman (1975), who noticed that cocultivation of T-lymphocytes with syngeneic spleen cells, the cell surface proteins of which have been conjugated with trinitrophenyl (TNP), endows the lymphocytes with the capacity to kill TNP-modified target cells. However, again this killing occurs only when the sensitized lymphocyte and the target share alleles at least at one of the two class I loci. And again, the effect is not restricted to TNP, but applies to a variety of other haptenic groups as well.

The third variant of the DZSB phenomenon was discovered by Bevan (1975) and by Gordon and co-workers (1975) during an *in vitro* study of minor H-loci involvement in the cell-mediated lymphocytotoxicity reaction. Thymus-derived lymphocytes sensitized *in vivo* against a particular minor

H antigen did kill *in vitro* target cells carrying the same antigen, provided that the responding, sensitizing, and target cells shared the same allele at the H-2K or H-2D loci.

The three discoveries are really a *thema con variazioni;* the three mechanisms apparently operate on the same principle and are a part of the same phenomenon, the Doherty-Zinkernagel-Shearer-Bevan or DZSB phenomenon. Its widespread occurrence suggests that the phenomenon probably plays some significant biological role. What might this role be? The DZ variant comes closest to hinting to the nature of this phenomenon's biological role. As pointed out by Doherty, Zinkernagel, and others, the phenomenon could be a part of a surveillance mechanism by means of which an organism recognizes and eliminates any aberrant cells with altered cell surfaces. However, exactly how the mechanism operates is a matter for speculation (see below). The attractiveness of the suggestion lies in the fact that, for the first time, it provides a dignified role for the class I regions, involving them critically in one of the most vital functions of the living body.

2.2.2 The KK Phenomenon

Although I have, with good conscience, placed the DZSB phenomenon in the "Facts" section, by placing the Kindred-Katz or KK phenomenon in the same section, I know that I am biasing the issue, because the latter is anything but established as a fact.

The triggering of a B-lymphocyte differentiation in the direction of antibody production has been known for some time to require T-cell help. Two laboratories (Kindred and Shreffler 1972; Katz et al. 1973) have reported that, under normal physiological conditions, this T,B-cell collaboration requires identity at the H-2 complex, more specifically at the I region of this complex. This observation is disputed by four other laboratories (Bechtol et al. 1974; von Boehmer et al. 1975; Heber-Katz and Wilson 1975; Waldmann et al. 1975), which could not find any evidence for a MHS restriction of T,B-cell collaboration. The whole T,B-cell collaboration field has become the Augean stable of immunology, and this most recent controversy does nothing in the way of clarifying it. However, no matter how the controversy will eventually be resolved, it will remain a fact that I region is somehow involved in T,B-cell collaboration. This statement is based on the fact that the I region contains the Ir genes and that the Ir genes influence the T,B-cell collaboration. The function of the I region (and class II region in general) could be, therefore, the regulation of the T,B-cell collaboration in antibody production. The exact mechanism of this regulation can be, however, again only speculated upon (see later sections).

2.3 Evolution

It may seem presumptuous to include under the heading "Facts" a discussion of MHS evolution. Is it not a fact that there are only a few facts known for certain about the phylogenetic origins of the MHS? That is obviously so, but the subject is of such importance for the understanding of the MHS physiology that one is obliged to make the most of the few facts that have been established so far.

The basic premise of this discussion will be the notion that "nothing in evolution is created *de novo*... each new gene must have arisen from an already existing gene" (Ohno 1970). It follows from this premise that ultimately the origin of each gene must be traceable to the most primitive organisms by climbing down the evolutionary scale. And this is precisely what I will attempt to do. What complicates such "biological paleontology" is the fact that the gene could have, of course, changed its function during the evolution so that the track one follows down the road may suddenly disappear. But it is unlikely that the gene changed its function so drastically that it could not be recognized in its new disguise. In searching for the invertebrate origins of the MHS one has to consider, therefore, several phenomena, at least some of which may eventually prove to have nothing to do with the MHS.

Comparative histogenetics, the discipline that strives to provide the description of phylogenetic origins of the MHS, is full of holes. Some groups of organism, among them many important ones, have not been studied at all, and in groups that have been studied, the study has often been limited to one or two species (out of thousands) that may happen to be totally unrepresentative of the group. Then there is the problem of experimental conditions. An experimenter working with an exotic species and getting negative results must always worry that the results are negative simply because he did not make the animal "happy" enough. All this, of course, complicates the situation so much that one can easily be misled in any attempt at generalization. But one must start somewhere!

2.3.1 Class I Regions

Histoincompatibility Reactions in Invertebrates. When tissues of two genetically disparate individuals come into contact, often reactions ensue that prevent fusion of the two tissues. These histoincompatibility reactions in the broadest sense occur in many phyla of multicellular organisms, including at least some phyla of plants. In invertebrates, the histoincompatibility reactions can occur in a variety of forms, some of which are briefly described below.

a. *Inhibition of specific cell aggregation.* This reaction is well developed in *Porifera,* but it has been also described for embryonic tissues of other Metazoa, including vertebrates.

Sponge tissues can easily be dissociated into cell suspensions by pressing them through a fine sieve. When the cells are then allowed to settle, they spontaneously adhere to one another, form aggregates, and often develop into miniature, functional sponges (Moscona 1973). The aggregation is, to a certain degree, species specific; i.e., when suspensions of two different species of sponge are mixed, the cells of each species sort out and form separate aggregates. How rapidly and how effectively they sort out depends on the combination of the two species. The recognition of nonself in this case is believed to be mediated by large (90 S), heat-labile glycoprotein molecules on the cell surface of sponges. The molecules can be released from the cell surface by exposure of cells to calcium- or magnesium-free water. There is no evidence of allorecognition (inhibition of aggregation of tissues from two genetically different individuals of the same species) or of any aggressive reaction resulting in cell damage or cell death in the mixes.

b. *Acute aggressive reactions*. These reactions are particularly well developed in certain *Coelenterata,* such as certain anemones (Francis 1973) and corals (Lang 1971, 1973). The response occurs within minutes or hours after tissue contact is established, and results in dissolution of one of the two tissues by extracoelenteric digestion. The reaction usually occurs between different species, and in each combination of species, the tissue of one species is the aggressor and the tissue of the other species the victim. Different species can thus be arranged into a hierarchy in which species in a higher position can attack species in a lower position but not vice versa (Ivker 1972).

c. *Encapsulation*. In some instances, the host surrounds the foreign tissue or organism by a wall of cells and intercellular matrix, which effectively isolates the intruder from the rest of the host's body. This encapsulation reaction frequently occurs in various orders of *Arthropoda* and *Mollusca*, where it serves as a protection mechanism against artificial xenografts (Cheng 1967).

d. *Histoincompatibility reactions sensu stricto*. These reactions are characterized by slow aggression of one tissue against another. The particular form the reactions assume depends on many variables, among them the particular species involved, the genetic difference between the tissues, the types of tissues establishing the contact, and general physiological and environmental conditions in which the contact occurs. Sometimes the tissues first fuse and remain united for many days or weeks before any signs of aggressive reaction appear. The aggressive reaction may destroy one tissue completely, or it may only destroy cells in the contact zone. Other times, the two tissues never establish a direct contact (e.g., the so-called avoidance reaction in corals, cf. Hildemann et al. 1975), remain separated by a narrow gap, and build a protective wall along the borders of the two incompatible tissues. Other species react to the presence of foreign tissue by hyperplastic growth, and there exist complex hierarchical relationships determining which of the two tissues in contact will respond by an overgrowth.

There is no reason to believe that the mechanism of the various forms of the histoincompatibility reactions described above is the same. More likely, different mechanisms are involved, ranging from tissue death because of different nutritional requirements, to a primitive, quasiimmunological attack by specialized cells in the tissue of the host. In no instance, however, has there been evidence obtained for memory similar to that observed in typical immunological reactions. Whether this negative observation is attributable to deficiencies in the experimental procedures or to the absence of memory in less advanced animals is not clear.

Such a variety of reactions as described above is unlikely to be controlled by a single genetic system. It is, therefore, surprising that the available genetic data on the control of histoincompatibility reactions in different invertebrate phyla *can* be interpreted as favoring a single chromosomal region (Du Pasquier 1974). Thus, in the marine sponge *Crambe crambe,* Van de Vyver (1970) observed 75 percent compatibility between larvae derived from the same mother (i.e., in 75 percent pairs, the two larvae fused and developed after metamorphosis into a single sponge). Because 100 percent fusion was observed between one mother and her progeny, Du Pasquier argues that a single allelic difference between two individuals does not suffice to prevent fusion of these individuals. If one accepts this thesis, and furthermore, takes into account the fact that progeny of a single mother do not necessarily have the same father, one can argue, as Du Pasquier (1974) does, that the 75 percent value is close enough to the 62.5 percent of compatible fusions that one would expect under these circumstances (single gene and six alleles, all parents heterozygous and carrying different alleles). However, if one postulates a different set of assumptions, one can also explain the same data as indicating multigenic control, and until genetically better-controlled experiments are carried out, it will not be possible to decide which interpretation is correct.

The most detailed genetic study of invertebrate histoincompatibility reaction is that of Hauenschild (1954, 1956) on *Hydractinia echinata,* a representative species of *Coelenterata.* Hauenschild determined the degree of tissue incompatibility between randomly selected individuals, between F_1 hybrids and parents, and within the F_2 generation. The data obtained are not easy to interpret, but Hauenschild favors the hypothesis that the histoincompatibility reactions in this species are controlled by a single locus with many alleles. Again, however, alternative interpretations are possible.

In other groups of *Coelenterata,* Kolenkine (1971) observed up to 60 percent of allograft compatibility in *Hydra,* but Theodor (1971) could not find two mutually compatible individuals among 25 individuals of *Gorgonians* collected in the same geographical area.

Clearly, genetics of histoincompatibility reactions in invertebrates has a long way to go before any definitive conclusions can be reached about the control of these reactions.

e. *Primitive allograft reaction.* True allograft reactions, i.e., reactions mediated by immunocytes capable of specific recognition and development of immunological memory, first appear in advanced invertebrates, notably in *Annelida* and *Echinodermata.*

Studies on earthworms as representative of the phylum *Annelida* (Valembois 1963; Duprat 1964; Cooper 1968, 1975) have led to the following conclusions. Orthotopic integument allografts between worms from the same geographical area often remain intact, whereas allografts between worms from different areas are often rejected. Xenografts exchanged between different genera and species of the same family, or between members of different families, are almost always rejected. The rejection of both allografts and xenografts is of the chronic type (some grafts survive for more than 250 days, and allografts usually survive longer than xenografts). According to Valembois (1973) the rejection process proceeds in two phases. In the first phase, about 2 days after transplantation, repressors, which normally control the production of lysosomal enzymes in grafted cells, are inhibited by the host tissue, large quantities of hydrolytic enzymes are released, and autolysis, accompanied by cell death and necrosis, follows. This phase is nonspecific and nonimmunological in nature. In the second phase, at about 12 days after transplantation, the degenerated musculature of the graft is infiltrated by coelomocytes, i.e., macrophage-like cells occurring freely in the coelomic fluid. Coelomocytes surround and eliminate the grafted tissues by engulfing autolysed cells. If a second graft is placed on the same recipient after the rejection of the first graft, it is often rejected in an accelerated manner, particularly in the case of xenografts. If coelomocytes are harvested after the rejection of the first allo- or xenograft and injected into an untreated recipient, this worm then rejects the graft derived from the coelomocyte donor in an accelerated fashion, typical of a second-set reaction. Grafts transplanted from F_1 hybrids onto parents are uniformly rejected (Duprat 1968), and this fact has been interpreted by Du Pasquier (1974) as indicating that *Annelida* reached an important phylogenetic step in that they can reject grafts differing from the host in only one histocompatibility allele.

Although there are reports that allografts and even xenografts in various species of sea stars *(Echinodermata)* can survive permanently (Truslé 1967), these results were almost certainly effected by inappropriately controlled experimental conditions. More recent studies on sea cucumber *(Cucumaria tricolor)* and sea star *(Protoreaster nodosus)* indicate that integumentary allografts are slowly rejected with survival times between 130 and 190 days (Hildemann and Dix 1972). Second grafts placed on recipients undergoing rejection of the first grafts are rejected in less than 60 days. The rejection is accompanied by infiltration of the graft with macrophages, granulocytes, and by what appear to be small lymphocytes. Nothing is known about the genetic control of the allograft reaction in *Echinodermata*.

The nature of the incompatibility reactions in *Tunicata* is not clear. In colonial ascidians such as *Botryllus,* when two pieces derived from the same colony are contraposed at the growing edges, they fuse completely and form a single colony within a common vasculatory system (Oka and Watanabe 1957; Tanaka and Watanabe 1972, 1973). On the contrary, when pieces from two different colonies are contraposed, one of the following two things can happen. In some species, the pieces do not fuse, the boundaries between them remain distinct, but no aggressive reaction is observed (reaction of indifference). In other species, the contact of the colonies results in necrosis at the contact zone (rejection reaction). Both nonfusion reactions appear to have a specific and nonspecific component, and the former appears to be mediated by a humoral factor or factors (Tanaka 1975). The fusibility appears to be controlled by a single genetic system with multiple alleles (Oka and Watanabe 1957, 1960). The single-system hypothesis requires most colonies to be heterozygous at the fusibility locus and postulates that colonies containing at least one allele in common are fusible with one another. In a natural population, the frequency of fusible colonies may vary from 5 to about 30 percent (Freeman 1970; Tanaka 1975).

In conclusion, some forms of histoincompatibility reactions probably exist in all phyla of invertebrates, but in some invertebrate groups the reactions are expressed more strongly than in other groups. Only in *Arthropoda* are the reactions difficult to demonstrate, and in some species of this phylum they may be completely lacking. For example, in *Drosophila,* allogeneic organ transplantations are routinely used in many embryological and genetic studies without any apparent complications caused by histoincompatibility reactions. In *Mollusca,* also, a clearcut demonstration of histocompatibility reactions has yet to be reported. In the more advanced invertebrates, such as *Annelida* and *Protochordata,* on the other hand, histocompatibility reactions come close to what one could call an allograft reaction. It is thus clear that in invertebrates, genetic systems exist that are good candidates for the function as predecessors of the vertebrate class I loci.

Allograft Reaction in Vertebrates. The capacity to mount a true allograft reaction is developed in all classes of vertebrates (for a review and references see Hildemann 1972, and Chapter 9). In some classes the reaction is of the chronic type; i.e., its onset is delayed often for many months and the rejection takes a long time, often several weeks, to complete. In other classes a new type of reaction emerges, namely the acute allograft reaction, which sets on shortly (1 to 3 weeks) after grafting and is extremely rapid (often completed within a few days). However, in classes capable of mounting acute allograft reaction, chronic reaction is also seen in some genetic combinations. Thus, the acute reaction is superimposed upon the chronic reaction.

The capacity to mount an acute allograft reaction first emerges in some advanced fishes, specifically the *Teleostei;* other fishes are capable only of chronic reaction. Similar situations exist in *Amphibia,* where only the *Anura* are capable of the acute allograft reaction, whereas the *Apoda* and *Urodela* reject grafts in a chronic fashion. Higher up on the evolutionary scale, the capacity to mount an acute allograft reactions appears to be completely lost in all *Reptilia* and emerges again in birds and mammals (Figure 10.2).

In all vertebrates, the allograft reaction is mediated by lymphocyte-like cells, which can adoptively transfer the reaction and which are always seen at the rejection site. Exposure of a recipient to a second graft of the same specificity results in an accelerated (but sometimes also delayed) onset of the second-set allograft reaction.

Wherever genetic data are available, they show that the acute reaction can be attributed to a single genetic system, in which even a single haplotype difference leads to rapid rejection. In species possessing the major system

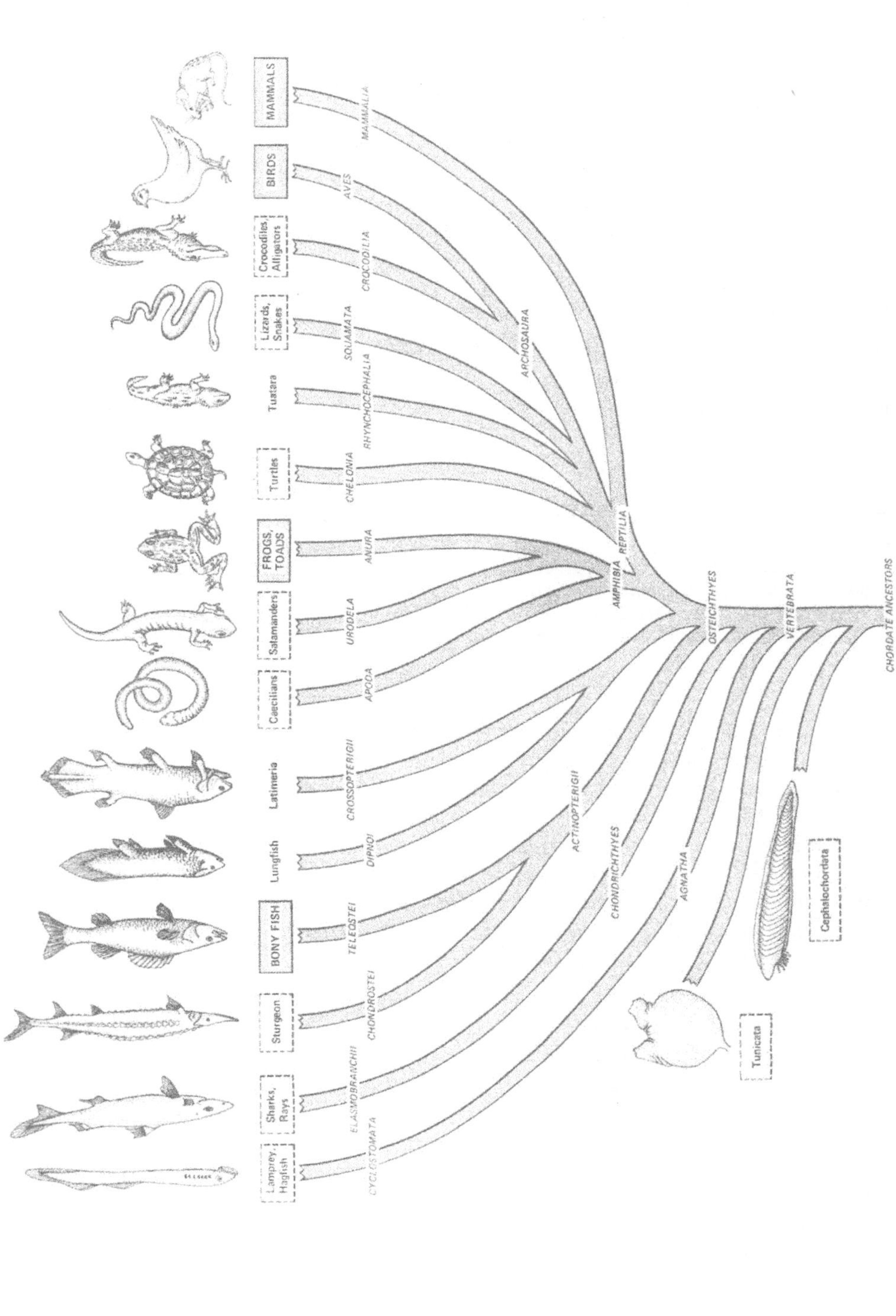

Figure 10.2. The occurence of the MHS among Chordata. Presence of the MHS in at least some species of a given class is indicated by a stippled box; absence is indicated by an empty box; absence of a box indicates that no MHS data are available for a given class

Table 10.1. Partial N-Terminal Amino Acid Sequences of Mouse (H-2) and Human (HLA)

		Position											
		1	2	3	4	5	6	7	8	9	10	11	12
Mouse transplantation antigens	H-2K^k	Met	Pro	His	.	Leu	Arg	Tyr	Phe	His	.	Ala	Val
	H-2K^b	—	Pro	His	.	Leu	Arg	Tyr	Phe	Val	.	Ala	Val
	H-2K^d	Met	—	His	.	—	Arg	Tyr	Phe	.	.	.	.
	H-2D^d	Met	Pro?	His	.	Leu	Arg	Tyr	—	Val	.	Ala	Val
	H-2D^b	—	Pro	—	.	—	—	Tyr	.	—	.	Ala	Val
Human transplantation antigens	HLA.2	Gly	Ser	.	Ser	Met	Arg	Tyr	Phe	Phe	Thr	Ser	Val
	HLA.7	Gly	Ser	.	Ser	Met	Arg	Tyr	Phe	Tyr	Thr	Ser	Val
	HLA.12	Gly	Ser	—	Ser	Met	Val	Tyr	Phe	Tyr	Thr	Ala	Val
β_2-microglobulin	Human	Ile	Gln	Arg	Thr	Pro	Lys	Ile	Gln	Val	Tyr	Ser	Arg
	Rat	Ile	Gln	Lys	Thr	Pro	Glx	Ile	Gln	Val	Tyr	Ser	Arg
	Mouse			Lys		Pro				Val	Tyr		

Dash indicates the absence of a particular amino acid found at that position in other proteins; points indicate that sequence information is not available at that position; boxes around the amino acids indicate sharing of these residues among products of different alleles or genes. For comparison, amino acid sequences of human, rat, and mouse β_2-microglobulin are also

for acute graft rejection, additional minor systems can be demonstrated, each of which leads to chronic rejection but which in multiple combinations can effect rapid graft rejection (a cummulative effect of minor loci). In *Teleostei,* 4 to 15 loci capable of causing graft rejection can be demonstrated, depending on the species, strain, and genetic cross; in birds the number is at least 15; and in mammals (mouse) it is at least 40. Thus, in conclusion, one can postulate the presence of class I-like regions in most advanced *Teleostei,* in *Anura,* birds, and mammals; all other vertebrate groups seem to lack these regions (Figure 10.2).

Homologies of Class I Regions. Until a short time ago, all conclusions about the evolution of class I regions have been based on the study of MHS-controlled traits (primarily the allograft reaction) in different classes of animals. Thus, they were indirect and not very convincing. Recently, however, the long-awaited day finally arrived when the first data on the primary structure of class I molecules became available and thus permitted, for the first time, a direct interspecies comparison of class I regions. The data obtained thus far are shown in Table 10.1. Because the data, although preliminary and perhaps unrepresentative, are such an important psychological booster for all who for so long have been involved in MHS studies, I shall discuss them in some detail.

Class I Antigens

Position														
13	14	15	16	17	18	19	20	21	22	23	24	25	26	27
.	Ile	Pro	.	Leu	.	Lys	Pro	Phe	Ala	.	.	.	.	Tyr
.	Arg	Pro	.	Leu	.	—	—	Arg	Tyr	.	.	.	.	Tyr
.	.	.	.	.	.	.	.	.	.	.	.	.	.	.
.	.	Pro	.	—	.	—	Pro	.	Tyr	.	.	.	.	.
.	Arg	Pro	.	Leu	.	—	Pro	Arg	Tyr	.	.	.	.	.
Ser	.	.	Gly	.	Gly	Glu	.	.	Phe	Ile	.	Val	.	.
Ser	Arg?	Pro	Gly	.	Gly	Glu	.	.	Phe	Ile	.	Val	.	.
Ser	Arg?	Pro	Gly	.	Gly	Glu	.	.	Phe	Ile	.	Val	.	.
His	Pro	Ala	Glu	Asn	Gly	Lys	Ser	Asn	Phe	Leu	Asn	Lys	Try	Val
His	Pro	Pro	Glu	Asn	Gly	Lys	Pro	Asn	Phe	Leu	Asn	Lys	Tyr	Val
.	Pro	Pro	.	.	.	Lys	Pro	.	.	Leu	.	.	Tyr	Val

shown. The sequences were obtained from the following sources: mouse H-2 (Ewenstein et al. 1976; Henning et al. 1976; Silver and Hood 1976; Vitetta et al. 1976b), human HLA (Terhorst et al. 1976), human $\beta_2\mu$ (Cunningham et al. 1973), rat $\beta_2\mu$ (Poulik et al. 1976), mouse $\beta_2\mu$ (Silver and Hood 1976a).

a. *Interallelic variation.* The data show, first of all, that an unusually high number of amino acid substitutions distinguishes allelic products of the same class I locus. Although most other allelic proteins differ in only one or two positions in the whole molecule, the H-2K^k and H-2K^b molecules differ in at least 7 positions of the first 18 N-terminal residues, and the H-2D^b and H-2D^d molecules differ in 4 of 14 residues. Thus, there are between 29 and 38 percent sequence differences between allelic H-2 products in the short stretch of the H-2 molecule examined. However, before one draws any far-fetched conclusions from these limited data, one should realize two important facts. First, the H-2^b haplotype is only distantly related to other H-2 haplotypes present in inbred strains (Klein 1975), including H-2^k and H-2^d. Although its origin cannot be reconstructed with as much detail as one would wish, this much is known that the C57-family of strains carrying the H-2^b haplotype was derived from Asiatic mice, most probably from a subspecies of *Mus musculus* distinct from the one that gave rise to most other inbred strains.[1] The comparison of H-2^b to other H-2 haplotypes, therefore, probably maximizes the allelic variability of class I loci.

[1] One should also keep in mind that the house mouse is an extremely variable species and that, therefore, some of its subspecies differences might actually be the beginning of a new set of species characteristics. The MHS might be one of such characteristics.

The second fact that one should keep in mind is the exceptional polymorphism of class I loci. To compare the sequence of two products of allelic MHS genes is not the same as to compare, for example, the sequence of two hemoglobin variants. The latter are usually the products of a recent mutation and normally would not be maintained in a natural population with an appreciable frequency. In contrast, alleles at MHS loci are maintained in the population for long periods of time and thus have an ample opportunity to accumulate multiple mutations. [2] The finding of multiple amino acid substitutions in allelic class I products should not, therefore, come as a surprise.

In general, the HLA class I molecules seem to display less interallelic variability than the H-2 molecules: Among the first 20 residues of the two allelic HLA-B products (HLA-B.7 and HLA-B.12), only two amino acid substitutions are found (sequence difference of 10 percent). This observation, if confirmed and extended to other alleles, would correlate well with the degree of MHS polymorphism in the two species. Limited data available seem to suggest that the H-2K and H-2D loci are far more polymorphic than the HLA-A and HLA-B loci (Klein 1974). It is tempting to speculate that the difference in the degree of H-2 and HLA polymorphism is influenced by the different population structure and/or evolutionary stability of the two species (the mouse population is divided into small inbreeding units or demes and the *Mus musculus* is a rather unstable species, cf. Klein 1975; the human population, on the other hand, is close to a Mendelian type and *Homo sapiens* is a relatively stable species).

b. *Interlocus variation within a species.* As discussed above, in man and mouse (as well as in other mammalian species), there are two class I loci, HLA-A and HLA-B (man[3]), H-2K and H-2D (mouse). In the latter species, long before the amino acid sequence data became available, Shreffler and co-workers (1971) postulated that the two ends of the H-2 complex arose by duplication from a common ancestral gene. The main reason for making this postulate was the serological cross-reactivity repeatedly observed between the products of the two loci. Similar cross-reactivity was also reported for the human HLA system, and there, too, it has been speculated that the A and B loci had a common origin. In both species the postulates have now been verified splendidly by the amino acid sequence data. In the mouse, the H-2K and H-2D molecules show between 63 and 85 percent sequence homology at the N-terminal ends; in man the two HLA loci show between 81 and 88 percent sequence homology. Clearly, the H-2K is homologous to H-2D, HLA-A is homologous to HLA-B, and the degree of homology between the individual loci is unexpectedly high. In the mouse, the degree of homology between the alleles of H-2K and H-2D is about the same as the degree of homology between the alleles of H-2K or alleles of H-2D. In other words, if in Table 10.1 someone were to erase the legend describing

[2] In fact, most of the $H\text{-}2K^k$–$H\text{-}2K^b$ amino acid substitutions are such that they require multiple base-pair substitutions at the DNA level, suggesting a sequence of mutations at each position.
[3] Although a third locus, *HLA-C*, has been reported in man (cf. Chapter 1), it is not clear whether it is homologous to the HLA-A and HLA-B loci.

the origin of the molecules, it would be impossible to distinguish whether a particular sequence were that of an H-2K or an H-2D molecule or that of allelic products of either H-2K or H-2D. Although this is a perplexing finding, it does not come unexpectedly, because Brown and co-workers (1974) reached the same conclusion some time ago on the basis of peptide mapping of H-2K and H-2D products.

There are a number of implications one can derive from this lack of "K-ness" and "D-ness" (Silver and Hood 1976b) (some of them will be discussed later).

c. *Interspecies variation of class I regions.* One of the more important conclusions that one can draw from the data in Table 10.1 concerns the homology of class I loci in man and mouse. Simple calculations indicate that the H-2 and HLA molecules share between 44 and 67 percent of their amino acids at their N-terminal ends. The class I loci in mouse and man, therefore, must be related by their origin from a common ancestral gene. The homology of human and murine MHS has been suspected for some time (David et al. 1973a) and it is, therefore, gratifying to see it finally confirmed.

2.3.2 Class II Regions

If tracing the phylogenetic origin of class I regions is difficult, tracing of class II regions is even more so, primarily because one does not know what to look for in the less advanced groups of animals. The most convenient assay for class II regions is the MLR, but it, too, has serious limitations. MLR, of course, cannot be done without lymphocytes, and that means that it is, for all practical purposes, restricted to vertebrates (Figure 10.3). Although the more advanced invertebrates most probably have lymphocyte-like cells, it is difficult to identify them, and further down the evolutionary scale it is outright impossible. There is also the problem of experimental conditions in the MLR assay. The vertebrate lymphocytes are tremendeously heterogeneous and must have undergone an evolution on their own. For this reacon, what applies to mammalian lymphocytes, with which the MLR assay has been worked out, does not necessarily apply to the lymphocytes of, for instance, shark or hagfish. A failure of a nonmammalian species to respond in MLR could, therefore, mean that the species lacks lymphocyte-activating determinants, but it could also mean that the experimenter failed to provide adequate conditions for the response. The opposite is also true: If one detects positive MLR in a particular species, the reaction does not have to be caused by MHS-associated determinants. Mammals (or at least the mouse) have a strong Lad locus (Mls, cf. Festenstein 1974) and, also, under slightly modified conditions, they can respond to a variety of non-MHS antigens (cf. Klein 1975). Similar situations may exist in nonmammalian vertebrates, and without genetic analysis one is never sure what caused the MLR.

When all these considerations are taken into account, it is not surprising to find the MLR data in the various phylogenetic groups confusing. In

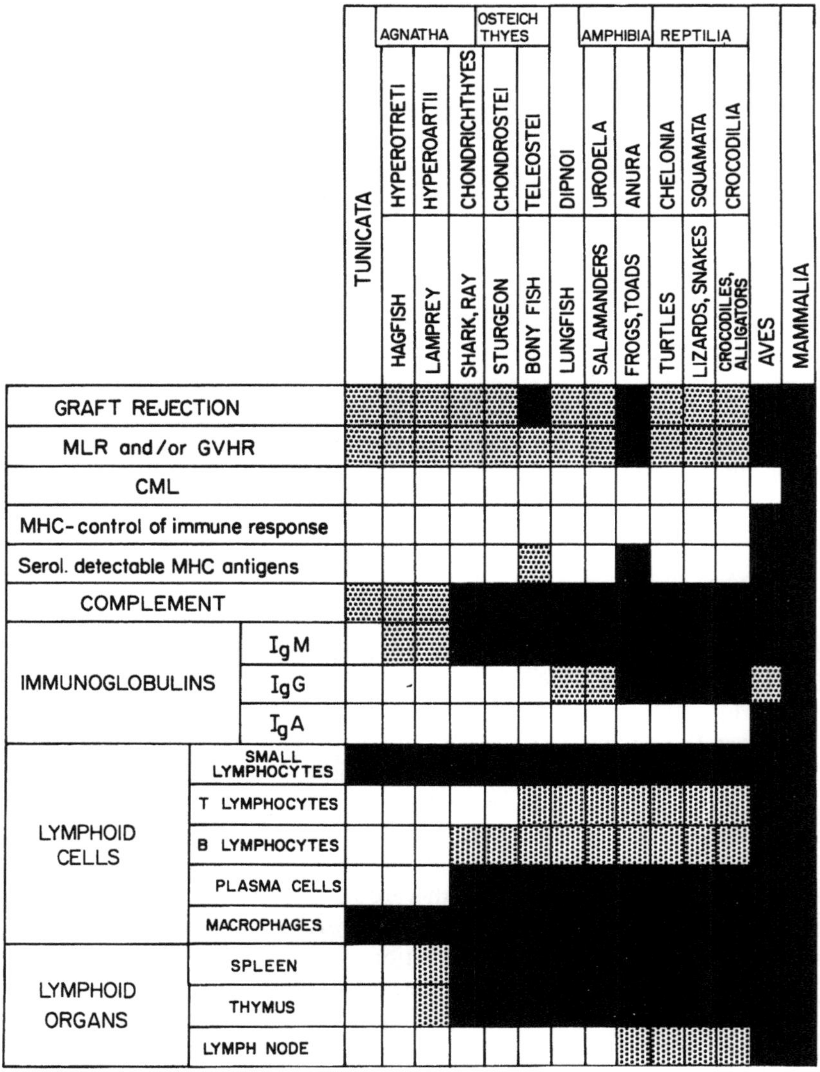

Figure 10.3. Evolution of immunologically important traits among *Chordata*. Full boxes indicate presence of typical and stippled boxes of atypical or not fully developed traits; empty boxes indicate either absence of traits or absence of knowledge about these traits in indicated species

many groups both positive and negative MLR results have been reported, sometimes even within the same species. However, to obtain positive results often required a modification of the classical MLR technique, for example, prolongation of the incubation period, alteration of the incubation temperature, addition of mitogens, etc. Perhaps one should be prepared for the possibility that in the end one form or another of MLR will be demonstrated in all vertebrate classes. However, if the ease with which MLR can be demonstrated were to be accepted as a criterion (admittedly not a very scientific one) for MHS-associated Lad's, then one could find a reasonable correspondence between the occurrence of acute allograft reaction and strong MLR. Strong MLR has been demonstrated in some but not in other representatives of *Teleostei,* and in representatives of *Anura,* birds, and mammals (for references see Chapter 9). How legitimate it is to generalize to the whole class from the results obtained with one or a few species is debatable. In mammals, it is probably not unreasonable to predict that all *Eutheria* will be shown to possess MHS-associated Lad's; whether *Prototheria* will also follow the suit is less certain. Birds are taxonomically such a homogeneous group[4] that one species may tell the story of the entire class. In *Anura* and *Teleostei,* additional species should be tested before one can confidently make any generalizations.

The information available about the other class II genes is even more scanty. MHS-associated Ir genes have been demonstrated in five species of mammals and one species of birds. No data are available on any of the subavian groups. Because the demonstration of Ir genes depends on the capacity of an organism to mount an IgG antibody response, and typical IgG antibodies do not appear until the *Amphibia* (Figure 10.3), it will probably be at this evolutionary stage that the Ir trail will disappear. One can, of course, attempt to follow the evolution of Ir genes by testing the capacity of the individual groups of animals to mount a delayed-type hypersensitivity, but such testing may prove to be technically difficult.

Ia-like antigens so far have been demonstrated only in mammals (man, mouse, rhesus monkey, guinea pig), and class II histocompatibility loci only in the mouse and guinea pig.

In all mammals tested so far, the Lad, Ir, and Ia loci always map in the same chromosomal region, distinct from regions occupied by class I loci. The relationship of the loci within the I-like region is unclear in any of these species.

In conclusion, typical class II MHS loci are almost certainly present in most mammals, probably in most birds, at least in some *Anura,* and in some *Teleostei.* No evidence is available for their presence in other vertebrate groups, and the nature of class II precursors in invertebrates is obscure.

2.3.3 Class III Regions

Complement activity has been demonstrated in a variety of vertebrate species and complement components are probably present in all vertebrates (Figure 10.3). Some evidence is also available for complement-like activity in more advanced invertebrates. The origin of the genes coding for the individual complement components, the presence, and the role of these components in the various vertebrate classes are largely unknown. The limited homology

---

[4] According to Romer (1959), "the differences between the orders making up the group (of birds) are no greater than those found within a single order of mammals".

observed between the human C3a component and Ig variable regions (D. J. Capra, *personal communication*) may suggest that the Ig genes and genes for at least some complement components could have shared a common evolutionary origin.

Linkage of complement-component genes to the MHS has so far been demonstrated in man, mouse, rhesus monkey, and guinea pig. Nothing is known about other mammals. Whether class III genes display any homology to class I and class II genes remains to be seen.

2.3.4 Occurrence of MHS Among Vertebrate Classes

Although ancestral MHS genes are probably present in all invertebrates, or at least in their most advanced forms, true MHS can be found only among vertebrates. If one were to accept as a main criterion of MHS the capacity to effect acute graft rejection and to cause strong allogeneic MLR, then, based on the current knowledge, one could conclude that the MHS is probably present in somee (but not other) *Teleostei,* in some *Amphibia,* in birds, and in mammals (Figure 10.2). Thus, distribution of MHS among vertebrates suggests that the evolution of the complex did not follow a single, uninterrupted line from more primitive to more advanced forms. For example, *Teleostei* are not on the direct evolutionary line leading to mammals, yet they appear to have come closer to developing an MHS than reptiles, which are direct ancestors of mammals. Also, there are differences in the occurrence of the MHS among closely related taxonomical groups. Thus, of the three orders of *Amphibia,* only one *(Anura)* appears to have developed a typical MHS. Similarly, birds and reptiles are closely related, yet the former developed an MHS, whereas the latter did not.

The occurrence of MHS in distantly related vertebrate classes could be an example of a convergent evolution, i.e., an independent development of the same trait in different taxonomical groups because of similarity in habits or environment. Apparently, all vertebrate classes possess the ancestral MHS genes and these genes can evolve into the MHS whenever there is a need for it. And, apparently, the need for the MHS has occurred repeatedly in different stages of evolution.

3. Speculations

3.1 Evolution and Function of MHS

3.1.1 Class I Regions

It has been said that Nature did not invent histocompatibility antigens to make life more difficult for transplant surgeons and that, therefore, tissue incompatibility could not be the true function of these antigens (Thomas 1959). The first part of this statement is undoubtedly correct; the second part may not be. Obviously, if one thinks of man or mouse, the idea that

H antigens of these species are here to prevent the fusion of tissues between individuals is preposterous. However, as I tried to point out in the preceding section, H genes probably did not arise with vertebrates; their ancestors must have existed already in the most primitive invertebrate forms. And if indeed the genes existed in the invertebrates, then the idea of their functioning as protectors of individuality is not so ridiculous any more. In general, invertebrates, with the exception of *Arthropoda,* are much less mobile than vertebrates. In fact, a majority of them lead a rather sedentary life, often crammed upon one another in very little space. Just think of all the sponges, corals, and sea anemones, all crowed onto one little rock! Or the parasites living inside other animals' bodies! Such living conditions provide ample opportunity for body contact, and the loss of individuality by tissue fusion becomes a real danger. To prevent a disaster, invertebrates must have developed a system that would recognize self from nonself and that would protect an organism against fusion with another individual (Burnet 1970). Evidence for the presence of such a system has been found in many invertebrates, from *Porifera* to *Protochordata* (cf. previous section).

In more advanced froms, particularly in the highly mobile chordates, the danger of losing individuality by direct, long-term contact subsided, because the opportunity for such a contact disappeared. However, the vertebrates face another danger. In addition to higher mobility, vertebrates differ from invertebrates in that they generally live longer. This prolongation of the individual's life-span means a higher risk that some somatic cell variants will appear capable of malignant growth and thus destruction of the organism from within. To control the outgrowth of variants, the vertebrates have to acquire a system that would recognize such aberrant cells and eliminate them. It seems possible that, rather than inventing a totally new defense system, the vertebrates adapted a new function to an old system that had become evolutionarily obsolete. So it might have happened that the original histoincompatibility system, designed by the organism for protection of its individuality, became a vehicle of surveillance and protection against somatic variants. The adaptation consisted of two main changes. The first change was the development of a more efficient recognition system—a system of specific cell receptors. The receptor system was developed for a different purpose (see next section) and the class I loci were merly hooked onto it (or more likely, the two systems coevolved in a parallel fashion). The second major adjustment was an improvement in killing efficiency. The rapid pace of life in vertebrates required fast action; the organism could no longer afford to spend months developing an aggressive reaction; the surveillance system had to act within days. The improvement was achieved by restricting the killer function to a single cell type—the lymphocyte—and by equipping this cell with a special property—memory, or the capacity to recall previous experience and mount an aggressive reaction.

To explain how class I antigens function in immune surveillance, I shall now return to the DZSB phenomenon and the role of class I loci in it. Two hypotheses have been proposed to explain the phenomenon (Doherty

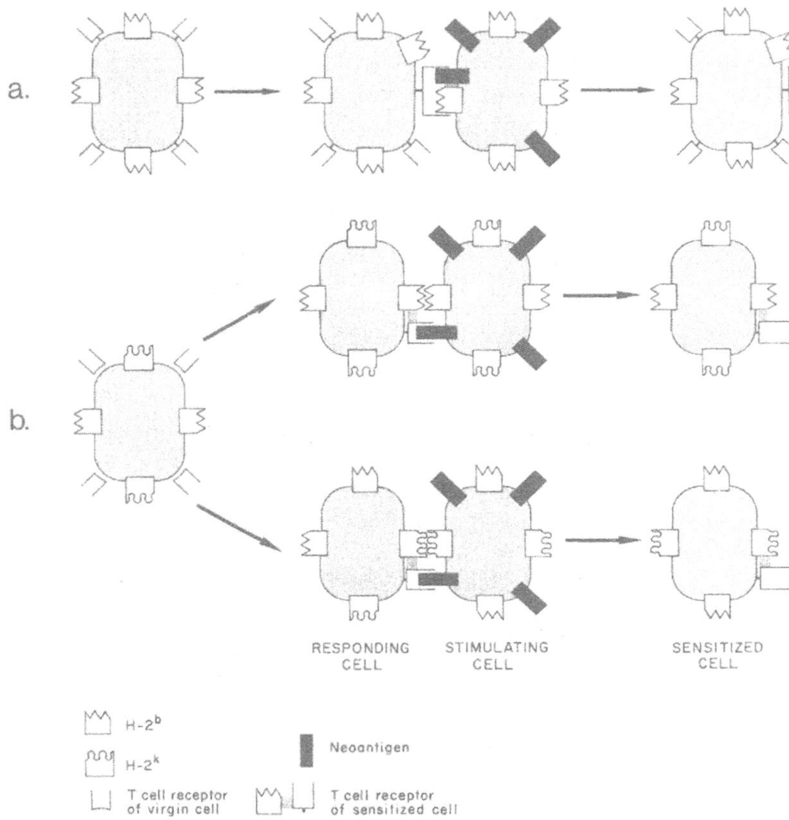

Figure 10.4. Two interpretations of the DZSB phenomenon. a. Altered-self interpretation. Neoantigen (virally induced, hapten-modified self-, or minor H antigen) associates on the stimulating cell with H-2K or H-2D antigens, the neoantigen-H-2 complex is recognized by the T-cell receptor of the responding cell, and the sensitized cell is then capable of killing any target cells carrying given neoantigen-H-2 supramolecular combination. b. Lock-in interpretation. Neoantigen is recognized by the T-cell receptor and at the same time like-like interaction occurs between H-2 antigens of stimulating and responding cells. The T-cell receptor then forms a supramolecular complex (is locked in) with the interacting H-2 molecule and the responding cell is thus sensitized against a given combination of neoantigen and H-2. When an H-2 heterozygous responding cell (as shown in the figure) is stimulated by a parental cell, it becomes, because of the locking-in process, sensitized against this but not the other parental strain.

et al. 1976). The first hypothesis (Figure 10.4a) postulates that the neoantigen (viral antigen, hapten, or minor H antigen) associates with MHS molecules on target cells, the antigen-MHS complex (altered-self antigen) is then recognized by the receptor on T-lymphocytes, and a cytotoxic reaction is triggered against the target cell (=altered-self hypothesis). The main difficulty with this hypothesis is how to explain the nature of the association between such a great variety of neoantigens and H-2. The second hypothesis postulates the existence of two receptors on the responding T-cell, one for the neoantigen and the other for the H-2 molecule (=dual-recognition hypothesis). The second receptor could be of the same class as the first one, or it could be the H-2 molecule itself. In the latter case, one must postulate the occurrence of like-like interactions between H-2 molecules. The main argument against the dual-recognition hypothesis, particularly against its version assuming like-like interactions, is the observation that F_1 hybrid (H-2 heterozygous) cells sensitized to a neoantigen present on one of the two parental cell types lyse neoantigen-carrying target cells of this but not of the opposite parent. To accommodate this observation, one would have to postulate clonal expression of the second receptor. However, in the case of H-2, there is no evidence for clonal expression; on the contrary, data are available indicating that H-2 antigens are nonclonally distributed in all cells, including effector T-cells (Davidson et al. 1976). As a way out of this contradiction, I suggested (Klein 1976b) a "locking-in" hypothesis depicted in Figure 10.4b. According to this version of the dual-recognition hypothesis, the recognition occurs in three steps: first, the T-cell receptor binds to the neoantigen on the target cell, then homologous H-2 molecules on the responding and the sensitizing cell interact in a like-like fashion, and finally, the H-2 molecules on the responding cell interact with the T-cell receptor and form a more or less stable supramolecular H-2—T-cell receptor complex (the receptor is "locked in" with the H-2 molecule). The formation of the complex "educates" the responding (effector) T-cell: From now on the cell can attack only those target cells that carry the same combination of the neoantigen and H-2 antigens. In the complex, the receptor is the recognition unit and the H-2 (or any other class I molecule) is the effector of, or at least a participant to, the cytotoxic mechanism. The original "locking-in" mechanism was proposed specifically to salvage the like-like interaction version of the dual-recognition hypothesis. However, the mechanism can be also applied to the nonlike version of the hypothesis; all one has to do, in this case, is to postulate locking in between the two types of T-cell receptors (rather than between the T-cell receptor and H-2). Furthermore, the locking-in mechanism does not necessarily have to be visualized as a physical bondage between the receptors; instead, one can also visualize that the same effect could be achieved by a selection during the induction phase of cells with a particular combination of receptors.

3.1.2 Class II and Class III Regions

In addition to the threat of losing its individuality on the outside, an organism is in a constant danger of being invaded from the inside by parasites of all kinds. To survive, it must develop a defense mechanism that will combat the invaders and neutralize their harmful effects. Some sort of an internal defense mechanism probably exists in all *Metazoa,* but its degree of sophistication depends on how serious the threat is. In invertebrates the loss of diseased individuals is probably compensated for by the large number of progeny these species produce. Consequently, most invertebrates can probably get by with a rather inefficient defense system, characterized by a relatively low degree of specificity, slowness, and only rudimentary, if any, memory.

With the emergence of vertebrates, the demands on the defense mechanism increased enormously. The evolutionary strategy of combating parasites by eliminating the diseased individuals was no longer feasible, because vertebrates in general produce only very few progeny. The defense mechanisms that served the invertebrates well were incapable of meeting the new needs of the vertebrates, and an urgent need for a solution pressured these advanced forms to develop a new system. The new defense mechanism had two vast improvements in comparison to the invertebrate mechanism: specificity and memory. [5] The defense mechanism thus became a true immunological system! The specificity of the immune response had been achieved by developing sets of clonally expressed receptors on both B- and T-lymphocytes, each receptor capable of reacting with only a limited range of antigens. The B-cell receptors are immunoglobulins (Ig); the nature of the T-cell receptor is still controversial, but here I shall take the stand that they, too, are molecules related to Ig. The origin of the receptor genes is not known. Some investigators would like to see them derived from ancestral MHS loci; alternatively, they may have been derived from primitive receptor loci of invertebrates or from some other, thus far unidentified group of genes. Primitive vertebrates might have possessed only one class of receptors and one class of lymphocytes; the T-B dichotomy probably developed later and probably represented additional improvement in the efficiency of the immune response. The mechanism of T,B-cell cooperation is unknown, but one way to visualize it is as follows (Klein 1975, 1976a). The Ig receptors bind the antigen and the antigen-Ig complex is recognized by the receptor on the T-cell which then gives the signal to the B-cell to differentiate and produce IgG antibodies. The signal could be mediated by the class II gene products, and the transmission of the signal can be hypothesized as operating on a similar principle as that involving class I gene products. As with the class I loci, there are two principal ways by which one can visualize the signal transmission. One way would be that the antigen-receptor complex on the B-cell associates with class II gene products, modifies these products, and the altered-self antigens are then recognized by T-cells. An alternative way is that the antigen-Ig complex is recognized by the T-cell and the triggering occurs because of like-like interaction between class II molecules on T- and B-cells. During this interaction, the class II molecules on T-cells associate with the T-cell receptor and form a supramolecular complex, very much like that formed by class I molecules (Figure 10.4b).

Nothing is known about the phylogenetic precursors of class II loci. Very attractive is the possibility of their being derived from class I loci by the

[5] This is not to say that invertebrate defense systems totally lacked these two properties. On the contrary, at least the most advanced invertebrates, such as *Annelida*, also possess systems that show some specificity and some memory. However, in vertebrates, these two properties have been improved to perfection.

loss of the killer function. Another possibility is that their precursors were some differentiation loci, perhaps those of the t group (see below). Finally, they may have existed all along but in a totally different functional capacity.

3.2 Organization of MHS

3.2.1 Why Bipartite Structure?

Class I loci in man, mouse, rhesus monkey, and guinea pig occur as doublets; i.e., each species has two such loci on each MHS chromosome. In other species, such as dog, pig, and rat, only one class I locus has been identified, but the reason for the lack of the second locus could be simply the lack of recombinants genetically separating the two loci. It would not be surprising if, in the end, all mammalian MHS were to be demonstrated to contain two class I loci.

The situation with the class II loci has not yet been clarified, but at this writing, and in the mouse at least, there appear to be two loci or two main clusters of loci in the I region.

The bipartite organization thus appears to be characteristic of the MHS loci, and the question arises of what is the biological significance of such an organization. Why does an organism need two loci that are apparently closely related and apparently perform the same function? Why is one not enough? To me, the most likely answer to these questions is that the bipartite organization is a way of achieving permanent heterozygozity at the MHS loci. Let us assume that when there was originally only one class I (or class II) locus, the heterozygotes at this locus were favored by selection. However, working against this heterozygous advantage was the mating system of many species. As mentioned earlier, in the mouse, and probably in many other species, natural populations are divided into small, relatively isolated breeding units (families or demes). The consequence of this organization is a relatively high degree of inbreeding within each unit. Inbreeding, of course, leads to homozygosity, a state not favored at the MHS loci. To escape the pressure of inbreeding, organisms used a trick that had proved to be useful many times before (Ohno 1970): They duplicated the originally single locus and thus achieved permanent heterozygozity, unaffected by inbreeding.

3.2.2 Why Clusters?

In all species that have been tested, the individual loci of the MHS are closely linked—they form a cluster. It is unlikely that this clustering could be explained by historical reasons only, i.e., by assuming that the entire MHS arose by tandem duplications and that the ensuing cluster, just by chance, had never been broken up. The improbability of such a notion becomes apparent when one considers the great number of chromosomal and genetic rearrangements accompanying the appearance of a new species. Even such closely related species such as the mouse and the rat have totally different karyotypes and very different chromosomal banding patterns. In fact, there are only a few cases of gene clusters being conserved during evolution. Most clusters are broken down or rearranged in a variety of ways. A classical example of this happening is the gene cluster controlling the pathway of tryptophan biosynthesis (Crawford 1975). Although the pathway is the same in all groups of organisms studied so far, prokaryotes and eukaryotes, there is a bewildering variety of arrangement of the genes controlling it. Nearly every major bacterial group studied has a distinctive arrangement of the genes for tryptophan biosynthesis. The genes probably have the same evolutionary origin (the corresponding enzymes show considerable sequence homology), and they originally formed a single cluster (the tryptophan operon). Yet, during evolution, the individual genes have been translocated to various positions and the cluster split up. Why did not the same thing happen to the MHS? Perhaps the MHS has remained a cluster for a similar reason for which the tryptophan cluster was disbanded. Geneticists believe that the disbanding of a cluster and translocation of its genes to a new position has the evolutionary advantage of providing an opportunity for the translocated genes to fall under the control of a different set of regulator genes and thus to respond differently to a selection in a changing environment. One can, therefore, also argue in the reverse, namely that the reason for the preservation of the MHS cluster is to retain its control under the same system of regulatory elements.

There is pitifully little known about the regulation of the MHS loci, and most of what is known is controversial anyway. In the H-2 system, for example, some data (Rajan et al. 1976) can be interpreted as indicating that the H-2K and H-2D loci share a common regulator gene, whereas other data (Boyse et al. 1968) seem to indicate just the opposite. A detailed discussion of the problem is beyond the scope of this communication. However, one point needs emphasizing. It need not be that the whole MHS cluster is controlled by a single regulator gene; for a cluster so large, this is unlikely. More probably there is a delicately balanced set of regulator genes, with different genes controlling different MHS regions. It could be this balance that favors conservation of the complex as a single gene cluster.

3.2.3 Is Murine MHS Organized Differently than the MHS of Other Mammals?

Figure 10.2 shows evolutionary relationships of those mammalian species in which a MHS has been described. It also summarizes what is known about the genetic organization of the MHS in these species. It can be seen that the mouse is the only species in which the class II regions are positioned between the two class I regions;[6] in all other species class II regions are

[6] Recently we obtained two recombinants that arose by crossing over between H-2 haplotypes of wild and inbred mice (Hauptfeld and Klein 1976). Genetic analysis of these recombinants indicates that in wild mice, as in inbred strains, class II and class III regions are positioned between the two class I regions.

outside of the genetic interval between the two class I regions. Even in the rat, a species closely related to the mouse, there is some preliminary evidence that its class II regions are not between the two class I regions (Gill and Kunz 1976).

Provided that this difference between the mouse MHS, on the one hand, and the MHS of other mammals, on the other hand, is not an artifact, one has to conclude that rearrangements *within* the MHS are apparently possible without seriously affecting the MHS function. In fact, it is surprising that more rearrangements have not been detected. If the two class I regions are, indeed, so closely related, as the preliminary sequence data indicate, one would expect that the high degree of homology between the two regions would lead to frequent mispairing, unequal crossing over, duplications, and deletions, and thus to rearrangements of the complex. The infrequency of such events could suggest the existence of a mechanism preventing genetic disruption of the complex. In the mouse, such mechanism could be the crossing over-suppression effect of the t factors, which is known to extend to the H-2 complex (Hammerberg and Klein 1975b). One can speculate that at some point in the history of *Mus musculus* a rearrangement occurred in a t-carrying chromosome that placed class II and class III regions between the two class I regions. Because of the association with a t haplotype, the rearrangement was rapidly disseminated throughout the entire mouse population and, as a consequence, all contemporary mice have it.

3.2.4 Is the MHS Evolutionarily Unstable?

The preliminary sequence data indicate that the two class I loci in man (HLA-A and HLA-B) are more closely related to each other than either of them is to the two class I loci in the mouse (H-2K and H-2D). This finding is rather unexpected, because until recently the commonly held view has been that the duplication of the ancestral gene giving rise to the two class I loci occurred long before the separation of the evolutionary branches leading to mouse and to man. The biochemical data contradict this assumption. There are several possible explanations of the maintenance of the close homology between the two class I loci after speciation, and these have been discussed extensively by Silver and Hood (1976b). To me, the most attractive one is the one assuming repeated duplications and deletions in the MHS portion of the chromosome. According to this hypothesis, the MHS is highly unstable and is subject to frequent rearrangements. Some of these rearrangements may reduce the number of class I regions from two to one, but later, duplication of the single region again restores the bipartite MHS structure. Thus, the MHS complex can be envisioned as oscillating between mono- and bi(multi)partite organization, with the bipartite organization being favored most by selection. This oscillation then results in the maintenance of the close homology between the class I loci within a single species, while the loci accumulate amino acid substitutions differentiating them from the MHS of other species.

3.3 Relationship of the MHS to Other Loci

3.3.1 Minor Histocompatibility Loci

In all mammals that have been studied, evidence has been obtained that, in addition to MHS, each species possesses a large number of minor H loci (in the mouse the number could be several hundreds), each of them capable of causing subacute or chronic graft rejection. Surprisingly, there is no evidence for the existence of homologous loci in invertebrates. In these species, the *sensu stricto* histocompatibility reactions can be explained as controlled by a single gene or a single chromosomal region, which may be the precursor of the MHS. What, then, were the precursors of the minor H loci? And are these loci in any way related to the MHS?

An interpretation that I would like to propose here is based on the Bevan variant of the DZSB phenomenon (see previous sections). Provided that Bevan's finding could be extended to the *in vivo* allograft reaction, then one can argue that the true function of minor H loci is not in any way related to histocompatibility reaction. The loci could code for enzymes, structural proteins, or hormones, and thus represent a very diverse group. The only feature the products of these loci could have in common is their presence on the cell surface. And it could be this latter property that makes the products histocompatibility antigens. Because of their expression in the cell membrane, any variant products of these loci are recognized as not-self by the MHS-dependent recognition system and a cytotoxic reaction is mounted against cells bearing the variants. They could thus be subject to the same surveillance as neoantigens. According to this hypothesis, minor H loci emerged as histocompatibility loci with the emergence of the MHS. Their involvement in histocompatibility has no physiological meaning; it is simply an artifact of transplantation. The loci have functions of their own, which are not related to the function of the MHS.

3.3.2 The t Complex

The t complex is comprised of a series of loci occupying regions of chromosome 17 between the H-2 complex and the centromere (for reviews, see Klein 1975; Bennett 1975). The wild-type alleles at these loci code for serologically detectable antigens on spermatozoa and on cells of embryonic tissues at specific stages of differentiation. The mutant alleles cause disturbances of normal development ranging from complete lethality to minor postnatal defects. The time of action of the mutant alleles coincides with the time of the appearance of antigens controlled by the corresponding wild-type alleles. Based on the periods at which they act and on the type of developmental disturbances they cause, t haplotypes can be divided into seven groups, with haplotypes in the earliest-acting group arresting blastogenesis and those in the latest-acting group affecting postnatal development. The classification of lethal factors into groups on the basis of their developmental effects coincides with their behavior in the genetic complementation test: Those alleles that are in the same group fail to complement each other in a heterozygous state, whereas those belonging to different groups permit an almost normal development of t^x/t^n heterozygous embryos (where t^x and t^n represent two different t haplotypes). In addition to their effect on development, t haplotypes may also cause segregation distortion (in a cross between a t/+ male and a +/+ female, the t haplotype is transmitted into the progeny with frequencies significantly departing from the expected 1:1 ratio), they may suppress crossing over in the centromeric arm of chromosome 17, and they may also lead to male sterility. A great majority of the known t haplotypes interact with a dominant mutation Brachyury (T), located near the centromeric end of chromosome 17. The T allele, in combination with wild-type allele (T/+), causes shortening of the tail; in combination with t haplotypes (T/t), a complete absence of the tail ensues.

Despite their deleterious effects, t haplotypes are found among wild mice with a relatively high frequency of some 20 percent. The haplotypes are distributed worldwide and are ubiquitous; populations lacking t haplotypes are rare. No convincing evidence has been obtained for the existence of t-like complexes in other species than the mouse. Amos and co-workers (1975) have suggested that the genes controlling the occurrence of spina bifida in man could be homologous to the murine t genes, but their evidence for linkage of this trait to HLA has been contradicted by the data of other investigators (Bobrow et al. 1975). It might be, however, that whereas homologous t genes exist in all mammals, the t complex as such is unique for the mouse. As discussed elsewhere (Hammerberg and Klein 1975a), the complex might have arisen as a genetic accident and has been perpetuated only because of the peculiar combination of characteristics of the genes locked into the complex (segregation distortion, suppression of crossing over, etc.). Therefore, to identify t homologues in other species, it might be more fruitful to search, for example, for sperm alloantigens coded for by loci linked to the MHS, rather than for MHS-linked developmental defects.

There are certain superficial resemblances between the t complex and the MHS of the mouse: Both complexes are carried by the same chromosome, both are clusters of apparently related loci, and both are expressed on the cell surface, and their products can function as antigens. Recently, much emphasis has been placed on the possible reciprocal relationship between the expression of t and H-2 antigens. It has been argued that t antigens are expressed on sperm and *early* embryos, but not in adult somatic tissues, whereas H-2 antigens are expressed on *late* embryonic and adult tissues (Artzt et al. 1974; Bodmer 1972; Nicolas et al. 1975). However, at present, there is no evidence that such a relationship exists. On the contrary, low levels of H-2 antigens have been detected by at least one technique as early as in the blastocyst stage (Searle et al. 1976), and by several techniques in 6- to 10-day-old embryos (for discussion and references, see Klein 1975). The fact that their concentration is lower in embryos than in adult mice may simply be due to the fact that lymphoid tissues, which in adult mice carry most of the H-2 antigens (Klein 1976a), are poorly developed in embryos. The reciprocity is also contradicted by the fact that many t factors act late in embryogenesis, and sometimes even postnatally, at a time when H-2 antigens are already present in a high concentration. The lack of t-H-2 reciprocity, however, does not detract from the possibility that the two complexes might be somehow related. In fact, recent data seem to support their relationship. Thus, the product of one t locus has been reported to be amazingly similar in its subunit structure and molecular weight to the products of class I H-2 loci (Vitetta et al. 1975); at the population level the H-2 and t loci are in a strong linkage disequilibrium (Hammerberg and Klein 1975a); and lethal t factors suppress recombination in the vicinity of H-2 (Hammerberg and Klein 1975b). Is it then possible that the t and H-2 complexes are homologous, as was first suggested by Gluecksohn-Waelsh and Erickson (1970) six years ago? We shall be able to determine the answer to this question only after sequence data on *t* products become available. In the meantime we can resort to conjecture. We can speculate, for example, that the precursors of the class I regions were coding for bifunctional molecules. In addition to the function discussed earlier (distinction of self from nonself), the molecules could also have acted as regulator genes in differentiation, providing signals for growth and stoppage of growth for the different tissues. There are a number of precedents for such a bifunctionality of genetic loci. For example, the incompatibility loci of the fungus *Schizophyllum commune* not only effect recognition of a proper mate but also function as regulator genes controlling the morphogenetic sequence of complete sexual progression (Koltin et al. 1972).

3.3.3 Immunoglobulin Loci

The hypothesis that MHS and Ig loci could be genetically related was first proposed by Gally and Edelman (1974). The evidence ususally cited as favoring this hypothesis is threefold. First, class I molecules are noncovalently associated with β_2-microglobulin molecules (Neauport-Sautes et al. 1974) and β_2-microglobulin is believed to be a free domain of the Ig molecule (Peterson et al. 1972). Second, *Staphylococcus aureus* protein A, known to bind to the Fc region of IgG, has been claimed to interact in a similar way with H-2 antigens (Peterson et al. 1975). And third, class I and Ig molecules have been claimed to have similar tertiary structure with each molecule composed of two light chains and two heavy chains (Peterson et al. 1975). Unfortunately, any one of these three types of experimental evidence could either be interpreted in a different way or is contradicted by results obtained in other laboratories. Furthermore, the preliminary amino acid sequence data of H-2 and HLA molecules do not indicate any extensive homology with immunoglobulin molecules. The situation could change when more sequence data become available, but the preliminary data already force one to conclude that if class I and Ig loci were to have evolved from common ancestors, the separation of the evolutionary branches must have occurred a long time ago.

3.3.4 The β_2-Microglobulin Locus

Among the loci that are not part of the MHS, yet appear to be somehow related to the MHS, the β_2-microglobulin locus is the strongest candidate for sharing common evolutionary origin with the class I loci. The β_2-microglobulin molecules are associated with class I molecules on the cell surface (Nakamuro et al. 1973; Grey et al. 1973; Peterson et al. 1974; Neauport-Sautes et al. 1974), and the amino acid sequence data indicate some questionable homology between the two types of molecules (Table 10.1). There are no clues available for the possible significance of the association between class I and β_2-microglobulin molecules.

4. Coda: The Temple of God?

In closing this book, I am once again tempted by the simile of the Tower of Babel. According to the legend, on the top of the mythical Tower of Babel, obscured by clouds, was to be the Temple of God. Here the tenants of the tower would gather to sing praises—under the guidance of the high priests—to the Almighty. But the Lord did not like the idea of people intruding into His quarters. He therefore punished the builders by making them speak different languages so that they could not understand one another. As a result, the builders stopped the construction of the Tower and scattered throughout the world....

Sometimes I wonder whether we, too, while attempting to build the Temple of GOD on the top of the MHS tower, have not reached the stage where we are beginning to speak different languages.

Acknowledgments. It is said that Molière owed much of the beauty of his prose to his cook. While working on a new comedy, he would read to her what he had written and she would tell him whenever his dialogue did not sound natural, the way common people spoke. I am not a Molière, my secretary is not my cook, and this communication is not a comedy (I hope!); but I owe Ms. JoAnne Tuttle much the same service as the great playwright owed to his servant.

My experimental work quoted in this communication was supported by grants AI11879, AI11650, AI12589, and CA17225.

References

Allen, F. H., Jr. Linkage of HLA and GBG. *Vox Sang. 27*:382–384, 1974.

Amos, D. B., Johnson, A. H., Ruderman, R. J., Mendell, N., and Yunis, E. J. *In* R. W. Cumley (ed.), *M. D. Anderson Symposium, New Concepts in Transplantation Immunity,* University of Texas, Houston, 1975.

Appleman, A. W. M., and Balner, H. Mixed leukocyte cultures in rhesus monkeys. *Transplant. Proc. 4*:17–20, 1972.

Artzt, K., Bennett, D., and Jacob, F. Primitive teratocarcinoma cells express a differentiation antigen specified by a gene at the T-locus in the mouse. *Proc. Natl. Acad. Sci. (USA) 71*:811–814, 1974.

Bach, F. H., and Amos, D. B. Hu-1: Major histocompatibility locus in man. *Science 156*:1506–1508, 1967.

Bach, F. H., Bach, M., and Sondel, P. M. Differential function of major histocompatibility complex antigens in T-lymphocyte activation. *Nature 259*:273–281, 1976.

Balner, H., Gabb, B. W., Dersjant, H., van Vreeswijk, W., and van Rood, J. J. Major histocompatibility locus of rhesus monkeys. *Nature 230*:177–180, 1971.

Balner, H., van Leeuwen, A., Dersjant, H., and van Rood, J. J. Defined leukocyte antigens of chimpanzees. Use of chimpanzee isoantisera for leukocyte typing in man. *Transplantation 5*:624–642, 1967.

Balner, H., van Vreeswijk, W., and Roger, J. H. Ia-like antigens of rhesus monkeys: Current state of serology and genetics.*Transplant. Rev. 30*:3–17, 1976.

Bechtol, K. B., Wegmann, T. F., Freed, J. H., Grumet, F. C., Chesebro, B. W., Herzenberg, L. A., and McDevitt, H. O. Genetic control of the immune response to (T,G)-A – L in C3H↔C57 tetraparental mice. *Cell. Immunol. 12*:264–277, 1974.

Bennett, D. The T-locus of the mouse. *Cell 6*:441–454, 1975.

Bevan, M. J. The major histocompatibility complex determines susceptibility to cytotoxic T cells directed against minor histocompatibility antigens. *J. Exp. Med. 142*:1349–1364, 1975.

Bobrow, M., Bodmer, J., Bodmer, W., McDevitt, H. O., Lorber, J., and Swift, P. The search for a human equivalent of the mouse T-locus – Negative results from a study of HL-A types in spina bifida. *Tissue Antigens 5*:234–237, 1975.

Bodmer, W. F. Evolutionary significance of the HL-A system, *Nature 237*:139–145, 1972.

Bogden, A. E., and Aptekman, P. M. The R-1 factor, a histocompatibility antigen in the rat. *Cancer Res. 20*:1372–1382, 1960.

Boyse, E. A., Stockert, E., and Old, L. J. Isoantigens of the H-2 and Tla loci of the mouse. Interactions affecting their representation on thymocytes. *J. Exp. Med. 128*:85–95, 1968.

Briles, W. E., McGibbon, W. H., and Irwin, M. R. Studies of the time of development of cellular antigens in the chicken. *Genetics 33*:97, 1948 (abstract).

Brown, J. L., Kato, K., Silver, J., and Nathenson, S. G. Notable diversity in peptide composition of murine H-2K and H-2D gene products. *Biochemistry 13*:3174–3178, 1974.

Touslé, J. Homogreffes et heterogreffes reciproques de entagument et ses gonades ches *Asterina gibbosa* et *Asterina panceri. Cah. Biol. Marine 8*:417, 1967.

Burnet, F. M. A certain symmetry: Histocompatibility antigens compared with immunocyte receptors. *Nature 226*:123–126, 1970.

Chai, C. K., and Lerner, C. P. Asymmetrical mixed lymphocyte reaction between inbred strain rabbit. *Immunogenetics 2*:363–368, 1975.

Chanh, T. C., Benedict, A. A., and Ablanalp, H. Association of serum hemolytic complement levels with the major histocompatibility complex in chickens. *J. Exp. Med. 144*:555–561, 1976.

Cheng, T. C. The compatibility and incompatibility concept as related to trematodes and molluscs. *Pacific Sci. 22*:141–160, 1967.

Cleton, F. J., Pousen, R., and van Rood, J. J. Leucocyte antigens in the dog. *In* E. S. Curtoni, P. L. Mattinz, and R. M. Tosi (eds.), *Histocompatibility Testing 1967*, pp. 277–280, Munksgaard, Copenhagen 1967.

Cooper, E. L. Transplantation immunity in earthworms. *Am. Zool. 8*:815–817, 1968.

Cooper, E. L. Characteristics of cell-mediated immunity and memory in annelids. *Adv. Exp. Med. Biol. 64*:127–136, 1975.

Cramer, D. W., Shonnard, J. W., and Gill, T. J., III Genetic studies in inbred rats. II. Relationship between the major histocompatibility complex and mixed lymphocyte reactivity. *J. Immunogenet. 1*:421–427, 1974.

Crawford, I. P. Gene rearrangements in the evolution of the tryptophan synthetic pathway. *Bacteriol. Rev. 39*:87–120, 1975.

Cunningham, B. A., Wang, J. L., Berggard, I., and Peterson, P. A. The complete amino acid sequence of β_2-microglobulin. *Biochemistry 12*:4811–4821, 1973.

Curman, B., Östberg, L., Sandberg, L., Malmheden-Eriksson, I., Stålenheim, G., Rask, L., and Peterson, P. A. H-2 linked Ss protein is C4 component of complement. *Nature* *258*:243–245, 1975.

Dausset, J. Iso-leuco-anticorps. *Acta Haematol. (Basel)* *20*:156–166, 1958.

David, C. S., Frelinger, J. A., and Shreffler, D. C. New lymphocyte antigens controlled by the Ir-IgG region of the H-2 gene complex. *Transplantation* *17*:121–125, 1974.

David, C. S., Hansen, T. H., and Shreffler, D. C. Studies on recombination within the mouse *H-2* gene complex. III. Further serological analysis of the $H\text{-}2^{t}$ haplotypes. *Tissue Antigens* *6*:353–365, 1975.

David, C. S., Klein, J., and Shreffler, D. C. Serologic homology between H-2 and HL-A systems. *Transplant. Proc.* *5*:461–466, 1973a.

David, C. S., Shreffler, D. C., and Frelinger, J. A. New lymphocyte antigen system (Lna) controlled by the *Ir* region of the mouse *H-2* complex. *Proc. Natl. Acad. Sci. (USA)* *70*:2509–2514, 1973b.

Davidson, W. F., Pang, T., Blanden, R. V., and Doherty, P. C. "Physiological interaction" does not explain the H-2 compatibility requirement of virus-infected cells. *Aust. J. Exp. Biol. Med. Sci. (in press)*, 1976.

Day, N. K., L'Esperance, P., Good, R. A., Michael, A. F., Hansen, J. A., Dupont, B., and Jersild, C. Hereditary C2 deficiency: Genetic studies and association with the HL-A system. *J. Exp. Med.* *141*:1464–1469, 1975.

Doherty, P. C., Blanden, R. V., and Zinkernagel, R. M. Specificity of virus-immune effector T-cells for H-2K or H-2D compatible interactions: Implications for H-antigen diversity. *Transplant. Rev.* *29*:89–124, 1976.

Dorf, M. E., Balner, H., deGroot, M. L., and Benacerraf, B. Histocompatibility-linked immune response genes in the rhesus monkey. *Transplant. Proc.* *6*:119–123, 1974.

Dorf, M. E., and Benacerraf, B. Complementation of H-2 linked Ir genes in the mouse. *Proc. Natl. Acad. Sci. (USA)* *72*:3671–3675, 1975.

DuPasquier, L. The genetic control of histocompatibility reactions: Phylogenetic aspects. *Arch. Biol. (Bruxelles)* *85*:91–103, 1974.

DuPasquier, L., Chardonneus, X., and Miggiano, V. C. A major histocompatibility complex in the toad Xenopus laevis (Daudin). *Immunogenetics* *1*:482–494, 1975.

Duprat, P. Mise en évidence de réactions immunitaires dans les homogreffes de paroi du corps chez le Lombricien *Eisenia foetida* typica. *C. R. Acad. Sci. (Paris)* *D*:4177–4180, 1964.

Duprat, P. Etudes des homogreffes de paroi du corps chez le Lombricien *Eisenia foetida* Sav. Aspects histologiques et immunitaries de la prise et de l'acceptation ou du refus des greffons. Thèse Doctorat ès Sciences Naturelles, Université de Bordeaux, 1968.

Ellman, L., Green, I., Martin, W. J., and Benacerraf, B. Linkage between the poly-L-lysine gene and the locus controlling the major histocompatibility antigens in strain 2 guinea pigs. *Proc. Natl. Acad. Sci. (USA)* *66*:322–328, 1970.

Ewenstein, B. M., Freed, J. H., Mole, L. E., and Nathenson, S. G. Studies on the localization of the papain cleavage site of H-2 glycoproteins. *Proc. Natl. Acad. Sci. (USA)* *73*:915–918, 1976.

Ferreira, L., and Nussenzweig, V. Genetic linkage between serum levels of the third component of complement and the H-2 complex. *J. Exp. Med.* *141*:513–517, 1975.

Festenstein, H. Pertinent features of M locus determinants including revised nomenclature and strain distribution. *Transplantation* *18*:555–557, 1974.

Finkelman, F. D., Shevach, E. M., Vitetta, E. S., Green, I., and Paul, W. E. Guinea pig immune response-related histocompatibility antigens. Partial characterization and distribution. *J. Exp. Med.* *141*:27–41, 1975.

Forman, J. On the role of the H-2 histocompatibility complex in determining the specificity of cytotoxic effector cells sensitized against syngeneic trinitrophenyl-modified targets. *J. Exp. Med.* *142*:403–418, 1975.

Francis, L. Intraspecific aggression and its effect on the distribution of *Anthopleura elegantissima* and some related sea anemones. *Biol. Bull.* *144*:73–92, 1973.

Freeman, G. Transplantation specificity in echinoderms and lower chordates. *Transplant. Proc.* *2*:236–239, 1970.

Frenzl, B., Křen, V., and Štark, O. Attempt to determine blood groups in rats. *Folia Biol. (Praha) 6*:121–126, 1960.

Friend, P. S., Handwerger, B. S., Kim, Y., Michael, A. F., and Yunis, E. J. C2 deficiency in man. Genetic relationship to a mixed lymphocyte reaction determinant (7A*). *Immunogenetics 2*:569–576, 1975.

Fu, S. M., Stern, R., Kunkel, H. G., Dupont, B., Hansen, J. A., Day, N. K., Good, R. A., Jersild, C., and Fotino, M. Mixed lymphocyte culture determinants and C2 deficiency: LD-7a associated with C2 deficiency in four families. *J. Exp. Med. 142*:495–506, 1975.

Gally, J. A., and Edelman, G. M. The genetic control of immunoglobulin systhesis. *Ann. Rev. Genet. 6*:1–46, 1974.

Geczy, A. F., de Weck, A. L., and Shevach, E. M. The major histocompatibility complex of the guinea pig. I. Serologic and genetic studies. *J. Immunol. 115*:1704–1710, 1975.

Gelfand, M. C., Sachs, D. H., Lieberman, R., and Paul, W. E. Ontogeny of B lymphocytes. III. H-2 linkage of a gene controlling the rate of appearance of complement receptor lymphocytes. *J. Exp. Med. 139*:1142–1153, 1974.

Gill, T. J., III, and Kunz, H. W. Genetic studies in inbred rats. VII. Tentative model for the major histocompatibility complex. *J. Immunogenet. 3*:139–143, 1976.

Gluecksohn-Waelsch, S., and Erickson, R. P. The *T*-locus of the mouse: Implications for mechanisms of development. *Curr. Top. Dev. Biol. 5*:281–316, 1970.

Gordon, R. D., Simpson, E., and Samelson, L. E. In vitro cell-mediated response to the male specific (H-Y) antigen in mice. *J. Exp. Med. 142*:1108–1120, 1975.

Gorer, P. A. The detection of a hereditary antigenic difference in the blood of mice by means of human group A serum. *J. Genet. 32*:17–31, 1936.

Götze, D. Serological characterization of Ia antigens of the $H\text{-}2^k$, $H\text{-}2^s$, and $H\text{-}2^k$ haplotype with antisera produced against skin, lymphocytes and lymphoblasts, their strain distribution pattern and relation to Ir-genes. *Immunogenetics 3*:139–156, 1976.

Greineder, D. K., and Rosenthal, A. S. Macrophage activation of allogeneic lymphocyte proliferation in the guinea pig mixed leukocyte culture. *J. Immunol. 114*:1541–1547, 1975.

Grey, H. M., Kubo, R. T., Colon, S. M., Poulik, M. D., Cresswell, P., Springer, T., Turner, M., and Strominger, J. L. The small subunit of HL-A antigens is β_2-microglobulin. *J. Exp. Med. 138*:1608–1612, 1973.

Günther, E., Balcarová, J., Hála, K., Rüde, E., and Hraba, T. Evidence for an association between immune responsiveness of chicken to (T,G)-A--L and the major histocompatibility system. *Eur. J. Immunol. 4*:548–553, 1974.

Günther, E., Rüde, E., and Štark, O. Antibody response in rats to the synthetic polypeptide (T,G)-A--L genetically linked to the major histocompatibility system. *Eur. J. Immunol. 2*:151–155, 1972.

Hammerberg, C., and Klein, J. Linkage disequilibrium between *H-2* and *t* complexes in chromosome 17 of the mouse. *Nature 258*:296–299, 1975a.

Hammerberg, C., and Klein, J. Linkage relationships of markers on chromosome 17 of the house mouse. *Genet. Res. (Camb.) 26*:203–211, 1975b.

Hauenschild, C. Genetische und Entwicklungsphysiologische Untersuchungen über Intersexualität und Gewebeverträglichkeit bei *Hydractinia echinata* Flenn. (Hydroz. Baugainvill). *Roux Arch. Entwicklungsmechanik 147*:1–41, 1954.

Hauenschild, C. Ueber die Vererbung einer Gewebestäglichkeits-Eigenschaft bei dem Hydroidpolypen *Hydractinia echinata. Z. Naturforsch. 11*:132–183, 1956.

Hauptfeld, M., and Klein, J. The *H-2* complexes of inbred and wild mice are organized in a similar fashion. *Immunogenetics 3*:603–607, 1976.

Hauptfeld, V., Klein, D., and Klein, J. Serological identification of an Ir-region product. *Science 181*:167–169, 1973.

Heber-Katz, E., and Wilson, D. B. Collaboration of allogeneic T and B lymphocytes in the primary antibody response to sheep erythrocytes in vitro. *J. Exp. Med. 142*:928–935, 1975.

Henning, R., Milner, R., Reske, K., Cunningham, B., and Edelman, G. Subunit structure, cell surface orientation and partial amino acid sequences of murine histocompatibility antigens. *Proc. Natl. Acad. Sci. (USA.) 73*:118–122, 1976.

Hildemann, W. H. Phylogeny of transplantation reactivity. *In* B. D. Kahan and R. A. Reisfeld (eds.), *Transplantation Antigens*, pp. 3–73, Academic Press, New York, 1972.

Hildemann, W. H., and Dix, T. G. Transplantation reactions in tropical Australian echinoderms. *Transplantation 15*:624–633, 1972.

Hildemann, W. H., Linthicum, D. S., and Vann, D. C. Transplantation and immunoincompatibility reactions among reef-building corals. *Immunogenetics 2*:269–284, 1975.

Humer, R. P., Keller, L. S., and Lee, K. D. Thymidine incorporation in mixed cultures of spleen cells from mice of differing H-2 types. *Transplantation 6*:706–715, 1968.

Ivker, F. B. A hierarchy of histocompatibility in *Hydractinia echinata. Biol. Bull. 143*:162–174, 1972.

Jaffe, W. P., and McDermid, E. M. Blood groups and splenomegaly in chick embryos. *Science 137*:984, 1962 (abstract).

Karakoz, I., Krejčí, J., Hála, K., Blaszczyk, B., Hraba, T., and Pekárek, J. Genetic differentiation of tuberculin hypersensitivity in chicken inbred lines. *Eur. J. Immunol. 4*:545–548, 1974.

Katz, D. H., Hamaoka, T., Dorf, M. E., and Benacerraf, B. Cell interactions between histoincompatible T and B lymphocytes. The *H-2* gene complex determines successful physiologic lymphocyte interactions. *Proc. Natl. Acad. Sci. (USA) 70*:2624–2628, 1973.

Katz, D. H., Graves, M., Dorf, M. E., Dimuzio, H., and Benacerraf, B. Cell interactions between histoincompatible T and B lymphocytes VII. Cooperative response between lymphocytes are controlled by genes in the I region of the H-2 complex. *J. Exp. Med. 141*:263–268, 1975.

Kindred, B., and Shreffler, D. C. H-2 dependence of co-operation between T and B cells in vivo. *J. Immunol. 109*:940–943, 1972.

Klein, J. Genetic polymorphism of the histocompatibility-2 loci of the mouse. *Ann. Rev. Genet. 8*:63–77, 1974.

Klein, J. *The Biology of the Mouse Histocompatibility-2 Complex.* Springer-Verlag, New York, 1975.

Klein, J. An attempt at an interpretation of the mouse *H-2* complex. *Contemp. Top. Immunobiol. 5*:297–336, 1976a.

Klein, J. Discussion. *In* D. H. Katz and B. Benacerraf (eds.), *The Role of Products of the Histocompatibility Gene Complex in Immune Response*, p. 213, Acadmic Press, New York, 1976b.

Klein, J., Chiang, C., Lofgreen, J., and Steinmuller, D. Participation of H-2 regions in heart-transplant rejection. *Transplantation 22*:384–390, 1976a.

Klein, J., and Forman, J. What can one learn about lymphocytes by studying H-2 mutations. *In* V. P. Eijsvoogel, D. Roos, and W. P. Zeijlemaker (eds.), *Leukocyte Membrane Determinants Regulating Immune Reactivity*, pp. 443–451, Academic Press, New York 1976.

Klein, J., Geib, R., Chiang, C., and Hauptfeld, V. Histocompatibility antigens controlled by the I region of the murine H-2 complex. I. Mapping of H-2A and H-2C loci. *J. Exp. Med. 143*:1439–1452, 1976b.

Klein, J., and Hauptfeld, V. Ia antigens: Their serology, molecular relationships, and their role in allograft reactions. *Transplant. Rev. 30*:83–100 1976.

Klein, J., Hauptfeld, M., and Hauptfeld, V. Evidence for a third, Ir-associated, histocompatibility region in the *H-2* complex of the mouse. *Immunogenetics 1*:45–56, 1974.

Klein, J., Merryman, C., Maurer, P., Hauptfeld, M., and Gardner, M. B. Histocompatibility-2 system in wild mice. IV. Ia and Ir typing of two wild mouse populations. *Cold Spring Harbor Symp. Quant. Biol.*, in press, 1976c.

Kolenkine, X. Les histoincompatibilites intra- et interspécifiques chez les Hydres d'eau douce. *Arch. Zool. Exp. Genet. 112*:63–72, 1971.

Koltin, Y., Stamberg, J., and Lemke, P. A. Genetic structure and evolution of the incompatibility factors in higher fungi. *Bacteriol. Rev. 36*:156–171, 1972.

Lachman, P. J., Grennan, D., Martin, A., and Démant, P. Identification of Ss protein as murine C4. *Nature 258*:242–243, 1975.

Lang, J. Interspecific aggression by scleractinian corals. 1. The rediscovery of *Scolymia culensis. Bull. Marine Sci. 21*:952–959, 1971.

Lang, J. Interspecific aggression by scleractinian corals. 2. Why the race is not only to the swift. *Bull. Marine Sci. 23*:260–279, 1973.

Levine, B. B., Stember, R. H., and Fotino, M. Ragweed hay fever: Genetic control and linkage to HL-A haplotypes. *Science 178*:1201–1203, 1972.
Levine, P., and Landsteiner, K. On immune isoagglutinins in rabbits. *J. Immunol. 18*:559–565, 1929.
Lieberman, R., Paul, W. E., Humphrey, W., Jr., and Stimpfling, J. H. H-2-linked immune response (Ir) genes. Independent loci for Ir-IgG and Ir-IgA genes. *J. Exp. Med. 136*:1231–1240, 1972.
Lindahl, K. F. Specificity of xenograft reactions in vitro. Thesis, University of Wisconsin, Madison, 1975.
Lonai, P., and McDevitt, H. The expression of *I* region gene products on lymphocytes. II. Genetic localization and cellular distribution of MLR determinants. *Immunogenetics (in press)*, 1976.
Marsh, D. G., Bias, W. B., Hsu, S. H., and Goodfriend, L. Association of the HL-A7 cross-reacting group with a specific reaginic antibody response in allergic man. *Science 179*:691–693, 1973.
McDevitt, H. O., and Chinitz, A. Genetic control of the antibody response: Relationship between immune response and histocompatibility (H-2) type. *Science 163*:1207–1208, 1969.
McDevitt, H. O., Deak, B. D., Shreffler, D. C., Klein, J., Stimpfling, J. H., and Snell, D. D. Genetic control of the immune response. Mapping of the *Ir-l* locus. *J. Exp. Med. 135*:1259–1278, 1972.
Meo, T., David, C. S., Rijnbeek, A. M., Nabholz, M., Miggiano, V. C., and Shreffler, D. C. Inhibition of mouse MLR by anti-Ia sera. *Transplant. Proc. 7*:127–129, 1975a.
Meo, T., Krasteff, T., and Shreffler, D. C. Immunochemical characterization of murine H-2 controlled Ss (serum substance) protein through identification of its human homologue as the fourth component of complement. *Proc. Natl. Acad. Sci (USA) 72*:4536–4540, 1975b.
Merryman, C. F., and Maurer, P. H. Characterization of a new *Ir-GLT* gene and its location in the *I* region of the *H-2* complex. *Immunogenetics 1*:549–449, 1975.
Miggiano, V. C., Birgen, J., and Pink, J. R. L. The mixed leukocyte reaction in chickens. Evidence for control by the major histocompatibility complex. *Eur. J. Immunol. 4*:397–401, 1974.
Moscona, A. A. Cell aggregation. *In* E. E. Bittar (ed.), *Cell Biology in Medicine*, John Wiley & Sons, New York, 1973.
Mozes, E. Expression of immune response *(Ir)* genes in T and B cells. *Immunogenetics 2*:397–140, 1975.
Nabholz, M., Young, H., Rynbeek, A., Boccardo, R., David, C. S., Meo, T., Miggiano, V., and Shreffler, D. C. *I*-region-associated determinants: Expression on mitogen-stimulated lymphocytes and detection by cytotoxic T cells. *Eur. J. Immunol. 5*:594–597, 1975.
Nakamuro, K., Tanigaki, N., and Pressman, D. Multiple common properties of human β_2-microglobulin and the common portion fragment derived from HL-A antigen molecules. *Proc. Natl. Acad. Sci. (USA) 70*:2863–2864, 1973.
Neauport-Sautes, C., Bismuth, A., Kourilsky, F. M., and Manuel, Y. Relationship between HL-A antigens and β_2-microglobulin as studied by immunofluorescence on the lymphocyte membrane. *J. Exp. Med. 139*:957–968, 1974.
Neefe, J. R., Vaal, L., Darrow, C. C. I. I., and Rogentine, G. N. Mixed lymphocyte reactivity in rhesus sibships. *Transplantation 15*:507–510, 1973.
Nicolas, J. F., Dubois, P., Jakob, H., Gaillard, J., and Jacob, F. Teratocarcinome de la souris: Differentiation en culture d'une lignee de cellules primitives and potentialites multiples. *Ann. Microbiol. (Inst. Pasteur) 126A*:3–22, 1975.
Ohno, S. *Evolution by Gene Duplication*. Springer-Verlag, Heidelberg, 1970.
Oka, H., and Watanabe, H. Colony-specificity in compound ascidians as tested by fusion experiments (a preliminary report). *Proc. Jap. Acad. 33*:657–659, 1957.
Oka, H., and Watanabe, H. Problems of colony-specificity in compound ascidians, *Bull. Marine Biol. Station Asamush. 10*:153–155, 1960.
Parish, C. R., Chilcott, A. B., and McKenzie, I. F. C. Low molecular weight Ia antigens in normal mouse serum. I. Detection and raising of a heterologous antiserum. *Immunogenetics 3*:113–128, 1976.

Peterson, P. A., Cunningham, B. A., Berggard, I., and Edelman, G. M. β_2-microglobulin—a free immunoglobulin domain. *Proc. Natl. Acad. Sci. (USA) 69*:1697–1701, 1972.

Peterson, P. A., Rask, L., and Linkblom, J. B. Highly purified papain-solubilized HL-A antigens contain β_2-microglobulin. *Proc. Natl. Acad. Sci. (USA) 71*:35–38, 1974.

Peterson, P. A., Rask, L., Sege, K., Klareskog, L., Anundi, H., and Ostberg, L. Evolutionary relationship between immunoglobulins and transplantation antigens. *Proc. Natl. Acad. Sci. (USA) 72*:1612–1616, 1975.

Poulik, M. D., Shennick, J. C., and Smithies, O. Partial amino acid sequences of rabbit and rat β_2-microglobulins. *Biochem. Biophys. Acta 56*:1221–1227, 1976.

Rajan, T. V., Nathenson, S. G., and Scharff, M.D. Regulatory variants for the expression of H-2 antigens. I. Isolation and characterization. *J. Natl. Cancer Inst. 56*:1221–1227, 1976.

Rogentine, G. N., Vaal, L., Ellis, E. B., and Marrow, C. C. I. I. Rhesus lymphocyte alloantigens. I. Identification of a major alloantigen system. *Transplantation 12*:267–270, 1971.

Romer, A. S. *The Vertebrate Story*. University of Chicago Press, Chicago, Ill., 1959.

Rudolph, R. H., Hered, B., Epstein, R. B., and Thomas, E. D. Canine mixed leukocyte reactivity and transplantation antigen. *Transplantation 8*:141–416, 1969.

Sato, W., and de Weck, A. L. Leucocyte typing in guinea pigs. *Z. Immunitaetsforsch. 144*:49–62, 1972.

Schierman, L. W., and Nordskog, A. W. Relationship of blood type to histocompatibility in chickens. *Science 134*:1008–1009, 1961.

Schirrmacher, V., Peña-Martinez, J., and Festenstein, H. Specific lymphocyte-activating determinants expressed on mouse macrophages. *Nature 255*:155–156, 1975.

Searle, R. F., Sellens, M. H., Elson, J., Jenkinson, E. J., and Billington, W. D. Detection of alloantigens during preimplantation development and early trophoblast differentiation in the mouse by immunoperoxidase labeling. *J. Exp. Med. 143*:348–359, 1976.

Serre, A., and Clot, J. Les tests d'histocompatibilité chez le chien en vue de L'experimèntation des greffes d'organes. *Rev. Fr. Etud. Clin. Biol. 13*:1019–1024, 1968.

Shearer, G. M., Rehn, T. G., and Garbarino, C. A. Cell-mediated lympholysis of trinitrophenyl-modified autologous lymphocytes. Effector cell specificity to modified cell surface somponents controlled by the H-2K and H-2D serological regions of the murine major histocompatibility complex. *J. Exp. Med. 142*:1348–1364, 1975.

Shevach, E. M., Frank, M. M., and Green, I. Linkage of the gene controlling the synthesis of the 4th component of complement to the major histocompatibility complex of the guinea pig. *Immunogenetics 3*:595–601, 1976.

Shreffler, D. C., and David, C. S. The *H-2* major histocompatibility complex and the *I* immune response region: Genetic variation function, and organization. *Adv. Immunol. 20*:125–195, 1975.

Shreffler, D. C., David, C. S., Passmore, H. C., and Klein, J. Genetic organization and evolution of the mouse *H-2* region: A duplication model. *Transplant. Proc. 3*:176–179, 1971.

Shreffler, D. C., Meo, T., and David, C. S. Genetic resolution of the products and functions of *I* and *S* region genes of the mouse *H-2* complex. *In* D. H. Katz and B. Benacerraf (eds.), *The Role of the Products of the Histocompatibility Gene Complex in Immune Response*, pp. 3–27, Academic Press, New York, 1976.

Silver, J., and Hood, L. Structure and evolution of transplantation antigens: Partial amino-acid sequences of H-2K and H-2D alloantigens. *Proc. Natl. Acad. Sci. (USA) 73*:599–603, 1976a.

Silver, J., and Hood, L. Preliminary amino acid sequences of transplantation antigens: genetic and evolutionary implications. *Contemp. Top. Mol. Immunol. (in press)*, 1976b.

Tanaka, K. Allogeneic distinction in *Botryllus primigenus* and in other colonial ascidians. *Adv. Exp. Med. Biol. 64*:115–124, 1975.

Tanaka, K., and Watanabe, H. Involvement of cellular and humoral factors in "nonfusion" reaction (NFR) of *Botryllus primigenus*, a compound ascidian. *Proceedings Second Annual Meeting of Japanese Society of Immunology*, pp. 101–103, 1972 (in Japanese).

Tanaka, K., and Watanabe, H. Allogeneic inhibition in a compound ascidian, *Botryllus primigenus Oka*. I. Processes and features of "nonfusion" reaction. *Cell. Immunol. 7*:410–426, 1973.

Terhorst, C., Parham, P., Mann, D., and Strominger, J. Structure of HLA antigens: Amino acid and carbohydrate compositions and N-terminal sequences of four antigen preparations. *Proc. Natl. Acad. Sci. (USA) 73*:910–914, 1976.

Theodor, J. Distinction between "self" and "non-self" in lower invertebrates. *Nature 227*:690–692, 1971.

Thomas, L. Discussion. *In* H. S. Lawrence (ed.), *Cellular and Humoral Aspects of the Hypersensitive States*, pp. 529–532, Cassell, London, 1959.

Tissot, R. G., and Cohen, C. Histocompatibility in rabbit. Linkage between RL-A, MLC, and the He blood group locus. *Transplantation 18*:142–149, 1974.

Vaiman, M., Renard, C., LaFage, P., Ameteau, J., and Nizza, P. Evidence for a histocompatibility system in swine (SL-A). *Transplantation 10*:155–164, 1970.

Valembois, P. Recherches sur la nature de la reaction antigreffe chez le Lombricien *Eisenia foetida* savigny. *C. R. Acad. Sci. (Paris) 257*:3489–3490, 1963.

Valembois, P. Quelques aspects phylogéniques de la réaction d'incompatibilité aux greffes chez les métazoaires. *Ann. Biol. 12*:1–26, 1973.

Valembois, P. Cellular aspects of graft rejection in earthworm and some other metazoa. *Contemp. Top. Immunobiol. 4*:121–126, 1974.

Van de Vyver, G. La non confluence intraspécifique chez les Spongiaires et la notion d'individu. *Ann. Embryol. Morphol. 3*:251–262, 1970.

Vitetta, E. S., Artzt, K., Bennett, D., Boyse, E. A., and Jacob, F. Structural similarities between products of the *T/t* locus isolated from sperm and teratoma cells, and H-2 antigens isolated from splenocytes. *Proc. Natl. Acad. Sci. (USA) 72*:3215–3219, 1975.

Vitetta, E. S., Capra, J. D., Klapper, D. G., Klein, J., and Uhr, J. W. The partial amino acid sequence of an H-2K molecule. *Proc. Natl. Acad. Sci. (USA) (in press)*, 1976b.

Vitetta, E. S., Poulik, M., Klein, J., and Uhr, J. W. Beta$_2$-microglobulin is selectively associated with H-2 and TL alloantigens on murine lymphoid cells. *J. Exp. Med. 144*:179–192, 1976a.

Von Boehmer, H., Hudson, L., and Sprent, J. Collaboration of histoincompatible T and B lymphocytes using cells from tetraparental bone marrow chimeras. *J. Exp. Med. 142*:989–997, 1975.

Wagner, H., Götze, D., Ptschelinzew, W., and Röllinghoff, M. Induction of cytotoxic T lymphocytes against *I*-region-coded determinants: In vitro evidence for a third histocompatibility locus in the mouse. *J. Exp. Med. 142*:1477–1487, 1975.

Waldmann, H., Pope, H., and Munro, A. Cooperation across the histocompatibility barrier. *Nature 258*:729–779, 1975.

Walford, R. L., Anderson, E. R., Carter, P. K., and Mihajlovic, F. Leucocyte antibodies in inbred strains of guinea pigs following first- and second-set skin homagrafts. *J. Immunol. 89*:427–433, 1962.

Wernet, P., Winchester, R., Kunkel, H. G., Wernet, D., Giphart, M., van Leeuwen, A., and van Rood, J. J. Serological detection and partial characterization of human MLC determinants with special reference to B-cell specificity. *Transplant. Proc. 7*:193–200, 1975.

Wolski, K. P., Schmid, F. R., and Mittal, K. K. Genetic linkage between the HL-A system and a deficit of the second component (C2) of complement. *Science 188*:1020–1022, 1975.

Würzburg, U. Correlation between the immune response to enzyme and histocompatibility type. *Eur. J. Immunol. 1*:496–497, 1971.

Zaleski, M., and Milgrom, F. Complementary genes controlling immune response to θ-AKR antigen in mice. *J. Immunol. 110*:1238–1244, 1973.

Ziegler, J. B., Alper, C. A., and Balner, H. Properdin factor B and histocompatibility loci linked in the rhesus monkey. *Nature 254*:609–610, 1975.

Subject Index

The following abbreviations were used: CML: cell-mediated cytotoxicity; GVH: graft versus host; Lad: lymphocyte activating determinants; MHS: major histocompatibility system; MLR: mixed lymphocyte culture reactivity; H: histocompatibility. Individual mouse inbred and congenic strains are not listed by their name in the index, but only tables listing them. Individual rat inbred strains are only listed by their name in the index if mentioned in the text too.

J. Klein
Biology of the Mouse Histocompatibility-2 Complex
Principles of Immunogenetic Applied to a Single System.
90 tables, 58 figures, XII, 620 pages. 1975.
ISBN 3-540-06733-7

Antineoplastic and Immunosuppressive Agents, Part 1
Editors: A.C. Sartorelli, D.G. Johns.
60 figures, XXIV, 762 pages. 1974.
(Handbook of Experimental Pharmacology, Vol. 38, Part 1)
ISBN 3-540-06402-8

Antineoplastic and Immunosuppressive Agents, Part 2
Editors: A.C. Sartorelli, D.G. Johns.
128 figures, XXXII, 1067 pages. 1975.
(Handbook of Experimental Pharmacology, Vol. 38, Part 2)
ISBN 3-540-06633-0

S. Shulman
Tissue Specificity and Autoimmunity
32 figures, XI, 196 pages. 1974.
(Molecular Biology, Biochemistry and Biophysics, Vol. 16)
ISBN 3-540-06563-6

E. Gurpide
Tracer Methods in Hormone Research
35 figures, XI, 188 pages. 1975.
(Monographs on Endocrinology, Vol. 8)
ISBN 3-540-07039-7

Th.E. Barman
Enzyme Handbook
(in 2 volumes, not available separately)
XI and III, 928 pages. 1969.
ISBN 3-540-04423-X
Distribution rights for Japan: Maruzen Co. Ltd. Tokyo

Th.E. Barmann
Enzyme Handbook—Supplement 1
1 figure, IV, 517 pages. 1974.
ISBN 3-540-06761-2
Distribution rights for Japan: Maruzen Co. Ltd. Tokyo

Advances in Biochemical Engineering

Vol. 1: Editors T. Ghose, A. Fiechter
70 figures, VII, 194 pages. 1971
ISBN 3-540-05400-6

Vol. 2: Editors: T.K. Ghose; A. Fiechter; N. Blakebrough
70 figures, V, 215 pages. 1972.
ISBN 3-540-06017-0

Vol. 3: T.K. Ghose; A. Fiechter; N. Blakebrough
119 figures, VI, 290 pages. 1974.
ISBN 3-540-06546-6

Vol. 4: Editors: T.K. Ghose, A. Fiechter; N. Blakebrough
87 figures, V, 172 pages. 1976.
ISBN 3-540-07747-2

Springer-Verlag Berlin Heidelberg New York

G. Mathé
Cancer Active Immunotherapy
Immunoprophylaxis and Immunorestoration
An Introduction
123 figures, 87 tables, XV, 405 pages. 1976.
(Recent Results in Cancer Research, Vol. 55)
ISBN 3-540-07601-8

Investigation and Stimulation of Immunity in Cancer Patients
Proceedings of the CNRS Colloquium, Paris, June 21–22, 1972
Editors: G. Mathé; R. Weiner
(Recent Results in Cancer Research, Vol. 47)
143 figures, IX, 501 pages. 1974.
ISBN 3-540-06771-X

M.R. Parwaresch
The Human Blood Basophil
Morphology, Origin, Kinetics, Function and Pathology
With a Foreword by K. Lennert
58 figures, some in color, XI, 235 pages. 1976.
ISBN 3-540-07649-2

J. van Lancker
Molecular and Cellular Mechanisms in Disease
411 figures, 68 tables, XX, 1168 pages. 1976.
(In 2 parts, not available separately)
ISBN 3-540-06932-1

Lymphocytes, Macrophages, and Cancer
Editors: G. Mathé; I. Florentin; M.-C. Simmler
53 figures, IX, 160 pages. 1976.
(Recent Results in Cancer Research, Vol. 56)
ISBN 3-540-07902-5

The Immune System
Editors: F. Melchers; K. Rajewsky
104 figures, XIV, 299 pages. 1976.
(27. Colloquium der Gesellschaft für Biologische Chemie
29. April–1. Mai 1976 in Mosbach/Baden)
ISBN 3-540-07976-9

www.ingramcontent.com/pod-product-compliance
Ingram Content Group UK Ltd.
Pitfield, Milton Keynes, MK11 3LW, UK
UKHW020952220926
475831UK00001B/47
* 9 7 8 3 6 4 2 9 5 2 9 5 1 *